D0203194

Ultrasound Physics
and
Instrumentation

Ultrasound Physics and Instrumentation

Wayne R. Hedrick, Ph.D.

Professor, Medical Radiation Biophysics,
Northeastern Ohio Universities College of Medicine, Rootstown, Ohio
Certified Diagnostic Radiological Physicist and Medical Nuclear Physicist,
American Board of Radiology,
Aultman Hospital, Canton, Ohio

David L. Hykes, Ph.D.

Assistant Professor, Medical Radiation Biophysics,
Northeastern Ohio Universities College of Medicine, Rootstown, Ohio
Certified Radiological Physicist, American Board of Radiology,
St. Joseph Hospital and Health Center, Lorain, Ohio

Dale E. Starchman, Ph.D.

Professor, Medical Radiation Biophysics,
Northeastern Ohio Universities College of Medicine, Rootstown, Ohio
Certified Radiological Physicist, American Board of Radiology,
Timken Mercy Medical Center, Canton, Ohio

THIRD EDITION

with 390 illustrations and 16 four-color plates

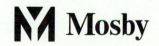 Mosby

St. Louis Baltimore Berlin Boston Carlsbad Chicago London Madrid
Naples New York Philadelphia Sydney Tokyo Toronto

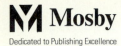

Managing Editor: Jeanne Rowland
Developmental Editor: Lisa Potts
Project Manager: John Rogers
Production Editor: George B. Stericker, Jr.
Designer: Renée Duenow
Cover Design: Jill Papke
Manufacturing Supervisor: Karen Lewis

THIRD EDITION
Copyright © 1995 by Mosby–Year Book, Inc.

Previous editions copyrighted 1985, 1992

All rights reserved. No part of this publication may be reproduced, stored in a retrieval system, or transmitted, in any form or by any means, electronic, mechanical, photocopying, recording, or otherwise, without prior written permission from the publisher.

Permission to photocopy or reproduce solely for internal or personal use is permitted for libraries or other users registered with the Copyright Clearance Center, provided that the base fee of $4.00 per chapter plus $.10 per page is paid directly to the Copyright Clearance Center, 27 Congress Street, Salem, MA 01970. This consent does not extend to other kinds of copying, such as copying for general distribution, for advertising or promotional purposes, for creating new collected works, or for resale.

Printed in the United States of America
Composition by Graphic World, Inc.
Printing/binding by Maple-Vail Book Mfg. Group, York

Mosby–Year Book, Inc.
11830 Westline Industrial Drive
St. Louis, Missouri 63146

Library of Congress Cataloging in Publication Data

Hedrick, Wayne R.
    Ultrasound physics and instrumentation / Wayne R. Hedrick, David
L. Hykes, Dale E. Starchman. — 3rd ed.
        p. cm.
    Rev. ed. of: Ultrasound physics and instrumentation / David L.
Hykes, Wayne R. Hedrick, Dale E. Starchman.
    Includes bibliographical references and index.
    1. Ultrasonic imaging. 2. Diagnosis, Ultrasonic—Instruments.
3. Medical physics. I. Hykes, David L. II. Starchman, Dale E.
III. Title.
    [DNLM: 1. Ultrasonics. 2. Ultrasonography—instrumentation. QT
34 H456 u 1994]
    RC78.7.U4H95 1994
    616.07′543—dc20
    DNLM/DLC   94-21585
    for Library of Congress   CIP

ISBN 0-8151-4246-3

95 96 97 98 99   /   9 8 7 6 5 4 3 2 1

DEC. 23 1994   C. I login   #33.96

To our wives
ANNE, LINDA, *and* JANE

Preface

This new edition continues to present ultrasound physics in an easy-to-understand and comprehensive manner for diagnostic ultrasound technology students and radiology residents. It will also benefit physicians and technologists in many medical specialties—including obstetrics, cardiology, vascular surgery, urology, general surgery, and veterinary medicine. In addition, medical physicists and engineers will find the principles of ultrasound physics and instrumentation that they need to know.

The field of medical diagnostic ultrasound has expanded rapidly over the past decade. Although the basic physical principles are unchanged, the operator's understanding of these principles and the factors affecting the presentation of data is more important than ever. If individuals who perform and/or interpret ultrasound scans are to obtain the highest quality of diagnostic information, they must understand the underlying physical principles. Because of this important fact, this text offers complete explanations of the physical principles one needs to understand to successfully perform diagnostic ultrasound examinations.

Significant advances in instrumentation have led to increased clinical use of diagnostic ultrasound. Motion-imaging techniques, particularly real-time and Doppler, have virtually eliminated static B-mode scanners. Duplex scanners that incorporate real-time imaging with nearly simultaneous Doppler capabilities are now commonplace. Computer processing techniques in color-flow imaging have enabled two-dimensional blood flow information to be superimposed on the real-time image. Due to the importance of this state-of-the-art technology, an entire new chapter has been added on color-flow imaging. Two additional chapters are also included. One, on hemodynamics, aids in the understanding of Doppler ultrasound and is particularly helpful in the interpretation of pulsed wave spectral analysis. The other, on vascular ultrasound, reflects the expanding clinical use of techniques in this area.

Now divided into 14 chapters, the book opens with a detailed presentation of the basic physical principles of ultrasound. Chapter 1 is vitally important because the physical principles it presents form the basis for understanding all ultrasonic scanning modes. These principles are dramatically different from those that apply to diagnostic x-ray imaging. Chapter 2, basic instrumentation, includes transducer and scanner design based on the echo-ranging principle. Static imaging modes (A, B, gated, and transmission) are discussed in Chapter 3. These instruments have been almost totally replaced by real-time imaging scanners, which are described in Chapters 4, 6, 7, and 9. Hemodynamics is presented in Chapter 5 ahead of the Doppler topics, including color-flow imaging (Chapters 6 and 7).

A knowledge of hemodynamics is essential for understanding Doppler scan data; thus clinical applications of ultrasound are illustrated in Chapters 8 (vascular) and 9 (echocardiology). Because computers have played an important role in the development of instrumentation, digital processing techniques are discussed in Chapter 10. The usual end product of ultrasonic scanning is an image recorded on film or other medium. An overview of image-recording devices is presented in Chapter 11. As do other imaging techniques, ultrasound deposits energy into the body and thus has the potential for causing biological effects. Chapter 12 reviews the literature concerning these biological effects and the clinical safety concerns associated with medical diagnostic ultrasound. The quality of the recorded image must be maintained at a high level via an appropriate quality-control program, as set forth in Chapter 13. The last chapter, Chapter 14, summarizes image artifacts that can seriously jeopardize the diagnostic interpretation.

This text fully prepares the reader, not only by explaining the necessary principles, but also by using analogies, incorporating sample problems throughout, presenting key terms, and providing review questions at the end of each chapter with answers at the back of the book. An extensive glossary of ultrasonic terms is included. The appendix contains a comprehensive mathematics review and a short discussion of Fourier analysis, a computer processing technique in Doppler scanning.

In addition, the accompanying practice examination booklet contains sample questions that will thoroughly test the working knowledge of readers in the physics and instrumentation of ultrasound, as well as vascular and cardiovascular techniques, thus helping them prepare for examinations given by the American Registry of Diagnostic Medical Sonographers. All the learning tools integrated within this text help make comprehension easier and more successful.

Wayne R. Hedrick
David L. Hykes
Dale E. Starchman

Acknowledgments

As with any undertaking of this type, the authors are indebted to a number of people who contributed their time and expertise.

A very special thanks to Cyndi Peterson, RDMS, Program Director, School of Diagnostic Medical Ultrasound, Aultman Hospital, Canton, Ohio, for her suggestions and comments and her help in obtaining ultrasonic images. The registered diagnostic medical sonographers at Aultman Hospital—Heather Elavsky, Sheri Tilton, Kathy Filicky, James Allman, Linda Welfley, Linda Metzger, Lisa Montini, Lori Conley, Amy Mitan, and Susan Schmidt—are a resource of technical expertise who create a challenging learning environment for residents and student sonographers.

David Baker, Christine Jankowski, Marsha Fritz, Terese Davis, Grace Brennan, and Regina Swearenger provided ultrasonic images. Tim Wedekamm performed the photographic work. We are grateful to Linda Hykes and Carol Beebe for their secretarial assistance. Linda Hykes also prepared many of the illustrations.

The comments and suggestions of the reviewers were very helpful and served to improve the manuscript. The thorough critique by John Parks, BA, RDMS, coordinator University of Wisconsin School of Diagnostic Medical Sonography, Madison, Wisconsin, is greatly appreciated.

Contents

Color Plates

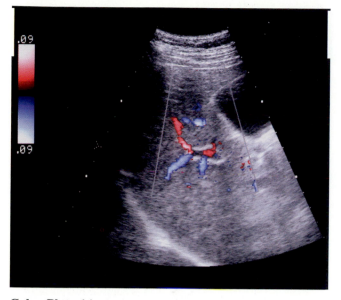

Color Plate 1A Color-flow image of the liver. The anterior right portal vein is shown in *red,* the posterior right portal vein in *blue.* (See Figure 7-2.)

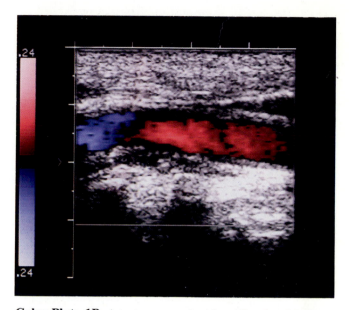

Color Plate 1B A tortuous vessel with unidirectional flow is depicted in changing colors, which erroneously suggests a reversal of flow. (See Figure 7-21.)

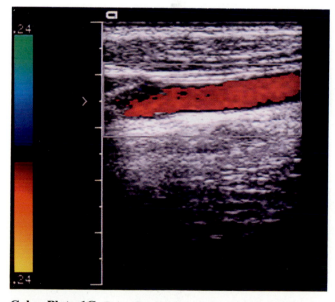

Color Plate 1C Color-flow image of the normal common carotid artery showing the velocity of flow throughout the vessel. (See Figure 8-7, *A.*)

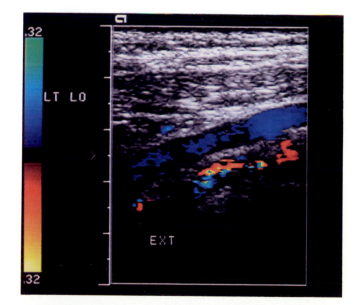

Color Plate 1D In this color-flow image the left external carotid shows moderately severe stenosis. The *blue* denotes an area of reduced flow velocity. (See Figure 8-7, *B.*)

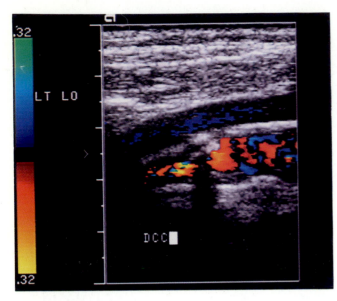

Color Plate 1E Shadowing by a calcified plaque obscures flow in the common carotid artery. (See Figure 8-8.)

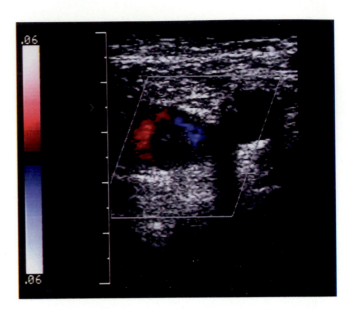

Color Plate 1F Color-flow image of the femoral vein with a clot. (See Figure 8-13.)

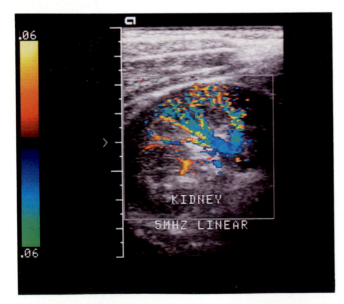

Color Plate 1G Color-flow image of a kidney. (See Figure 8-14.)

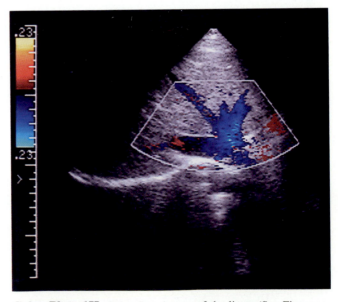

Color Plate 1H Color-flow image of the liver. (See Figure 8-15.)

CHAPTER 1

Basic Ultrasound Physics

SOUND WAVES

Sound is mechanical energy that is transmitted through a medium. Periodic changes in the pressure of the medium (air or water or iron) are created by forces acting on the molecules, causing them to oscillate about their mean or average positions. Since the motion of the molecules is repetitive, the term *cycle* is used to describe this sequence of changes in molecular motion (displacement, density, pressure, and particle velocity) that recurs at regular intervals.

The *frequency* of a wave is the number of vibrations that a molecule in it makes per second or the number of times the cycle is repeated per second. For comparative purposes high frequency means that the cyclic motion is executed at a faster rate and more cycles are completed in the 1-second interval than at low frequency. Frequency is discussed in the section "Properties" later in this chapter. Sound waves are those pressure changes that the human ear can detect. They oscillate at frequencies of 20 to 20,000 cycles/second (c/s), also referred to as *hertz* (Hz).

Propagation

The periodic changes in pressure when vibrating molecules interact with neighboring molecules are conveyed from one location to another. The term *propagation* describes this transmittal to distant regions remote from the sound source.

Sound waves are mechanical in nature, but they are not restricted to transmission through air. They require, however, an elastic deformable medium for propagation, which can be gas, liquid, or solid. A solid is deformable because increased pressure applied to it causes a change in its shape. Elasticity is demonstrated by a return to the original shape when the pressure is lowered to its initial value. Sound waves are not electromagnetic radiation, as are light and x rays. Electromagnetic radiation consists of alternating electrical and magnetic fields that are at right angles to each other and that propagate through a vacuum at the speed of light. Sound transmission cannot occur in a vacuum because no molecules are available to transfer the vibrations.

Ultrasound is defined as high-frequency mechanical waves that humans cannot hear; they are mechanical waves with frequencies of greater than 20,000 Hz, or 20 kHz ($k = 10^3$). *Infrasound* refers to mechanical waves with frequencies of less than 20 Hz, which humans also cannot hear. Sound, ultrasound, and infrasound have the same properties, and thus these terms are often used interchangeably in the description of physical interactions.

Wave equation. A pendulum having a small angle of displacement moves back and forth, displaying simple harmonic motion. Its movement can be represented as a sinusoidal wave (Fig. 1-1). The location as a function of time can therefore be described using the wave equation

1-1

$$A = A_0 \sin(2\pi ft)$$

where A is the amplitude at time t, A_0 the peak amplitude, f the frequency, and π a constant with the value of 3.1416. The peak amplitude is the maximum distance from the rest position.

Compression and rarefaction. Sound waves are pressure or mechanical waves that result in movement of the particles of a medium across or through their mean positions

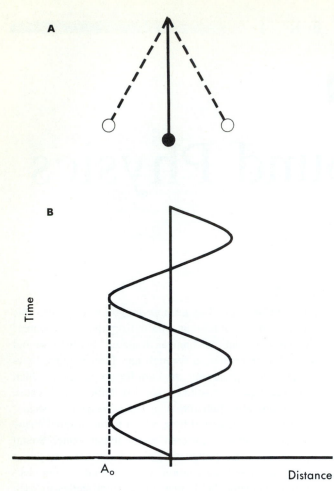

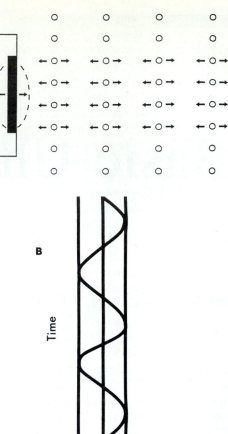

Figure 1-1 Pendulum motion. **A,** Oscillatory displacement. **B,** Plot of the displacement with time. Maximum displacement from the position at rest is designated A_0.

Figure 1-2 Concept of molecular motion. **A,** Oscillation of air molecules produced by a piston. **B,** Plot of molecular displacement with time.

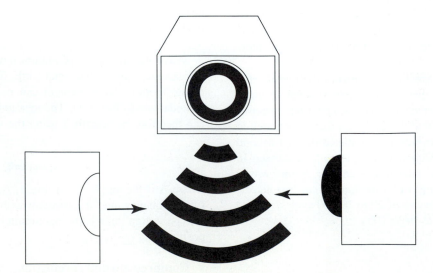

Figure 1-3 Molecular motion induced by a speaker. Zones of rarefaction *(open areas)* alternate with zones of compression *(shaded areas)*.

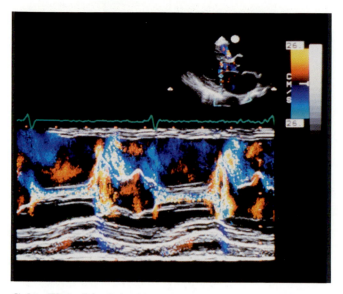

Color Plate 2A Color M-mode trace of aortic insufficiency and mitral valve regurgitation. (See Figure 9-6.)
Courtesy Hewlett-Packard Imaging Systems, Andover Mass.

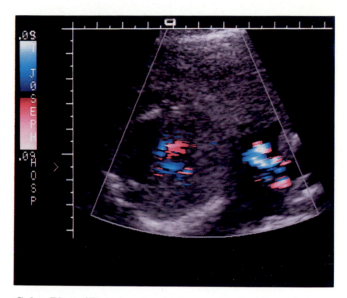

Color Plate 2B Color Doppler image of a fetal heart (color area on the *left*) and umbilical cord (color area on the *right*). (See Figure 9-10.)

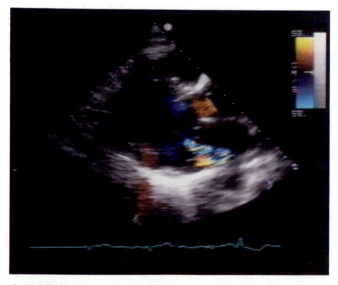

Color Plate 2C Color Doppler image of mitral valve regurgitation *(blue)*. (See Figure 9-11, *C*.)

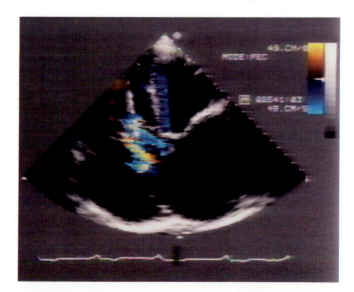

Color Plate 2D Color Doppler image (apical four-chamber view) of tricuspid valve regurgitation (*mosaic* pattern). (See Figure 9-12, *A*.)

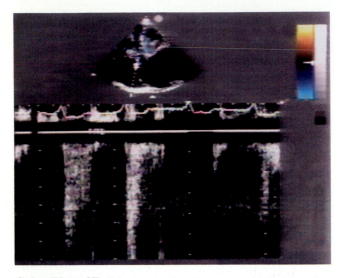

Color Plate 2E Pulsed-wave Doppler spectrum of tricuspid valve regurgitation demonstrating reverse flow. (See Figure 9-12, *B*.)

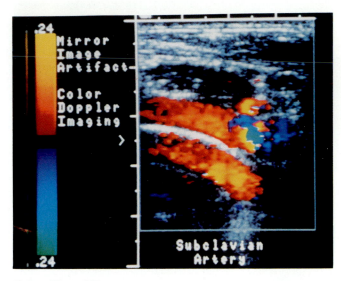

Color Plate 2F Color Doppler mirror-image artifact of the subclavian artery. (See Figure 14-21.)
Courtesy Rob Steins, Acusonic, Mountain View Calif.

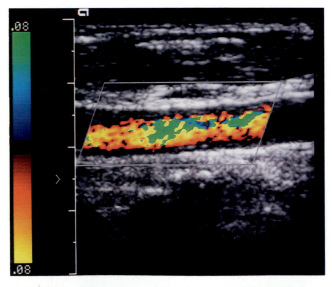

Color Plate 2G Color Doppler aliasing. Note the improper color progression—*red* to *yellow* to *green* to *blue*. If reverse flow were present, *red* and *blue* would be separated by a black region. (See Figure 14-22, *A*.)

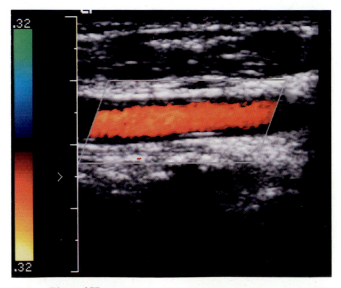

Color Plate 2H Increasing the velocity range removes the aliasing artifact. (See Figure 14-22, *B*.)

(Fig. 1-2). This movement is described mathematically by the wave equation (Equation 1-1) and can be illustrated by looking at the movement of an audio speaker. An electronic signal causes the mechanical movement of the speaker. The speaker mechanically vibrates or oscillates at the frequency of the sound being produced (Fig. 1-3).

The motion of the speaker can be visualized as a piston. When the speaker front moves forward, the air molecules immediately in front are pushed together, producing a region of increased air density, characterized by a small zone of increased pressure. The term *compression* describes the formation of the high-pressure region (Fig. 1-4). When the speaker front is pulled back, a zone of decreased molecular density results. The term *rarefaction* describes the creation of this low-pressure region (Fig. 1-4).

The speaker alternately compresses the air on a forward thrust and rarefies the air on a backward thrust. The regions of compression and rarefaction are passed through the medium by molecular interactions. The originally affected molecules collide with adjacent molecules to propagate the action of the speaker. Thus the transmission of mechanical energy through the medium creates regions of varying particle density or pressure. Compression zones alternate with rarefaction zones. Between the adjacent compression zones particle density decreases to a minimum in the rarefaction zone and then increases back toward a maximum. If the action of sound propagation is frozen in time, a plot of the particle density as a function of distance exhibits a wave pattern (Fig. 1-5, *A*). At a later instant the wave pattern of density variation is maintained (Fig. 1-5, *B*). The compression and rarefaction zones have shifted to new locations, however. Particle density is not constant at a particular position but fluctuates with a certain time dependence imposed by the frequency of the sound wave.

The molecules vibrate back and forth through their mean positions (a distance of only several microns). A micron is equal to 10^{-6} meter. Molecules do not travel from one end of the medium to the other; there is no flow of particles. Rather, the effect is transmitted over long distances because of neighbor-to-neighbor interactions. This molecular motion is necessary for sound transmission, which explains why sound cannot be transmitted through a vacuum.

Sound transmission is usually portrayed by showing the compression zones. A compression zone is often considered the leading portion of the sound wave and hence is called the *wavefront*. Wavefronts are helpful in illustrating the direction sound travels (perpendicular to the compression zone) and the region over which sound transmission takes place (the ultrasonic field).

Types

Waves are divided into two basic types: longitudinal and transverse. Longitudinal waves are those in which particle motion is along the direction of the wave energy propagation; that is, the molecules vibrate back and forth in the same direction as the wave is traveling (Fig. 1-6). Sound waves are longitudinal.

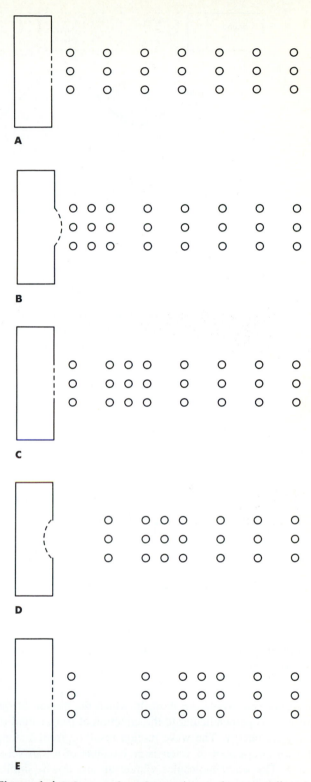

Figure 1-4 Influence of speaker motion on the surrounding air molecules. **A,** Undisturbed medium (no speaker motion). **B,** Speaker moving outward, compressing the medium. **C,** Speaker returning to its original position as a region of compression advances. **D,** Speaker moving inward, creating rarefaction in the medium. **E,** Speaker returning to its original position as the regions of compression and rarefaction advance.

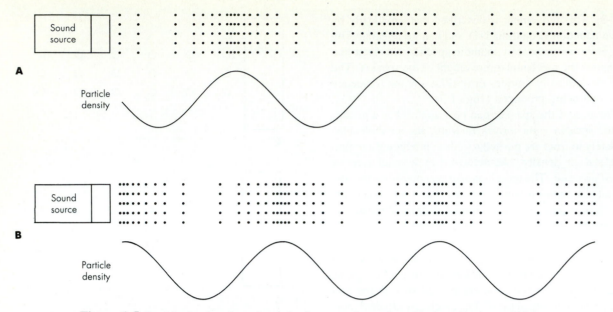

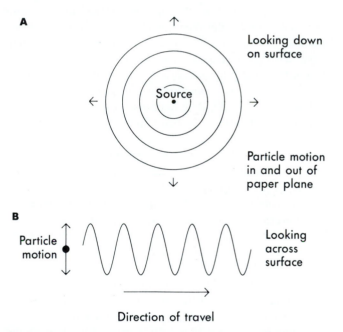

Figure 1-5 Particle density along the path of propagation varies with time. Regions of high and low density alternate (as shown by the *sinusoidal curves*). **A,** Initial observation. **B,** After a short time the regions of high and low density are displaced to the right.

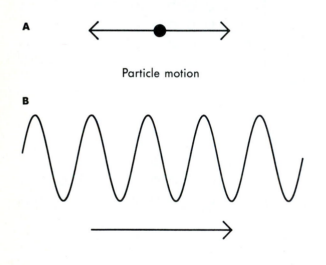

Figure 1-6 Longitudinal wave. **A,** Molecular (particle) motion. **B,** Direction of travel of the wave.

Figure 1-7 Transverse wave. The direction of travel of the wave is radially outward from the sound source, **A,** which produces particle motion perpendicular to the direction of travel, **B.**

Transverse waves are those in which the motion of the particles is perpendicular to the direction of propagation of the wave energy. The wave motion resulting from a stone thrown into a pool of water is an example of a transverse wave. The water molecules vibrate up and down, similar to a cork floating on the water, as the wave moves away from the point of origin across the surface of the water. An example of a transverse wave is shown in Figure 1-7.

Bone is the only biological tissue that can cause the production of transverse waves, which are sometimes referred to as shear waves or stress waves.

Properties

Waves have certain physical characteristics that are used to describe them. Table 1-1 lists common descriptors and the corresponding symbols that are used in this text. Each descriptor will be introduced and discussed in the chapter.

Physical quantities are measured in terms of a numerical value and a unit. A unit is a standard of measurement usually expressed in length, time, mass, charge or some combination of these. Table 1-2 lists common units and the corresponding symbols that are used throughout the text.

Wavelength. Wavelength is the extent of one complete wave cycle (Fig. 1-8). A cycle is a sequence of changes in

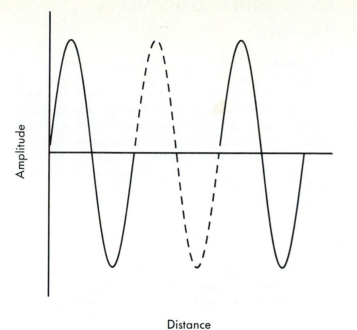

Figure 1-8 Amplitude of particle density as function of distance of wave travel. The wavelength is equal to the distance between successive maxima or minima. It is also defined as the distance needed to complete one wave cycle *(dotted line)*.

■ **Table 1-1** List of Physical Descriptors and Symbols

Descriptor	Symbol
Absorption coefficient	α
Acoustic impedance	Z
Acoustic power	W
Acoustic pressure	p
Attenuation coefficient	a
Bulk modulus	β
Compressibility	K
Density	ρ
Distance	z
Frequency	f
Instantaneous intensity	i
Intensity attenuation coefficient	μ
Particle displacement	s
Particle velocity	u
Percentage reflection	%R
Percentage transmission	%T
Period	τ
Reflection coefficient	ϕ_r
Elapsed time	t
Time-averaged intensity	I
Transmission coefficient	α_τ
Velocity of sound	c
Wavelength	λ

amplitude that recur at regular intervals. When particle density is plotted against distance, *amplitude* describes the variation in density. Wavelength is the distance between two successive density zones (i.e., two compression zones or two rarefaction zones) and is expressed in units of a meter (m), centimeter (cm), or millimeter (mm).

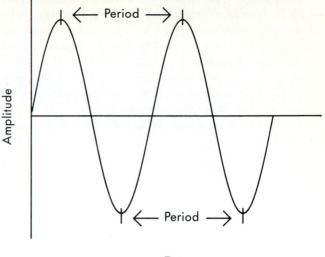

Figure 1-9 Variation in particle density at one point in the ultrasound field as a function of time. The period is equal to the time between successive maxima or minima. It is also defined as the time to complete one wave cycle.

■ **Table 1-2** List of Units and Symbols

Unit	Symbol
Meter	m
Centimeter	cm
Millimeter	mm
Micron (or micrometer)	μm
Kilogram	kg
Gram	g
Second	s
Millisecond	ms
Microsecond	μs
Hertz	Hz
Kilohertz	kHz
Megahertz	MHz
Joule	J
Watt	W
Pascal	Pa
Atmosphere	atm
Newton	Nt
Pound	lb
Volt	V
Coulomb	C
Degree Celsius	°C

Amplitude. Amplitude is the change in magnitude of a physical entity. The term can be applied to pressure in the medium or to particle density, particle displacement, or particle velocity in the medium. It has other applications, such as to characterize the size of a voltage pulse delivered to or induced within the crystal of the transducer (discussed later). When the amplitude is plotted as a function of time, the period of the wave (τ) is defined as the time necessary for one complete cycle or the time between two successive compression zones or rarefaction zones (Fig. 1-9). The unit of the period is the second (s).

Frequency. The frequency of a wave (f) is the number of cycles (pressure oscillations) occurring at a given point in one unit of time (usually 1 second). It corresponds to the inverse of the period ($1/\tau$). The unit of frequency is the *hertz,* which is equal to 1 cycle per second (c/s). Cycle is not a standard of measurement but is used as a descriptor to clarify the concept of frequency. Often frequency is expressed in units of inverse time only ($1/s$ or s^{-1}).

The following equations define the relationship between period and frequency:

1-2

$$\tau = \frac{1}{f}$$

and

1-3

$$f = \frac{1}{\tau}$$

■ **Example 1-1**

Calculate the period of a wave whose frequency is 4,000,000 or 4×10^6 cycles per second.

$$\tau = \frac{1}{f}$$

$$= \frac{1}{4,000,000 \ 1/s}$$

$$= 2.5 \times 10^{-7} \ s$$

■ **Example 1-2**

Calculate the frequency of a wave whose period is 5×10^{-7} second.

$$f = \frac{1}{\tau}$$

$$= \frac{1}{5 \times 10^{-7} \ s}$$

$$= 2.0 \times 10^6 \ s^{-1}$$

Examples 1-1 and 1-2 illustrate the inverse relationship between frequency and period. When the period is doubled (from 2.5×10^{-7} to 5.0×10^{-7} s), the frequency is halved (from 4×10^6 to 2×10^6 c/s).

Acoustic velocity. The speed at which a wave propagates through the medium is called the acoustic velocity (c). The velocity of sound is determined by the rate at which the wave energy is transmitted through the medium, which depends on the density and compressibility of the medium. Note that the acoustic velocity is not the same as the particle velocity (u), which refers to the speed at which the particles vibrate back and forth across their mean positions.

SOUND-PROPAGATION MEDIA

Properties

Elasticity. Elasticity refers to the ability of an object to return to its original shape and volume after a force is no longer acting on it. When a force is applied to the object (steel bar or soft tissue), a change in shape or volume (distortion) is induced. The amount of this distortion depends on the strength of the force and the elastic properties of the object. The latter is determined by molecular interactions.

An ultrasound wave traveling through soft tissue causes elastic deformations by the separation and compression of neighboring molecules.

Density. Density is the mass of a medium per unit volume. If all other physical properties of the medium are maintained unchanged, then an increase in density will impede the rate of sound propagation through the medium. As the density increases, more mass is contained within a given volume. For particles with increasingly larger mass, more force is required to produce molecular motion; and once the molecules are moving, more force is required to stop them. This is true for the rhythmic starting and stopping required to produce sound transmission. Thus, on the basis of density alone, we would expect sound (ultrasound) to have a greater velocity in air (low density) than in bone (high density).

Quantitatively, the velocity of sound in a medium is inversely proportional to the square root of the density of the medium ($\sqrt{\rho}$):

$$c \propto \frac{1}{\sqrt{\rho}}$$

where c is the velocity and ρ is the density of the medium.

Compressibility. Another physical characteristic of a medium, compressibility (K), affects the velocity of sound through the medium. Compressibility indicates the fractional decrease in volume when pressure is applied to the material. The easier a medium is to reduce in volume, the higher is its compressibility.

The velocity of sound through a medium is also inversely proportional to the square root of the compressibility of the medium ($\sqrt{K}$):

$$c \propto \frac{1}{\sqrt{K}}$$

However, the parameter relating the elastic properties of a medium to the velocity of sound through it is usually expressed as the reciprocal of the compressibility, termed the *bulk modulus* (β):

$$\beta = \frac{1}{\text{Compressibility}} = \frac{1}{K}$$

Thus velocity is directly proportional to the square root of β:

$$c \propto \sqrt{\beta} \propto \frac{1}{\sqrt{K}}$$

A dense material (e.g., bone or other solid) is very difficult to reduce in volume when pressure is applied to it. This low compressibility predicts the high velocity of sound in bone. By contrast, air is easily reduced in volume because the gas molecules are far apart and can be easily brought closer together (compressibility is high). The velocity of sound in air is low. Based on density and compressibility differences, the velocity of sound in bone is much greater than that in air.

Bulk modulus. The bulk modulus (β) is often defined as the negative ratio of stress and strain. Stress is the force per unit area (or pressure) applied to an object. Strain is the fractional change in volume of the object. The negative sign is required since a positive pressure causes a decrease in volume. Large values for the bulk modulus indicate that a material is resistant to change in its volume when force is applied.

As the bulk modulus increases—and the compressibility decreases—the velocity of sound in the medium increases. Some authorities refer to this property as the "stiffness" of the medium.

Influences on Acoustic Velocity

Combining compressibility and density into one equation, we can determine the acoustic velocity for a particular medium:

1-4

$$c = \frac{1}{\sqrt{K\rho}}$$

or

$$c = \frac{\sqrt{\beta}}{\sqrt{\rho}}$$

If the density can be increased without affecting the compressibility, then Equation 1-4 predicts that the speed of sound will decrease. Compressibility and density of a particular substance are interdependent; a change in density is often coupled with a larger and opposing change in compressibility. Because compressibility varies more rapidly, it becomes the dominant factor in Equation 1-4. The overall effect is commonly summarized by the statement that, as density increases, the velocity of sound through a medium increases. Although exceptions can be cited, for materials of interest to the sonographer (air, lung, fat, soft tissue, plastic, bone) this statement is generally true.

As shown in Table 1-3, the velocity of sound in air is 330 meters per second (m/s) whereas in bone it is 4080 m/s. Bone is more dense than air; but compressibility is the key factor in determining the relative acoustic velocities, because bone is less compressible than air.

Another comparison of density and compressibility effects can be made by looking at two liquids. Water has a density of 1 gram per cubic centimeter (1 g/cm³), and mercury a density of 13.6 g/cm³. On the basis of density alone, water would have a velocity of sound $\sqrt{13.6}$ times greater

Table 1-3 Properties of Different Media

Material	Density (kg/m³)	Velocity (m/s)	Acoustic Impedance (kg/m²/s × 10⁻⁶ or g/cm²/s × 10⁻⁵)
Air	1.2	330	0.0004
Water (20° C)	1000	1480	1.48
Mercury	13,600	1450	20.0
Soft tissue			
Average*	1060	1540	1.63
Liver	1060	1550	1.64
Muscle	1080	1580	1.70
Fat	952	1459	1.38
Brain	994	1560	1.55
Kidney	1038	1560	1.62
Spleen	1045	1570	1.64
Blood	1057	1575	1.62
Bone	1912	4080	7.8
Lung	400	650	0.26
PZT†	7650	3791	29.0
Lens	1142	1620	1.85
Aqueous humor	1000	1500	1.50
Vitreous humor	1000	1520	1.52
Lucite	1180	2680	3.16
Polystyrene	1060	2350	2.49
Castor oil	969	1477	1.43

*Average tissue (e.g., abdomen).
†Lead zirconate titanate.

than mercury. The compressibility of water is 13.4 times that of mercury (water is more easily compressed). Differences in compressibility and density between the two liquids cancel, so the velocities for water and mercury are similar (Table 1-3). For liquids in general, density and compressibility offset each other and consequently different liquids tend to transmit ultrasound at nearly the same velocity. In the transmission of sound, soft tissue behaves similarly to liquid; the acoustic velocities for various tissue types do not vary by more than a few percentage points.

In general, because their compressibility is low, more dense media (most solids) have greater velocities than do less dense media (liquids or gases). This is one of the reasons (the other will soon become evident) why, in old western movies, cowboys and Indians would put their heads to the ground or to a railroad track to hear stampeding buffalo or an approaching train. *Sound travels faster in media that are denser than air,* because of reduced compressibility.

The average velocity of ultrasound in tissue is 1540 m/s. A slight dependence on temperature of the medium and on sound frequency is exhibited; the velocity of ultrasound waves in water at 20° C is 1480 m/s but rises to 1570 m/s in water that is 37° C. For a few degrees' shift in temperature, the change in velocity through water is small. Thus room temperature fluctuations are not a problem with respect to clinical applications; the body maintains a nearly constant temperature. Sound propagation in phantoms, however, is very dependent on temperature. To mimic tissue, a mixture of 8% ethanol and water at room temperature can be used. A change of 1° in a phantom significantly alters the velocity of sound through the mixture.

The dependence of velocity or other physical parameter on frequency is called dispersion. The change in velocity with frequency is small (less than 1%) over the frequency range used in diagnostic ultrasound, which is 1 to 20 megahertz (MHz) (M = 10^6). The velocity of sound in different materials (e.g., blood versus soft tissue) has a varying frequency dependence, but these small differences have no importance in clinical imaging.

FREQUENCY, WAVELENGTH, AND VELOCITY

The velocity of sound or ultrasound remains constant for a particular medium. The velocity (c) is equal to the frequency (f) times the wavelength (λ). Stated mathematically:

1-5

$$c = f\lambda$$

This is probably the most important equation used in diagnostic ultrasound. Because the velocity is constant for a particular medium, increasing the frequency causes the wavelength to decrease. This phenomenon is demonstrated by Examples 1-3 and 1-4.

■ Example 1-3

Using Equation 1-5, we can determine the wavelength in tissue for a 1.5 MHz frequency ultrasound source as follows:

$$c = f\lambda$$

$$\lambda = \frac{c}{f}$$

$$= \frac{1540 \text{ m/s}}{1.5 \times 10^6 \text{ c/s}}$$

$$= \frac{1.54 \times 10^3 \text{ m/s}}{1.5 \times 10^6 \text{ c/s}}$$

$$= \frac{1.54 \times 10^3 \times 10^{-6} \text{ m}}{1.5}$$

$$= 1.03 \times 10^{-3} \text{ m}$$

$$= 1.03 \text{ mm} \ (1 \text{ mm} = 10^{-3} \text{ m})$$

If the frequency is increased to 3 MHz, the wavelength must decrease to half the value of 1.03 mm, because the frequency has doubled. Thus

$$\lambda = \frac{1540 \text{ m/s}}{3 \times 10^6 \text{ c/s}}$$

$$= \frac{1.54 \times 10^{-3} \text{ m/s}}{3 \times 10^6 \text{ c/s}}$$

$$= 5.1 \times 10^{-4} \text{ m}$$

$$= 0.51 \text{ mm}$$

When going from a medium with one acoustic velocity to a medium with another, the frequency of the sound beam

■ Table 1-4 Frequency, Wavelength, and Period for Ultrasound Waves in Soft Tissue

Frequency (MHz)	Wavelength (mm)	Period (μs)
1.0	1.54	1.00
2.5	0.62	0.40
3.5	0.44	0.29
5.0	0.31	0.20
7.5	0.21	0.13
10	0.15	0.10
15	0.10	0.07
20	0.08	0.05

remains constant. This means that a change in the wavelength of the sound beam must accompany the velocity shift, as expressed by Equation 1-5.

■ Example 1-4

The wavelength of an ultrasonic beam in tissue generated by a 1 MHz transducer is

$$\lambda = \frac{1540 \text{ m/s}}{1 \times 10^6 \text{ c/s}}$$

$$= 1.54 \times 10^{-3} \text{ m}$$

$$= 1.54 \text{ mm}$$

or 1.54 mm in tissue. If the sound beam is then transmitted into a layer of bone, the wavelength becomes

$$\lambda = \frac{4080 \text{ m/s}}{1 \times 10^6 \text{ c/s}}$$

$$= 4.08 \times 10^{-3} \text{ m}$$

$$= 4.08 \text{ mm}$$

Table 1-4 lists the wavelength and period of an ultrasound wave in soft tissue as the frequency is varied.

We will see in Chapter 2 that the wavelength of ultrasound affects the axial resolution of an ultrasound system. The term *resolution* describes the ability to distinguish separate entities that are located close together.

INTERACTIONS OF ULTRASOUND WITH TISSUE

In diagnostic radiography the beam of x rays is produced outside the patient's body; the x rays are subsequently attenuated (absorbed and scattered) as they pass through the patient's tissues. Ultimately, the transmitted photons are recorded on film. (For diagnostic ultrasound the recorded image is typically based on reflected rather than transmitted energy.) The single device that generates the ultrasound wave and, subsequently, detects the reflected energy is the transducer. An ultrasound wave is directed into the body to interact with tissues in accordance with the characteristics of the targeted tissues. The results of these interactions are recorded for diagnosis in the form of reflected ultrasound waves. The types of interactions that occur are similar to the wave behavior observed with light: reflection, refrac-

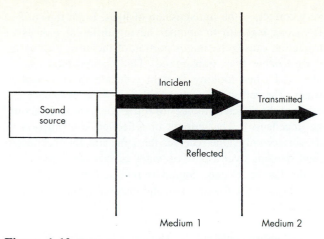

Figure 1-10 Reflection caused by a sound wave striking a large smooth interface at normal incidence. The interface is larger than the beam width and acts as a specular reflector. The relative intensities of the transmitted and reflected waves are determined by the acoustic impedances of the media that compose the interface.

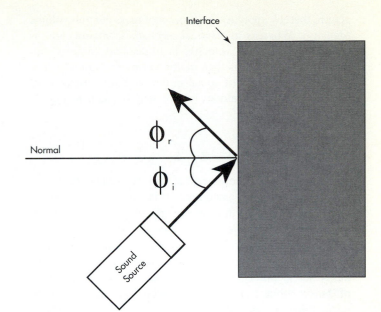

Figure 1-11 Reflection caused by a sound wave striking a specular reflector at an angle. The resulting angle of reflection (ϕ_r) equals the angle of incidence (ϕ_i).

tion, scattering, diffraction, divergence, interference, and absorption. With the exception of interference, all these interactions reduce the intensity of the beam, termed *attenuation*. Interference may increase or decrease the intensity. In practice, reflection is often treated separately from attenuation; in other words, all interactions that decrease the intensity of the beam except for reflection are included in the attenuation process.

Reflection

The major interaction of interest for diagnostic ultrasound is reflection. If a sound beam is directed at right angles (called normal incidence) to a smooth interface (e.g., the boundary between different tissue types) larger than the width of the beam, it will be partially reflected toward the sound source (Fig. 1-10). These interfaces, called specular reflectors, are responsible for the major organ outlines seen in diagnostic ultrasound examinations. The diaphragm and pericardium are examples of specular reflectors.

The angle of reflection of a sound beam is equal to the angle of incidence (Fig. 1-11). These angles are defined relative to a line drawn perpendicular to the surface of the interface (normal incidence). To obtain maximum detection of the reflected signal, we must orient the transducer (which sends and receives) so the generated sound beam will strike the interface perpendicularly.

What conditions result in a reflection of energy? A useful analogy would be throwing a baseball against a brick wall; not much energy will be transferred to the wall. Conservation of energy would permit the ball to transfer all its energy to the wall and simply stop at the surface of the wall, but conservation of momentum prevents this from occurring because of the differences in mass. Only a small portion of the energy will be transferred to the wall. Most will be retained by the baseball, which will return with

almost the same velocity as when it struck the wall.

Similarly, if a Mack truck rams into a Volkswagen, very little energy will be transferred to the Volkswagen. The truck will continue at almost the same velocity as it originally had. Most of its energy will be retained, although a great deal of damage will be done to the Volkswagen. Energy cannot be transmitted readily from large objects to small ones or from small objects to large ones. If massive transfers of kinetic energy are required, collisions between objects of equal mass must occur. For example, to slow down a baseball, the maximum amount of energy transfer will result if it collides with another baseball. To transfer energy from a Mack truck by the maximum amount, it would have to collide with another Mack truck. Vibrating molecules behave in a similar manner. As long as they are transmitting energy to identically sized molecules, maximum transfer will occur. If there is a difference in the masses of the molecules, less energy will be transferred and the energy that is not transferred will be reflected.

This analogy can be carried further by looking at the transfer of ultrasonic energy through a layer of water on top of a pool of mercury. At the water-mercury interface the small water molecules (similar to baseballs or Volkswagens) are inefficient in transferring energy to the large mercury molecules (similar to the wall or a Mack truck). They bounce off the mercury molecules, indicating that most of their energy is reflected back into themselves, with very little being transferred into the mercury. This reflection is determined by the conservation of momentum.

Acoustic impedance. In ultrasound the quantity analogous to momentum is acoustic impedance. Here we are looking not at individual molecules but at their concerted action, thereby applying the concept of mass per unit volume (density). Whereas in classical mechanics "momentum" is equal to mass times velocity, in ultrasound "density" replaces the mass and is then multiplied by the velocity. The velocity used is that of sound in the medium. The product of density (ρ) times velocity (c) is called the *acoustic impedance* (Z):

1-6

$$Z = \rho c$$

This quantity is a measure of the resistance to sound passing through the medium. It is similar to electrical resistance, which is the degree of difficulty experienced by electrons in traversing a specific type of material. Acoustic impedance is expressed as kilograms per square meter per second ($kg/m^2/s$) or grams per square centimeter per second ($g/cm^2/s$) and is the product of the units of density times velocity. The combination of units in the meter-kilogram-second (mks) system is given a special name, the rayl.

■ Example 1-5

What is the acoustic impedance of castor oil (which has a density of 969 kg/m^3)? Assume the velocity of sound in castor oil to be 1477 m/s.

$$
\begin{aligned}
Z &= \rho c \\
&= (969 \text{ kg/m}^3)\,(1477 \text{ m/s}) \\
&= 1.43 \times 10^6 \text{ kg/m}^2/\text{s}
\end{aligned}
$$

High-density materials give rise to high-velocity sound waves and therefore high acoustic impedances. Similarly, low-density materials such as gases have low acoustic impedances. Table 1-3 lists the acoustic impedances for several materials of interest.

Impedance mismatch. If the acoustic impedance is the same in one medium as in another, sound will be readily transmitted from one to the other. A difference in acoustic impedances causes some portion of the sound to be reflected at the interface. It is primarily the change in acoustic impedance at a biological interface (a discontinuity or an impedance mismatch) that allows visualization of soft tissue structures with an ultrasonic beam.

Watching late-night western movies teaches that one does not listen for the train or for buffalo in a normal standing position. Every youngster learned from old westerns that you put your ear to the rail or to the ground. The late John Wayne most likely would not have said, "Put your ear to the ground because that way you will eliminate the acoustic impedance mismatch and thus get a better sound transfer," but he should have, for that is the case.

Thus we have the second reason for placing one's ear on a solid surface. Whereas the transfer of sound from rail to air and then from air to ear is very inefficient, *with direct contact the transmission from rail to air is eliminated and vibrations pass readily across a solid-solid interace.*

Another analogy that might be used, and that would be very correct, is the transmission of light. Light transmitted from one medium to another having different indices of refraction causes the major portion of the energy to be reflected rather than transmitted. This phenomenon can be observed when looking at light reflected from a pool of water. The reflection occurs at the air-water boundary because of the different indices of refraction (similar to acoustic impedance). The amount of reflection is a function of the surface only. One receives the same amount of reflected light standing over a pool of water as over the deepest part of the Pacific Ocean. Sound is reflected at the interface regardless of the thickness of the material from which it is reflected.

Reflection coefficient. The reflection coefficient for intensity is expressed as follows:

1-7

$$\alpha_R = \left(\frac{Z_2 - Z_1}{Z_2 + Z_1}\right)^2$$

where α_R is the reflection coefficient, Z_2 the acoustic impedance of medium no. 2, and Z_1 the acoustic impedance of medium no. 1. Multiplying this relation by 100 gives the percentage reflection (%R):

1-8

$$\%R = \left(\frac{Z_2 - Z_1}{Z_2 + Z_1}\right)^2 \times 100$$

Transmission coefficient. The percentage transmission (%T) is 100 minus the percentage reflection (%R), and the transmission coefficient is 1 minus the reflection coefficient. The transmission coefficient (α_T) is calculated directly by the formula

1-9

$$\alpha_T = \frac{4\,Z_1 Z_2}{(Z_2 + Z_1)^2}$$

Multiplying the right-hand side of Equation 1-9 by 100 gives the percentage transmission through the interface:

1-10

$$\%T = \frac{4\,Z_1 Z_2}{(Z_2 + Z_1)^2} \times 100$$

Interface composition. It does not matter which impedance is the larger or smaller for two materials composing the interface, the difference between them squared gives the same number. Thus the same percentage of reflection occurs at the interface, whether sound is going from a high acoustic impedance to a low acoustic impedance, and vice versa. If the acoustic impedance difference is small, the magnitude of the reflected wave will be small. Because the same device transmits and receives the sound waves, maximum detection of the reflected echo occurs when the sound beam strikes the interface with normal incidence. If the acoustic impedance difference is large, such as in bone compared to soft tissue (see Example 1-6), a large fraction of sound will be reflected; little of the transmitted beam will penetrate structures behind the bone, and much will return to the detector. Consequently, for examinations involving the head, ultrasound is restricted to relatively simple non-invasive studies (echoencephalography). To visualize the liver, which is largely positioned under the ribs, one must look either through the intercostal spaces (between the ribs) or under the ribs and back up at the liver.

■ Example 1-6

Calculate the percentage reflection (%R) for a bone-tissue interface using the acoustic impedance values listed in Table 1-3:

$$\%R = \left(\frac{Z_B - Z_T}{Z_B + Z_T} \right)^2 \times 100$$

$$= \left(\frac{(7.8 \times 10^6) - (1.63 \times 10^6)}{(7.8 \times 10^6) + (1.63 \times 10^6)} \right)^2 \times 100$$

$$= 43\%$$

where Z_B is the acoustic impedance in bone and Z_T the acoustic impedance in tissue.

■ Example 1-7

Calculate the percentage transmission (%T) for a soft tissue–bone interface using the acoustic impedance values listed in Table 1-3:

$$\%T = \frac{4 \, Z_B Z_T}{(Z_B + Z_T)^2} \times 100$$

$$= \frac{4 \, (7.8 \times 10^6) \, (1.63 \times 10^6)}{((7.8 \times 10^6) + (1.63 \times 10^6))^2} \times 100$$

$$= 57\%$$

Note that the result for percentage reflection at the soft tissue–bone interface determined in Example 1-6 can be used to calculate the percentage transmission at this interface:

$$\%T = 100\% - \%R$$

$$= 100\% - 43\%$$

$$= 57\%$$

This is one of the reasons why bone is usually avoided during an ultrasound examination. The acoustic impedance difference is also large for an air-tissue interface, which causes most of the beam to be reflected.

■ Example 1-8

Calculate the percentage reflection (%R) for an air-tissue interface using the acoustic impedance values listed in Table 1-3:

$$\%R = \left(\frac{Z_T - Z_A}{Z_T + Z_A} \right)^2 \times 100$$

$$= \left(\frac{(1.63 \times 10^6) - (0.0004 \times 10^6)}{(1.63 \times 10^6) + (0.0004 \times 10^6)} \right)^2 \times 100$$

$$= 99.9\%$$

where Z_T is the acoustic impedance in tissue and Z_A the acoustic impedance in air.

If the acoustic impedance values are expressed with the same power of 10, the effects of 10 raised to the same exponent will cancel in the calculation for percentage reflection. Thus we can ignore the factors with a base of 10 in calculating for percentage reflection.

Table 1-5 lists the percentage reflections at interfaces of varying composition. The acoustic impedances used to calculate these values were obtained from Table 1-3. Note that the thickness of the medium is not considered in the calculations; only the impedance mismatch at the interface is of concern.

Even if the air layer between a transducer and the patient is extremely thin, nearly total reflection occurs at the air-tissue interface. During scanning, coupling gel is used to eliminate this. The gel also serves to reduce friction between the transducer and the skin.

Remember: When the heart or other thoracic structures are being studied, the lungs must be avoided because of the large amount of reflection that occurs at the multiple interfaces within them. Acoustic impedance differences at fat–soft tissue interfaces produce relatively strong echoes compared with echoes from parenchyma. Reflections from these interfaces are primarily responsible for the organ outlines seen in imaging. As an exercise, the reader should calculate the percentage reflection from a fat–soft tissue interface.

Echo-induced signals. When a device that produces and detects ultrasonic waves (i.e., a transducer) scans a patient, multiple interfaces are encountered along the path of travel of the ultrasound beam. A percentage of the incident beam intensity is reflected and transmitted at each interface. A series of echoes is subsequently detected (Fig. 1-12). If losses by reflection only are considered, the relative intensities of these echoes depend on the acoustic impedance mismatch at the interface that originally created the echo and on the transmission of sound energy through the interfaces along the path of travel to and from the transducer. On the return path each interface allows a fraction of the echo energy to pass through toward the transducer.

Reflections occur at the crystal-tissue interface because these materials are not perfectly matched. The acoustic impedance of the crystal is usually much greater than that of tissue. Poor transmission across the crystal-tissue interface inhibits the detection of weakly reflecting interfaces.

■ Table 1-5 Percentage Reflection at Different Interfaces

Interface	Reflection Percent
Soft tissue–air	99.9
Soft tissue–lung	52
Soft tissue–bone	43
Aqueous humor–lens	1.1
Fat–liver	0.79
Soft tissue–fat	0.69
Soft tissue–muscle	0.04
Water–Lucite	13
Castor oil–soft tissue	0.43

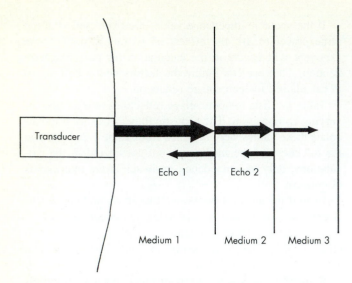

Figure 1-12 Sound beam incident on a phantom consisting of three tissue types (or media). A fraction of the incident sound energy is reflected at each boundary between the media (labeled *Echo 1* and *Echo 2*).

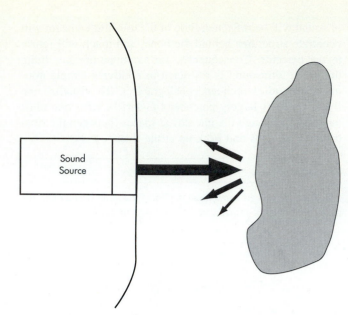

Figure 1-13 Diffuse reflection. When a sound beam is incident on an irregular interface *(shaded area)*, it is reflected in multiple directions.

In the next chapter we will consider methods to decrease this effect.

Remember: In diagnostic ultrasound, reflected echoes are detected by conventional systems. Small signals are generated if the acoustic impedances are nearly the same (soft tissue to soft tissue), but strong signals occur if the difference in acoustic impedances is large (air and soft tissue). Much weaker echoes are produced by diffuse reflection and scattering.

Diffuse reflection. The large smooth surface of a specular reflector acts as a mirror to form a well-defined redirected beam. A large rough-surfaced interface deflects the ultrasound beam in multiple directions (Fig. 1-13). Since the interface is not flat, the sound beam strikes the interface with various angles of incidence, which gives rise to differing angles of reflection. This is called *diffuse reflection*. The loss of coherence in the reflected beam weakens the echo returning to the transducer.

Before the bathroom mirror becomes fogged when you take a shower, it provides a true representation of objects placed in front of it. After you shower, the buildup of water on its surface causes it to act as a diffuse reflector and the images of objects are less well defined. Water particles roughen its surface, reducing the coherence of reflected light.

Scattering

Another important interaction between ultrasound and tissue is scattering, or nonspecular reflection, which is responsible for providing the internal texture of organs in the image. The scattering occurs because the interfaces are small, less

than several wavelengths across. Each interface acts as a new separate sound source, and sound is reflected in all directions (Fig. 1-14). Scattering by small particles in which the linear dimensions are smaller than the wavelength is called Rayleigh scattering. These nonspecular reflections have a strong frequency dependence (f^2 to f^6), which may make them useful in characterizing tissue. Tissue characterization involves the absolute determination of tissue type via some physical measurement obtained by noninvasive means. When the frequency is changed, the altered scattering of the sound beam may provide important information for differentiating tissue types.

Reflectivity

Many factors influence the fraction of incident intensity that is reflected at an interface toward the transducer — the acoustic impedance mismatch, the angle of incidence, the size of the structure compared with the wavelength, the shape of the structure, and the texture of the surface of the interface. The combination of these factors is described by the term *reflectivity*.

Differences in reflectivity are partially responsible for the patient-to-patient variations that sonographers observe when performing a particular type of examination. Ultrasound imaging systems are capable of detecting extremely small changes in reflectivity on the order of one in a million.

Refraction

Another interaction that occurs between ultrasound and tissue is refraction. If the ultrasound beam strikes an interface

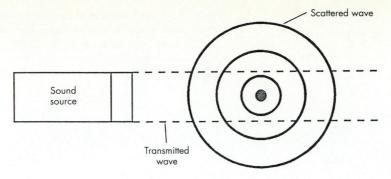

Figure 1-14 Nonspecular reflection. The scattered wave is emitted in all directions, shown here in two dimensions only.

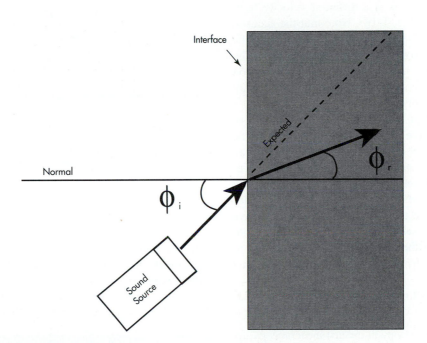

Figure 1-15 Refraction. The velocity of a sound beam in the incident medium is greater than that in the transmitted medium, causing the beam to be bent toward the normal ($\phi_i > \phi_t$).

between two media at an angle of 90 degrees (normal incidence), a percentage will be reflected back to the first medium and the rest will be transmitted into the second medium without a change in direction. If the beam strikes the interface at an angle other than 90 degrees, however, the transmitted part will be refracted or bent away from the straight-line path (Fig. 1-15).

Snell's law. Refraction of sound waves obeys Snell's law, which relates the angle of transmission to the relative velocities of sound in the two media. (Note that this relationship is not based on acoustic impedance.) Snell's law is given by

$$\frac{\text{Sin } \phi_i}{\text{Sin } \phi_t} = \frac{c_i}{c_t} \qquad \text{1-11}$$

where ϕ_i is the incident angle, ϕ_t the transmitted angle, c_i the velocity of sound in the incident medium, and c_t the velocity of sound in the transmitted medium. In Snell's law the angles ϕ_i and ϕ_t are defined with respect to a line drawn perpendicular to the interface.

■ **Example 1-9**

Calculate the transmitted angle if an ultrasound beam is directed at an interface composed of soft tissue and fat. The angle of incidence is 10 degrees. Assume that the sound beam is moving from soft tissue into fat.

$$c_i = 1540 \text{ m/s}$$

$$c_t = 1459 \text{ m/s}$$

$$\phi_i = 10 \text{ degrees}$$

$$\frac{\text{Sin } \phi_i}{\text{Sin } \phi_t} = \frac{c_i}{c_t}$$

$$\frac{\text{Sin } 10 \text{ degrees}}{\text{Sin } \phi_t} = \frac{1540 \text{ m/s}}{1459 \text{ m/s}}$$

$$\frac{0.174}{\text{Sin } \phi_t} = 1.056$$

$$\text{Sin } \phi_t = 0.165$$

$$\phi_t = 9.5 \text{ degrees}$$

This bending occurs because the portion of the wavefront in the second medium travels at a different velocity from that in the first medium (Fig. 1-16). Note that the acoustic velocity in medium *2* is less than that in medium *1* (the spacing between successive wavefronts is smaller). The wavefront is continuous across the interface, but the portion of the wavefront in medium *2* is moving at a slower velocity than the rest and lags behind.

To illustrate this shift in wavefronts, imagine successive rows of four wheel–drive vehicles traveling through the Sahara Desert. As the vehicles cross a boundary between flat smooth terrain and sandy terrain, their velocity is reduced. If the drivers who enter the sandy terrain stubbornly maintain their alignment, the advance of this row of vehicles will be slowed compared to that of the drivers who have not yet encountered the sandy terrain. For the vehicles to continue to advance so the row remains perpendicular to their direction of travel, the drivers in the sandy terrain must turn slightly to the right.

Three situations regarding Snell's law should be considered:

Case 1 refraction: The velocity in the first medium is greater than that in the second medium. The angle of transmittance bends toward the normal from the expected straight-line path (Fig. 1-15). For example, this occurs at a bone-tissue interface.

Case 2 refraction: The velocity in the first medium is less than that in the second medium. The angle of transmittance is bent away from the normal (Fig. 1-17). For example, this occurs at a tissue-bone interface.

Case 3 refraction: This is a special extension of case 2 refrac-

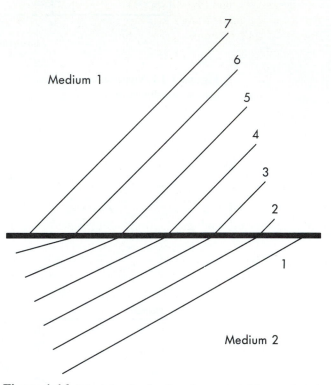

Figure 1-16 Principle of refraction demonstrated by numbered wavefronts striking an interface between two media having different velocities.

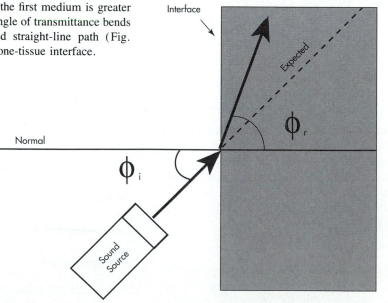

Figure 1-17 Case 2 refraction. The velocity of a sound beam in the incident medium is less than that in the transmitted medium, causing the beam to be bent away from the normal ($\phi_i < \phi_t$).

tion. If the velocity in the first medium is less than that in the second medium and if the angle of incidence is beyond the so-called critical angle, the refracted beam travels along the interface and no energy enters the second medium. This is called total reflection and occurs at an incident angle of greater than 22 degrees when the interface is composed of tissue and bone.

The critical angle (ϕ_c) is determined by Snell's law, in which the transmitted angle is assigned a value of 90 degrees. Since sin 90 equals 1,

$$\sin \phi_c = \frac{c_i}{c_t}$$

or

$$\phi_c = \text{Arcsin} \frac{c_i}{c_t}$$

For soft tissue and bone

$$\sin \phi_c = \frac{1540 \text{ m/s}}{4080 \text{ m/s}}$$
$$= 0.377$$

and

$$\phi_c = 22.2 \text{ degrees}$$

If the velocity of sound is the same in the two media, no refraction (bending) occurs, although the acoustic impedances may be different. Nor does refraction occur at normal incidence, regardless of the relative velocities in the two media (Fig. 1-10).

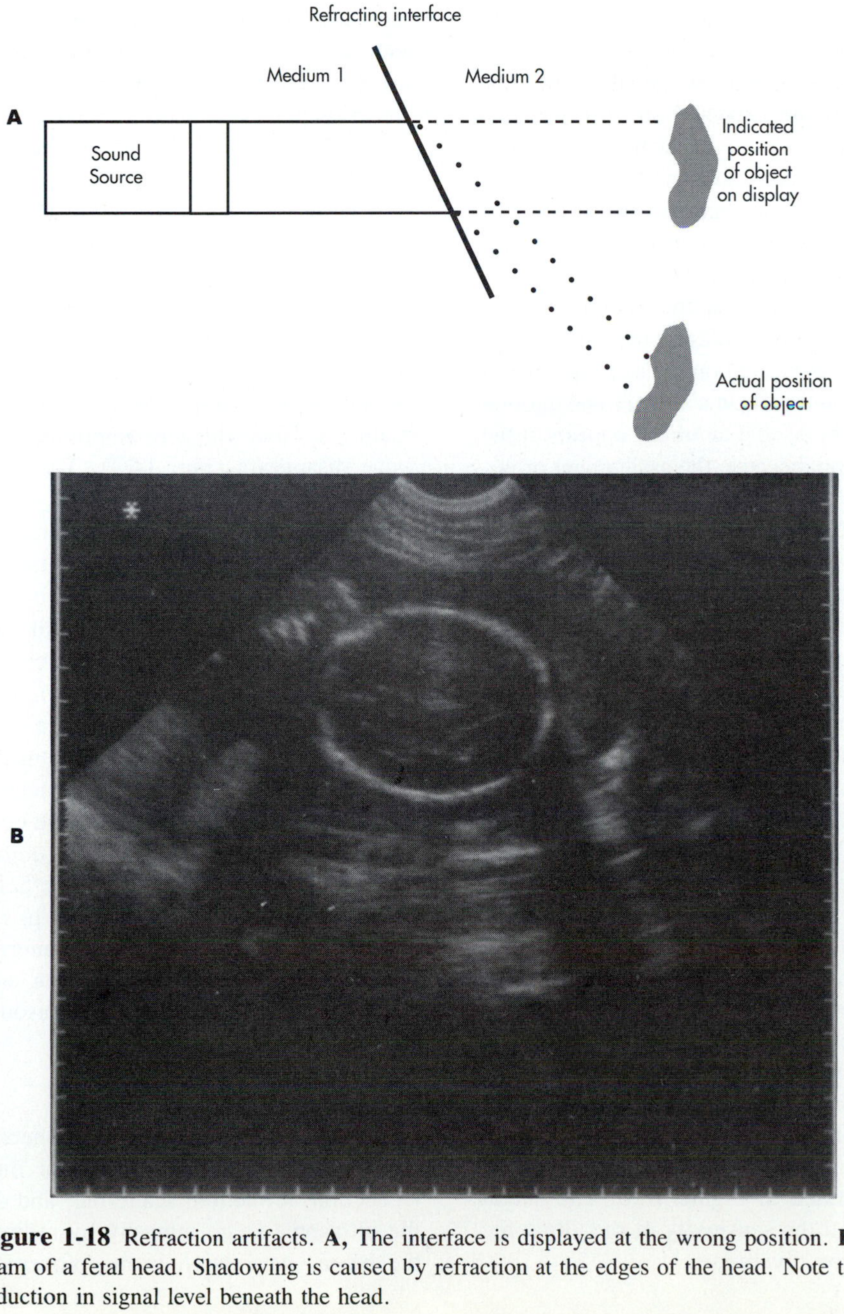

Figure 1-18 Refraction artifacts. **A,** The interface is displayed at the wrong position. **B,** Sonogram of a fetal head. Shadowing is caused by refraction at the edges of the head. Note the reduction in signal level beneath the head.

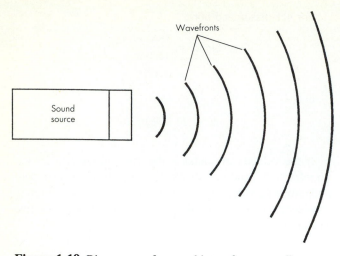

Wavefronts

Sound source

Figure 1-19 Divergence of a sound beam from a small source.

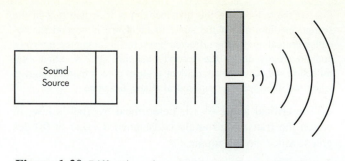

Sound Source

Figure 1-20 Diffraction of a sound beam after passing through a small aperture.

Misregistration. As indicated by Snell's law, the amount of deviation from the expected straight-line path changes with the angle of incidence and with the velocities in the associated media. This does not generally present any difficulty in diagnostic ultrasound because the velocity of ultrasound in soft tissue is relatively constant (Table 1-3). Although refraction is not a major problem in diagnostic ultrasound, under certain conditions the bending of the sound beam can cause artifacts in diagnostic images. The formation of the image is predicated on the assumption that the ultrasound beam always travels in a straight line through tissue. Note in Figure 1-18, *A,* that an object appears at the wrong location in the image because the assignment of position is based on the projected straight line path of the beam whereas the true location of the object is actually offset from the assumed path.

A similar effect caused by the refraction of light is seen when an object under water is viewed from above. If one reaches for the object through the water, the misregistration becomes immediately apparent. Misregistration of interfaces can also result from reflections caused by ultrasonic side lobes, as discussed in Chapters 2, 4 and 14. In addition, refraction may account for the distortion of an object seen on the monitor (Fig. 1-18, *B*).

Diffraction

Diffraction causes the ultrasound beam to diverge or spread out as the waves more farther from the sound source (Fig. 1-19). The rate of divergence increases as the size (diameter) of the sound source decreases. Diffraction also occurs after the beam with planar wavefronts passes through a small aperture on the order of one wavelength. Because the wave is blocked everywhere but in the area of the aperture, the aperture acts as a small sound source and the beam diverges rapidly. This is demonstrated in Figure 1-20. The lateral resolution of the beam and the sensitivity of the ultrasonic system are both affected by divergence.

Interference

Sound waves demonstrate interference phenomena or the superposition of waves (algebraic summation). If waves with the same frequency are in phase, they undergo constructive interference. Waves are in phase if crossing and inflection points are matched along the distance or time axis (Fig. 1-21). Constructive interference results in an increased amplitude.

If waves with the same frequency are out of phase, they undergo destructive interference; that is, a decrease in amplitude results because the peaks are not matched in the same position (Fig. 1-22). Completely destructive interference occurs when the waves are of the same frequency and amplitude and are completely out of phase (i.e., the trough of one wave corresponds to the peak of the other). The result is a wave with zero amplitude; hence, the summation wave disappears (Fig. 1-23). The effect of one wave is countered by the opposite effect of the other wave. For example, when a soccer ball is approached by two opposing players, the player who kicks it first controls the direction of travel. If both players kick the ball simultaneously with equal force, the forces applied will cancel each other and the ball will not move toward either goal.

Every combination—from completely constructive to completely destructive interference—can occur, resulting in a complex wave summation. Figure 1-24 shows the result when waves with differing frequencies create interference. This interference is important in the design of an ultrasonic transducer because it affects the uniformity of the beam intensity throughout the ultrasonic field. (See Chapter 2.) Focusing of the ultrasound beam in real time imaging is based on the principle of wave interference (Chapter 4). Waves of similar frequency, when combined, produce a "beat" that is used in Doppler ultrasound (Chapter 6).

Absorption

Absorption is the only process whereby sound energy is dissipated in a medium. All other modes of interactions (reflection, refraction, scattering, and divergence) decrease the ultrasonic beam intensity by redirecting the energy of the beam. Absorption is the process whereby ultrasonic

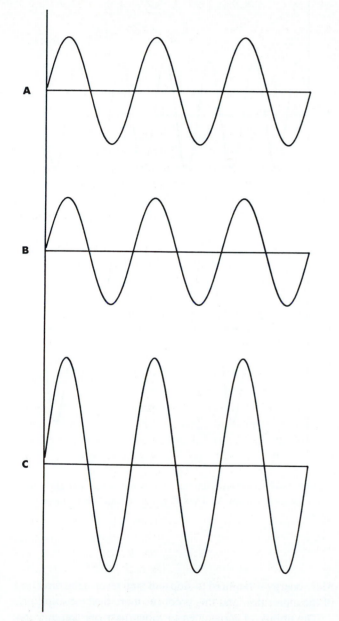

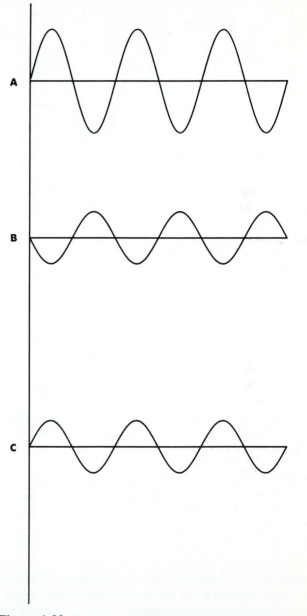

Figure 1-21 Constructive interference or superposition (algebraic summation) of waves. **C,** The resultant wave, is the sum of waves **A** and **B.**

Figure 1-22 Destructive interference. The resultant wave, **C,** is the sum of waves **A** and **B** and is reduced in amplitude because the waves are out of phase.

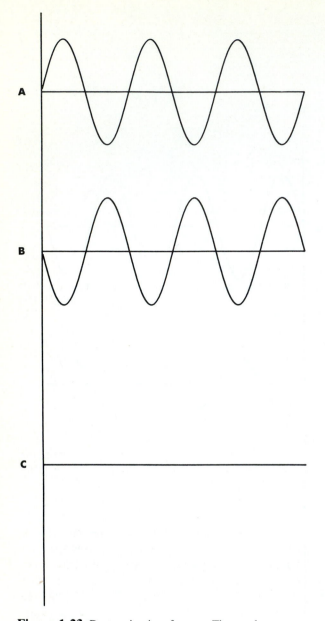

Figure 1-23 Destructive interference. The resultant wave, **C,** is zero because waves **A** and **B** are completely out of phase and have the same amplitude.

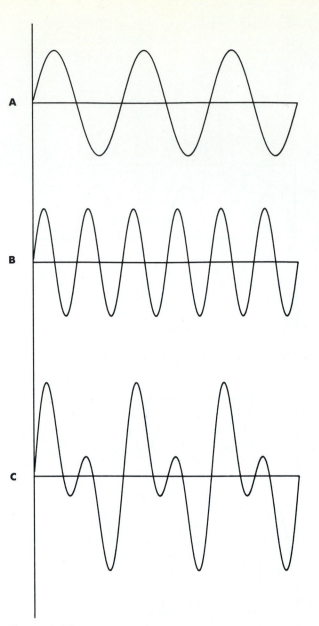

Figure 1-24 Wave interference. Note that **B** has a slightly different frequency from **A.** Thus C is the summation of these two waves.

energy is transformed into other energy forms, primarily heat. It is responsible for the medical applications of therapeutic ultrasound (physiotherapy).

Factors influencing absorption. The absorption of an ultrasonic beam is related to the beam's frequency and to the viscosity and relaxation time of the medium. The relaxation time describes the rate at which molecules return to their original positions after being displaced by a force.

If a substance has a short relaxation time, the molecules return to their original positions before the next wave compression arrives. If it has a long relaxation time, however, the molecules may be moving back toward their original positions as the wave crest (compression) strikes them.

More energy is required to stop and then reverse the direction of the molecules, and this produces more heat (absorption).

The ability of molecules to move past one another determines the viscosity of a medium; high viscosity provides great resistance to molecular flow. For instance, a low-viscosity fluid (water) flows more freely than a viscous one (maple syrup). The frictional forces must be overcome by vibrating molecules, and thus more heat is produced in the maple syrup.

The frequency also affects absorption in relation to both the viscosity and the relaxation time. If the frequency is increased, the molecules must move more often, thereby generating more heat from the drag caused by friction (viscosity). Also, as the frequency is increased, less time is

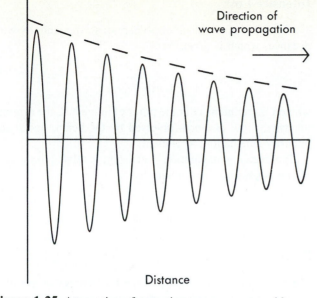

Figure 1-25 Attenuation of acoustic pressure as a sound beam penetrates the medium. The *dashed curve* demonstrates an exponential decrease of the peak acoustic pressure.

available for the molecules to recover during the relaxation process. Molecules remain in motion, and more energy is necessary to stop and redirect them, again producing more absorption. The rate of absorption is directly related to the frequency. If the frequency doubles, the rate of absorption (as specified by the absorption coefficient, α) also doubles.

Consider the mechanical action of rubbing one's hands together. The movement produces heat. If the hands are rubbed together more rapidly (higher frequency), increased warming occurs. If lotion is placed between the palms so the resistance is decreased (lower viscosity), less heat will be generated.

Mathematical description. The peak amplitude of acoustic pressure (mm Hg [torr], pascals, or atmospheres), particle density (kg/m^3 or g/cm^3), particle displacement (m, cm, mm), and particle velocity (m/s, cm/s, mm/s) all decrease as the wave traverses a homogeneous medium. In Figure 1-25 the absorption of the ultrasonic beam follows an exponential function:

1-12

$$A = A_0 \exp(-\alpha z)$$

where A is the peak amplitude of the beam at distance z, A_0 the original peak amplitude of the beam, α the absorption coefficient, and z the distance traversed by the beam.

At a particular location within a continuous single-frequency ultrasonic field, the variations of pressure with time demonstrate an oscillatory behavior, the greatest deviations occurring during maximum pressure (p). The decrease in maximum pressure as the ultrasound energy is absorbed is described by Equation 1-12.

Rewriting Equation 1-12 with the notation for pressure shows that the initial maximum value (p_0) decreases exponentially (to p) as the beam penetrates the medium:

Table 1-6 Attenuation of Human Tissues at 1 MHz

Material	Np/cm
Blood	0.021
Fat	0.069
Kidney	0.115
Muscle (across fibers)	0.380
Muscle (along fibers)	0.138
Brain	0.098
Liver	0.103
Lung	4.6
Skull	2.3

1-13

$$p = p_0 \exp(-\alpha z)$$

The maximum particle velocity (u) and the maximum particle displacement (s) are related to the maximum pressure:

1-14

$$u = \frac{p}{\rho c}$$

and

1-15

$$s = \frac{p}{2\pi f c \rho}$$

As the maximum pressure is reduced, a corresponding decrease in particle velocity and particle displacement occurs.

Attenuation

Attenuation includes the effects of both scattering and absorption in the characterization of amplitude reduction as the ultrasound wave propagates through a medium. Attenuation is also described by an exponential function. Thus the form of Equation 1-12 remains unchanged, but the absorption coefficient is replaced by the attenuation coefficient (a)

1-16

$$A = A_0 \exp(-az)$$

The attenuation coefficient is given by the sum of the scattering coefficient (a_s) and the absorption coefficient (α):

1-17

$$a = a_s + \alpha$$

The various coefficients quantitate the respective fractional losses in amplitude per unit length from absorption, scattering, and both processes together. The special unit for these coefficients is the neper (Np) per centimeter. The attenuation coefficients at 1 MHz for various tissue types are presented in Table 1-6. The effect of frequency must be included in any specification of attenuation coefficient. In a first approximation the attenuation coefficient increases linearly with frequency. For example, the coefficient for fat at 3.5 MHz is estimated by multiplying the value in Table 1-6 (0.069 Np/cm) by 3.5 to obtain 0.24 Np/cm.

INTENSITY

The intensity of an ultrasonic beam is the physical parameter that describes the amount of energy flowing through a cross-sectional area per second. Simply, it is the rate at which the energy is transmitted by the wave over a small area.

When characterizing audible acoustics, we use the term *intensity* to describe the loudness of sound. For ultrasound, increasing intensity means the distribution of particles within the compression regions becomes more dense, acoustic pressure is higher, length of particle oscillation increases, and maximum particle velocity is greater. The intensity of an ultrasound beam decreases as the beam propagates through tissue. The transmitted intensity and the rate of itensity loss influence the ability of a scanner to observe weakly reflecting structures. (Frequency, wavelength, and velocity of an ultrasonic beam are not affected by a change in intensity.)

The study of potential biological effects is linked to intensity. Since the particle velocity and length of displacement are dictated by intensity, a high-intensity ultrasound wave is more disruptive than a low-intensity ultrasound wave is to living systems. The biological effects of ultrasound are examined in Chapter 12.

Traditionally, acoustic intensity is expressed in mixed units of watts per centimeter squared or milliwatts per centimeter squared (a combination of meter kilogram second [MKS] and centimeter gram second [CGS] system units). In other areas of physics this is considered bad form. One watt is equal to one joule per second.

Intensity Descriptors

The intensity of an ultrasound beam is proportional to the square of the pressure amplitude, particle-displacement amplitude, or particle-velocity amplitude ($I \propto A^2$). For example, the equation for instantaneous intensity (i) is given by

$$1\text{-}18$$

$$i = \frac{p_i^2}{\rho c}$$

where p_i is the instantaneous acoustic pressure, c the velocity of sound, and ρ the density. Acoustic pressure is expressed in pascals (Pa) in the MKS system. Pressure is the force exerted on a small area; thus a pascal is equivalent to a newton per meter squared (nt/m^2). One atmosphere equals 10^5 pascals.

Often the time-averaged intensity (I) is of interest. At any point through which an ultrasound beam passes, the pressure oscillates between high and low values. The greatest deviation from average pressure during a cycle is the maximum-pressure or peak-pressure amplitude (p). Since the pressure is fluctuating as a function of time, the instantaneous intensity is also oscillating between high and low values. By averaging the instantaneous intensity over one cycle it is possible to find the time-averaged intensity:

$$1\text{-}19$$

$$I = \frac{p^2}{2 \rho c}$$

Intensity Loss

The intensity of the beam also decreases exponentially with distance, which is given by:

$$1\text{-}20$$

$$I = I_0 \exp(-\mu z)$$

where I is the intensity at the point of interest, I_0 the original intensity, z the distance traversed by the beam, and μ the intensity attenuation coefficient.

The intensity attenuation coefficient is related to the amplitude attenuation coefficient by

$$1\text{-}21$$

$$\mu = 2a$$

Power

The power (W) is a measure of the total energy transmitted per unit time summed over the entire cross-sectional area of the beam:

$$1\text{-}22$$

$$W = \text{Intensity} \times \text{Area}$$

The emitted power from the transducer assembly is not constant, but fluctuates over the wave cycle. Ultrasonic power, averaged over a time period, is referred to as the temporal average power. The unit of power is the watt.

Decibel

Absolute values of the power and intensity of an ultrasonic beam are difficult to measure. This is particularly true of pulsed diagnostic beams, for which both temporal and spatial properties must be considered (Chapter 12).

Although no standard reference intensity for ultrasound has been established, a useful method for determining the reduced intensity of a beam is to make relative measurements that compare the value at one point with a reference intensity at another point. The following analogy may help illustrate the concept: Johnny owns 25 marbles, Tommy 50. To find out how much Johnny's marbles weigh in ounces, we lay them on a scale. If we are interested only in the relative weights of the marbles, we say one batch is "half as heavy as the other." The absolute weight in ounces is not known but can be described with respect to a standard (Tommy's marbles).

Relative measurements are usually made and given in decibels (dB). The intensity variation or level expressed in decibels is

$$1\text{-}23$$

$$\text{Level (dB)} = 10 \log_{10}\left(\frac{I}{I_0}\right)$$

where I is the intensity at the point of interest and I_0 is the original or reference intensity.

One advantage of decibels is that they enable a wide range of intensity and power levels to be expressed in a compact form. (See "Mathematics Review" in Appendix A for further discussion.) Decibels are not restricted to the parameters of power and intensity, however. They can also be used to describe relative measurements for amplitude, noise level, percentage reflection, and many other quantities. In Equation 1-23, I_0 and I are replaced by the reference value and the value for the parameter of interest respectively.

■ Example 1-10

Assume that the intensity at a particular point is reduced to half the original and that at a second point is $1/10,000$ of the original. Convert these relative intensity measurements to decibels.
For point 1:

$$\text{Level (dB)} = 10 \log_{10} \left(\frac{1/2\, I_0}{I_0} \right)$$

$$= 10 \log_{10} 0.5$$

$$= (10)\,(-0.301)$$

$$= -3.01$$

For point 2:

$$\text{Level (dB)} = 10 \log_{10} \frac{(1/10,000)\, I_0}{I_0}$$

$$= 10 \log 0.0001$$

$$= 10(-4)$$

$$= -40$$

The comparison of ratios for both points requires a range of 2 to 10,000 in intensity whereas a range of only -3 to -40 dB units is needed to express this same relation. The negative sign indicates that the intensity of the beam has decreased from the reference point to the point of interest. Further examples are cited in Table 1-7.

Another advantage of the decibel notation is that decibel changes along the beam path are additive. Consider the situation illustrated in Figure 1-26, in which the intensity at point 1 is one tenth the original intensity and the intensity at point 2 is half the intensity at point 1 or one twentieth the original. By using the decibel methodology, the change in decibels can be found:

dB change from transducer to point 1

$$\text{Level (dB)} = 10 \log (I_1/I_0)$$

$$= 10 \log (0.1\, I_0/I_0)$$

$$= -10$$

dB change from point 1 to point 2

$$\text{Level (dB)} = 10 \log (I_2/I_1)$$

$$= 10 \log (0.5\, I_1/I_1)$$

$$= -3.01$$

dB change from transducer to point 2

$$\text{Level (dB)} = 10 \log (I_2/I_0)$$

$$= 10 \log (0.05\, I_0/I_0)$$

$$= -13.01$$

The sum of the decibel changes between points along the path is equal to the decibel change for the entire path. The intensity of the detected echo is often compared with the intensity of the transmitted ultrasound wave. If the relative intensity of the returning echo is 50 dB less than that of the transmitted wave, Equation 1-23 demonstrates that the echo will be a small fraction $(1/100,000)$ of the transmitted intensity:

$$-50 = 10 \log \frac{I}{I_0}$$

$$-5 = \log \frac{I}{I_0}$$

$$\frac{I}{I_0} = \text{Antilog}\ (-5)$$

$$= 0.00001$$

■ Table 1-7   Intensity Ratio Versus Decibels

I/I_0	dB
10,000	40
1000	30
100	20
10	10
1	0
0.1	−10
0.01	−20
0.001	−30
0.0001	−40

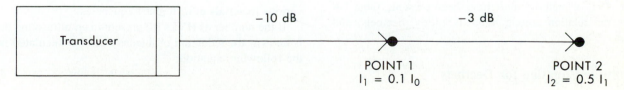

Figure 1-26 Decibel notation. Intensity losses along the path are additive. Thus the change of intensity from the *Transducer* to *point 2* is -13 dB.

The attenuation expressed in nepers equals the attenuation coefficient times the distance traversed. The conversion to nepers for attenuation loss expressed in decibels is given as

1-24

$$\text{Attenuation (Np)} = 0.115 \times (\text{dB loss})$$

The conversion to decibels for attenuation loss expressed in nepers is given as

1-25

$$\text{Attenuation (dB)} = 8.686 \times (\text{Np loss})$$

The attenuation coefficient expressed in dB/cm or Np/cm can be converted from one unit to the other in a similar fashion.

■ Example 1-11

Find the attenuation loss in nepers and decibels for a 1 MHz ultrasound beam traversing 7 cm of liver. From Table 1-6 the attenuation coefficient for liver can be seen to be 0.103 Np/cm. A thickness of 7 cm causes a loss of 0.721 Np (0.103 Np/cm × 7 cm). The decrease in maximum pressure amplitude is calculated by using Equation 1-13:

$$p = p_0 \exp(-az)$$
$$= p_0 \exp(-0.721)$$
$$= 0.486\, p_0$$

Intensity is directly proportional to the square of the maximum pressure amplitude.

$$I = 0.236\, I_0$$

The decibel loss is calculated using Equation 1-23.

$$\text{Level (dB)} = 10 \log(I/I_0)$$
$$= 10 \log(0.236\, I_0/I_0)$$
$$= 10 \log(0.236)$$
$$= 10(-0.627)$$
$$= -6.27$$

Note that the loss in decibels (6.27)—when multiplied by the factor 0.115 as defined by Equation 1-24—equals the loss in nepers of 0.721.

Half-Value Layer

A half-value layer (HVL) of material is the thickness that will reduce the intensity to half its original value. Note in Example 1-10 that a reduction in intensity by a factor of 2 results in 3 dB loss. A decrease in intensity by 3 dB indicates that 1 HVL of material must have been present. Table 1-8 shows the relation among intensity ratios, decibels, and HVLs.

Amplitude Equation for Decibels

Equation 1-23 defines decibel using the ratio of the intensities at two different points. Another equation using the ratio

■ Table 1-8 Relation Among Intensity Ratios, Decibels, and Half-Value Layers

Percent of Sound Remaining	I/I_0	dB	Half-Value Layer
100	1	0	—
50	0.5	−3.01	1.00
25	0.25	−6.02	2.00
10	0.1	−10.00	3.32
5	0.05	−13.01	4.32
1	0.01	−20.00	6.64
0.1	0.001	−30.00	9.96
0.01	0.0001	−40.00	13.29
0.001	0.00001	−50.00	16.61

of the amplitudes may be employed to calculate intensity changes in decibels. Recall that the square of the amplitude is proportional to the intensity. Consequently

1-26

$$\left(\frac{A}{A_0}\right)^2 = \frac{I}{I_0}$$

where A_0 is the original peak amplitude of the beam and A is the peak amplitude at the point of interest. Substituting for I/I_0 in Equation 1-23:

1-27

$$dB = 10 \log_{10}\left(\frac{A}{A_0}\right)^2$$

or

$$dB = 20 \log_{10}\left(\frac{A}{A_0}\right)$$

Table 1-9 lists several examples of amplitude ratio and the corresponding decibel, calculated using Equation 1-27.

A reduction in amplitude by a factor of 2 or half-amplitude (A = 0.5 A_0) results in a 6 dB loss. This reduction is equivalent to a reduction of intensity by a factor of 4, or 2 HVLs. One HVL corresponds to a change in amplitude by a factor of 1.414 (A = 0.707 A_0). The term *half-power* describes a reduction of intensity by a factor of 2 (which corresponds to a 3 dB loss).

Decibels and HVLs

A 9 dB reduction in intensity is expected from a thickness of material composed of 3 HVLs—that is, 9 dB divided by 3 dB/HVL equals 3 HVLs. Table 1-10 lists HVLs for various materials at different frequencies.

If the number of HVLs (n) present in an ultrasound beam is known, the reduction of intensity can be calculated from the following equation:

1-28

$$I = \frac{I_0}{2^n}$$

■ **Table 1-9** Amplitude Ratio Versus Decibels

A/A₀	dB
100	40
10	20
2	6
1	0
0.5	−6
0.1	−20
0.05	−26
0.01	−40

■ **Table 1-10** Half-Value Layers (in Centimeters) at Different Frequencies

Material	Frequency			
	1 MHz	2 MHz	5 MHz	10 MHz
Air	0.25	0.06	0.01	—
Water	1360.0	340.0	54.0	14.0
Blood	17.0	8.5	3.0	2.0
Bone	0.2	0.1	0.04	—
Brain	3.5	2.0	1.0	—
Fat	5.0	2.5	1.0	0.5
Liver	3.0	1.5	0.5	—
Muscle	1.5	0.75	0.3	0.15
Tissue (average)	4.3	2.1	0.86	0.43

■ **Example 1-12**

Suppose a 2 MHz transducer is used to image a patient's abdomen at a depth of 15 cm. If the incident intensity is known to be 5 mW/cm², the intensity at 15 cm can be determined from Equation 1-28. The first step is to find the HVL for the tissue at 2 MHz, which Table 1-10 lists as 2.1 cm. In this case the number of HVLs is 7.14 because the thickness of material (15 cm) divided by the HVL (2.1 cm) equals 7.14. The intensity at 15 cm is given as

$$I = \frac{5 \text{ mW/cm}^2}{2^{7.14}}$$

$$= \frac{5 \text{ mW/cm}^2}{141}$$

$$= 0.035 \text{ mW/cm}^2$$

The same result could be obtained using Equation 1-23, which gives the relative intensities in decibels. The change in intensity corresponds to −21.49 dB (7.14 HVL × −3.01 dB/HVL). Substituting and solving for I gives

$$-21.49 = 10 \log \frac{I}{5 \text{ mW/cm}^2}$$

$$-2.149 = \log \frac{I}{5 \text{ mW/cm}^2}$$

$$\text{Antilog } (-2.149) = \frac{I}{5 \text{ mW/cm}^2}$$

$$0.007 = \frac{I}{5 \text{ mW/cm}^2}$$

$$I = 0.035 \text{ mW/cm}^2$$

The attenuation of an ultrasound beam is a measure of the decrease of power or intensity as the beam traverses a medium. All the interactions of ultrasound with tissue (reflection, refraction, scattering, divergence, and absorption) cause a decrease in beam intensity and contribute to the overall attenuation of the beam. Only absorption results in energy transfer to the tissue; all other interactions with tissue cause a redirection of ultrasonic energy.

CALCULATION OF ATTENUATION LOSS

The intensity loss in decibels caused by attenuation as the ultrasound beam passes through a medium is calculated by the equation

1-29

$$\text{Loss (dB)} = \mu f z$$

where μ is the intensity attenuation coefficient expressed in dB/cm/MHz, f is the frequency of the ultrasound wave expressed in MHz, and z is the distance traveled in the medium expressed in cm.

A loss of intensity relative to the reference intensity (Equation 1-23) is denoted by a negative sign. The negative sign is not included in Equation 1-29, because attenuation always causes decreased intensity as the ultrasound beam penetrates a medium. The descriptor "loss" and the negative sign would be redundant. However, if the result is used in Equation 1-23 to calculate an absolute intensity expressed in W/cm², intensity loss by attenuation must include the negative sign. The intensity attenuation coefficient is tissue specific and accounts for differences in the attenuation rate for various tissue types. Rapid attenuation is indicated by high values of the intensity attenuation coefficient.

As an approximation, the attenuation (neglecting reflection) of an ultrasound beam propagating through soft tissue is 1 dB/cm/MHz. The actual value is closer to 0.8 dB/cm/MHz. For a 1 MHz ultrasound beam approximately 20% of the energy is absorbed after 1 cm of travel in soft tissue. The decreased intensity expressed in decibels is directly proportional to both the depth of penetration and the frequency of the ultrasound beam. This can be seen more clearly by citing an example.

■ **Example 1-13**

Calculate the intensity loss in decibels for a 2.5 MHz ultrasound beam after traversing 6 cm of soft tissue.

$$\mu = 0.8 \text{ dB/cm/MHz}$$

$$f = 2.5 \text{ MHz}$$

$$z = 6 \text{ cm}$$

$$\text{Loss} = \mu f z$$

$$= (0.8 \text{ dB/cm/MHz}) (2.5 \text{ MHz}) (6 \text{ cm})$$

$$= 12 \text{ dB}$$

■ **Table 1-11** Attenuation of Human Tissues and Other Media at 1 MHz

Material	dB/cm
Blood	0.18
Fat	0.6
Kidney	1.0
Muscle (across fibers)	3.3
Muscle (along fibers)	1.2
Brain	0.85
Liver	0.9
Lung	40.0
Skull	20.0
Lens	2.0
Aqueous humor	0.022
Vitreous humor	0.13
Water	0.0022
Castor oil	0.95
Lucite	2.0

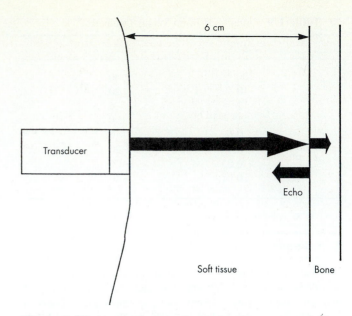

Figure 1-27 An echo is created at an interface composed of soft tissue and bone after the sound wave penetrates 6 cm of soft tissue.

Penetration

High-frequency sound waves are attenuated faster than low-frequency sound waves. Thus the ability to penetrate tissue is reduced at higher frequencies. In addition, a reflector positioned at progressively greater depths generates progressively lower-intensity returning echoes. A method whereby the strength of the received signal is increased by amplification as a function of depth, called *time gain compensation* (TGC), is presented in Chapter 2. Table 1-11 shows some intensity attenuation factors for human tissues at a frequency of 1 MHz. Refer to Table 1-10 and note that the HVLs of some materials do not vary linearly with frequency. For example, muscle exhibits a linear change in HVL with frequency, but this is not the case for water.

DETERMINATION OF ECHO INTENSITY

Soft Tissue–Bone Interface

Figures 1-27 and 1-28 depict the ultrasound beam striking an interface composed of soft tissue and bone. An echo is created at the interface that returns toward the transducer. The thickness of the soft tissue is 6 cm, and that of the bone 0.5 cm. In Figure 1-27 the sound wave must traverse 6 cm of tissue before striking the soft tissue–bone interface. In Figure 1-28 the order of the media is reversed: the sound wave must traverse 0.5 cm of bone before striking the interface. These figures will be utilized to illustrate the change in intensity of a sound beam after undergoing various interactions, specifically attenuation and reflection.

From Example 1-13, the intensity loss in decibels for a 2.5 MHz ultrasound beam after traversing 6 cm of soft tissue can be seen to be 12 dB. The intensity loss for a 2.5 MHz ultrasound beam after traversing 0.5 cm of bone is calculated in an identical manner and found to be 25 dB.

A small thickness of bone is very effective at reducing the intensity of the ultrasound beam, as indicated by the

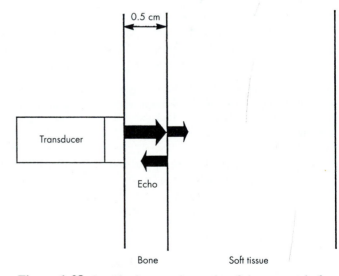

Figure 1-28 An echo is created at an interface composed of bone and soft tissue after the sound wave penetrates 0.5 cm of bone.

high intensity-attenuation coefficient. The large reduction attributed to attenuation in bone is the major reason why bone is generally avoided during an ultrasound examination. Additionally, there is a large amount of reflection at any soft tissue–bone interface.

In ultrasound imaging the transducer sends out a pulsed wave and subsequently detects the returning echo. Intensity loss occurs by attenuation of the transmitted wave going out to the interface and also by attenuation of the reflected wave coming back toward the transducer from the interface. The rate of attenuation depends on tissue type and wave frequency. The intensity of the detected echo from an interface is diminished by increasing the distance of travel.

HAHNEMANN UNIVERSITY LIBRARY

■ Example 1-14

Calculate the relative intensity in decibels for an echo generated at a bone–soft tissue interface that is 6 cm deep in soft tissue. The transducer operates at a frequency of 2.5 MHz. Neglect the contribution of reflection at the interface.

The loss as the ultrasound beam strikes the interface is the same as in Example 1-13 (i.e., 12 dB). Since the echo must repeat the path back to the transducer, the total intensity loss is twice this amount (24 dB).

Similarly, the total intensity loss of an echo returning from the bone–soft tissue interface after traveling a total distance of 1 cm in bone is 50 dB. If the frequency of the transducer is increased, the rate of attenuation between soft tissue and bone will be even more pronounced. For example, operating at a frequency of 7.5 MHz, the attenuation loss is tripled (to 72 dB and 150 dB).

Attenuation and Reflection Losses

We will now consider the combined effect of attenuation and reflection on the intensity of a detected echo. *Attenuation* refers to all processes (except reflection) that act to reduce ultrasound intensity. Losses from attenuation and reflection must be expressed in the same units, usually decibels. To convert percentage reflection into decibels, we modify Equation 1-23 by replacing I_0 with 100 and I with the percentage reflection and inverting the fraction within the logarithmic function (to eliminate the negative sign):

1-30

$$\text{Loss (dB)} = 10 \log \frac{100}{\%R}$$

The negative sign is not included, because the descriptor "loss" indicates that reflection always causes a reduction of intensity. Furthermore, losses from attenuation and reflection expressed in decibels are additive and can be easily combined. The following examples illustrate the total effect of attenuation and reflection on the intensity of the detected echo. Figures 1-27 and 1-28 are reexamined to include the contribution of reflection.

■ Example 1-15

Calculate the relative intensity in decibels for an echo generated at a bone-tissue interface that is 6 cm deep in soft tissue. The transducer operates at a frequency of 2.5 MHz. Include the contribution of reflection at the interface.

For the transmitted wave

$$\text{Loss} = \mu fz$$
$$= (0.8 \text{ dB/cm/MHz}) (2.5 \text{ MHz}) (6 \text{ cm})$$
$$= 12 \text{ dB}$$

For the returning echo

$$\text{Loss} = 12 \text{ dB}$$

For the reflection at this soft tissue–bone interface (i.e., the percentage reflection, 43%) which must be converted into decibels

$$\text{Loss (dB)} = 10 \log \frac{100}{\%R}$$

$$= 10 \log \frac{100}{43}$$
$$= 3.7 \text{ dB}$$

The total loss from attenuation and reflection

$$\text{Loss} = 12 \text{ dB} + 12 \text{ dB} + 3.7 \text{ dB}$$
$$= 27.7 \text{ dB}$$

■ Example 1-16

Calculate the relative intensity in decibels for an echo generated at a bone-tissue interface that is 0.5 cm deep in bone. (The transducer operates at a frequency of 2.5 MHz.) Include the contribution of reflection at the interface.

For the transmitted wave

$$\text{Loss} = \mu fz$$
$$= (20 \text{ dB/cm/MHz}) (2.5 \text{ MHz}) (0.5 \text{ cm})$$
$$= 25 \text{ dB}$$

For the returning echo

$$\text{Loss} = 25 \text{ dB}$$

For the loss from reflection at this soft tissue–bone interface (i.e., the percentage reflection, 43%), which must be converted into decibels

$$\text{Loss (dB)} = 10 \log \frac{100}{\%R}$$

$$= 10 \log \frac{100}{43}$$
$$= 3.7 \text{ dB}$$

The total loss from attenuation and reflection

$$= \text{Loss (going out)} + \text{Loss (returning)} + \text{Loss (reflection)}$$
$$= 25 \text{ dB} + 25 \text{ dB} + 3.7 \text{ dB}$$
$$= 53.7 \text{ dB}$$

In general, absorption has a greater effect than reflection on the overall loss of beam intensity. Comparing the results from the previous two examples demonstrates that the intensity of the echo at the transducer associated with a soft tissue–bone interface varies according to the attenuation along the path. Structures with the same reflectivity are not always depicted with the same signal level.

Calculation of Intensity

Once the total attenuation from all sources (i.e., absorption, reflection, refraction, and scattering) in decibels is found, the intensity ratio can be calculated. For a loss of 30 dB, Equation 1-23 demonstrates that the original intensity is reduced by a factor of 1000:

$$-30 = 10 \log \frac{I}{I_0}$$
$$-3 = \log \frac{I}{I_0}$$
$$\frac{I}{I_0} = \text{Antilog} (-3)$$
$$= 0.001$$

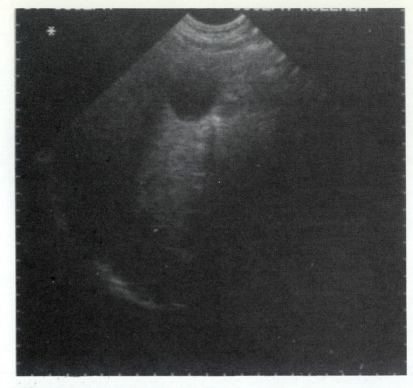

Figure 1-29 Sonogram of a liver with a cyst. There is acoustic enhancement behind the liquid-filled structure.

The intensity ratio can be used to calculate the actual intensity value for I or I_0 if one of them is known. For example, if I_0 is 10 mW/cm^2, the intensity at the point of interest (I) will be 0.01 mW/cm^2. An understanding of decibel notation and the various intensity parameters is essential when biological effects of ultrasound are being discussed. (See Chapter 12.)

■ Example 1-17

Calculate the intensity in watts per square centimeter for the detected echo in Example 1-15. (The transmitted intensity is 5 W/cm^2.)

$$\text{Level (dB)} = -27.7$$

$$I_0 = 5 \text{ W/cm}^2$$

$$\text{Level (dB)} = 10 \log \frac{I}{I_0}$$

$$-27.7 = 10 \log \frac{I}{5 \text{ W/cm}^2}$$

$$-2.77 = \log \frac{I}{5 \text{ W/cm}^2}$$

$$\text{Antilog} \,(-2.77) = \frac{I}{5 \text{ W/cm}^2}$$

$$0.0017 = \frac{I}{5 \text{ W/cm}^2}$$

$$I = 0.0085 \text{ W/cm}^2 \text{ or } 8.5 \text{ mW/cm}^2$$

■ Example 1-18

Calculate the intensity in watts per square centimeter for the detected echo in Example 1-15. (The transmitted intensity is 5 W/cm^2.)

$$\text{Level (dB)} = -53.7$$

$$I_0 = 5 \text{ W/cm}^2$$

$$\text{Level (dB)} = 10 \log \frac{I}{I_0}$$

$$-53.7 = 10 \log \frac{I}{5 \text{ W/cm}^2}$$

$$-5.37 = \log \frac{I}{5 \text{ W/cm}^2}$$

$$\text{Antilog} \,(-5.37) = \frac{I}{5 \text{ W/cm}^2}$$

$$0.0000043 = \frac{I}{5 \text{ W/cm}^2}$$

$$I = 0.000022 \text{ W/cm}^2 \text{ or } 0.022 \text{ mW/cm}^2$$

Solid masses can be differentiated from cysts by examining the transmission of the beam through the structure. Solids attenuate the beam more rapidly than cystic (liquid-like) structures do. Liquids (blood, water, or cystic structures) are transonic or sonolucent and do not sharply attenuate. They are said to be anechoic. A liquid creates en-

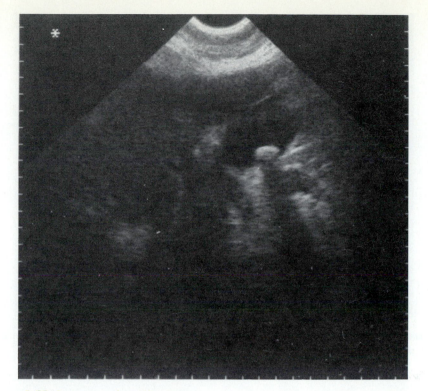

Figure 1-30 Sonogram of a gallbladder. There is acoustic shadowing behind the strongly attenuating structure.

hancement beyond the structure, compared with the surrounding more attenuating structures, as illustrated in Figure 1-29. Shadowing (characterized by diminished signal levels) may occur behind sharply attenuating structures such as gallstones. Structures that create shadowing are called echogenic (Fig. 1-30). Shadowing may also occur at the edges of both solid and cystic structures induced by refraction artifacts, as demonstrated in Figures 1-18, *B*, and 1-31.

ECHO RANGING

In diagnostic ultrasound, reflections of the sound beam from interfaces along the ultrasonic path are of primary interest. An ultrasound wave is transmitted into the body, strikes an interface (acoustic mismatch between two media), and is partially reflected to the transducer, as determined by the percentage reflection formula. The reflected waves arising from the various acoustic impedance mismatches result in ultrasonic detection of interfaces within the body.

The distance (z) traveled by the sound beam is specified by the formula

1-31

$$z = ct$$

where c is the velocity and t the time of travel.

If the velocity of ultrasound in the medium and the elapsed time from the original send pulse to the detection of the return echo are known, the distance to an interface is determined from Equation 1-31.

The following calculation demonstrates the time necessary to travel distances that are of clinical interest. The average velocity of ultrasound in tissue is 1540 m/s. For an interface exactly 1 cm away, the total time for the sound wave to travel out to the interface and back to the transducer is calculated by using Equation 1-31 and by solving for t (Fig. 1-32). The total distance out and back is 2 cm, or 0.02 m (1 cm = 0.01 meter). Because the velocity is 1540 m/s in tissue, the elapsed time is

$$t = \frac{0.02 \text{m}}{1540 \text{ m/s}}$$

$$= \frac{2 \times 10^{-2} \text{ m}}{1.54 \times 10^{3} \text{ m/s}}$$

$$= 13 \times 10^{-6} \text{ s}$$

$$= 13 \text{ } \mu\text{s}$$

Only 13 μs are required for the sound beam to travel 1 cm and return 1 cm in tissue. Each centimeter of travel beam takes 6.5 μs.

◼ **Example 1-19**

A pulsed ultrasound wave is transmitted through soft tissue toward an interface composed of soft tissue and bone. The elapsed time between the transmitted pulse and the detected echo is 74 μs. What is the depth of the interface?

$$z = \frac{t}{13 \text{ } \mu\text{s/cm}}$$

$$= \frac{74 \text{ } \mu\text{s}}{13 \text{ } \mu\text{s/cm}}$$

$$= 5.7 \text{ cm}$$

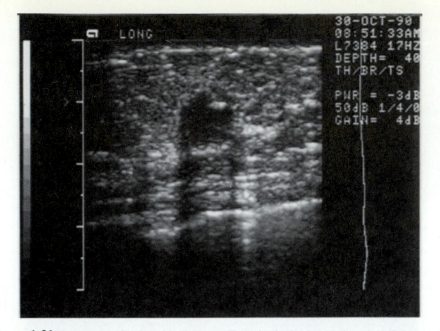

Figure 1-31 Sonogram of a thyroid adenoma. There is shadowing at the edge of the anechogenic structure.

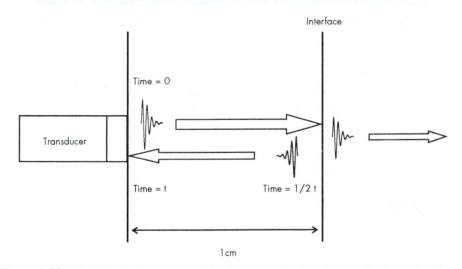

Figure 1-32 Principle of echo ranging. The distance to the interface can be determined by measuring the time between the transmitted pulse and the received echo. A constant velocity in the medium must be assumed.

The distance to an interface is determined by the elapsed time; in other words, the time of travel to and from the interface at a constant velocity is set by the distance of travel. As the depth to the interface increases, the elapsed time increases. For an interface 10 cm away, 130 μs between the transmitted pulse and the returning echo are required.

A system that can generate an ultrasonic pulsed wave and detect the reflected echo after a measured time permits the distance to an interface (i.e., the depth of the interface) to be determined. This technique is called echo-ranging, a concept that formed the basis of sonar (sound navigation and ranging) developed during World War II.

For echo ranging to delineate the position of an interface correctly, certain conditions must hold: (1) the ultrasound wave must travel directly to the interface and back to the transducer along a straight-line path and (2) the velocity of sound must remain constant along the path of travel.

SUMMARY

An understanding of the physics of ultrasound is essential to the successful clinical application of diagnostic ultrasonographic techniques. The types and properties of sound waves and the interaction of those waves with tissues (reflection, refraction, scattering, interference, absorption, and attenuation) influence the collection and interpretation of scan data. The technique of echo ranging forms the basis of most ultrasonic scanning modes. This chapter provides a foundation for understanding the principles of all scanning modes and their associated instrumentation.

REVIEW QUESTIONS

1. The velocity of ultrasound is directly proportional to the compressibility of the medium.
   a. True
   b. False

2. For an ultrasound beam incident on a large smooth interface, the angle of reflection is equal to the angle of incidence.
   a. True
   b. False

3. The wavelength is directly proportional to the frequency.
   a. True
   b. False

4. If the frequency of an ultrasound beam is increased, its penetration in soft tissue is enhanced.
   a. True
   b. False

5. Reflection is the major cause for the loss of intensity of an ultrasound beam in a continuous homogeneous medium.
   a. True
   b. False

6. Constructive interference is the superposition of waves that causes the resultant wave to increase in amplitude.
   a. True
   b. False

7. Absorption causes energy to be transferred from the ultrasound beam to the medium.
   a. True
   b. False

8. The bending of an ultrasound beam by refraction depends on the acoustic impedances of the two media forming the interface.
   a. True
   b. False

9. The period of an ultrasound wave is directly proportional to the frequency.
   a. True
   b. False

10. Ultrasound waves are electromagnetic waves.
    a. True
    b. False

11. Particle density and acoustic pressure are not influenced by ultrasound beam intensity.
    a. True
    b. False

12. A half-value layer is the amount of material required to reduce the intensity of an ultrasound beam by a factor of 2.
    a. True
    b. False

13. Absorption is the only process that redirects an ultrasound beam.
    a. True
    b. False

14. If an ultrasound beam is directed at an interface at a 15 degree angle of incidence and the velocity in medium 1 is greater than that in medium 2, the beam will be bent toward the normal.
    a. True
    b. False

15. Ultrasound waves in soft tissue are transverse waves.
    a. True
    b. False

16. Find the period of a wave whose frequency is 5 MHz or 5×10^6 cycles per second.

17. Find the frequency of a wave whose period is 4×10^{-7} second.

18. What is the wavelength of a 3.5 MHz sound wave in soft tissue?

19. What is the acoustic impedance of Lucite (whose density is 1190 kg/m³)? Assume the velocity of sound in Lucite to be 2680 m/s.

20. What is the acoustic impedance of fat, whose density is 950 kg/m³? Assume the velocity of sound in fat to be 1460 m/s.

21. Calculate the percentage reflection (%R) for a large smooth interface composed of Lucite and water. Use the acoustic impedance values in Table 1-3.

22. Calculate the percentage reflection (%R) for a smooth interface composed of aqueous humor and the lens. Use the acoustic impedance values in Table 1-3.

23. Calculate the percentage transmission (%T) for a large smooth interface composed of fat and soft tissue. Use the acoustic impedance values listed in Table 1-3.

24. The acoustic impedance of air is 0.0004×10^5 kg/m²/s, and that of tissue is 1.63×10^5 kg/m²/s. What are the percent reflection and the percent transmission at an interface composed of air and soft tissue?
    a. 99.95%, 0.05%
    b. 0.1%, 99.9%
    c. 99.9%, 0.1%
    d. None of the above

25. The acoustic impedance of bone is 7.8×10^5 kg/m²/s, and that of tissue is 1.63×10^5 kg/m²/s. What are the reflection coefficient and the transmission coefficient at an interface composed of bone and soft tissue?
    a. 0.345, 0.655
    b. 0.655, 0.345
    c. 0.428, 0.572
    d. None of the above

26. Calculate the transmitted angle if an ultrasound beam is directed at a large interface composed of soft tissue and bone. The angle of incidence is 20 degrees. Assume the sound beam to be moving from soft tissue into bone.

27. Calculate the transmitted angle if an ultrasound beam is directed at a large interface composed of bone and soft tissue. The angle of incidence is 20 degrees. Assume that the sound beam is moving from bone into soft tissue.

28. The attenuation of ultrasound propagating through soft tissue is approximately _____ dB/cm/MHz.

29. What is the attenuation loss in decibels for an ultrasound beam traversing 2 cm of fat? Assume the frequency to be 3 MHz, the acoustic velocity 1460 m/s, and the attenuation coefficient 0.6 dB/cm/MHz.

30. If an ultrasound beam has a transmitted intensity of 4 W/cm² and the detected echo has an intensity of 0.005 W/cm², what is the relative intensity in decibels?

31. Calculate the relative intensity in decibels for an echo generated at a soft tissue–bone interface that is 4 cm deep. The ultrasound beam travels through soft tissue before being reflected at the interface. The transducer frequency is 3.5 MHz.

32. Calculate the relative intensity in decibels for an echo generated at a bone−soft tissue interface that is 0.4 cm deep. The ultrasound beam travels through bone before being reflected at the interface. The transducer frequency is 3.5 MHz.

33. Calculate the relative intensity is decibels for an echo generated at a fat−soft tissue interface that is at a depth of 2 cm. The ultrasound beam travels through fat before being reflected at the interface. The transducer frequency is 7.5 MHz.

34. Calculate the relative intensity in decibels for an echo generated at a soft tissue−lung interface that is at a depth of 5 cm. The ultrasound beam travels through soft tissue before being reflected at the interface. The transducer frequency is 5.0 MHz.

35. Calculate the returning echo intensity as a fraction of the transmitted intensity if the intensity of the detected echo is described as 25 dB below the transmitted intensity.

36. The elapsed time between the transmitted pulse and the detected echo is 39 μs. How far is the interface from the transducer?

37. The distance of a tissue interface is 2 cm from the face of the transducer. How much time elapses between the transmitted ultrasound pulse and the detected echo?

38. How far away is an interface in tissue if the elapsed time for the sound wave to travel out and back is 260 μs?
    a. 20 mm
    b. 40 mm
    c. 20 cm
    d. 40 cm

39. What is the velocity of ultrasound in a medium if the wavelength is 0.03 cm and the frequency is 5 MHz?
    a. 3×10^6 m/s
    b. 1.5×10^3 m/s
    c. 3×10^3 m/s
    d. 1.5×10^6 m/s

40. What is the wavelength of ultrasound in a medium if the velocity is 4080 m/s and the frequency is 2.5 MHz?
    a. 1.63 cm
    b. 0.00163 m
    c. 163 mm
    d. 1.63 km

41. What is the frequency of ultrasound in a medium if the velocity is 333 m/s and the wavelength is 1 mm?
    a. 3.33×10^5 Hz
    b. 3.33×10^6 Hz
    c. 3.33×10^{-6} Hz
    d. 3.33×10^7 Hz

42. As the thickness of the two materials forming an interface is increased, the intensity of the reflected echoes _____.
    a. Becomes greater
    b. Remains unchanged
    c. Becomes smaller

43. The percent reflection at an interface between two media having different acoustic impedances will _____ when a sound beam moves from the low-impedance medium to the high-impedance medium compared with when it moves in the opposite direction.
    a. Increase
    b. Decrease
    c. Remain the same

44. If intensity is decreased by a factor of 2, this corresponds to a decible change of _____.
    a. −6 dB   c. −12 dB
    b. −3 dB   d. −9 dB

45. For an examination of the breast the sonographer replaces the 5 MHz transducer with a 10 MHz one. The wavelength of the ultrasound wave in soft tissue will be _____ times that exhibited by the previous transducer and the attenuation rate will be _____ times that with the previous transducer.

46. Refraction does not occur under the conditions of?
    a. Normal incidence   d. a and b
    b. $C_1 = C_2$ e. a and c
    c. $Z_1 = Z_2$

47. Specular reflection occurs when the interface is _____ than the width of the ultrasound beam.

48. Match the letter with the correct number.
    a. Nonspecular
    b. Wavelength
    c. Period
    d. Frequency
    e. Velocity
    f. Intensity
    g. Acoustic impedance
    h. Absorption
    i. Interference
    j. Longitudinal wave

    1. Algebraic summation of waves
    2. Power per unit area
    3. Reciprocal of period
    4. Rayl
    5. Time to complete one cycle
    6. Distance to complete one cycle
    7. Rate of travel of sound through a medium
    8. Dissipates energy in a medium
    9. Scattering
    10. Ultrasound

BIBLIOGRAPHY

Avecilla LS: The physics and instrumentation of diagnostic ultrasound: a review. I, *Med Ultrasound* 3:11, 1979.

Bushong SC: *Radiologic science for technologists: physics, biology, and protection,* ed 5, St Louis, 1993, Mosby.

Carlsen EN: Ultrasound physics for the physician: a brief review, *J Clin Ultrasound* 3:69, 1975.

Curry TS III, Dowdey JE, Murry RC Jr: *Christensen's Physics of diagnostic radiology,* ed 4, Philadelphia, 1990, Lea & Febiger.

Devey GB, Wells PNT: Ultrasound in medical diagnosis, *Sci Am* 5:98, 1978.

Hagen-Ansert S: *Textbook of diagnostic ultrasonography,* ed 3, St Louis, 1989, Mosby.

Hendee WR, Ritenour ER: *Medical imaging physics,* ed 3, St Louis, 1992, Mosby.

Kremkau FW: *Diagnostic ultrasonics: physical principles and exercises,* ed 3, Philadelphia, 1988, WB Saunders.

McDicken WN: *Diagnostic ultrasonics: principles and use of instruments,* ed 3, Edinburgh, 1991, Churchill Livingstone.

Powis, RL: *Physics for the fun of it,* Denver, 1978, Unirad Corporation.

Rose JL, Goldberg BB: *Basic physics in diagnostic ultrasound,* New York, 1979, John Wiley & Sons.

Sarti DA, Sample WF: *Diagnostic ultrasound: text and cases,* Boston, 1980, GK Hall.

Smith SW, Lopez H: A contrast-detail analysis of diagnostic ultrasound imaging, *Med Phys* 9:4, 1982.

Wells PNT: *Physical principles of ultrasonic diagnosis,* New York, 1969, Academic Press.

Wells PNT: *Biomedical ultrasonics,* New York, 1977, Academic Press.

Woodcock JP: *Ultrasonics,* Bristol, 1979, Adam Hilger.

CHAPTER 2

Basic Ultrasound Instrumentation

K E Y   T E R M S

Axial resolution
Backing material
Bandwidth
Cathode ray tube
Duty factor
Dynamic range
Far field
Focusing
Lateral resolution
Matching layer
Near field

Noise
Piezoelectric
Pulse duration
Pulse repetition frequency
Pulse repetition period
Q value
Sensitivity
Signal processing
Signal to noise ratio
Spatial pulse length

Ultrasound as a clinical modality began in the mid-1950s with the use of A-mode scanning for examination of the eye and for echoencephalography. In the early to mid-1970s ultrasound instrumentation changed significantly with the advent of analog and digital scan converters, which made two-dimensional static B-mode gray-scale imaging possible. The development of ultrasound instrumentation continued with the introduction of real-time scanners in the late 1970s, followed by Doppler and color Doppler units in the 1980s.

A better understanding of the design criteria for transducers—coupled with such developments as the miniaturization of electronics, the formation of computer-based signal processing, and the creation of flexible microprocessor-driven instrumentation, along with the lack of demonstrated adverse biological effects—has contributed to this dramatic increase in the clinical applications of medical diagnostic ultrasound. It is important that the functions of the basic scanner discussed here be understood, to serve as a prerequisite for understanding the modifications that have been made in each scanning mode discussed in the following chapters.

• • •

The information obtained from ultrasound scanning depends in large part on the beam characteristics, which in turn are governed by transducer design and instrument settings. Numerous parameters are used to describe the ultrasound sampling process. Physical descriptors and the corresponding symbols introduced in this chapter are listed in Table 2-1.

GENERAL REQUIREMENTS

There are three requirements for diagnostic medical ultrasound: generation of a beam, reception of the returning echo, and processing of the signal for display. All types of ultrasonic scanning equipment have these basic features. Changes in the reception and in the processing, analysis, and display of returning echo signals differentiate one scanning mode from another.

Any discussion of ultrasonic instrumentation must include the basic A-mode scanner, from which all other scanning systems are derived by incorporating various modifications. A-mode scanning is an echo-ranging technique in which an ultrasound beam is directed along a single path into the body. Detected echoes from interfaces along this path are displayed as a series of spikes. The position of the spikes along the horizontal display axis denotes the depth of the interface; the height of the spikes denotes the strength of the echo. The A-mode scanner is used here as a model to demonstrate the fundamentals of equipment design.

Although the basic scanner is electronically complex, a block diagram (Fig. 2-1) describes the main system components and operation of the unit. The block diagram shows an electroacoustic conversion device connected to the transmitter-receiver section of the scanner. This component, called the transducer, is responsible for the generation of an ultrasound beam and the detection of returning echoes. Once

■ **Table 2-1** Physical Descriptors and Symbols

Bandwidth	Δf
Beam width	w
Center frequency	f_c
Degree of focusing	κ
Diameter	d
Duty factor	DF
Far field divergence	ϕ
Focal length	F
Maximum pulse repetition frequency	PRF_m
Near field depth	D
Number of cycles	n
Pulse duration	PD
Pulse repetition frequency	PRF
Pulse repetition period	PRP
Radiofrequency	RF
Radius	r
Range of scanning	R
Signal to noise ratio	SNR
Spatial pulse length	SPL
Transducer factors	
Dielectric constant	ϵ
Electromechanical coefficient	k
Mechanical coefficient	Q
Reception coefficient	g
Transmission coefficient	h

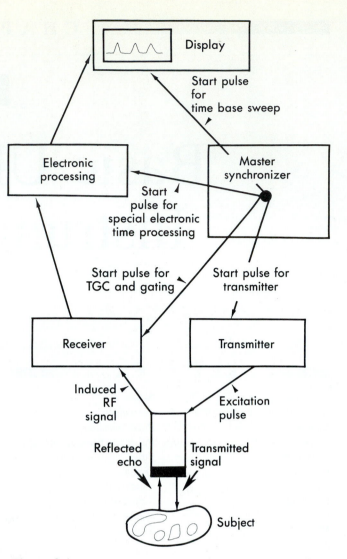

Figure 2-1 Basic scanner. The master synchronizer controls all components.

an echo is received, the induced signal is electronically processed to enhance the signal for viewing purposes. The displayed signal must be related to interaction that has taken place in the body.

All the subsystems are controlled by a master synchronizer. An electronic signal from the master synchronizer to the transmitter initiates the process. A pulsed ultrasound beam is generated and sent into the body. It undergoes various interactions (discussed in Chapter 1), and when an interface is encountered, a fraction of the beam's energy is reflected back toward the transducer. The transducer, acting as a receiver rather than a transmitter, converts the ultrasound wave (returning echo) to an electronic signal that is processed and displayed. To correlate the amplitude of the induced signal with the depth of the interface, the time interval between the time that an ultrasound pulse leaves the transducer and the time the echo returns must be known. Any special amplification based on elapsed time, such as time gain compensation (TGC) and gating applied to the detected signals, also requires knowledge of the exact time of travel for the pulse. All these subsystems must be activated simultaneously by the master synchronizer to ensure proper timing. For each system the clock in the master synchronizer measures the elapsed time from generation of the ultrasound pulse to reception of the echoes.

FREQUENCY DETERMINATION

The first requirement of an ultrasonic scanner is that a sound wave at ultrasonic frequencies (greater than 20 kHz) be generated. The primary objectives are to produce a unidi-

rectional beam (analogous to a flashlight beam versus a porch light) that is of uniform intensity and limited physical dimensions so that good spatial resolution is obtained. As a practical matter, the spatial variation of beam intensity can be manipulated but is not completely eliminated (a totally uniform beam is impossible). For positional information, a short burst is required and thus the sound beam must be turned on and off rapidly.

Spatial Resolution and Frequency

In echo detection, reflected mechanical vibrations are recorded. The time is measured for short pulses (which may be a single vibration) to travel from the point of sound origin to the object and back to the receiver. For example, if a Chinese gong were allowed to move only once after being struck and then were cushioned with a pillow to shorten the duration of the vibration, a single-cycle sound wave would be produced that would move out to some distant object and return toward the listener. In such circumstances, when we are listening as sound waves come back from the en-

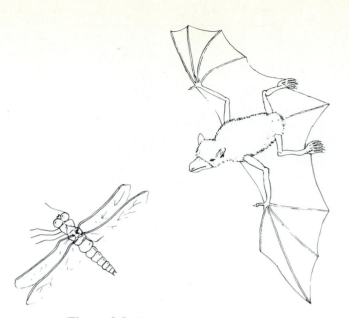

Figure 2-2 Transducer using bat power.

vironment, we are actually hearing an integral number of vibrations (10 or 15 or 50) return as echoes. Since the position of any object in space can be determined only to an accuracy of about one wavelength (or a quarter wavelength if special equipment capable of measuring high-pressure or low-pressure points is used), this limitation on resolvability is imposed by wavelength. (The ability to distinguish two objects separated by a small distance is called *axial resolution*.) Because frequency and wavelength are inversely related, it can be readily appreciated that shorter wavelengths, which produce finer resolution, correspond to higher frequencies. The question then becomes what frequencies are needed to produce the resolution required in diagnostic ultrasound.

Wavelength of Sound Sources

The human ear can detect sound waves from approximately 20 Hz to 20 kHz. Assume that the smallest objects resolvable are one wavelength in size. A 20 Hz sound source produces a sound wave with a 77-meter (m) wavelength in tissue (the velocity of sound in tissue is 1540 m/s):

$$c = f\lambda$$

$$\lambda = \frac{c}{f}$$

$$= \frac{1540 \text{ m/s}}{20 \text{ c/s}}$$

$$= 77 \text{ m}$$

This may be suitable for detection of aircraft carriers or submarines, but it is not appropriate for the fine resolution needed in medical diagnostic ultrasound.

In nature, bats and certain other animals (porpoises, moles, and some grasshoppers) generate ultrasound waves having frequencies of around 100 kHz. In medicine, if we had to rely on bats as a source of ultrasound, we would need first a device to contain them and then a supply of bugs

to activate (or stimulate) them; then, each time a signal was needed, a new bug would be released and the bat (if it were hungry) would generate an ultrasound wave to locate it (Fig. 2-2). Aside from the impracticality of this arrangement, there would be another problem: with a frequency of 100 kHz, the wavelength produced is 1.54 cm, which is much too long for the accurate location of small objects.

$$c = f\lambda$$

$$\lambda = \frac{c}{f}$$

$$= \frac{1540 \text{ m/s}}{100 \times 10^3 \text{ c/s}} = 0.0154 \text{ m} = 1.54 \text{ cm}$$

Although suitable for locating objects in the dark, it would not be adequate for medical diagnostic ultrasound, in which objects with dimensions on the order of 1 mm (1/1000 m) or less often need to be identified.

Frequency Requirement

If one wavelength is a good approximation of the smallest detectable object, what frequency is required for a resolution of 1 mm in tissue? Using the relationship $c = f\lambda$ and solving for the frequency, we find that

$$f = \frac{c}{\lambda}$$

$$= \frac{1540 \text{ m/s}}{0.001 \text{ m}} = 1.54 \times 10^6 \text{ 1/s} = 1.54 \text{ MHz}$$

For medical diagnostic ultrasound it is evident that megahertz frequencies are necessary.

PIEZOELECTRIC PROPERTIES

Dipole Alignment

Nothing in nature can be readily adapted to transmit ultrasonic energy in the megahertz frequency range. Consequently, the transducer must be manufactured. The construction of such a device relies on a phenomenon first studied by Pierre and Marie Curie before the turn of the century and known as the piezoelectric (pressure electric) effect. This effect is commonly found in crystalline materials that have dipoles (regions of positive and negative charge) on each molecule. Dipolar molecules are positive at one end and negative at the other, as shown in Figure 2-3. In the normal crystalline lattice structure these randomly arranged dipoles cannot migrate (Fig. 2-4). If the material is heated above a temperature called the Curie temperature, however, the molecules are released and can move freely. When a pair of charged plates (one positive and one negative) is placed across the material, the negative region of each molecule points toward the positive plate and the positive region toward the negative plate (opposite charges attract, like charges repel). The positive and negative regions of the molecules do not align directly with the electrical field produced by the plates because of thermal motion. If the material is then cooled below the Curie temperature

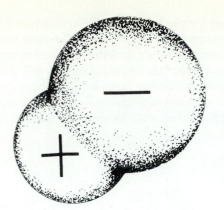

Figure 2-3 Molecular dipole. There are regions of net positive and net negative charge on the molecule.

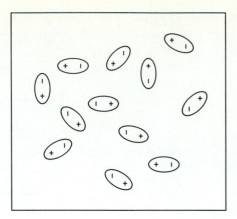

Figure 2-4 Random arrangement of dipoles (natural state).

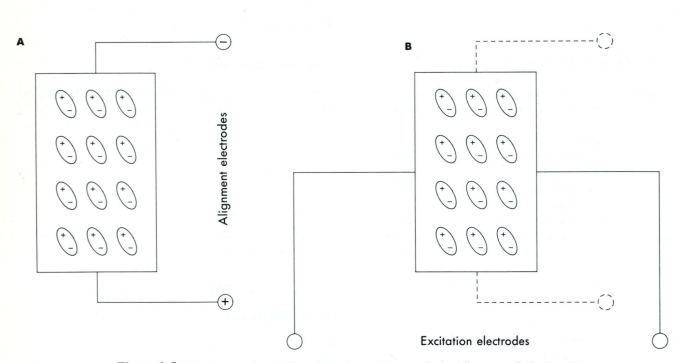

Figure 2-5 Alignment and excitation electrodes on the crystal. **A,** Alignment of dipoles with an externally applied electrical field during heating of the crystalline material. **B,** Placement of excitation electrodes following removal of the alignment electrodes *(dashed lines).*

while the charged plates are still applied, the molecules will maintain their orientations (Fig. 2-5, *A*). Ultrasound transducers should not be autoclaved, because this destroys the piezoelectric properties of the material by raising its temperature above the Curie temperature and returning the dipoles to their random arrangement.

Once the material is cooled below the Curie temperature, the charged plates used for alignment are removed without altering the configuration of the dipoles. The molecular arrangement of the dipolar molecules gives piezoelectric materials their unique properties. Conducting plates are placed on the opposite faces of the crystal adjacent to the positions of the original alignment electrodes (Fig. 2-5, *B*). When a voltage is applied to the conducting plates, the molecules twist to align themselves with the electrical field (positive

molecules toward the negative electrode, negative molecules toward the positive electrode), thereby thickening the crystal (Fig. 2-6). If the plates are reversed in polarity, the molecules will twist back in the opposite direction, creating a decrease in the crystal thickness (Fig. 2-6). The actual movement is only a few microns (10^{-6} m), although in Figure 2-6 this change in thickness has been exaggerated for clarity. The flipping back and forth of the polarity causes expansion and contraction of the crystal, which creates mechanical vibrations. When the expanding and contracting crystal is placed on the body, sound waves (mechanical vibrations or pressure waves) are passed into the body. Thus a voltage applied across the piezoelectric material creates mechanical motion (sound waves). In the crystal this phenomenon (the converse piezoelectric effect) allows an ultrasound beam to be generated by the transducer.

Alternatively, the piezoelectric effect enables the same transducer to receive an ultrasonic echo (high-frequency pressure wave). Ultrasound waves returning from interactions with interfaces in the body strike the crystal and induce electrical signals. These are processed and ultimately displayed.

Natural Vibrational Frequency

If left alone, the transducer would ring in a manner similar to a tuning fork. Note that if a tuning fork is to ring at 2000 Hz it does not have to be struck 2000 times each second to maintain the sound (although this is a possibility, particularly for continuous wave generation). Instead, a natural vibrational frequency occurs in which the wave is transmitted back and forth (from prong to prong) at a set frequency that depends on wave interference. If a crystal suspended in air is struck with a voltage pulse, ultrasound waves are generated. Multiple wavefronts are formed: forward from the front face, backward into the crystal from the front face, into the crystal from the back face, and away from the crystal at the back face. These waves undergo constructive and destructive interference within the crystal, depending on the crystal thickness. The ultrasound moves from one face of the crystal to the other, undergoing reflection between the two crystalline surfaces. The crystal has a natural vibrational frequency (just as the tuning fork does) that is related to the distance between those two surfaces. To have constructive interference so a single wave moves back and forth across the crystal, the distance from one surface to the other must be equal to half the wavelength (Fig. 2-7). These crystals are extremely thin.

■ **Example 2-1**

What thickness of piezoelectric material is required to produce an ultrasound wave with a frequency of 1.5 MHz? (The velocity of sound in the piezoelectric material is 4000 m/s.)

$$c = f\lambda$$

$$\lambda = \frac{4000 \text{ m/s}}{1.50 \times 10^6 \text{ c/s}} = 2.7 \times 10^{-3} \text{ m}$$

$$= 2.7 \text{ mm}$$

$$\text{Crystal thickness} = \frac{\lambda}{2} = \frac{2.7}{2} = 1.35 \text{ mm}$$

Note that the 1.5 MHz transducer produces an ultrasound beam having a wavelength of 1 mm in tissue.

$$\lambda = \frac{1540 \text{ m/s}}{1.50 \times 10^6 \text{ c/s}} = 1 \times 10^{-3} \text{ m} = 1 \text{ mm}$$

Frequency does not change when the ultrasound wave enters one medium from another. The difference in wavelength between the crystal and the tissue arises from velocity differences in the two media (1540 m/s for tissue and approximately 4000 m/s for the crystal). A transducer should never be dropped, because the thin crystal cracks easily.

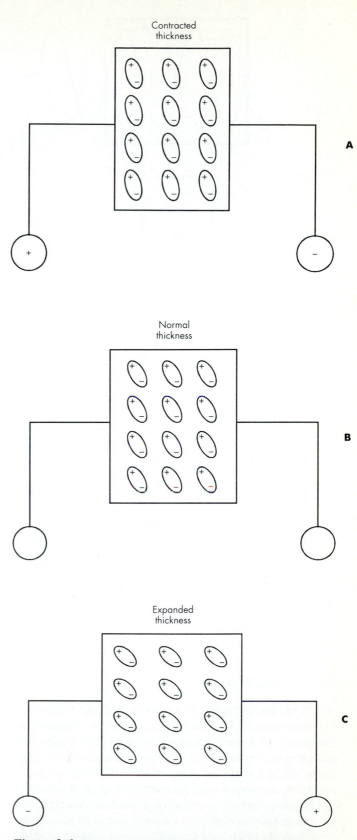

Figure 2-6 Crystal response to voltage applied across the excitation electrodes. **A,** Contraction of the crystal caused by movement of the dipoles trying to align with an applied electrical field. **B,** Normal thickness with no applied electrical field. **C,** Expansion of the crystal caused by movement of the dipoles trying to align with an applied electrical field. The polarity is reversed from that depicted in **A.**

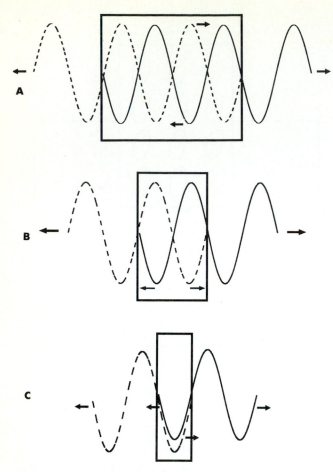

Figure 2-7 Determination of crystal thickness using superimposition of waves. Waves generated at the back of the crystal *(dashed line)*. Waves generated from the front of the crystal *(solid line)*. *Arrows* indicate the direction of wave motion. **A,** Crystal thickness greater than one wavelength produces destructive interference if the thickness is not an odd-integer multiple of one half wavelength. **B,** Complete destructive interference occurs when the crystal thickness is equal to one wavelength. **C,** Complete constructive interference occurs when the crystal thickness is equal to one half wavelength or odd multiples of a half wavelength.

Piezoelectric Materials

To change the frequency of a transducer requires changing the transducer itself (with some exceptions, discussed in Chapter 4). A higher-frequency transducer that produces a shorter wavelength has an even thinner crystal. For diagnostic medical applications the almost universally used material in transducers is lead zirconate titanate (PZT). Barium lead titanate, barium lead zirconate, lead metaniobate, and lithium sulfate have also been used. Crystals of polyvinylidene fluoride (PVF_2) are being developed with an acoustic impedance closer to that of tissue; thus matching layers applied to the crystal face to increase the fraction of ultrasonic energy that enters the body are not needed.

Quartz is a naturally occurring substance that can be made to have piezoelectric properties. It was the material studied by the Curies. Quartz is used in therapeutic ultrasound transducers because of its excellent transmission properties.

TRANSDUCER CONSTRUCTION

The major component of a transducer is a crystal of piezoelectric material with electrodes on opposite sides of it that create the changing polarity. The electrodes are formed by plating a thin film of gold or silver on the crystal surface. To improve the transfer of energy to and from the patient, the matching layer is located next to one of the electrodes. Crystal ringing is diminished by the introduction of the backing material that adjoins the surface electrode further from the patient. The entire crystal assembly, including the electrodes, matching layer, and backing material, is housed in an electrically insulating casing (usually some type of plastic). This casing also provides structural support. An acoustic insulator, made of rubber or cork, prevents the transmission of ultrasound energy into the casing. Figure 2-8 is a cross-sectional view of a transducer.

The transducer is sensitive to electromagnetic interference, which contributes to the noise level (i.e., signals that do not correspond to physical interactions of sound waves with tissue). High noise levels prohibit the detection of weak echoes. To reduce the electromagnetic interference, a radiofrequency shield composed of a hollow metallic cylinder is placed around the crystal and backing material and electronically grounded to the front electrode surface. The acoustic insulating layer coats the inner surface of the radiofrequency shield to prevent reverberations.

The backing material indicated in the diagram (Fig. 2-8) depends on whether the transducer is designed for therapeutic purposes or diagnostic imaging. For ultrasonic therapy the objective is to deliver the maximum amount of energy in the form of heat (caused by absorption of the ultrasound) to the patient. This is achieved by a continuous output of ultrasound waves from the transducer (Fig. 2-9). Maximum output results if natural ringing (resonance) occurs in the crystal, in which case the backing material should have an acoustic impedance different from that of the crystal. Maximum reflection at the backing material–crystal interface causes the crystal to ring. Air is commonly employed as the backing material for therapy transducers. Alternatively, the crystal may be driven by an alternating voltage source of the correct frequency to induce continuous wave output. This is the usual method used for therapeutic continuous wave ultrasound transducers, which also has applications in Doppler scanning. A crystal producing continuous wave output cannot receive reflected ultrasound waves.

For imaging, the transducer sends out a short burst of ultrasound (preferably one cycle) followed by a period of silence to listen for returning echoes (receiving mode) before another burst is generated. This is called a pulsed system (Fig. 2-10), and the design is based on the echo-ranging principle discussed at the end of Chapter 1. Ideally the backing material should absorb all the energy, except for one cycle of sound produced from the front face of the transducer. For maximum transfer of energy to occur (from crystal to backing material), the backing material must have an acoustic impedance identical to that of the crystal. An epoxy resin and tungsten powder combination is used for the backing material in diagnostic transducers to damp

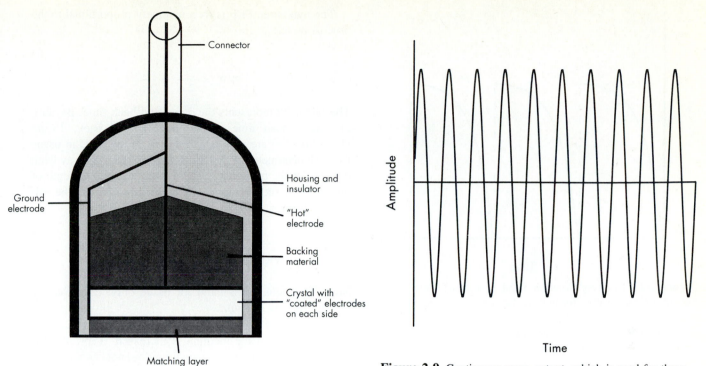

Figure 2-8 labels: Connector, Housing and insulator, "Hot" electrode, Backing material, Crystal with "coated" electrodes on each side, Ground electrode, Matching layer

Figure 2-8 Single-element transducer.

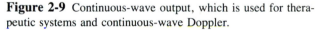

Figure 2-9 Continuous-wave output, which is used for therapeutic systems and continuous-wave Doppler.

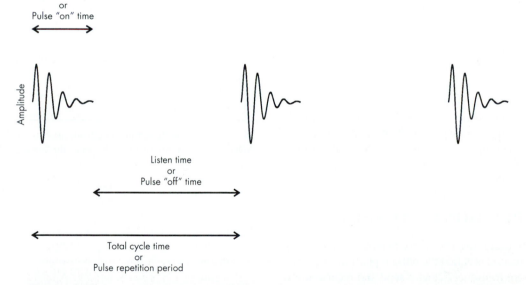

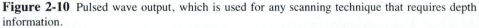

Pulse duration or Pulse "on" time

Listen time or Pulse "off" time

Total cycle time or Pulse repetition period

Figure 2-10 Pulsed wave output, which is used for any scanning technique that requires depth information.

(shorten) the ultrasonic pulse. The rear surface of the backing material is slanted to prevent reflection of sound energy into the crystal. The sensitivity (ability to detect weakly reflecting interfaces) of the transducer decreases with increased damping because damping lowers the intensity of the output ultrasound wave from the transducer.

Dynamic Damping

Dynamic damping is an electronic means to suppress ringing. A voltage pulse of opposite polarity is applied to the crystal immediately following the excitation pulse. This counteracts the expansion and contraction of the crystal stimulated by the first pulse, and ringing is inhibited.

Pulsed-Wave Output

In echo-ranging systems the transducer must pause after transmitting the sound wave to "listen" for the returning echoes. Because the crystal cannot send and receive simultaneously, it must be pulsed for transmission after an appropriate listening time has elapsed. The master synchronizer sends an electronic signal to a pulser or transmitter

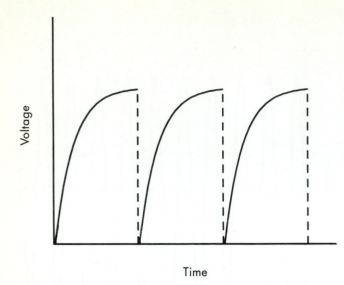

Figure 2-11 Charging *(solid line)* and discharging *(dashed line)* of a capacitor used for pulsing the crystal in a transducer.

to initiate the process. The start command is, in turn, relayed to the transducer to generate a short burst of ultrasound. There are two methods by which the transmitter can work.

In the first the output from a sine-wave generator is gated to apply a rapidly alternating voltage to the crystal. If the gate is switched on for a long period, a continuous wave is produced. If it is switched on for a short period, a short pulse is created.

The second transmitter pulsing method uses a charged capacitor (a device that stores electrical charge). This is discharged through the piezoelectric crystal, which is stimulated to vibrate at the resonance frequency as previously discussed. The capacitor is recharged while the crystal is waiting for returning echoes (Fig. 2-11). The discharge time of the capacitor, in conjunction with the crystal damping and frequency, determines the pulse length (related to the number of cycles in the pulse burst). The recharge time is set to coincide with the listening time.

PULSE REPETITION FREQUENCY

The number of times the crystal is pulsed or electrically stimulated per second is called the pulse repetition frequency (PRF). Because a transducer cannot send and receive ultrasound at the same time, a limit exists with respect to the rate at which it can be pulsed. The maximum pulse repetition frequency (PRF_m) is limited by the maximum depth (R) to be sampled and by the velocity of ultrasound (c) in the medium, as shown in the following equation:

2-1

$$PRF_m = \frac{c}{2\,R}$$

The factor 2 accounts for the distance down to the interface and back to the transducer. The time (t) necessary for the wave to travel to depth R is given as

2-2

$$R = ct$$

The maximum PRF is then inversely proportional to the time of travel:

2-3

$$PRF_m = \frac{c}{2\,ct} = \frac{1}{2\,t}$$

The factor 2 t represents the down-and-back time. Because of wave transit time to the reflector and back, 13 μs (13×10^{-6} s) are required to detect an interface in tissue for each centimeter of depth that the interface is away from the face of the transducer. Thus, if the maximum depth of interest in tissue is known, the maximum PRF can be calculated from

2-4

$$PRF_m = \frac{1}{(13 \times 10^{-6}\ \text{s/cm})\ (R\ \text{cm})}$$

Note: This equation is valid for tissue only; Equation 2-1 is valid for any medium.

Equation 2-1 illustrates that the PRF_m can be increased if the velocity in the medium is increased. Typically, the velocity of ultrasound in the medium does not change (being nearly constant for all types of tissue) and velocity is not adjustable by the sonographer. Equation 2-1 also indicates that the PRF_m can be increased if the depth of interest is decreased. Depth is the only potential parameter capable of being changed by the operator. In designing their systems, however, manufacturers often vary the PRF with the depth. The PRF set by the manufacturer is normally not a selectable parameter by the operator. These concepts are illustrated by the following three examples.

■ **Example 2-2**

Assume that the maximum depth of interest in tissue is 10 cm. What is the maximum PRF? Express the answer using three significant figures.

$$PRF_m = \frac{c}{2\,R} = \frac{1540\ \text{m/s}}{2\ (0.1\ \text{m})} = 7700\ \frac{\text{pulses}}{\text{s}}$$

or

$$PRF_m = = \frac{1}{(13.0 \times 10^{-6}\ \text{s/cm})\ (10\ \text{cm})} = 7690\ \frac{\text{pulses}}{\text{s}}$$

Note the difference in the two answers. This discrepancy occurs because the travel time is rounded off to 13 μs per centimeter (actual time, 12.987 μs) in Equation 2-4.

■ **Example 2-3**

Assume that the maximum depth of interest in tissue is increased to 20 cm. What is the maximum PRF?

$$PRF_m = \frac{1540\ \text{m/s}}{2\ (0.2\ \text{m})} = 3850\ \frac{\text{pulses}}{\text{s}}$$

or

$$PRF_m = \frac{1}{(13 \times 10^{-6}\ \text{s/cm})\ (20\ \text{cm})} = 3850\ \frac{\text{pulses}}{\text{s}}$$

For deep-lying structures to be visualized, the PRF_m must be reduced.

■ Example 2-4

Suppose that bone replaces tissue. What is the maximum PRF allowed to sample a depth of 10 cm?

$$PRF_m = \frac{c}{2\ R} = \frac{4080\ m/s}{2\ (0.1\ m)} = 20400\ \frac{pulses}{s}$$

A high velocity enables the PRF_m to be increased dramatically.

Pulse repetition frequencies range from 200 to 2000 per second for typical A-mode and B-mode transducers. Higher PRFs are used for real-time and Doppler units. The PRF is often expressed in units of kHz (corresponding to 1000 pulses per second).

PULSE REPETITION PERIOD

The time required to transmit a pulsed ultrasound wave plus the time devoted to listening for the returning echoes from that wave is called the pulse repetition period (PRP). It is equal to the reciprocal of the pulse repetition frequency:

2-5

$$PRP = \frac{1}{PRF}$$

■ Example 2-5

What is the PRF if a pulsed sound wave is emitted every 500 μs?

The time between pulses is given as 500 μs, which is equal to the PRP. Using Equation 2-5

$$PRF = \frac{1}{PRP}$$

$$= \frac{1}{500 \times 10^{-6}\ s}$$

$$= 2000\ pulses/s$$

■ Example 2-6

What is the PRP if the PRF is 1 kHz?

Using Equation 2-5 and substituting a value of 1000 pulses per second for the PRF

$$PRP = \frac{1}{PRF}$$

$$= \frac{1}{1000\ pulses/s}$$

$$= 0.001\ s$$

SPATIAL PULSE LENGTH

Ideally, for each pulse, a short packet of ultrasound energy of the appropriate frequency (i.e., 3.5 MHz for a 3.5 MHz transducer) is directed into the body. In practice, the pulse is composed of a range of different frequencies described by the bandwidth. The length of this short-duration pulse can be estimated and is called the spatial pulse length (SPL). It is calculated from the wavelength (λ) and the number of cycles (n) in the pulse:

2-6

$$SPL = \lambda n$$

Assume that a 3 MHz transducer produces a pulse that is 3 cycles in duration. The wavelength is determined from Equation 1-5:

$$\lambda = \frac{c}{f} = \frac{1540\ m/s}{3 \times 10^6\ c/s} = 5.13 \times 10^{-4}\ m = 0.513\ mm$$

With n = 3, the SPL is calculated to be

$$\lambda n = (0.513\ mm)\ (3) = 1.54\ mm$$

The SPL influences a scanner's effectiveness at depicting spatial detail. Axial resolution is the ability to distinguish as separate images two objects that are close to each other along the direction of propagation. To improve axial resolution, a pulse of short duration is desirable. To shorten the pulse spatially, the number of cycles must be reduced or the frequency must be increased to decrease wavelength. Often the pulsed wave is two to five cycles in duration.

Pulse Duration

The pulse duration (PD), or temporal pulse length, is the time interval for one complete pulse. It describes the actual time that the transducer is generating the ultrasonic pulse. A more formal definition is the elapsed time from initiation of the pulse to a point 20 dB below the maximum peak-to-peak pressure amplitude of the wave (Fig. 2-12). An alternative definition is the number of half cycles in which the peak amplitude is greater than 25% of the maximum amplitude in the pulse. The effectiveness of the backing material in damping the pulse is indicated by this parameter.

The axial resolution, and thus the ability to visualize superficial structures, depends on the PD (or spatial pulse length). The PD is calculated from the number of cycles in the pulse (n) and the period (τ) of the wave:

2-7

$$PD = n\tau$$

Consider, once more, a three-cycle pulse (at -20 dB) from a 3 MHz transducer. The following analysis can be made:

$$\tau = \frac{1}{f} = \frac{1}{3 \times 10^6\ Hz} = 3.3 \times 10^{-7}\ s$$

$$PD = (3\ cycles/pulse)\ (3.3 \times 10^{-7}\ s)$$

$$= 9.9 \times 10^{-7}\ s \simeq 1 \times 10^{-6}\ s \simeq 1\ \mu s$$

The SPL varies directly with the pulse duration, the constant of proportionality being equal to the velocity in the medium:

2-8

$$SPL = (c)\ (PD)$$

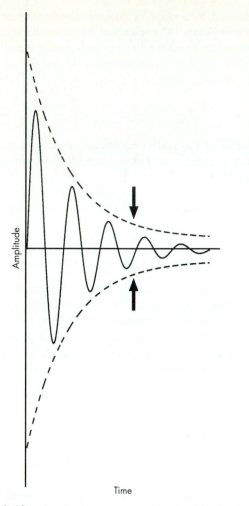

Figure 2-12 Pulse duration or temporal pulse length. Because of damping and friction, the pressure peak amplitude decreases with time after the crystal is excited. The pulse duration is determined by the cutoff point *(arrows)* defined at 20 dB below the maximum pressure amplitude.

Given a pulse duration of 1.0×10^{-6} s and a velocity of 1540 m/s,

$$\text{SPL} = (1540 \text{ m/s}) (1 \times 10^{-6} \text{ s}) = 1.54 \times 10^{-3} \text{ m} = 1.54 \text{ mm}$$

which is the same answer as obtained using Equation 2-6.

Duty Factor

A typical unit with a pulse duration of 1 μs and a PRF of 1 kHz is transmitting only 0.1% of the time. By far, most of its time (99.9%) is spent in a receive mode. The duty factor (DF) is the fraction of time the unit is active and is calculated by obtaining the ratio of the pulse duration and the pulse repetition period:

2-9

$$\text{DF} = \frac{\text{PD}}{\text{PRP}}$$

Both the PD and the PRP are expressed in units (either seconds or microseconds), but the DF has no units. It is merely the ratio of time that the pulse is on to the time between pulses. It is important in determining some intensity parameters used to quantitate the dose response for various biological effects.

■ **Example 2-7**

Calculate the duty factor for a 3 MHz transducer that produces three cycles per pulse. The PRF is 1500 per second.

The pulse duration is 1 μs, and the PRP 6.7×10^{-4} second (670 μs). From Equation 2-9

$$\text{DF} = \frac{\text{PD}}{\text{PRP}}$$

$$= \frac{1 \text{ μs}}{670 \text{ μs}} = 0.0015$$

TRANSDUCER FACTORS

Several factors or parameters influence the overall performance of a transducer.

- k—electromechanical coupling coefficient
- h—transmission coefficient
- g—reception coefficient
- ε—dielectric constant
- Z—acoustic impedance
- Q—mechanical coefficient

The electromechanical coupling coefficient (k) describes how efficiently the transducer converts electrical stimuli from the transmitter into ultrasonic energy and recieved ultrasound energy into electrical signals. The transmission coefficient (h) indicates the fraction of electrical energy that is converted into acoustic energy. The fraction of returning acoustic echo energy that is converted into electrical energy is given by the reception coefficient (g). The product of the transmission coefficient and the reception coefficient yields the electromechanical coupling coefficient.

2-10

$$k = hg$$

The mechanical and electrical properties of the transducer are partially characterized by the dielectric constant (ε), which is also related to the transmission and reception coefficients. The dielectric constant describes the relative strain (movement) that the crystal undergoes when an electrical stress is applied to it and the induced voltage when it is strained. Two conditions are established to evaluate the dielectric constant: unrestricted movement and restricted (clamped) movement. This corresponds to the crystal in a free state and the crystal placed in a transducer assembly with backing and facing materials. A high dielectric constant is desirable during reception of low-megahertz frequencies because it minimizes electronic noise from cabling and receiver amplifiers. In fact, a high dielectric constant may be more desirable than a high reception coefficient.

The acoustic impedance (Z) of the crystal, defined in Chapter 1 as the product of velocity times density, influences the energy transfer across the crystal-tissue interface. Matching the Z values of tissue and crystal enhances the transmission of ultrasound into the body. The mechanical coefficient (Q) characterizes the frequency response of the transducer. It is a major consideration when selecting a transducer for a particular application.

SENSITIVITY

Sensitivity, although not formally defined, describes the ability of an ultrasound system to distinguish low-reflectivity objects with nearly the same acoustic properties at specific locations in the medium. All the transducer factors mentioned previously influence it. Other considerations, in addition to the transducer factors, affect the sensitivity of an ultrasound system.

Conversion Efficiencies

Of all the transducer factors, conversion efficiencies (electrical energy to acoustic energy, and vice versa) are most important in dictating the sensitivity of a transducer. To a first approximation, transducer sensitivity is given by the product of the transmission coefficient and the reception coefficient. A transducer that converts 100% of the electrical energy into acoustic energy, but only 1% of the acoustic energy to electrical energy, uses 1% of the available energy. If the transmission coefficient and reception coefficient were both 0.25, then 6.25% ($0.25 \times 0.25 \times 100\%$) of the available energy would be used. The latter case permits detection of weaker signals; the sensitivity is thus increased by a transducer with a high electromechanical coupling coefficient.

Circuit Impedance

The electrical impedance matching of the transducer to the initiating pulser and to the receiver also affects the sensitivity. Electrical impedance mismatch at the pulser decreases the amount of electrical energy delivered to the transducer in the generator circuit, thereby creating a lower-intensity ultrasonic pulse. If there is an electrical impedance mismatch at the transducer-receiver, electrical energy is reflected into the transducer and a smaller signal is available for processing. Again, the sensitivity of the system is reduced. The electrical impedance mismatch also causes deterioration in the axial resolution by creating a longer pulse length. Electrical impedance matching depends partially on the dielectric constant.

Matching Layers

The acoustic impedance matching of the transducer to the object scanned is another important factor that affects sensitivity. As demonstrated in Chapter 1, an acoustic impedance (Z) mismatch at an interface causes partial reflection of the ultrasonic energy. The acoustic impedance of the crystal is large (30×10^5 g/cm²/s) compared with that of the tissue (1.6×10^5 g/cm²/s), which results in a large reflection (81%) at the crystal-tissue interface. Only 19%

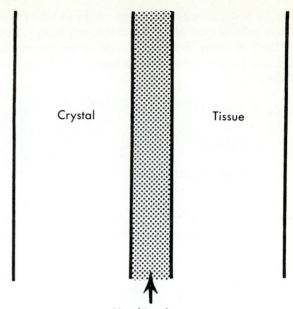

Crystal

Tissue

Matching layer

Figure 2-13 Matching layer (facing material) between crystal and tissue. The objective is to reduce the impedance mismatch between the crystal and the tissue.

of the ultrasonic energy enters the tissue (percent transmission):

$$\%T = 100 - \%R$$
$$= 100 - \left[\left(\frac{Z_c - Z_t}{Z_c + Z_t}\right)^2 \times 100\right]$$

where Z_c is the acoustic impedance of the crystal and Z_t the acoustic impedance of tissue.

$$\%T = 100 - \left[\left(\frac{30 \times 10^5 - 1.6 \times 10^5}{30 \times 10^5 + 1.6 \times 10^5}\right)^2 \times 100\right]$$
$$= 100 - 81 = 19\%$$

The introduction of facing materials or matching layers between the crystal and the tissue partially eliminates this problem (Fig. 2-13). The facing material of proper acoustic impedance provides a better match between the crystal and the tissue (i.e., reduces the acoustic impedance mismatch by interposing a material with intermediate acoustic impedance between the crystal and tissue). The transfer of sound energy from the crystal to soft tissue, and vice versa, is enhanced. Matching layers are composed of aluminum powder in an epoxy resin. The concentration of aluminum determines the acoustic impedance of the matching layer.

The acoustic impedance of the matching layer is selected to reduce the amount of reflection at the crystal–matching layer and matching layer–tissue interfaces. This is accomplished by taking an arithmetic or a geometric mean of the acoustic impedances for the crystal and tissue. The geometric mean is defined as the antilogarithm of the average of the logarithms for each acoustic impedance. The following equation illustrates this concept:

2-11

$$Z_{ml} = \text{Antilog}\left(\frac{\log Z_c + \log Z_t}{2}\right)$$

where Z_{ml} is the acoustic impedance of the matching layer, Z_c the acoustic impedance of the crystal, and Z_t the acoustic impedance of tissue. For example, the acoustic impedance of the matching material is calculated for PZT and tissue as follows:

$$Z_{ml} = \text{Antilog} \left(\frac{\log (30 \times 10^5) + \log (1.6 \times 10^5)}{2} \right)$$

$$= \text{Antilog} \left(\frac{6.477 + 5.204}{2} \right)$$

$$= \text{Antilog} (5.841)$$

$$= 6.9 \times 10^5$$

Another method of obtaining the geometric mean is to take the square root of the product of the acoustic impedances:

2-12

$$Z_{ml} = \sqrt{Z_c Z_t}$$

The acoustic impedance of the matching layer is recalculated using Equation 2-12.

$$Z_{ml} = \sqrt{(30 \times 10^5)(1.6 \times 10^5)}$$

$$= \sqrt{48 \times 10^{10}}$$

$$= 6.9 \times 10^5$$

To calculate the improvement in energy transfer from the crystal through the matching layer to the tissue involves a two-step process.

First, from the crystal ($Z = 30 \times 10^5$ g/cm²/s) to the matching layer ($Z = 6.9 \times 10^5$ g/cm²/s) the percentage of transmission is found:

$$\%T = 100 - \%R$$

$$= 100 - \left[\left(\frac{30 \times 10^5 - 6.9 \times 10^5}{30 \times 10^5 + 6.9 \times 10^5} \right)^2 \times 100 \right]$$

$$= 61\%$$

Next, the percentage of transmission through the matching layer to the tissue ($Z = 1.6 \times 10^5$ g/cm²/s) must be calculated:

$$\%T = 100 - \left[\left(\frac{6.9 \times 10^5 - 1.6 \times 10^5}{6.9 \times 10^5 + 1.6 \times 10^5} \right)^2 \times 100 \right] = 61\%$$

Thus, of the total sound energy generated, 61% passes from the crystal to the matching layer and 37% (the product of transmission coefficients) is transferred into the tissue. The improvement above 19% transmission without the matching layer is evident.

Optimizing Matching Layer Performance

The acoustic impedance of the matching layer should be optimized to give the best axial resolution (shortest pulse possible) with maximum transmitted beam intensity. Optimizing the facing material may result in an acoustic impedance that is not the geometric mean of the crystal and tissue acoustic impedances.

A specific thickness of the facing material is also necessary. A thickness equal to integer multiples of the quarter

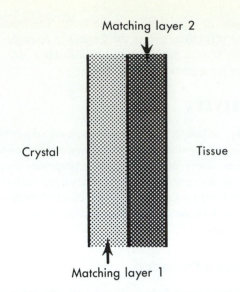

Figure 2-14 Multiple matching layers between crystal and tissue. The objective is to transfer nearly 100% of the generated acoustic energy into the tissue (i.e., to minimize the impedance mismatch between crystal and tissue).

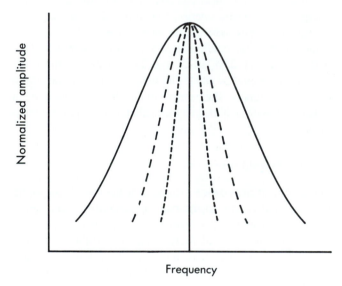

Figure 2-15 Frequency spectrum produced by various transducers: Ideal transducer *(solid line)*; single matching layer *(short dashed line)*; multiple matching layers *(long dashed line).*

wavelength provides maximum reinforcement of the ultrasound wave reflected from the crystal-facing material interface. This enhances the intensity of the ultrasound wave transmitted into the body. Because pulsed systems produce ultrasound waves of many frequencies (broad bandwidth) and each frequency has its own associated wavelength, the optimal system for transmission or reception is difficult to design. Normally, the one-quarter layer (which causes less attenuation than a three-quarter layer or any other quarter multiple) is adjusted for the center frequency of the transducer. A transducer with a quarter-wavelength matching layer is referred to as a quarter-wavelength transducer.

Additional improvement in performance can be achieved

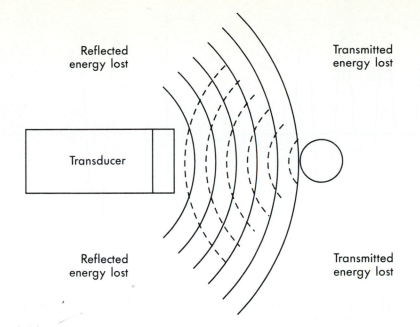

Figure 2-16 Energy loss due to divergence. Energy is lost in both transmitted *(solid lines)* and received *(dashed lines)* directions.

by using multiple matching layers on the face of a transducer (Fig. 2-14). The multiple matching layers alter the frequency distribution (Fig. 2-15) toward a broader bandwidth. The increased bandwidth enhances the sensitivity of the transducer, which results in improved image quality. The axial resolution is enhanced because the larger bandwidth normally means a shorter spatial pulse length. Short spatial pulse length allows the echoes from close objects to be processed separately. To form a short spatial pulse, multiple frequency components are necessary. A wide frequency distribution provides a better opportunity to match the crystal to the rest of the ultrasonic system. The low-frequency components of the spectrum can be controlled to decrease the far field divergence. The angular divergence of the far field is inversely proportional to the frequency (discussed at greater length later in this chapter).

Focusing

Divergence of the ultrasonic beam causes a decrease in the intensity with increasing distance from the transducer. This is easily understood by considering a constant amount of energy spread over a larger and larger area. The amount of energy incident on a unit area reflector will decrease as the distance between the reflector and the transducer increases. The reflected beam will also diverge, returning to the transducer and creating a partial "miss" of the ultrasound wave at the transducer (Fig. 2-16). Thus divergence is responsible for intensity loss for both the transmitted and the reflected beam.

The ultrasound beam can be focused, which concentrates the acoustic energy over a small area at a specific distance from the transducer. Compared with a nonfocused beam, the focused beam produces a stronger echo reflected to the transducer for detection. This is true only for structures within the focal zone of the transducer, however, where less divergence occurs.

Damping

The damping characteristics (methods of reducing pulse length) of the transducer affect the sensitivity. They are partially controlled by the backing material placed next to the crystal in the transducer. In therapeutic systems air is used for maximum reflection and reinforcement to produce a long pulse whereas in imaging systems the acoustic impedance of the backing material is made to equal the acoustic impedance of the crystal to obtain maximum transmission into the backing material and produce a short pulse.

Tissue Variations

Several nontransducer related variables influence the overall sensitivity of the system. The intensity of the sound beam is not spatially uniform as the beam leaves the face of the transducer. The intensity of the beam incident on an interface depends on the location of the interface. Because a fraction of the incident energy is reflected, the position of the reflecting interface affects the intensity of the returning echo. In addition, the beam is attenuated with depth; that is, the medium transmitting the sound removes acoustic energy from the beam. Recall from Chapter 1 that the attenuation for tissue is approximately 1 dB/cm/MHz (the more accurate value being 0.8 dB/cm/MHz). The composition, shape, and size of structures in the medium also contribute to the reflectivity and thus to the sensitivity. When scanning human subjects, the operator cannot control characteristics of the medium. A transducer can be selected, however, that will have properties conducive to the diagnostic information desired from the portion of the body to be scanned.

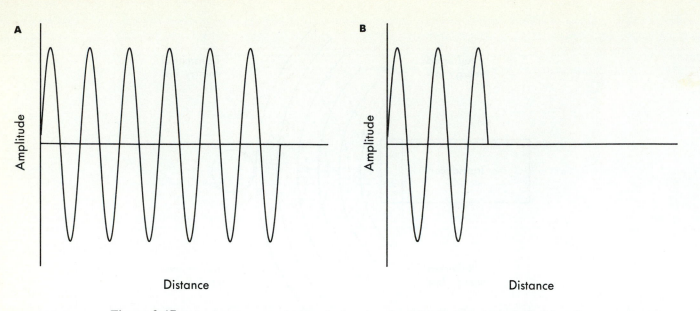

Figure 2-17 Pulse length versus ringing. **A,** 6-cycle pulse (high Q, long ringing); **B,** 2.5-cycle pulse (low Q, short ringing).

Q VALUE

The Q value, or mechanical coefficient, assesses two essential characteristics of the pulsed ultrasound beam—axial resolution and bandwidth. The Q value can thus be thought of as having two separate definitions relating to the two affected beam characteristics. These definitions are

2-13

$$Q = \frac{\text{Energy stored per cycle}}{\text{Energy lost per cycle}}$$

and

2-14

$$Q = \frac{\text{Center frequency}}{\text{Bandwidth}}$$

A high-Q transducer stores energy in the crystal and therefore loses very little each cycle. After being stimulated by the voltage pulse, it vibrates (rings) for an extended duration, producing a long pulse. A low-Q transducer, on the other hand, generates a short pulse after excitation because most of its energy is lost during the first few vibrations (Fig. 2-17). Diagnostic pulsed-wave ultrasound uses low-Q transducers, the Q value being typically 2 to 3. High-Q transducers (700 or greater) are good for continuous-wave ultrasound. Quartz, with a Q value of 25,000, is advantageous for therapeutic applications.

AXIAL RESOLUTION

The Q of a transducer—in conjunction with the backing material used for damping and the frequency of the transducer—determines the pulse length, which in turn limits the axial resolution of the transducer. The axial resolution specifies how close together two objects can be along the axis of the beam and yet still be detected as two distinct entities. Axial resolution also specifies the smallest object

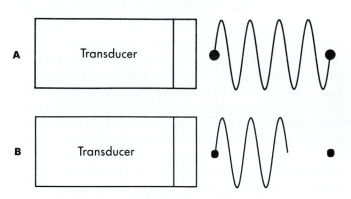

Figure 2-18 Pulse length versus axial resolution. **A,** A 4-cycle pulse includes both objects *(dots)* within the spatial pulse length. **B,** A 2.5-cycle pulse, which has a shorter SPL, can resolve objects located more closely together.

detectable along the axis of the beam. For a constant wavelength, as the pulse is shortened the axial resolution improves (Fig. 2-18).

For diagnostic ultrasound imaging, the resolution (minimum object size detectable) should be on the order of 1 mm. Commonly, the spatial pulse length is used as a specifier for the axial resolution. The best possible axial resolution is the spatial pulse length divided by 2. Figure 2-19 illustrates this concept. The beam leaves the transducer with a spatial pulse length of SPL and is directed toward two interfaces spaced SPL/2 apart. The beam strikes the first interface, which causes a fraction of the ultrasonic energy to be reflected toward the transducer. The remaining energy of the pulse is transmitted through the interface and progresses to the second interface, at which point some of the energy is again reflected. The echo with the pulse length of SPL leaving the first interface has traveled a distance of SPL/2 when the transmitted pulse strikes the second interface. As the reflected sound wave from the second interface moves toward the first interface, the echo from the first

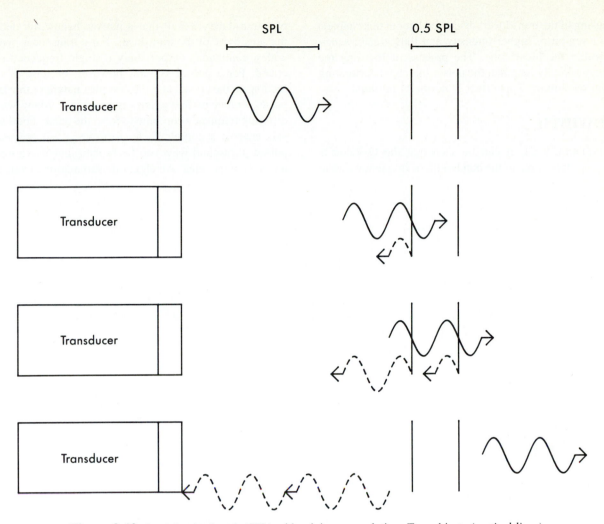

SPL   0.5 SPL

Figure 2-19 Spatial pulse length (SPL) with minimum resolution. Two objects *(vertical lines)* are separated by 0.5 SPL. The echo from each interface is shown by *dashed lines*. The objects are just resolvable.

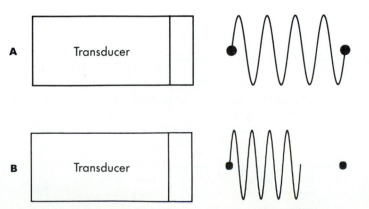

Figure 2-20 Pulse length shortened by increasing the frequency. **A,** The 4-cycle pulse from a low-frequency transducer includes both objects *(dots)* within the spatial pulse length. **B,** The 4-cycle pulse from a high-frequency transducer has a shorter spatial pulse length and can resolve objects located more closely together.

interface is moving toward the transducer. When the echo from the second interface arrives at the first interface, the first echo has moved a distance of SPL and therefore the echoes from the two interfaces are separated in both distance and time when detected by the transducer.

In addition to the transducer Q value, several other factors influence axial resolution (pulse length). The backing material absorbs the ultrasound beam from the back surface of the crystal and thereby damps the pulse length (fewer number of cycles). The more efficient the transfer of energy into the backing material (Z of the backing approaching Z of the crystal), the shorter the pulse will be. As the pulse composition becomes more complex, however (i.e., frequency components increase), the rate of damping is increased.

The spatial pulse length also depends on the frequency of the transducer. For a constant number of cycles, as the frequency is increased, the shortened wavelength decreases the spatial pulse length and improves the axial resolution (Fig. 2-20). Note that a trade-off occurs. Although the resolution is enhanced at higher frequencies, the depth of penetration is decreased because of the frequency dependence of the attenuation coefficient.

Focusing of the transducer (discussed later in this chapter) creates a region of higher intensity and thus greater sensitivity within the focal zone. The process of focusing the beam may actually lengthen the pulse, thereby deteriorating the axial resolution. This effect is normally minimal.

BANDWIDTH

From Equation 2-14, it can be seen that the Q value is indirectly proportional to the bandwidth or frequency spread of a transducer. Recall that a narrow bandwidth decreases the sensitivity of the transducer. For a transducer operating with a continuous output, only a single frequency is generated. For a pulsed system, however, because of imperfections in the crystal and the complex nature of the damped pulse, a range of frequencies is generated. Many waves of differing frequency combine to form the pulse. Fourier analysis enables a complex waveform (e.g., square wave or pulsed ultrasound wave) to be broken into its various frequency components. An algebraic summation of sine waves

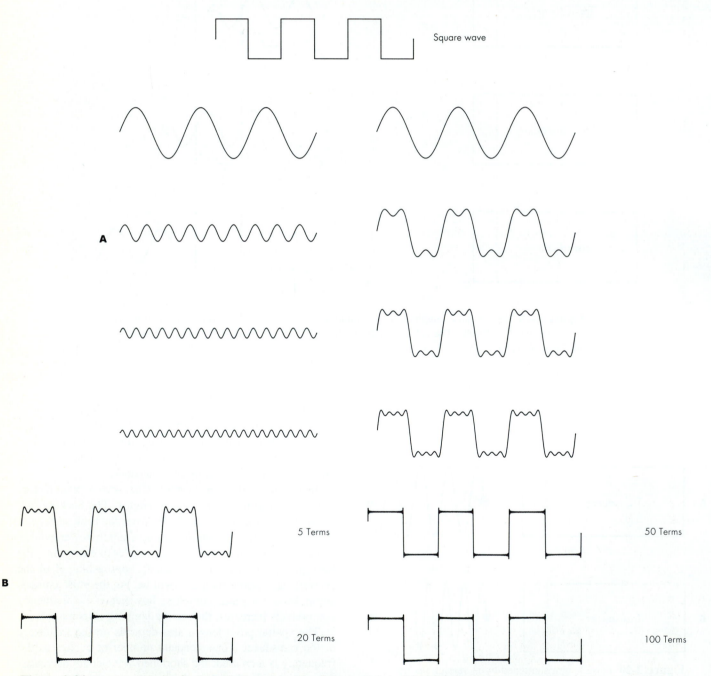

Figure 2-21 Fourier analysis of a "complex" square wave. Representation of the square wave as a summation of sine waves with varying frequency. Each single-frequency sine wave is added to other sine waves yields a waveform that approximates the square wave. **A,** The first four sine waves are shown individually with their effect on the composite waveform. **B,** As more sine waves with different frequencies and amplitudes are added together, the shape more closely represents the square wave (5 to 100 terms).

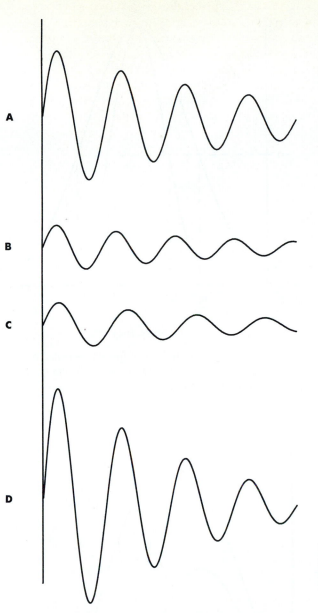

Figure 2-22 **A** to **C,** Three component frequencies derived from Fourier analysis of a pulsed ultrasound wave, **D.** The amplitude of each sine wave is assumed to decrease at the same rate because of damping.

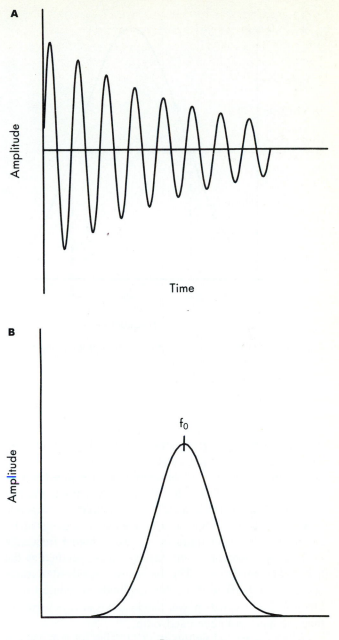

Figure 2-23 Relationship between pulse length and the frequency spectrum. **A,** Amplitude versus time illustrating pulse length. **B,** Relative importance of various frequencies present in the pulse. The center frequency (f_0) is the dominant component. The component frequencies are determined by Fourier analysis.

of varying frequency (Figs. 2-21 and 2-22) yields the original waveform; in other words, any complex waveform can be considered a series of sine waves with different frequencies and amplitudes. (A more complete discussion of Fourier analysis is presented in Appendix B.)

The frequency spectrum can be analyzed by measuring the amplitude versus the time signal induced by an echo returning from a flat steel target located a fixed distance from the transducer. With Fourier analysis, the signal waveform is converted from the time domain to the frequency domain. *Frequency domain* is a mathematical term meaning that the various frequency components of the signal are identified. Amplitude plotted against frequency shows a spectrum of values, with the center frequency (f_0) having the greatest amplitude (Fig. 2-23). Amplitude in this instance indicates

the relative importance of each frequency in the ultrasound pulse. The amplitude represents the fraction of the pulse composed of waves of a particular frequency.

The center frequency is the primary operating frequency or the natural resonance frequency of the transducer, which depends on the crystal thickness. Rewriting Equation 2-14 with symbols:

2-15

$$Q = \frac{f_0}{\Delta f}$$

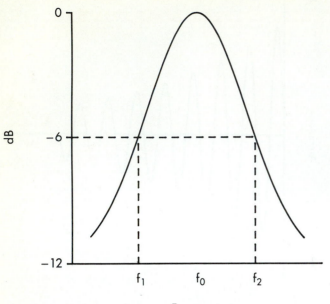

Figure 2-24 Determination of bandwidth by subtracting f_1 from f_2. The limits f_1 and f_2 correspond to one half the center frequency amplitude.

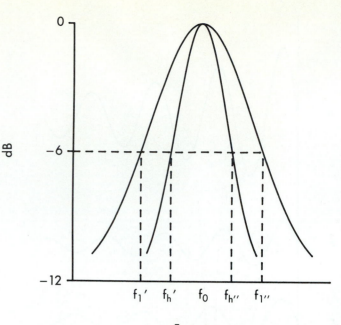

Figure 2-25 Comparison of frequency spectra generated by low-Q and high-Q transducers: low Q, broad bandwidth $(f_1''\text{-}f_1')$ versus high Q, narrow bandwidth $(f_h''\text{-}f_h')$.

where Δf is the bandwidth between the 6 dB points on each side of the center frequency (f_0).

A 6 dB loss occurs if the amplitude is reduced to half its original value. From the frequency spectrum, the frequency corresponding to a 6 dB loss is marked on each side of the center frequency. The bandwidth is calculated by subtracting the lower frequency from the higher frequency (Fig. 2-24). Sometimes the bandwidth is specified as the half-power bandwidth. The half-power bandwidth corresponds to a 3 dB loss, or the amplitude is reduced by a factor of $2^{1/2}$. The half-power bandwidth is always narrower than the half-amplitude bandwidth.

When the second definition of Q value for a transducer is used, it becomes evident (as stated by Equation 2-15) that a high-Q transducer has a very narrow bandwidth whereas a low-Q transducer has a broad bandwidth (Fig. 2-25).

As the beam is transmitted through matter, ultrasound waves of higher frequency are absorbed more rapidly than those of lower frequency, causing a shift in the frequency spectrum toward a lower range (Fig. 2-26). This is similar to the shift toward higher energies as an x-ray beam penetrates the body, because low energies are absorbed more readily. The preferential absorption of the high-frequency components influences the sensitivity of the system. A broadband transducer (as opposed to one with a narrow bandwidth) has greater sensitivity as the sound beam penetrates tissue. A transducer with a broad frequency spectrum is also easier to match electronically with the rest of the ultrasound system, which allows the receiver to be tuned to variable frequencies to maximize the sensitivity at various depths.

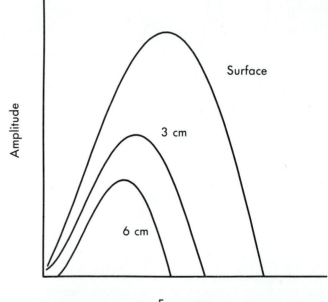

Figure 2-26 Effect of attenuation on the frequency distribution, illustrating the need for a low-Q (broad bandwidth) transducer.

To summarize: A low-Q transducer has a short pulse length (easily damped) and a broad bandwidth. A high-Q transducer has a long pulse length (from crystal ringing) and a narrow bandwidth (Fig. 2-27). In diagnostic ultrasound imaging, trade-offs exist between good reception and good transmission but generally low-Q transducers are desirable.

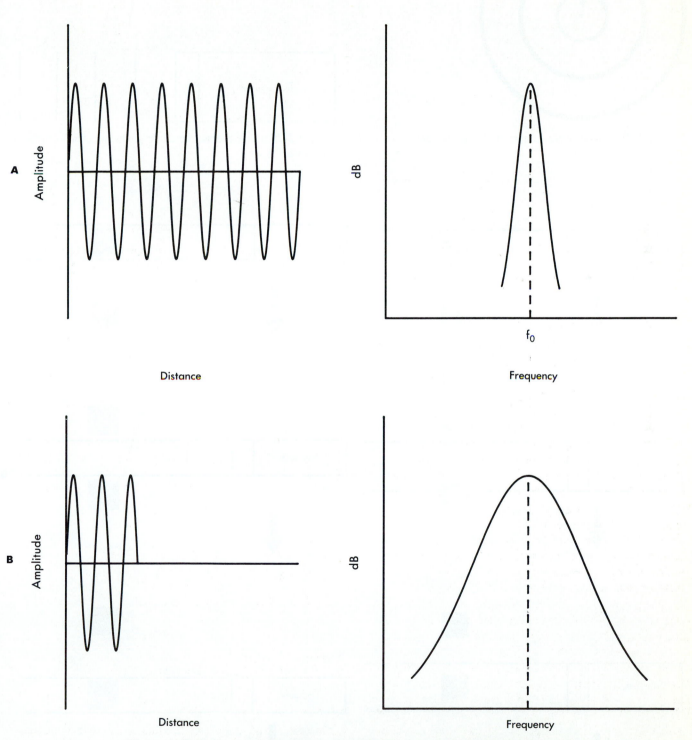

Figure 2-27 Summary of high-Q versus low-Q transducers. **A,** High Q yields a long pulse length and narrow bandwidth. **B,** Low Q yields a short pulse length and broad bandwidth.

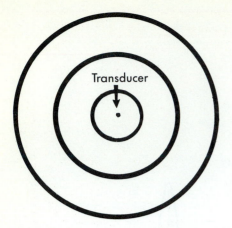

Figure 2-28 Spherical wavefronts produced by a point source of sound.

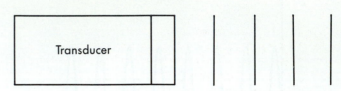

Figure 2-29 Large-radius transducer producing planar (directional) wavefronts.

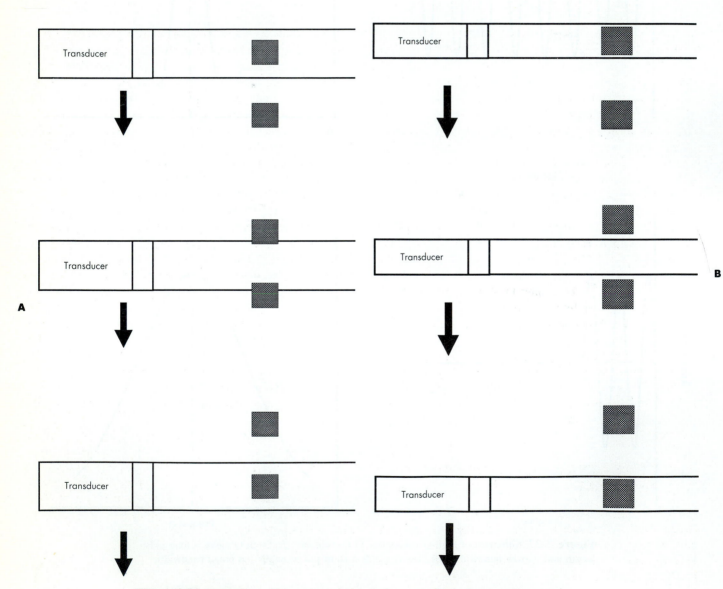

Figure 2-30 Dependence of lateral resolution on beam width. **A,** Two objects are not resolved with a wide beam. **B,** Two objects can be resolved with a narrow beam when the beam is scanned across the objects.

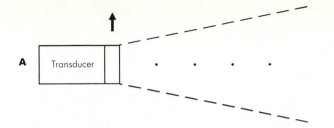

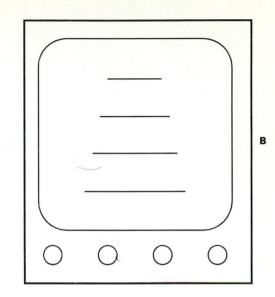

Figure 2-31 Displayed object size versus beam width. **A,** Sound source scanning small spherical reflectors. **B,** The size of an object represented on the display is equivalent to the beam width at the depth of the object. When an object is included within the beam, an echo is produced. A two-dimensional image shows each spherical reflector as a line rather than a dot. The size of the object is misrepresented because the beam width is larger than the object size.

BEAM WIDTH AND LATERAL RESOLUTION

One of the original objectives in designing a device for ultrasound production was to generate a beam that would be directional (similar to a flashlight beam) rather than nondirectional (e.g., light from a light bulb). If a point source of sound is used, waves are emitted in all directions (Fig. 2-28). The beam from a large-diameter transducer is unidirectional, with planar wavefronts and the lateral extent of the beam nearly the same as the diameter of the crystal (Fig. 2-29).

Lateral resolution describes the ability to resolve two objects adjacent to each other that are perpendicular to the beam axis (Fig. 2-30). It also refers to the ability of the ultrasound beam to detect single small objects across the width of the beam. Decreasing the beam width improves the lateral resolution by allowing objects close together to be resolved and by providing a more accurate presentation of small objects. A single object smaller than the sound beam width produces a signal the entire time it is within the beam; thus the object appears to be the same size as the width of the beam (Fig. 2-31). A small beam width enables small objects to become distinguishable. Lateral resolution is a major factor in the quality of diagnostic ultrasound images.

THE ULTRASONIC FIELD: NEAR FIELD AND FAR FIELD

Another objective in designing a device for ultrasound production was to generate a beam of uniform intensity. A circular sound source with a diameter equal to one wavelength produces spherical wavefronts originating from the face of the crystal. The beam diverges rapidly from the crystal face, and the lateral resolution deteriorates. In addition, regions of rarefaction and compression create a nonuniform beam (Fig. 2-32). If the diameter of the sound source is increased to a value of several wavelengths, each small area (one wavelength in size) is considered to be an individual vibrating sound source and thus to produce its own spherical wavefronts. These wavefronts undergo constructive and destructive interference, resulting in a very complex wave pattern (Fig. 2-33), in accordance with Huygens' principle. A nonuniform beam intensity exists in the near field (area of nondivergence) and a uniform beam is present in the far field (area of divergence, in which lateral resolution is poor). The far field is called the Fraunhofer zone, and the near field the Fresnel zone (Fig. 2-34).

If the acoustic pressure along the axis of the beam is measured (axial pressure profile) for a high-Q transducer (continuous wave, single frequency), the pressure alternates between a maximum value and zero in the near field and then slowly decreases after the last maximum, which is the beginning of the far field (Fig. 2-35). Cross-sectional intensity measurements (transverse pressure profiles) also reveal a nonuniform beam in the near field (Fig. 2-36). Low-intensity side lobes (adjacent to, but angled away from, the main beam axis) may be produced from these interference phenomena. The side lobes create artifacts in an image by the incorrect placement of an interface. This is particularly true for real-time ultrasound, which is discussed in Chapter 4.

A low-Q transducer (broad bandwidth, short pulse length) produces many frequencies rather than just a single frequency. The presence of multiple frequencies tends to make the near field more uniform. Every frequency has a different interference pattern and, when these patterns are superimposed on each other, the result is a smoothing of the overall intensity pattern (Fig. 2-37).

Near-Field Depth

For a nonfocused transducer the depth of the near field (D), or the distance that the near field extends into the patient, is dependent on the diameter and frequency (or wavelength

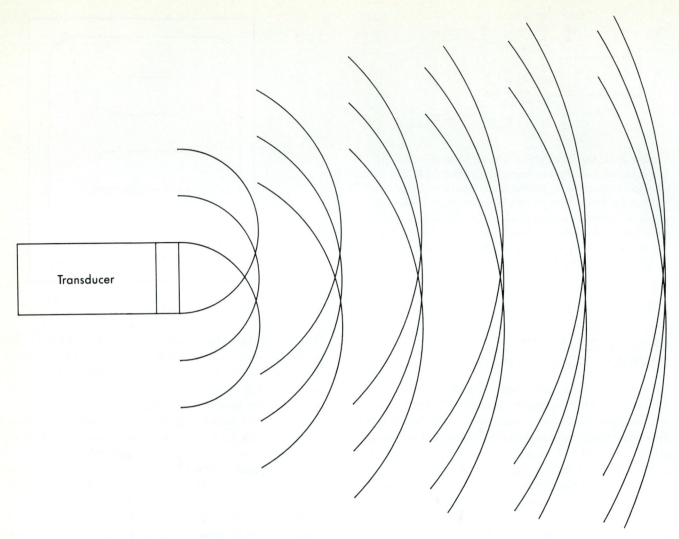

Figure 2-32 Wavefronts produced from a sound source whose diameter is equal to one wavelength.

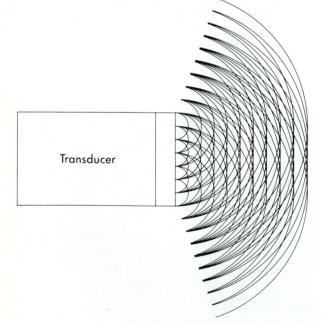

Figure 2-33 A large sound source acting as multiple, single wavelength sound sources produces a complex pattern of wavefronts.

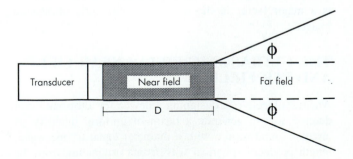

Figure 2-34 Beam pattern showing the near field (Fresnel zone) and far field (Fraunhofer zone). Distance D indicates the depth of the near field. Angle ϕ characterizes the divergence of the far field.

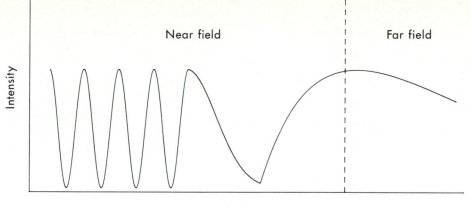

Figure 2-35 Axial intensity (or pressure) profile from a high-Q transducer. Note the large variation of intensity in the near field.

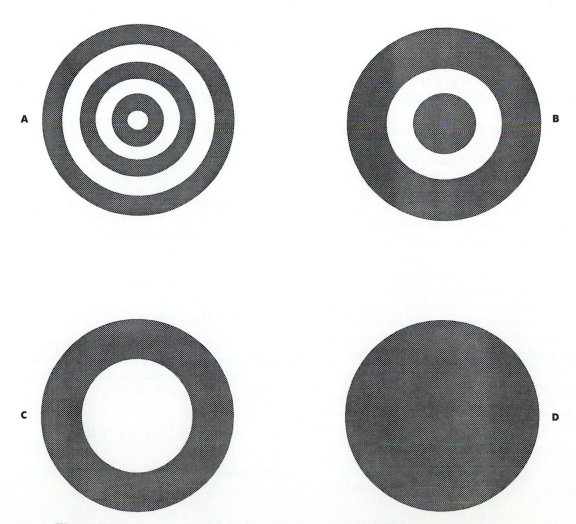

Figure 2-36 Transverse (cross-sectional) intensity (or pressure) profiles. The profiles are shown at various locations along the axis of the beam. **A,** Depth in the near field in which the axial pressure profile is minimal. **B,** Depth in the near field in which the axial pressure profile is maximal. **C,** Depth of the last minimum in the near field. **D,** Depth in the far field.

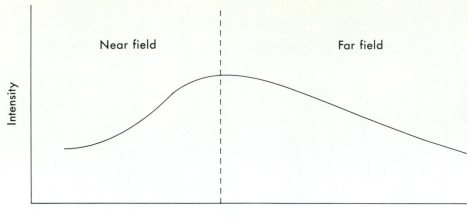

Figure 2-37 Axial intensity (or pressure) profile from a low-Q transducer. The broad frequency components cause the near field to have less intensity fluctuation.

via $c = f\lambda$) of the transducer according to the following formula:

$$\text{2-16}$$

$$D = \frac{d^2 f}{4\,c} = \frac{d^2}{4\,\lambda} = \frac{r^2}{\lambda}$$

where f is the frequency of the transducer, d the diameter of the transducer, c the velocity of ultrasound in the medium, λ the wavelength of the ultrasound, and r the radius of the transducer.

As the frequency increases (with the wavelength decreasing), the depth of the near field increases. In theory, by increasing the frequency, the region of best lateral resolution would be extended. This is illustrated by Example 2-8 below. In practice, higher frequencies are absorbed more rapidly as the beam propagates through tissue and, consequently, deep structures may not be visualized because the reflected ultrasound waves are too weak. At high frequencies lateral resolution associated with narrow beam width in the near field is maintained at increased depth.

Equation 2-16 also indicates that the depth of the near field (area of nondivergence) increases rapidly as the diameter of the transducer increases. Example 2-9 demonstrates this effect. The lateral resolution at shallow depths, however, is sacrificed as the crystal diameter is made larger.

■ **Example 2-8**

Calculate the near-field depth (D) for transducers with frequencies of 1, 2, and 5 MHz. Assume a constant diameter of 20 mm (0.02 m). Using Equation 2-16, $D = \dfrac{d^2 f}{4\,c}$,

$$(1\ \text{MHz})\ D = \frac{(0.02)^2\,(1 \times 10^6)}{(4)\,(1540)} = 0.065\ \text{m} = 6.5\ \text{cm}$$

$$(2\ \text{MHz})\ D = \frac{(0.02)^2\,(2 \times 10^6)}{(4)\,(1540)} = 0.13\ \text{m} = 13.0\ \text{cm}$$

$$(5\ \text{MHz})\ D = \frac{(0.02)^2\,(5 \times 10^6)}{(4)\,(1540)} = 0.325\ \text{m} = 32.5\ \text{cm}$$

This example illustrates that, for a constant-diameter transducer, if the frequency increases (causing the wavelength to decrease) the depth of the near field increases. This extends the useful area of best lateral resolution to greater depths.

■ **Example 2-9**

Calculate the depth of the near field (D) for transducers with diameters of 10, 20, and 30 mm. Assume a constant frequency of 1 MHz. Solve using the same formula as in Example 2-8.

$$(10\ \text{mm})\ D = \frac{(0.01)^2\,(1 \times 10^6)}{(4)\,(1540)} = 0.016\ \text{m} = 1.6\ \text{cm}$$

$$(20\ \text{mm})\ D = \frac{(0.02)^2\,(1 \times 10^6)}{(4)\,(1540)} = 0.065\ \text{m} = 6.5\ \text{cm}$$

$$(30\ \text{mm})\ D = \frac{(0.03)^2\,(1 \times 10^6)}{(4)\,(1540)} = 0.146\ \text{m} = 14.6\ \text{cm}$$

This example illustrates that, for a constant frequency, as the diameter increases the depth of the near field increases. The increasing beam diameter (i.e., beam aperture, as discussed for real-time scanners in Chapter 4) increases the depth of the near field.

Far-Field Divergence

Beyond the near field is the region called the far field (Fraunhofer zone), where the ultrasound beam begins to diverge. The angle ϕ, a measure of the beam's divergence for a nonfocused transducer, is given as

$$\text{2-17}$$

$$\sin \phi = \frac{0.61\,\lambda}{r} = \frac{1.22\,\lambda}{d} = \frac{1.22\,c}{df}$$

Therefore

$$\text{2-18}$$

$$\phi = \text{Arcsin}\ \frac{0.61\,\lambda}{r} = \text{Arcsin}\ \frac{1.22\,\lambda}{d} = \text{Arcsin}\ \frac{1.22\,c}{df}$$

These formulas predict that, as the frequency is increased (or wavelength is decreased), the angle of divergence becomes smaller.) This is demonstrated by Example 2-10. Also, as the diameter is increased, the beam diverges less rapidly. Example 2-11 illustrates this point.

■ Example 2-10

Calculate the angle of divergence (ϕ) for transducers with frequencies of 1 and 2 MHz. Assume a constant diameter of 20 mm. Using equation 2-18, solve for ϕ.

$$(1 \text{ MHz}) \ \phi = \text{Arcsin} \ \frac{(1.22)(1540)}{(0.02)(1 \times 10^6)} = 5.4 \text{ degrees}$$

$$(2 \text{ MHz}) \ \phi = \text{Arcsin} \ \frac{(1.22)(1540)}{(0.02)(2 \times 10^6)} = 2.7 \text{ degrees}$$

This example illustrates that the angle of divergence for nonfocused transducers with a constant diameter decreases as the frequency increases. The result is improved lateral resolution in the far field.

■ Example 2-11

Calculate the angle of divergence (ϕ) for transducers with diameters of 10 and 20 mm. Assume a constant frequency of 1 MHz. Using Equation 2-18, solve for ϕ.

$$(10 \text{ mm}) \ \phi = \text{Arcsin} \ \frac{(1.22)(1540)}{(0.01)(1 \times 10^6)} = 10.8 \text{ degrees}$$

$$(20 \text{ mm}) \ \phi = \text{Arcsin} \ \frac{(1.22)(1540)}{(0.02)(1 \times 10^6)} = 5.4 \text{ degrees}$$

This example illustrates that, if the diameter of nonfocused transducers can be increased (for a constant frequency), the angle of divergence decreases. This results in improved lateral resolution in the far field.

The influence of crystal size and operating frequency on near-field depth and far-field divergence is further demonstrated by the calculated results from Equations 2-17 and 2-18 (which are listed in Table 2-2).

The lateral resolution deteriorates in the far-field region because of divergence of the beam. Therefore scanning areas of interest should be confined to the near field if possible. An exception to this practice may occur when scanning large patients.

Transducer Selection

The depth of the structures of interest is a primary consideration when selecting the optimum transducer. The objective is to enhance lateral resolution by scanning the area of interest with a narrow beam. Evaluation of the near-field depth and far-field divergence indicates that transducers with high frequencies and large diameters maintain beam shape to greater depths. Although large-diameter transducers have a large near-field beam width and thus provide poor lateral resolution at shallow depths, the near field extends to greater depths in the body compared with a smaller diameter transducer. The divergence of the beam in the far field is less, which makes the larger transducer preferable for deep-lying structures (Fig. 2-38).

A similar effect is observed with frequency; that is, with

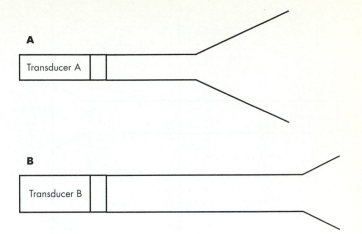

Figure 2-38 Effect of transducer diameter on lateral resolution. **A,** A small-diameter transducer can maintain a narrow beam width only at shallow depths. **B,** At greater depths the large-diameter transducer has a smaller beam width and better lateral resolution.

■ **Table 2-2** Near-Field Depth and Far-Field Divergence as a Function of Crystal Diameter and Center Frequency

Frequency (MHz)	Transducer Diameter (mm)	Near-Field Depth (cm)	Far-Field Divergence (degrees)
1	8	1.0	13.6
1	10	1.6	10.8
1	15	3.6	7.2
1	20	6.5	5.4
2	8	2.1	6.7
2	10	3.2	5.4
2	15	7.3	3.6
2	20	13.0	2.7
3.5	8	3.6	3.8
3.5	10	5.7	3.1
3.5	15	12.8	2.0
3.5	20	22.7	1.5
5	8	5.2	2.7
5	10	8.1	2.2
5	15	18.3	1.4
5	20	32.5	1.1
7.5	8	7.8	1.8
7.5	10	12.2	1.4
7.5	15	27.4	1.0
7.5	20	48.7	0.7
10	8	10.4	1.4
10	10	16.2	1.1
10	15	36.5	0.7
10	20	64.9	0.5

other factors constant, an increased frequency results in a deeper near field and a less diverging far field. This may compensate for the loss in penetration (Fig. 2-39).

If shallow structures and irregular surfaces are of interest, a small-diameter high-frequency transducer should be used.

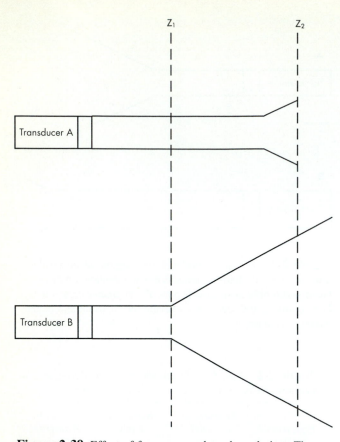

Z_1 Z_2

Transducer A

Transducer B

Figure 2-39 Effect of frequency on lateral resolution. The region between depths z_1 and z_2 is sampled with better lateral resolution when a high-frequency transducer (A) is used. The region beyond z_2 is not probed by high-frequency sound waves because of rapid attenuation of the beam. A low-frequency transducer (B) must be used to sample this region.

Abdominal studies usually entail medium-frequency medium-diameter transducers, whereas larger patients or harder to penetrate areas may require low-frequency large-diameter transducers. Various methods to enhance sensitivity permit the use of a higher frequency transducer.

Self-Focusing Effect

Before we leave this topic, the assumption that, in the near field, the beam width is equal to the transducer crystal diameter should be clarified. The nonfocused single-crystal transducer has a self-focusing effect so the beam width actually decreases to a minimum value at the transition point between the near field and far field and then begins to diverge. In fact, the beam width at the transition point is equal to half the diameter of the crystal (Fig. 2-40). The maximum acoustic pressure actually occurs at the transition point because the same power is distributed over a smaller area (Fig. 2-41). At a distance equal to twice the near-field depth, the beam diameter diverges to a size equal to the crystal diameter. The following formula describes the near-field beam width (w_N) and the far-field beam width (w_F).

2-19

$$w_N = d - \frac{2\lambda z}{d}$$

2-20

$$w_F = \frac{2\lambda z}{d}$$

where d is the crystal diameter, λ the wavelength of the ultrasound, and z is the depth of interest.

Two special cases are considered in the following examples.

■ **Example 2-12**

Calculate the beam width at the transition point, where z = D, the depth of the near field:

$$w_N = d - \left(\frac{2\lambda z}{d}\right) \text{ and } z = \frac{d^2}{4\lambda}$$

Therefore

$$w_N = d - \left(\frac{2\lambda d^2}{4\lambda d}\right) = d - \left(\frac{d}{2}\right) = \frac{d}{2}$$

This example illustrates that the beam width at the transition zone is half the crystal diameter, rather than equal to the crystal diameter as is normally assumed.

■ **Example 2-13**

Calculate the beam width at a distance in the far field that is equal to twice the near-field depth, where z = 2D.

$$w_F = \frac{2\lambda z}{d} \text{ and } z = 2D = \frac{2d^2}{4\lambda}$$

Therefore

$$w_F = \frac{2\lambda 2d^2}{4\lambda d} = \frac{4\lambda d^2}{4\lambda d} = d$$

This example demonstrates that the beam width in the far field is less than or equal to the crystal diameter up to a distance of twice the near field depth.

Thus the lateral resolution, based on beam width, is better than normally expected for nonfocused transducers. Typically, however, the beam shape changes in the presence of an attenuating medium, and therefore the beam width is assumed equal to the crystal diameter in the near field.

SIDE LOBES

The discussion of side lobes must now be completed. Side lobes are secondary projections of ultrasonic energy that radiate away from the main ultrasound beam (Fig. 2-42). Immediate echoes (reverberations at the transducer-tissue interface), pulse shape, transducer design, and radial mode vibration (Fig. 2-43) all contribute to the formation of side lobes. The position (angle) and intensity of side lobes can be predicted from directivity functions obtained by solving the wave equation. The intensity of side lobes is normally 60 to 100 dB below that of the main ultrasound beam, which usually does not pose significant problems. If present at high intensity levels, however, side lobes create artifacts (presentation of off-axis structures) and noise in the image.

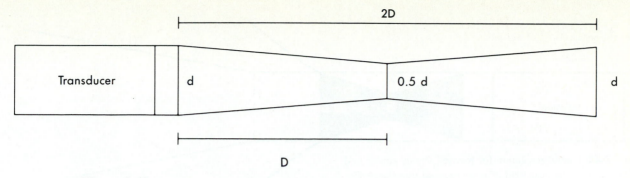

Figure 2-40 Actual beam width for a nonfocused transducer in the presence of a nonattenuating medium. A beam width of half the crystal diameter occurs at the limit of the near field and increases to equal the crystal diameter at twice the near-field depth.

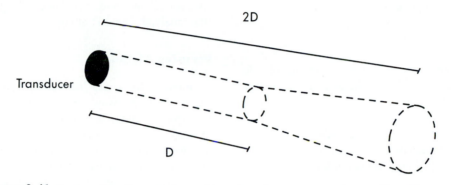

Figure 2-41 Beam pattern for a nonfocused transducer in a nonattenuating medium. The same power is delivered throughout the ultrasonic field. The intensity is maximal at the transition zone (near field to far field) because of the decreased beam size. Ultrasonic field intensity is changed when an attenuating medium is present.

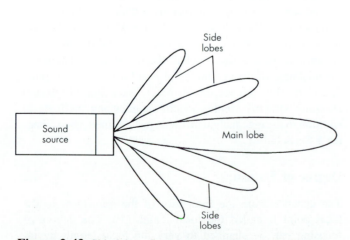

Figure 2-42 Side lobes. Sound energy radiates in multiple directions. The intensity of the side lobes is less than that of the main lobe.

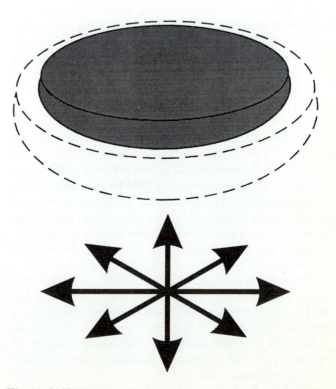

Figure 2-43 Radial mode vibrations of a circular transducer contribute to side lobe formation.

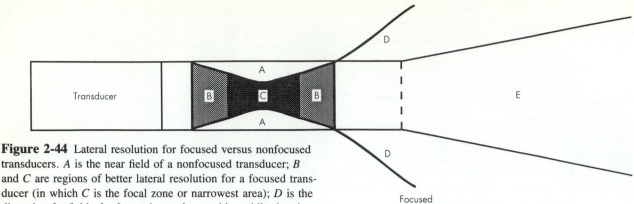

Figure 2-44 Lateral resolution for focused versus nonfocused transducers. *A* is the near field of a nonfocused transducer; *B* and *C* are regions of better lateral resolution for a focused transducer (in which *C* is the focal zone or narrowest area); *D* is the diverging far field of a focused transducer with rapidly deteriorating lateral resolution; and *E* is the far field for a nonfocused transducer indicating the area of better lateral resolution compared to that for a focused transducer.

Clutter, a type of acoustic noise, consists of low-amplitude signals from weak echoes that originate from secondary lobes striking off-axis structures.

Broad bandwidth (low-Q) transducers create fewer and less intense side lobes than do high-Q transducers, although the main lobe intensity pattern is widened. (A further discussion of secondary ultrasonic energy lobes is presented in Chapter 4.)

FOCUSING

Lateral resolution (a major consideration for diagnostic ultrasound imaging) can be improved by focusing the transducer crystal (Fig. 2-44). Focusing limits the useful near-field depth because the beam diverges rapidly beyond the focal zone. The focal zone is defined as the region where intensity has a value within 3 dB of the maximum along the transducer axis. Manufacturers may also quote a larger focal zone based on intensity measurements within 6 dB of the maximum. The focal zone or focused area is closer to the face of the transducer than the nonfocused near-field depth, provided the transducers are of equal diameter and frequency. This is demonstrated by Figure 2-44. The focal zone may not be symmetrical around the focal point, which is the point of maximum intensity. The beam is most narrow at the focal point. The intensity of an ultrasound beam at the focal point is expected to be greater than that for the same diameter of nonfocused transducer because the cross-sectional area of the beam is less for the focused than for the nonfocused beam.

The magnitude of an intensity increase produced by focusing may be as high as a factor of 100. Attenuation will shift the maximum intensity from the transition point to a location closer to the face of the nonfocused transducer. Attenuation may also dramatically affect the intensity of focused beams. When a patient is being scanned, the lack of tissue uniformity may have a dramatic effect on the position of the focal zone compared with that observed in a uniform phantom. The axial resolution may be somewhat

worse for the focused beam in the focal zone because the stronger echoes are detected over a lengthened time interval (the received signal is elongated).

Focusing Methods

To improve the lateral resolution, a transducer can be focused in several ways. Sound follows many of the same principles as light. It can be focused by a special acoustic mirror (Fig. 2-45, *A*) or by an acoustic lens (Fig. 2-45, *B*) that works in a manner similar to a light lens. These are examples of external focusing methods.

Acoustic mirrors are made of tungsten-impregnated epoxy resin. Acoustic lenses are formed from polystyrene, nylon, or aluminum. The velocity of sound in the lens is greater than that in tissue; thus sound waves are bent toward a point in tissue (principle of refraction). The most common form of focusing for transducers with frequencies of less than 5 MHz uses a curved crystal (Fig. 2-45, *C*), which is an internal focusing method. For frequencies above 5 MHz, external focusing methods are normally used because the crystals become extremely thin and are difficult to form into curved shapes of proper uniformity without breaking. With a velocity of 4000 m/s for PZT, a 5 MHz crystal has a wavelength of 0.8 mm and a 10 MHz crystal 0.4 mm. The crystal thickness is equal to half the wavelength. Therefore the thickness of the crystal is 0.4 mm for the 5 MHz transducer and 0.2 mm for the 10 MHz. Real-time ultrasound scanning systems employ electronic focusing methods in addition to the mechanical methods just outlined. (See Chapter 4 for details.)

Degree of Focusing

The distance from the front face of the transducer to the focal point is called the focal length (F). The degree of focusing can be changed to vary the focal length by increasing the radius of curvature of the crystal (Fig. 2-46) or by increasing the curvature of the acoustic lens or mirror. This allows transducers with the same frequency to be made with focal zones at different depths, depending on the degree of focusing (Fig. 2-46). As the degree of focusing becomes stronger, the beam width is made more narrow but the focal zone is drawn closer to the face of the transducer.

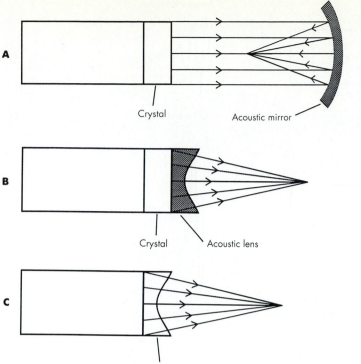

Figure 2-45 Methods of focusing transducers. **A,** Acoustic mirror; **B,** acoustic lens; **C,** curved crystal. The first two methods are called external focusing, and the third is termed internal focusing.

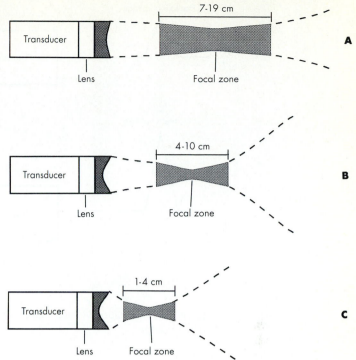

Figure 2-46 As the focusing is made stronger, the beam width decreases, the focal zone moves closer to the face of the transducer, and the intensity increases in the focal zone. **A,** Weak or long focusing; **B,** medium focusing; **C,** strong or short focusing.

The degree of focusing (κ) is expressed quantitatively as the ratio of near-field depth to focal length.

$$\kappa = \frac{r^2/\lambda}{F} \qquad \text{2-21}$$

or

$$\kappa = \frac{r^2}{\lambda F} \qquad \text{2-22}$$

In this scheme weak focusing has a value of less than 6, medium focusing a value of 6 to 20, and strong focusing a value greater than 20.

■ **Example 2-14**

Calculate the degree of focusing (κ) for a 3 cm diameter crystal operating at a frequency of 3 MHz if the focal length is 7 cm.

$$\kappa = \frac{r^2}{\lambda F}$$

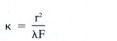

$$= \frac{(15 \text{ mm})^2}{(0.51 \text{ mm})(70 \text{ mm})}$$

$$= 6$$

Weak-focused transducers (also called long-focused) composed of a single element have a focal length of 7 to 19 cm, medium-focused transducers a focal length of 4 to 10 cm, and strong-focused (short-focused) transducers a focal length of 1 to 4 cm. Focusing, particularly for real-time scanners, has been one of the major reasons why ultrasound is so widely accepted today as a clinical imaging modality. (Methods of checking the transducer focus are discussed in Chapter 13.)

RECEPTION

A system has been devised in which a transducer is used to generate an ultrasound beam via the converse piezoelectric effect and then to direct that beam into the body. As the ultrasound wave strikes various interfaces in the body, some of the energy is transmitted and some is reflected, in accordance with the reflection formula (Equation 1-7). The reflected echo returns toward the transducer.

Transmit Gain

Most ultrasound units include an output, power, or transmit gain control that adjusts the voltage spike to the transducer to produce an acoustic pulse of higher intensity. This results in a stronger echo (Fig. 2-47). The typical excitation voltage pulse ranges from 300 to 600 V but may be as high as 900 V. Frequently the control is adjustable in 3 dB (50%) increments.

Increased sound wave intensity enhances the detectability

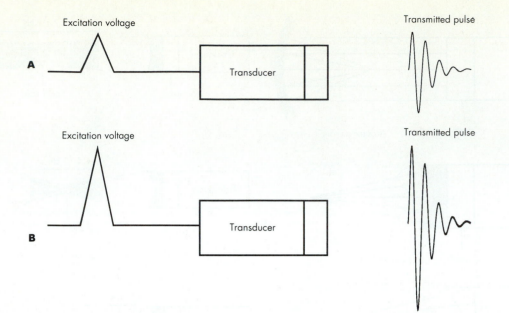

Figure 2-47 Excitation voltage regulates the transmitted beam intensity. **A,** Low voltage. **B,** High voltage.

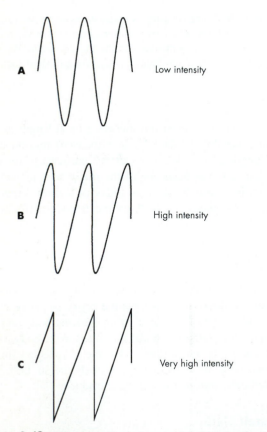

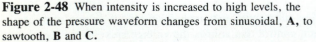

Figure 2-48 When intensity is increased to high levels, the shape of the pressure waveform changes from sinusoidal, **A,** to sawtooth, **B** and **C.**

of weak reflectors. However, higher intensity levels increase patient exposure and unlimited power gain does not continue to improve sensitivity. In addition, high intensity distorts the sinusoidal pressure wave, altering both the propagation and the reception of sound waves (Fig. 2-48).

Amplification

The echo, in the form of waves, strikes the crystal and induces a radiofrequency (RF) signal via the piezoelectric effect (Fig. 2-49). The waveform of the RF signal mimics the ultrasound waveform, since the voltage variations are in response to pressure-induced thickness changes in the crystal. The microvolt or millivolt RF signal is amplified to 1 V to 10 V for processing and display purposes. Combinations of linear, exponential, logarithmic, and variable amplifications can be used.

The most common type of receiver gain is logarithmic. The amount of amplification or gain is adjustable by the operator. Weak signals undergo greater amplification than do strong signals. The disparity between weak and strong reflectors is diminished. Dynamic range (usually expressed in decibels) is the ratio of the largest to the smallest signal that can be accommodated by a system component. Logarithmic amplification reduces the dynamic range of the induced RF signals. Decreasing the dynamic range is called compression.

Most gain controls adjust only the amplification of the received signals and have no effect on the intensity of the generated ultrasound beam. The improved sensitivity in these cases is the result of extra amplification only and possible tuning of the receiver to allow detection of weaker signals.

Time Gain Compensation

One problem that must be considered is the attenuation of an ultrasonic beam with depth. Equally reflective interfaces produce different signal levels, depending on their relative distances from the transducer. It is often advantageous to display reflectors of similar size, shape, and reflection co-

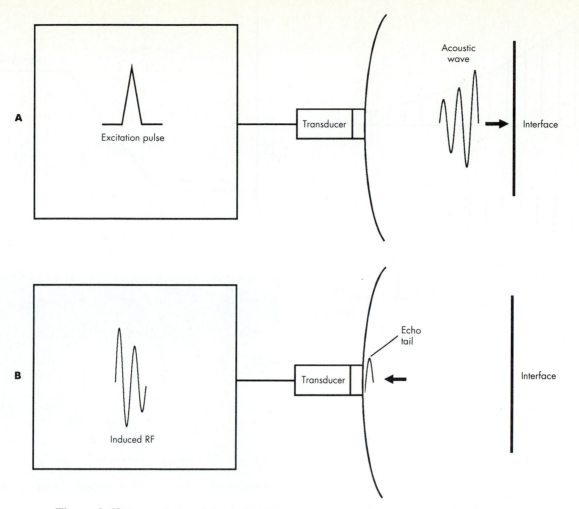

Figure 2-49 Transmission and reception of signals. **A,** Acoustic wave initiated by the excitation pulse applied to the transducer striking an interface. **B,** The echo on return to the transducer induces the radiofrequency signal.

efficients with equal signal strengths or brightness levels. Exponential amplification is used to correct the signals for attenuation. This can be easily demonstrated:

Assume that a phantom is composed of alternating layers of water and gelatin (Fig. 2-50) that are very similar in acoustic impedance. Each layer is 1 cm thick. A small fraction of the incident beam is reflected at each interface, and the percentage reflected is constant for every interface in the phantom. Recall that the reflection formula (Equation 1-7) does not distinguish which medium contains the incident beam.

Because of attenuation, however, the display shows exponentially decreasing signal strengths (Fig. 2-51, *A*) rather than signals of equal amplitude. To compensate for this attenuation, a time gain compensation (TGC) control is used to increase the amplitude of processed signals with time or depth (Fig. 2-51, *B*). The amplification could be a reverse exponential function, because the signals decrease exponentially (Fig. 2-51, *C*). TGC also contributes to signal compression. When the liver is scanned with TGC, all echoes should be of nearly the same amplitude, unless an abnormality is present or vessels are observed. Other terms for TGC include *depth gain compensation* (DGC), swept

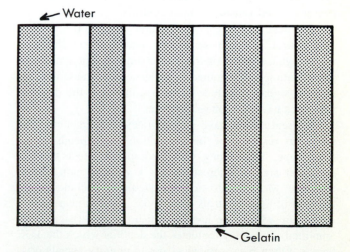

Figure 2-50 Phantom composed of alternating layers of water and gelatin.

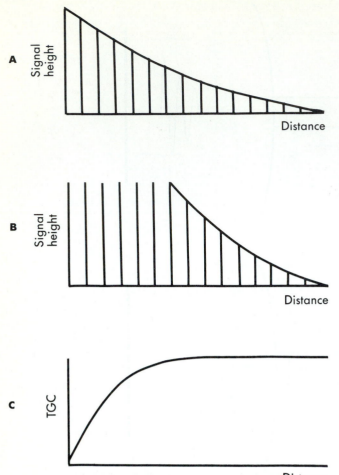

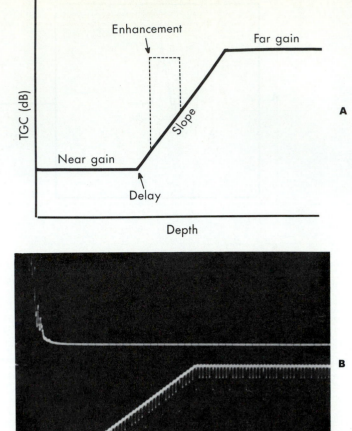

Figure 2-51 Effect of time gain compensation. **A,** Signal amplitude versus depth without TGC. **B,** Signal amplitude versus depth with TGC. **C,** Reverse exponential TGC used to obtain the signal levels in **B.**

Figure 2-52 Time gain compensation. **A,** Possible control adjustments. **B,** Instrument display of the TGC slope with no enhancement.

gain control, depth-varied gain, distance-attenuation compensation, and sensitivity-time control.

Automatic TGC (also called adaptive gain control, auto–gain control, and auto–sensitivity control) adjusts the time-varying gain without operator intervention. The amount of amplification is determined by the general decrease in echo-induced signal amplitude. This assumes that the detected structures have similar reflectivities.

Different tissues have varying rates of attenuation. The frequency response of the attenuation rate depends on the tissue type. This, along with the capability to enhance a particular area of interest, makes a variable gain control desirable. Most diagnostic ultrasound units include a combination of TGC controls (Fig. 2-52, *A*). The near gain or mean gain adjusts the level at which the initial signals are amplified. The delay regulates the depth at which the TGC begins. Often it is convenient not to amplify signals originating close to the transducer because they have high amplitude levels. The slope of the TGC indicates the amount of compensation that is applied with depth. Some ultrasound units have a completely variable gain control, permitting

a particular area of interest to be enhanced beyond that provided by TGC. The far gain represents the maximum amount that signals can be amplified. In this zone the signals are amplified by a constant amount, but they exhibit an exponential decrease because of attenuation (Fig. 2-52, *B*).

The variable TGC controls permit adjustable compensation for different frequency transducers, allowing greater amplification when high frequencies are used. Remember: Attenuation in soft tissue is frequency dependent. As the frequency is increased, more amplification is required to counteract the accelerated loss of beam intensity.

Flexibility in the TGC controls enables higher quality images to be obtained. Nevertheless, the sonographer must be more aware of the functions of the different controls; furthermore, he or she must also interact more with the system during scanning. A scanner with selectable TGC controls can produce poor quality images when operated by an inexperienced individual. Automation of the TGC controls provides more consistent images, but they are often poorer in overall quality.

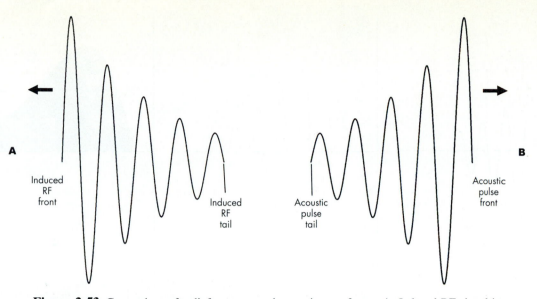

Figure 2-53 Comparison of radiofrequency and acoustic waveforms. **A,** Induced RF signal in a crystal. **B,** The acoustic wave.

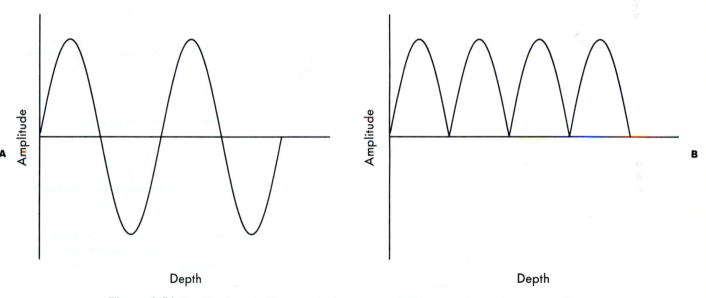

Figure 2-54 Rectification. **A,** The crystal response to an incident sound wave induces a radiofrequency signal in the receiver circuit. **B,** In the rectified signal negative components are flipped to become positive.

SIGNAL PROCESSING

The radiofrequency (RF) signal induced in the transducer by the returning echoes could be amplified and then displayed, but it would then appear similar to the acoustic pulse sent out (Fig. 2-53). If numerous interfaces are present, the interpretation of the received signals becomes confusing. For viewing ease, the goal is to process the signal before displaying it. The processing lowers the information content (smaller dynamic range) while, at the same time, facilitating the association of final output with physical structures.

The normal processing procedure involves rectification (converting the negative portion of the RF signal to positive)

after the signal has been amplified and has undergone TGC amplification (Fig. 2-54). Alternatively, the negative component of the RF wave can be eliminated rather than flipped to positive. The peaks of the RF waves are "electronically" surrounded or enveloped, resulting in a processed signal that could be further amplified for display purposes (Fig. 2-55). Enveloping is often referred to as demodulation and is generally accomplished by passing the signal through a circuit with a slow time response. The overall outline of the pulse is retained, but the internal fast oscillations are lost. This is not the true meaning of demodulation, but it shows how the term is used in this context. Demodulation normally involves removing a signal that has undergone interference

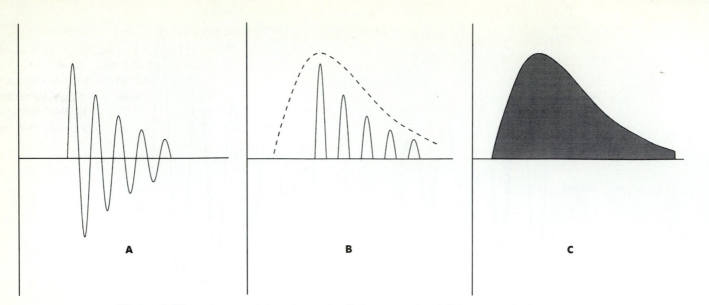

Figure 2-55 Enveloping. **A** is an induced radiofrequency signal; **B** is the enveloping (i.e., an electronic surrounding of the peaks); **C** is the resultant enveloped signal.

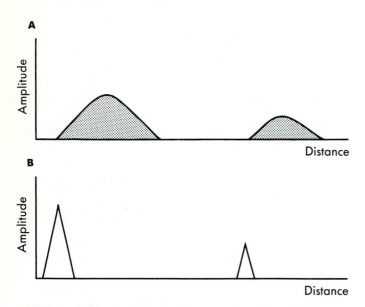

Figure 2-56 Integration. **A** is two enveloped signals; **B** is the area under each enveloped signal (represented as a *spike*).

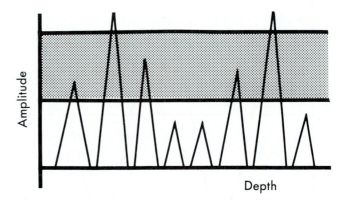

Figure 2-57 Reject processing. The three signals within the range between the upper and lower levels *(shaded area)* are processed and ultimately displayed; the others, above and below the *shaded area*, are not.

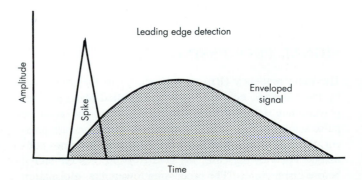

Figure 2-58 Leading edge detection. The leading edge of the enveloped signal *(shaded area)* is represented as a *spike*. Normally this technique is used with other processing techniques (e.g., integration) to define the interface position more accurately.

with a carrier wave, which is important in Doppler ultrasound (as discussed in Chapter 6).

Usually the area under the enveloped signal is electronically measured. Determination of the area is called integration. This area is then represented as a spike for A-mode scanning or as a dot for other scanning techniques (Fig. 2-56). An increase in the amplitude of the induced RF signal results in a larger area under the curve and therefore an increase in the height of the spike or brightness of the dot. A reject control (also called threshold or suppression control) may be added to eliminate peaks below or above a certain level, as selected by the operator (Fig. 2-57). The

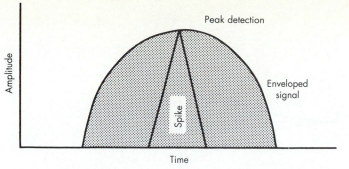

Figure 2-59 Peak detection. The peak of the enveloped signal *(shaded area)* is represented as a *spike*. Unless combined with leading-edge processing, peak detection can create a small position error of the interface.

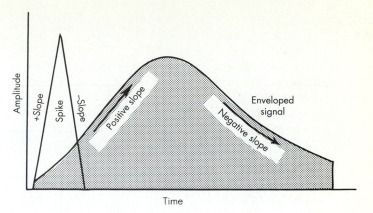

Figure 2-60 Differentiation. The *spike* represents the positive and negative slopes of the enveloped signal.

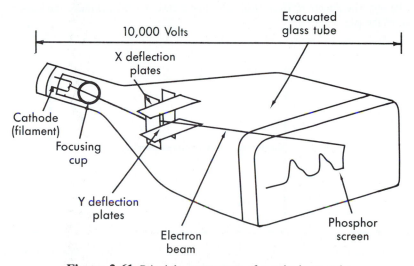

Figure 2-61 Principle components of a cathode ray tube.

reject control is similar to the lower level (or upper level) discriminator used in radiation counting systems. Rejection of signals decreases the dynamic range.

Other techniques can be incorporated into signal processing. These include (1) leading edge detection—representing the *beginning* of the RF pulse as a spike or dot (Fig. 2-58); (2) peak detection—representing the *maximum height* of the enveloped signal as a spike or dot (Fig. 2-59); and (3) differentiation—representing the *slope* of the enveloped signal as a spike or dot (Fig. 2-60). Usually integration is employed in conjunction with leading edge detection.

DISPLAY

A cathode ray tube (CRT) is the simplest output device used for display purposes. It is a large evacuated (low-pressure) glass tube with a potential difference of 10,000 V from back to front. This voltage difference accelerates electrons emitted from the cathode (filament) at the back of the CRT toward the screen (Fig. 2-61). A special focusing cup near

the filament confines the electrons to a narrow beam and prevents them from spreading out over a wide area. The glass envelope maintains the vacuum. The glass screen on the front of the CRT is covered with a phosphorescent material (usually zinc sulfide, zinc sulfate, or potassium iodide) that produces light when struck with electrons. Two sets of special electrical or magnetic plates control the position of the electron beam on the X (across the screen) and Y (up and down the screen) axes of the tube face. Electrical fields are produced when a voltage difference is applied to one set of plates. If no voltage is applied, no electrical field is present and the electrons travel along a straight-line path to the center of the screen. Applying a positive voltage to one plate in the set, however, and a negative voltage to the other (i.e., creating a potential difference across the plates) deflects the beam toward the positive plate; and reversing the voltage deflects it in the opposite direction (Fig. 2-62). The two sets of plates allow the beam to be positioned anywhere on the CRT screen.

Applying a linear voltage change to the plates causes the beam to move across the screen—to the Y plates

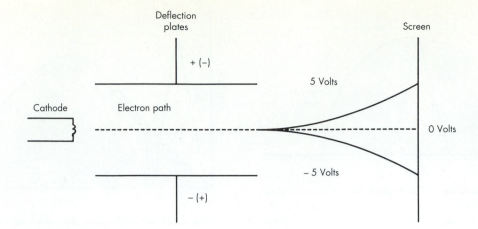

Figure 2-62 Vertical deflection of the electron beam in a cathode ray tube. If no voltage is applied to the deflection plates, the electrons travel in a straight-line path *(dashed line)*. A voltage applied to the deflection plates alters the electron path. Reversing the polarity deflects the beam in the opposite direction. Horizontal deflection plates *(not shown)* move the electron beam in and out of the page.

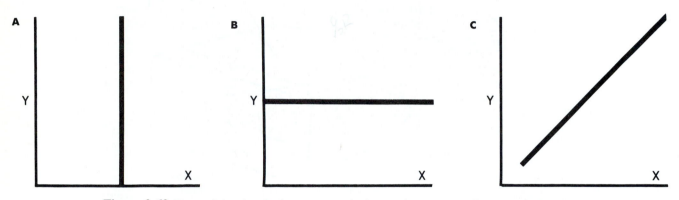

Figure 2-63 Trace of the electron beam on a cathode ray tube screen. A linear voltage applied to the Y deflection plates moves the beam upward or downward, **A,** to the X plate moves it horizontally, **B,** and to both plates simultaneously moves it diagonally, **C.**

moves it up or down, to the X plates moves it horizontally, and to both pairs of plates moves it diagonally (Fig. 2-63).

For the simplest scanning system (A-mode) a voltage to the X plates moves the time base sweep across the display at a constant rate that correlates with the speed of ultrasound in tissue. The sweep, which must advance the equivalent of 1 cm on the distance scale for every 13 μs, is initiated by a pulse from the master synchronizer; and as it progresses across the display, the signal detected for each interface is amplified and sent to the Y plates to control the electron beam's vertical position.

For example, assume that an interface generates a 5-volt pulse to the Y plates. This would deflect the electron beam upward. Because the duration of the induced pulse is short, the voltage on the Y plates would return to zero and the beam would move back to the baseline in but a fraction of a second (Fig. 2-64). The beam would again be deflected vertically when the next interface was encountered and the signal would be sent to the display. This whole process occurs repeatedly many times per second for the

line of sight which thus defines the direction of sampling.

As long as the transducer is directed along the same line of sight (scan line), the displayed signals remain unchanged because the scan is repeated many times each second. The sampling rate is equal to the PRF of the unit (200 to 2000 times per second). If the transducer is positioned toward a new line of sight, the displayed signals change in accordance with the interfaces encountered along this line. Once again, the scan is displayed at the rate of the PRF. Figure 2-65 is a typical A-mode display showing a plot of echo amplitude versus time or depth.

DYNAMIC RANGE

The dynamic range, which is a measure of the signal magnitudes that can be identified and handled by various components of the ultrasound system, needs to be considered in more detail. Echo amplitudes may be as much as 100 to 150 dB (or a factor of 10^{10} to 10^{15}) below the original intensity sent into the body depending on the depth of sampling and frequency of the transducer. This wide range of

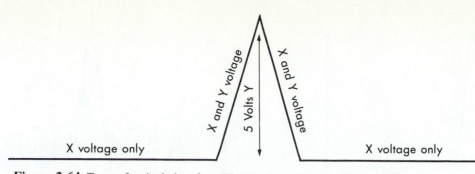

Figure 2-64 Trace of a single interface. The X voltage corresponds to a time base sweep of 1 cm for every 13 μs; the Y voltage remains constant until an interface is encountered.

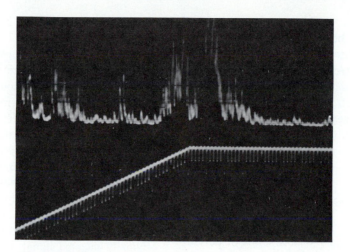

Figure 2-65 A-mode display of the liver *(top curve)* with the accompanying time gain compensation *(lower curve)*.

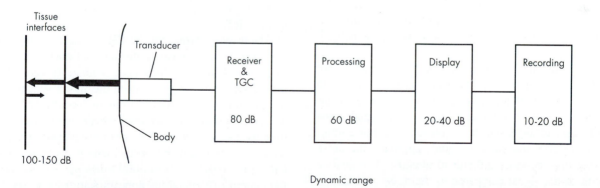

Figure 2-66 Dynamic range associated with the various components of an ultrasound system.

echo strengths is also present in the induced signals from the receiver section.

TGC and logarithmic amplification reduce the dynamic range to about 80 dB. Depending on the processing method and storage device (analog or digital), the dynamic range may be further reduced. The output device (CRT or TV) decreases the dynamic range to 20 to 40 dB. The signals normally undergo greatest compression in the display system. The recording device reduces the useful range even further, to 10 to 20 dB. Figure 2-66 summarizes the compression of information.

Compression by TGC and thresholding is desirable because these signal-processing steps attempt to correlate displayed signal level with reflectivity. Compression is necessary, however, between detection and display because system components have limited capacity to preserve the range of signal magnitudes. The best example of this limitation is the brightness levels available on a CRT. Suppose eight brightness levels are available. The entire dynamic range of signals must then be depicted as one of eight values when the echo data are displayed. Ultimately, signals must be combined in groups so they can be managed by the CRT.

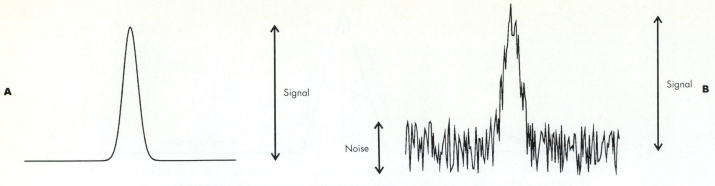

Figure 2-67 Effect of noise on the processed signal. **A,** Ideal signal (no noise). **B,** Noise masking the true signal.

If the original data could be maintained without loss, then noninvasive tissue characterization might be possible. Much research has been devoted to reducing data compression and increasing the dynamic range of ultrasound systems. Fourier analysis, as well as special feature analysis using multiple frequency images, may play a major role in tissue characterization. The ultimate aim is to identify malignant, benign, and normal tissues without surgical intervention.

NOISE

If a reflector is probed repeatedly with a series of pulsed ultrasound waves, each wave creates an echo characteristic of the object. The returning echoes are detected by the transducer. Under these conditions induced signals of equal strength are expected. In practice, however, the signal amplitude is not constant but fluctuates from one measurement to the next. This variation is known as noise (or random noise).

Noise is inherent in the measurement process and cannot be totally eliminated. System electronics also contributes to it. External sources of noise include environmental RF interference and power line voltage fluctuations. Signals must be processed and displayed in the presence of noise (Fig. 2-67). As weaker and weaker signals approach the noise level, they become more difficult to identify. The relative amplitude of the signal compared to the noise variation is delineated by the signal to noise ratio (SNR).

High SNRs indicate strong signals, which are easily detected. A minimum SNR of 3 to 5 is necessary to distinguish weak echoes from the noise. The sensitivity of an ultrasound instrument is often quantified by measuring the SNR from a well-defined reflector.

Improvements in equipment design have reduced the noise level and improved the sensitivity of modern scanners. Since noise is random, signal processing cannot isolate the signal from the noise; that is, mathematical corrections applied to the detected signal to eliminate the noise are not possible. When averaged together, however, the induced signals from multiple samplings of an interface increase the SNR. This is called frame averaging or persistence (and is discussed in Chapter 10).

SUMMARY

A piezoelectric material is electronically stimulated to produce an ultrasonic pressure wave via the converse piezoelectric effect. The ultrasound wave enters the patient's body, and a small portion is reflected at the various interfaces in accordance with the percentage reflection relation presented in Chapter 1. Returning echoes strike the transducer and, because of the piezoelectric effect, induce a voltage (RF signal). The RF signals undergo both amplification and TGC, the latter compensates for attenuation of the sound wave with depth. The electronically amplified and processed signal is represented as a voltage spike on the CRT. The height of the spike is proportional to the amplitude of the originally detected signal. The master synchronizer initiates the excitation voltage pulse to the transducer as well as the start signals to activate the timer mechanisms for TGC and special electronic processing. It also provides electronic signals for gating purposes and initiates the time base sweep of the CRT.

The display format for the CRT consists of amplitude in the vertical direction versus distance or time in the horizontal direction. A linearly increasing voltage is applied to the horizontal deflection plates from the master synchronizer so the electron beam moves at a rate of 1 cm every 13 μs. All electronic trigger signals must occur at exactly the same time for the correct depth (time) measurement (of each interface) to be displayed on the screen. Sweeps across the CRT are repeated 200 to 2000 times per second, and thus the pattern of deflections appears stationary to the human eye. This pattern can also be recorded on film.

■■■■■■■ **R E V I E W   Q U E S T I O N S** ■■■■■■■

1. What is the main controlling subsystem of the ultrasound unit?
   a. Transmitter
   b. Receiver
   c. Master synchronizer
   d. Display
2. What are the primary objectives when generating an ultrasound beam?
   a. Unidirectional
   b. Uniform intensity
   c. Small physical dimensions
   d. All of the above

3. Assume the best resolution of an ultrasound imaging system to be one wavelength. What frequency is required to detect a 0.5 mm object in tissue?
   a. 0.5 MHz
   b. 3.1 MHz
   c. 5.0 MHz
   d. 30.0 MHz

4. A dipolar molecule contains separate regions of positive and negative charge.
   a. True
   b. False

5. The Curie temperature is the temperature at which dipolar molecules produce radiation.
   a. True
   b. False

6. The piezoelectric effect of a crystal allows the conversion of electrical energy to ultrasound waves.
   a. True
   b. False

7. The converse piezoelectric effect of a crystal allows the conversion of electrical energy to ultrasound waves.
   a. True
   b. False

8. A transducer is any device that converts one form of energy into another.
   a. True
   b. False

9. A voltage pulse is used to excite the piezoelectric crystal so mechanical vibrations (pressure waves) are produced.
   a. True
   b. False

10. What thickness of piezoelectric crystal (c = 5000 m/s) is required to produce a resonant frequency of 5 MHz?
    a. 0.1 mm
    b. 0.5 mm
    c. 1.0 mm
    d. 5.0 mm

11. The wavelength in tissue for the crystal in Question 10 is?
    a. 0.150 mm
    b. 0.308 mm
    c. 1.5 mm
    d. 3.08 mm

12. PZT is the most commonly used piezoelectric material for diagnostic imaging applications.
    a. True
    b. False

13. Quartz is commonly used as a transducer crystal in therapeutic ultrasound.
    a. True
    b. False

14. The acoustic impedance of the crystal must equal the acoustic impedance of the backing material to produce a long pulse.
    a. True
    b. False

15. A 2 MHz alternating voltage applied continuously drives the crystal so that a 2 MHz continuous ultrasound wave is produced.
    a. True
    b. False

16. The maximum pulse repetition frequency (PRF) is directly proportional to the maximum depth of penetration and inversely proportional to the velocity of ultrasound in a medium.
    a. True
    b. False

17. Assume the depth of interest to be 15 cm. What is the maximum PRF?
    a. 510 pulses/s
    b. 770 pulses/s
    c. 5100 pulses/s
    d. 7700 pulses/s

18. What is the pulse repetition period (PRP) corresponding to the maximum PRF calculated in Question 17?
    a. 2 ms
    b. 1.3 ms
    c. 0.2 ms
    d. 0.13 ms

19. What is the spatial pulse length (SPL) for a 2.5 cycle pulse if the frequency is 5 MHz?
    a. 0.308 mm
    b. 0.770 mm
    c. 3.08 mm
    d. 7.7 mm

20. Determine the pulse duration (PD) for the transducer in Question 19.
    a. 0.5 μs
    b. 1.0 μs
    c. 5.0 μs
    d. 7.7 μs

21. The duty factor is important in determining certain intensity parameters related to dose response for various biological effects.
    a. True
    b. False

22. Calculate the duty factor for a 5 MHz transducer that produces 2.5 cycles per pulse. The pulse repetition frequency is 1000 per second.
    a. 0.0002
    b. 0.0005
    c. 0.002
    d. 0.005

23. Echo detection is an important parameter for therapeutic ultrasound systems.
    a. True
    b. False

24. Matching layers increase the ultrasonic energy transferred from the piezoelectric crystal to the patient and vice versa.
    a. True
    b. False

25. Calculate the acoustic impedance of a matching layer assuming $Z_{crystal}$ is 40×10^5 kg/m²/s and Z_{tissue} is 1×10^5 kg/m²/s.
    a. 40×10^5 kg/m²/s
    b. 20.5×10^5 kg/m²/s
    c. 6.3×10^5 kg/m²/s
    d. 1×10^5 kg/m²/s

26. Calculate the increase in percentage of transmission for the crystal–matching layer and matching layer–tissue interfaces compared to the crystal-tissue interface alone in Question 25.
    a. 9.5%
    b. 12.5%
    c. 22.0%
    d. None of the above

27. A high-Q transducer has a short pulse and a narrow bandwidth.
    a. True
    b. False

28. A low-Q transducer has a short pulse and a broad bandwidth.
    a. True
    b. False

29. The lateral resolution improves as the beam width is made smaller.
    a. True
    b. False

30. The acoustic pressure along the beam axis in the near field is constant for a high-Q transducer.
    a. True
    b. False

31. Calculate the depth of the near field for a 20 mm diameter, nonfocused, 3 MHz transducer.
    a. 195 cm.
    b. 19.5 m
    c. 19.5 cm
    d. 19.5 mm

32. Calculate the far field divergence for a 20 mm diameter, nonfocused, 3 MHz transducer.
    a. 5.4 degrees
    b. 2.7 degrees
    c. 1.8 degrees
    d. 0.9 degrees

33. The near-field depth is directly proportional to the frequency and the square of the diameter.
    a. True
    b. False

34. The far-field divergence is directly proportional to the frequency and the diameter.
    a. True
    b. False

35. Focusing the sound beam improves the lateral resolution.
    a. True
    b. False

36. Mirrors, lenses, and curved crystals are all internal focusing methods.
    a. True
    b. False

37. Assume focused and nonfocused transducers to have the same diameter and operating frequency. The focal zone is located at a depth that is beyond the near field for the nonfocused transducer.
    a. True
    b. False

38. Time gain compensation corrects acoustic signal levels for attenuation (which occurs with depth).
    a. True
    b. False

39. Rectification and enveloping are processing techniques applied to the induced RF signals before display.
    a. True
    b. False

40. The amplitude of the processed signal is determined by integrating the enveloped signal.
    a. True
    b. False

41. *Dynamic range* refers to the variation in signal amplitudes that can be represented (or preserved) by the various components of an ultrasound system.
    a. True
    b. False

42. Which of the following signal-processing techniques contributes to compression (decreases the dynamic range)?
    a. Logarithmic amplification
    b. TGC
    c. Thresholding
    d. All of the above

43. In A-mode scanning the amplitude of the processed signal controls the vertical deflection plates in the CRT.
    a. True
    b. False

44. Echo-induced radiofrequency signals can be detected and processed without interference from noise.
    a. True
    b. False

45. *Sensitivity* refers to be the ability of an ultrasound instrument to detect weak echoes in presence of noise.
    a. True
    b. False

BIBLIOGRAPHY

Bushong SC: *Radiologic science for technologists: physics, biology, and protection,* ed 5, St Louis, 1993, Mosby.

Curry TS III, Dowdey JE, Murry RC Jr: *Christensen's Physics of diagnostic radiology,* ed 4, Philadelphia, 1990, Lea & Febiger.

Kremkau FW: *Diagnostic ultrasonics: physical principles and exercises,* ed 3, Philadelphia, 1988, WB Saunders.

McDicken WN: *Diagnostic ultrasonics: principles and use of instruments,* ed 3, Edinburgh, 1991, Churchill Livingstone.

Powis RL: *Physics for the fun of it,* Denver, 1978, Unirad Corporation.

Rose JL, Goldberg BB: *Basic physics in diagnostic ultrasound,* New York, 1979, John Wiley & Sons.

Wells PNT: *Physical principles of ultrasonic diagnosis,* New York, 1969, Academic Press.

Wells PNT: *Biomedical ultrasonics,* New York, 1977, Academic Press.

Woodcock JP: *Ultrasonics,* Bristol, 1979, Adam Hilger Ltd.

Static Imaging Principles and Instrumentation

━━━━━━━━   K E Y   T E R M S   ━━━━━━━━

A-mode

B-mode

C-mode

ECG gating

Line of sight

Position generator

Raster scanning

Registration arm

Scan converter

Speckle

Transmission mode

Two-dimensional image

Sonar (sound navigation and ranging) played a major role in the development of medical diagnostic ultrasound instrumentation, particularly in A-mode scanning. The previous chapter has described the fundamentals of equipment design. This chapter discusses the modifications and refinements required to convert the basic unit into systems that are used for static imaging techniques. A-mode instrumentation is considered only briefly because the basic unit described in Chapter 2 is the typical A-mode scanner. Static B-mode gray-scale imaging and specific gated scanning techniques are the main subjects of this chapter, along with transmission-mode scanning, the only technique that does not rely on the echo-ranging principle. Most static imaging systems have now been replaced by real-time, Doppler, and M-mode scanning techniques, which are the subjects of subsequent chapters.

A-MODE SCANNING

A-mode (amplitude-mode) scanning is based on the echo-ranging principle, similar to sonar. A pulsed ultrasound wave is directed into the patient's body, and the echoes generated at various interfaces are detected. Only structures that lie along the direction of propagation are interrogated. This sampling according to the beam path is called the line of sight or scan line.

Display of Detected Echoes

The term *amplitude* refers to the strength of a detected echo signal. A-mode displays the amplitude of the signal as a spike in the vertical dimension versus depth or time of the signal in the horizontal dimension. (Depth and time are interchangeable because they are directly proportional.) An increase in the amplitude or strength of the signal gives rise to an increase in the height of the spike. This variation in signal strength is due to the reflectivities of different interfaces and the attenuation of the beam as the ultrasound wave travels to and from the various interfaces. Time gain compensation attempts to correct for attenuation loss. Strong reflectors far from the transducer may produce greater-amplitude signals than weak reflectors nearer the transducer. The A-mode scan also contains spatial information; that is, it registers the distance between interfaces.

Multiple interfaces encountered along the sampling direction are detected by a series of echoes. Figure 3-1 shows three interfaces as three separate spikes. Interface *I* generates a larger signal than interface *II* or interface *III*. This A-mode scan also preserves the spatial relationship of the observed structures. Interface *II* is located closer to interface *III* than to interface *I*.

System Components

Figure 3-2 is a block diagram of the A-mode scanner. The master synchronizer initiates the scanning process by commanding the transmitter to send a voltage pulse to the transducer. The excitation of the crystal generates a pulsed ultrasound wave (via the converse piezoelectric effect) that is directed into the body. Coincidentally, the master synchronizer sends a command to activate the clock that measures the elapsed time from transmission of the ultrasound pulse

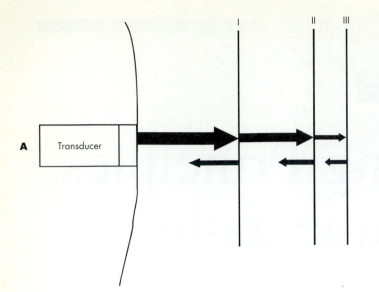

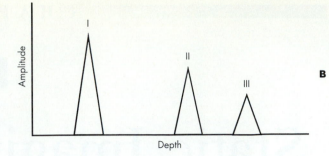

Figure 3-1 A-mode scan and display. **A,** Three interfaces (I, II, and III). **B,** Corresponding display of the interfaces.

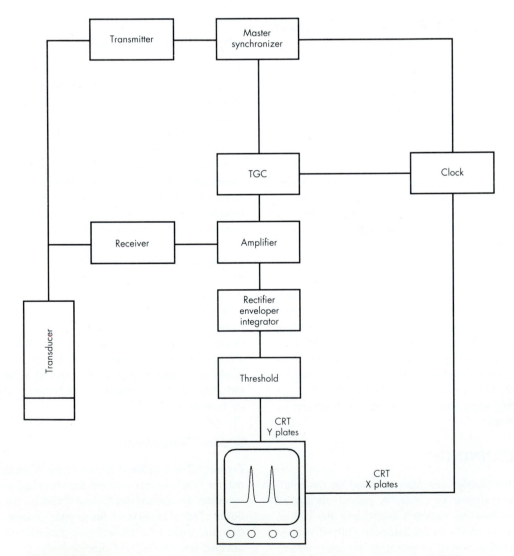

Figure 3-2 The A-mode scanner modified to show the signal processing steps of TCG, amplification, integration, and thresholding before display.

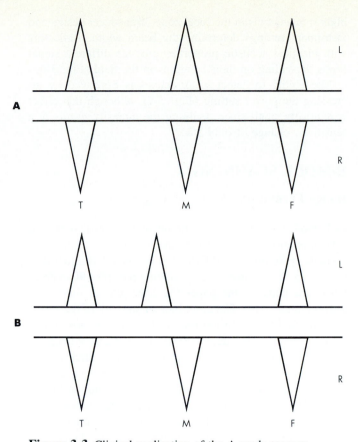

Figure 3-3 Clinical application of the A-mode scanner. **A,** Normal echoencephalogram showing a similar pattern from the left (L) and right (R) sides. T, Transducer; M, midline; F, far side. **B,** Abnormal echoencephalogram with the midline spikes not aligned.

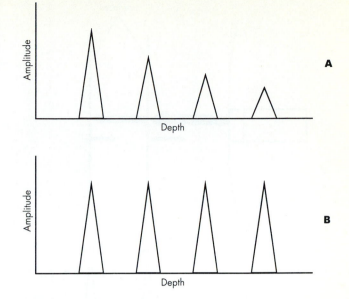

Figure 3-4 Signals from identical reflectors located at different depths. **A,** No time gain compensation. **B,** TGC applied during signal processing.

to reception of the echo. This time determines the depth of the interface based on the constant velocity of ultrasound in tissue (1540 m/s). When the transducer is excited, the master synchronizer sends a command to the display to begin moving the electron beam (time base sweep) across the screen of the cathode ray tube (CRT). The sweep rate corresponds to 1 cm every 13 μs. As the ultrasound pulse propagates away from the transducer, part of the energy is reflected at each interface encountered along the beam path. This sampling is restricted laterally by the width of the beam. The reflected energy returns toward the transducer in the form of an echo. As the echo strikes the transducer, an electrical signal is induced in the crystal (piezoelectric effect) and this is processed for display. The processed signal is applied to the deflection plates in the CRT to shift the electron beam upward during the time base sweep. The height of the deflection indicates the strength of the received echo; the position along the horizontal denotes the depth of the interfaces.

The A-mode "image" is a one-dimensional portrayal of the amplitude of the signal versus depth. A narrow beam samples the structures along the line of sight. Only one line can be observed at any given instant on the display. As long as the transducer and detected interfaces are stationary, the trace appears unchanged because the CRT screen is refreshed at the rate of the pulse repetition frequency. For a different line of sight to be observed, the transducer must be moved to a different position.

Applications

A-mode scanning is used in echoencephalography for detection of midline shift (Fig. 3-3) and for the localization of foreign bodies in the eye. A-mode information may be valuable for tissue characterization because the detected echoes can be displayed in unaltered form (signal processing can be bypassed). A greater dynamic range of signals is preserved compared with other imaging techniques. Identification of cysts in the breast is occasionally facilitated by A-mode scanning. Nonmedical applications include nondestructive testing in industry.

Illustrative A-Mode Scans

The A-mode scan can be used to illustrate the concepts of time gain control, axial resolution, focusing, and sensitivity introduced in the last chapter. Without TGC, identical reflectors at different depths have exponentially decreasing signal levels as the beam path is increased. TGC provides variable amplification based on elapsed time; thus the displayed signal level for each reflector is equal regardless of the depth of the reflector (Fig. 3-4).

When the interfaces are located close together, the spikes in the display overlap (Fig. 3-5). The two echoes appear as one spike, which is consequently interpreted as a single interface. Echoes are more likely to be resolved if the spatial pulse length is kept short (high frequency, few cycles).

Focusing alters the intensity in the ultrasound field. The

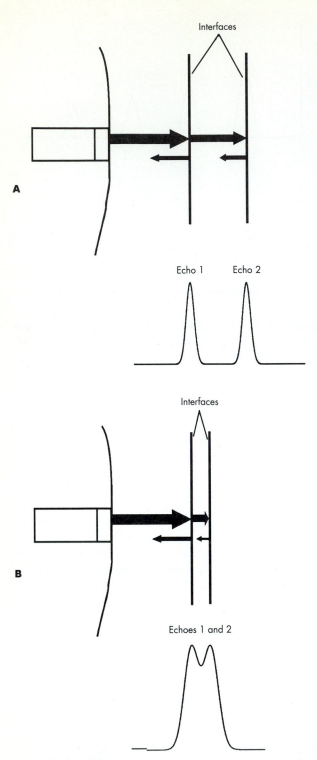

Figure 3-5 Axial resolution in A-mode scanning. **A,** Interfaces separated by a distance greater than half the spatial pulse length are depicted as two distinct spikes. **B,** When interfaces are located close together, the time intervals during which each returning echo strikes the transducer overlap. The signals are combined into one spike.

highest intensity is in the focal zone. Transducer design and instrument settings determine the beam width. Reflectors with identical acoustic properties produce different signal levels depending on their locations in the field (Fig. 3-6).

The ability to detect weak echoes is improved by increasing the power setting (Fig. 3-7), although this effect is relatively small since doubling the intensity results in a sensitivity change of only 5%.

B-MODE SCANNING

Image Formation

In B-mode imaging the amplitude of the signal (detected echo strength) is represented by the brightness of a dot. The A-mode spike on the CRT display is converted into a dot, which can be demonstrated by rotating the spike 90 degrees out of the plane of the paper (i.e., the axis of rotation is the horizontal axis). The amplitude or strength of the signal is designated by the brightness of the dot. The position of the dot represents the depth (time) of the interface from the transducer (Fig. 3-8). Normally we are interested in constructing a two-dimensional image of the area of interest rather than acquiring data from a single scan line or line of sight. This is accomplished by compound B-scanning, whereby multiple sets of dots are combined to delineate the echo pattern from internal structures within the body. The patient is scanned from many different directions. The superimposition of multiple scan lines creates a composite two-dimensional image, which has the advantage of portraying the general contour of the patient and the internal organs (Fig. 3-9). Compound B-mode scanning produces a static image that can be envisioned as a stop-action photograph of the reflecting surfaces.

Scanning Requirements

Two problems with B-mode scanning not present with A-mode are registration (i.e., the two-dimensional placement of an echo's origin) and storage of the scan-line information. A knowledge of transducer position is essential to the proper placing of dots from different scan lines at the correct locations within the image. To build up the image, information about previous scan lines must be retained in some manner.

Registration. For the accurate localization of an interface (i.e., the origin of its echo), the horizontal and vertical position of the transducer, and also its angulation, must be known. Thus the transducer is mounted on a special scanning or registration arm (Fig. 3-10) that indicates its precise location so the time-of-flight (depth) measurements along the beam axis can be accurately displayed. Because the transducer changes its orientation frequently during scanning, this arm must be flexible; however, at the same time, it must be stable to accurately correlate collected information within the image.

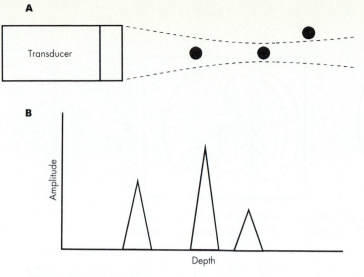

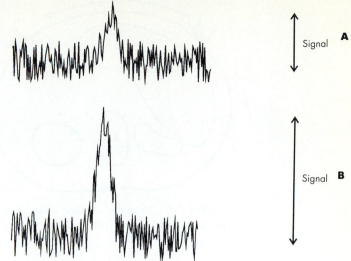

Figure 3-6 Nonuniform beam intensity causes variation in signal level. **A,** Three identical reflectors located in the ultrasonic field of a focused transducer. **B,** A-mode scan of the reflectors. Note that the highest signal corresponds to the focal zone and that intensity does not immediately decrease to zero at the boundary of the ultrasonic field. The lowest signal is generated by a reflector located outside the indicated beam width (designating regions where the intensity is within 6 dB).

Figure 3-7 Effect of transmitted power on the signal-to-noise ratio. **A,** Signal from a weak reflector at a low power setting. **B,** Signal from the same reflector at a high power setting. The signal-to-noise is increased, and sensitivity improved. The change in signal has been exaggerated to illustrate this effect.

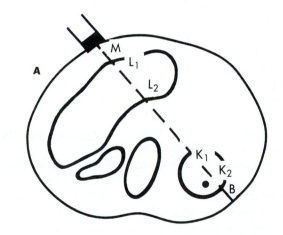

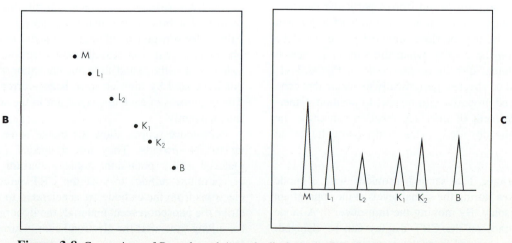

Figure 3-8 Comparison of B-mode and A-mode displays. **A,** The transducer position defines the line of sight sampled. **B,** In B-mode the interfaces are represented as dots of varying brightness along the line of sight. **C,** In A-mode they are represented as spikes of varying height.

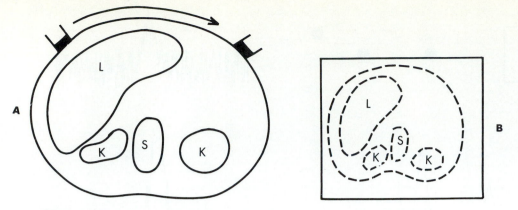

Figure 3-9 Compound B-mode scanning. **A,** The transducer is moved to probe the patient along several lines of sight. **B,** In the display the interfaces are formed as a composite of dots along the lines of sight.

The interface location (dot) on the display is moved to the appropriate location by biasing the X and Y deflection plates with voltages from the position generator. Sensors mounted in the registration arm define the position of the transducer with respect to a reference point established at the time of scanning. This information is communicated to the position generator, which calculates the appropriate X and Y voltages as a function of elapsed time. Registration arms can be mechanical in nature, using voltage signals obtained through potentiometers to indicate the position of the transducer. A change in position of one segment of the registration arm is sensed by a change in resistance within the potentiometer, which alters the voltage sent to the position generator. Registration arms can be made using electromagnetic or optical arrangements that do not require moving electrical contacts. Some systems are computer controlled for more precise determination of transducer position.

Multiple images of the entire pelvis and abdomen in any plane (transverse, longitudinal, or sagittal) can be acquired in this manner. The registration arm is responsible for ensuring that the echo information from a particular interface is displayed at the same location, regardless of transducer orientation; that is, the interface should be in exactly the same location on the display when the subject is viewed from many different directions, as shown in Figure 3-11. This arm should be checked periodically to ensure that echo data are displayed properly with respect to position. Otherwise, false placement of interface position can cause the image to become distorted. (This is discussed further in Chapter 13.)

Signal storage. The second problem with B-mode scanning involves storing the signal levels at the appropriate locations for display. By moving the transducer in A-mode scanning, the trace on the CRT display can be changed. The information obtained from the previous transducer po-

sition is not retained on the screen. To maintain the trace, the transducer must be kept in the same position—pointed along a single line of sight. The display is continually updated with the same information (i.e., the scan is repeated over and over at the rate of the pulse repetition frequency, PRF). If a scan were acquired all the way around a patient, as is the case for B-mode scanning, the initial traces would disappear from the screen before the total scan was completed (10 to 20 seconds are required to perform a B-mode scan). Indeed, as soon as the ultrasound beam is directed along a new line of sight, the prior trace is lost. In addition to the scanning arm modifications already discussed, a modification in the display system is necessary.

Cathode Ray Tubes

A-mode scan information is limited to depth and signal level only. B-mode, however, has three variables—vertical and horizontal dimensions and the signal level. The X and Y deflection plates within the CRT are responsible for positioning the dot in two dimensions on the screen. The number of electrons striking the screen controls the brightness of the dot. The processed signal is routed to the cathode (also called electron gun or filament). As the amplitude of the processed signal is increased, more electrons are permitted to leave the cathode and strike the phosphor screen. A bright dot is created by high electron beam current (Fig. 3-12). The brightness of each displayed dot in the scan is adjusted independently.

Persistence scopes allow the image to be displayed for up to 20 seconds. They use a special phosphorescent material (i.e., potassium iodide, barium lead sulfate, or cadmium sulfide) to coat the CRT screen. When the electrons from the cathode are accelerated to the screen and strike the phosphorescent material, the light produced glows for a long time after the electron beam is turned off (persistence).

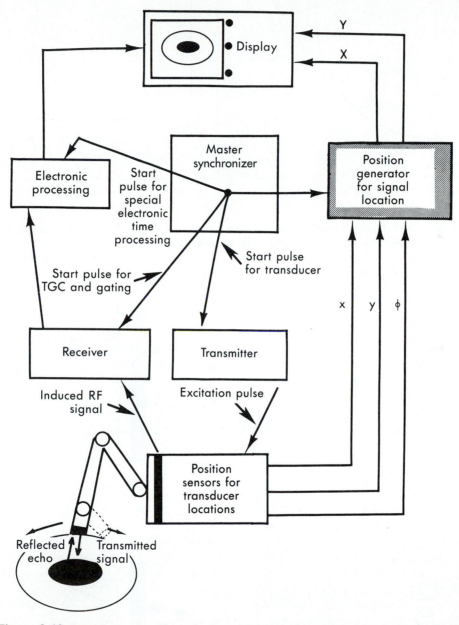

Figure 3-10 B-mode scanner. The basic A-mode scanner (from Chapter 2) modified to include a scanning arm, position generator, and storage display.

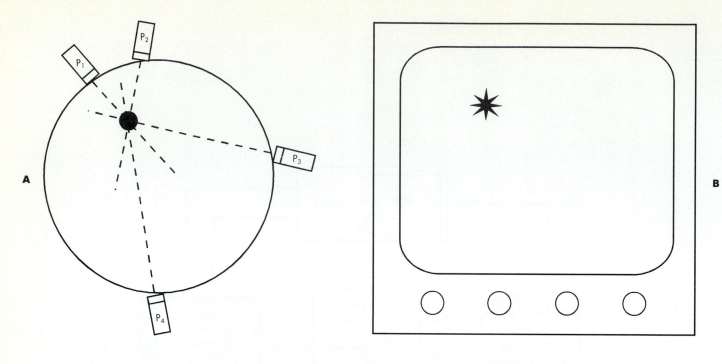

Figure 3-11 Registration of an interface with compound B-mode. **A,** Scan of the interface from four positions (P_1, P_2, P_3, and P_4). **B,** Display of the interface.

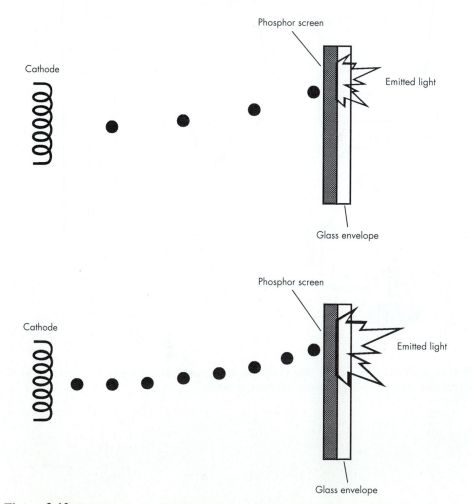

Figure 3-12 Cathode ray tube brightness is controlled by the number of electrons striking the phosphor screen. **A,** Low beam current. **B,** High beam current.

Special CRTs that enable the image to be stored have also been developed. They use a storage mesh placed next to the phosphor material (Fig. 3-13). The amplitude of the signal controls the stream of electrons that are accelerated from the cathode toward the storage mesh. These electrons crash into the storage mesh, knocking out additional electrons and creating regions of positive charge. The number of incident electrons (dictated by the amplitude of the signal controlling the filament) determines the amount of positive charge left on the storage mesh. Detected interfaces correspond to these positively charged areas. For the interface information contained on the storage mesh to be visualized, it must be transferred to the phosphorescent screen. This is accomplished by reading the mesh with medium-energy electrons from a separate flood gun (Fig. 3-13). The electrons are accelerated through the positively charged regions of the storage mesh to the phosphor material. A constant output of electrons from the flood gun permits continuous display of the image for viewing and recording. The image is erased by bombarding the mesh with low-energy electrons captured in the regions of positive charge on the mesh.

These CRTs exhibit only an "on" or "off" mode. If the detected signal is strong enough, a positively charged region is created on the storage mesh and displayed as a light-emitting area on the phosphorescent screen. Otherwise, weakly charged regions are read as no signals and no light is emitted from the corresponding areas on the screen. This produces the so-called bistable image (Fig. 3-14). Most of the internal detail of organs is absent, however. Because the nonspecular reflections lost in a bistable image (i.e., when the amplitude is too low to be recorded) would be helpful in analyzing normal and abnormal tissues, a system has been developed that is capable of showing the finer detail of internal structures. It is called the analog scan converter.

Analog Scan Converter

Druing the early 1970s special systems were developed with gray-scale displays for B-mode scanning. Called analog scan converters, these devices enabled different echo amplitudes (i.e., detected signal strengths) to be displayed in varying shades of gray so the fine internal structure of various organs could be visualized (Fig. 3-15). They represented a major innovation in the evolution of ultrasound.

The analog scan converter is similar to a CRT, except that the phosphor face is completely replaced by a wafer of silicon called the dielectric matrix (Fig. 3-16). The scan converter consists of an evacuated glass tube with a high voltage applied between the filament (cathode or source of

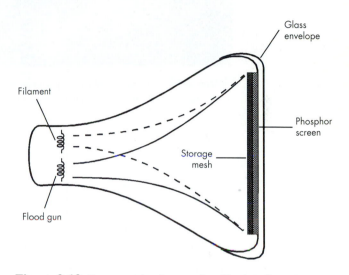

Figure 3-13 Storage cathrode ray tube. The interfaces are recorded on the storage mesh as positively charged regions. Electrons from the electron flood gun are accelerated through these areas and strike the phosphor screen, producing a visible image.

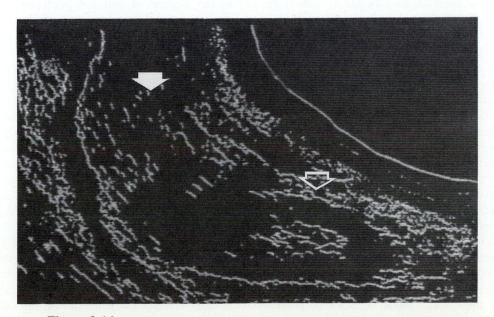

Figure 3-14 Bistable image of a kidney *(open arow)* and the liver *(solid arrow)*.

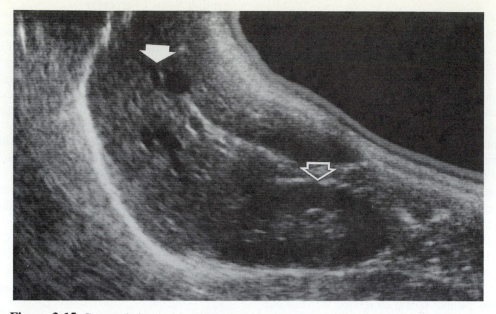

Figure 3-15 Gray-scale image of a kidney *(open arrow)* and the liver *(solid arrow)*. Note the increased detail of these structures in this image compared with those in the bistable image (Fig. 3-14).

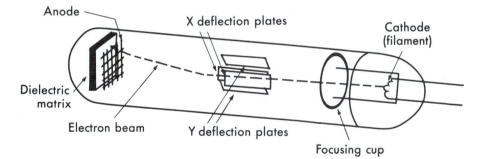

Figure 3-16 Analog scan converter. Note its similarity with the cathode ray tube (Chapter 2).

electrons) and a wire mesh (anode) located in front of the dielectric matrix. The dielectric matrix is biased, with a positive potential less than that applied to the anode. The number of electrons emitted by the filament is controlled by the amplitude of the processed signal. The accelerated electrons from the cathode pass through the wire mesh at high velocities and are slowed in the region between the wire mesh and the dielectric matrix. They strike the dielectric matrix and knock electrons out of that material, leaving a positive charge on the matrix. The ejected electrons drift back to the anode (wire mesh) and are collected. The positive charge left on the dielectric matrix is proportional to the number of electrons striking the matrix, which in turn is proportional to the amplitude of the processed signal used to control the cathode.

Data collected on the dielectric matrix are distributed in a well-defined spatial pattern; that is, position sensors in the registration arm communicate with the position generator, which controls the X and Y deflection plates of the scan converter during the "write" mode. Regions of positive charge are arranged on the dielectric matrix and correspond

to the location of detected interfaces. Variations in the amount of positive charge represent changing signal strengths. In essence, an image of echo measurements is imprinted on the dielectric matrix in the form of the charge distribution that is present. This is similar to the latent image on an x-ray film, which cannot be visualized until the film is chemically processed.

For the gray-scale image to be read, medium-energy electrons are accelerated through the positively charged regions of the dielectric matrix and collected by a signal plate located behind the matrix. This forms the output signal from the scan converter. The beam current is modulated by the amount of positive charge deposited in the matrix during the write mode. After passing through the matrix, the electron beam carries information regarding the relative signal amplitudes. Note that the magnitude of the beam current depends on the dielectric area sampled by the electron beam. A large-diameter beam striking areas with both high and low charge densities creates an intermediate beam current. A more accurate assessment of charge density is obtained by a small-diameter electron beam interrogating each small region sequentially. The diameter of the electron beam also affects the size of the observed dot on the phosphor screen. A raster scan moves the electron beam across the dielectric matrix. The same filament (electron source) used to generate the original charge distribution during the write mode also supplies the electrons for the read mode—except in the case of a dual-head scan converter. Dual-head scan converters have separate electron filaments for reading and writing. Excess electrons from the read scanning are collected by the anode and are removed from the tube.

Video Signal

In raster scanning the X deflection plate voltage is changed to sweep the electron beam horizontally from left to right across the display. This trace forms one raster line. The voltage to the Y deflection plate is changed to drop the trace down one line as the electron beam is positioned back to the left side of the display (change in the X voltage) to begin the next raster line (Fig. 3-17). To avoid spurious signals, the electron beam is actually turned off during the retrace. This is similar to reading a book, in which you start at the top left-hand corner and move across to the end of the line before dropping down one line to return to the left-hand side, where a new line is read.

It is also essentially how a television works. The difference is that—whereas in reading, each line is scanned in sequence—in the television, odd-numbered raster lines are traced first followed by the even-numbered lines. The two sets of tracings (called fields) are interlaced to form one frame. Frames composed of 525 lines are displayed 30 times per second. The interlacing of fields doubles the image update rate and allows flicker-free viewing, though with some sacrifice of spatial resolution. The output, in the form of an electron beam current resulting from the raster scan of the dielectric matrix in the scan converter, is connected to the cathode of a television and is synchronized with the raster scan of the television to produce the observed image (Fig. 3-18); that is, the brightness of light on the television screen is dictated by the level of the input signal, and the position is governed by the raster scanning sequence. Because raster scanning of the dielectric matrix and raster scanning of the television screen are synchronized, the charge distribution on the dielectric matrix—and therefore the echo measurements—is converted into a visual image.

By repeating the raster scan of the dielectric matrix thirty times a second, the image is continuously refreshed but appears stationary to the human eye; thus prolonged viewing and hardcopy recording of the image are now possible.

The information obtained by raster scanning of the dielectric matrix is assembled in a standard format called the video signal. This format is based on the line-by-line readout of the image data and is the same as that described for television. The frame rate and number of lines that compose a frame depend on the national television industry (30 frames per second and 525 lines in the United States, 25 frames per second and 625 lines in England). Synchronization voltage pulses are added during readout to mark horizontal (new line) and vertical (new field) positioning. The communication of image data between scan converter and display monitor or hardcopy device is often accomplished by the video signal.

Image Viewing

Rapid alternating between the read (display) mode and the write (collect) mode enables the image to be viewed as it is being formed; that is, the scan converter switches back

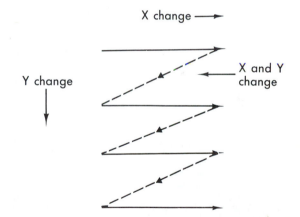

Figure 3-17 Raster scanning. Voltage changes on the X deflection plates cause the electron beam *(solid line)* to be swept across the screen. The beam is turned off during repositioning *(broken line)*.

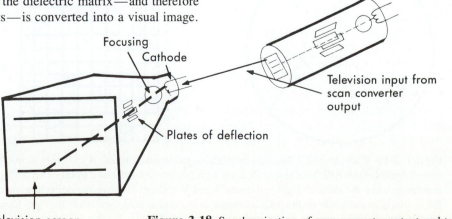

Figure 3-18 Synchronization of scan converter output and television input.

and forth from line by-line-acquisition during collection to raster by raster scanning during display. This characteristic is responsible for the name of the device—the scan converter. Once the data are collected, the image can be viewed by operating the device in a continuous read mode.

Images may be stored for several hours when using scan converters. Some deterioration occurs, however, with the loss of positive charge (absorption of free electrons) on the matrix. In addition, analog scan converters have a tendency to drift over long periods, creating inconsistent images from day to day. The resolution is excellent for analog scan converters because the size of the electron beam can be made very small (sharply focused to a fine point).

The scan converter tube is erased by applying low-energy electrons from the filament, which neutralize the positive charges on the dielectric matrix. Because the matrix has no regions of varying charge, an image of uniform intensity is displayed on the television screen. The scan converter is now ready to store a new image.

Digital Scan Converter

More recently (during the mid-1970s), digital scan converters were developed. These systems are essentially solid-state computer memories that have proved to be inexpensive, reliable, and versatile. Because they do not use evacuated tubes, drift associated with the analog systems is eliminated. Prolonged viewing of acquired image data is now possible. Digital scan converter resolution is superior to the resolution obtained from analog systems. Spatial resolution, however, is determined primarily by the ultrasound beam width and the raster scanning readout.

The area scanned is divided into small rectangular or square picture elements called pixels, which make up a two-dimensional matrix. Each pixel contains a digital number to represent the amplitude of the received echo. The placement of echo amplitudes within the matrix is designated by the position generator (Fig. 3-19). The out-of-plane width of the sound beam means that each pixel actually signifies a three-dimensional volume of tissue, called a voxel. The matrix size denotes the number of rows and columns in the pictorial representation. For example, a 512×512 matrix has 512 rows and 512 columns. The image is composed of 262,144 individual pixels. The physical extent of each pixel is typically less than 0.5 mm. The output of the computer memory (digital scan converter) is read in a raster fashion and converted back into an analog signal, which provides the input to the television cathode for display.

Signal Processing

Another feature of the scan converter system is the overwrite-protect circuit. Each interface is scanned from many orientations or directions during a B-mode acquisition. A variety of signal levels is detected for each pixel depending on the transducer orientation. When a signal is received, the appropriate location in the scan converter is identified via sensors in the registration arm and the position generator. The scan converter adds the new signal amplitude to the value that already exists in memory if the overwrite-protect system is not present. Overwrite-protect processing permits maximum-strength signals to be displayed while not recording low-amplitude signals.

The overwrite-protect circuit works in the following manner: When the interface is scanned for the first time, the associated signal level is stored in the scan converter. As the scan continues, the ultrasound wave's approach to the interface may be closer to normal incidence, resulting in a stronger detected signal. This signal level replaces the first in the scan converter for that pixel. At another scan line the interface may yield a lower signal level, which is discarded because a higher value has previously been recorded for that location. Thus an image is generated in which the maximum

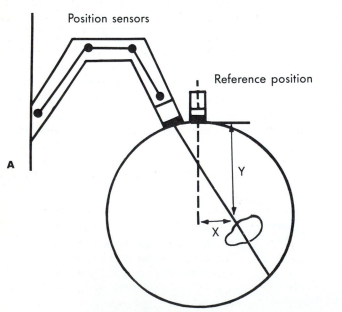

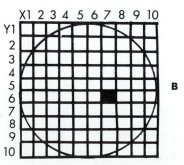

Figure 3-19 Placement of a detected interface in the storage device. **A,** Sensors in the registration arm determine the transducer location with respect to a reference point. The position generator, using the time of flight, produces X and Y voltages to drive the deflection plates in the analog scan converter or the address maker in the digital scan converter. **B,** Pixel location for the digital scan converter, or position on the dielectric matrix for the analog scan converter.

signal level is recorded for each pixel. A buildup of signal levels, which would result in an all-black or all-white image is prevented; if not, contrast would be decreased because most pixels would contain the same numerical value for the echo amplitude.

Many other algorithms are possible for manipulating the incoming signal levels to determine the numerical value placed at a particular pixel location. These preprocessing techniques are applied before data storage. The presentation of the image on the display also can be manipulated via various postprocessing techniques (see the discussion in Chapter 10).

Spatial Resolution

The digital scan converter and television system may degrade the spatial resolution beyond the limits imposed by pulse length and beam width. For example, assume that a patient measures 20 cm in the anterior-posterior dimension and 30 cm in the lateral dimension. This area (20 × 30 cm) is represented by a 20 × 20 digital matrix (400 pixels). The physical dimensions depicted by each pixel are 10 × 15 mm. If the pixel size is compared with the axial resolution and beam width (1.5 and 10 mm) obtained with a nonfocused transducer (3 MHz, 10 mm diameter, 3 cycles per pulse), the computer matrix size becomes the limiting factor in the image resolution.

■ Example 3-1

Calculate the total number of pixels (n) in a matrix that is 512 × 512.

$$n = \text{No. in row} \times \text{No. in column}$$
$$= 512 \times 512$$
$$= 262{,}144$$

■ Example 3-2

Calculate the pixel size (χ) if the 20 × 30 cm field of view is digitized using a 512 × 512 matrix:

$$\chi = \frac{\text{Length} \times \text{Unit conversion}}{\text{No. of pixels}}$$

$$= \frac{(20 \text{ cm})(10 \text{ mm/cm})}{512} = 0.4 \text{ mm depth}$$

and

$$= \frac{(30 \text{ cm})(10 \text{ mm/cm})}{512} = 0.6 \text{ mm width}$$

A matrix size of 512 × 512 decreases the pixel size to 0.4 × 0.6 mm. The ultrasound beam is now the major determinant of image resolution. Some manufacturers improve the resolution of their digital scan converters by using an asymmetrical matrix; that is, the number of pixels in each direction are not equal (i.e., 512 × 750).

A single television frame consists of 525 lines. The limit imposed on the resolution of the imaging system is similar to that contributed by the digital scan converter. This means that the vertical direction cannot depict spatial detail finer than the physical dimensions of each line.

Character Generator

The display monitor also contains a character generator, which is a device that translates coded electrical signals into light patterns that form characters on the screen. The placement of text with image data on the screen is a valuable aid in the identification of patient and the scan parameters.

Temporal Resolution

One major problem with B-mode (and other static imaging techniques) is the poor temporal resolution. Moving interfaces create blurred B-mode images. The inability of static B-mode scanning to rapidly update the displayed image with new scan data has caused the almost total replacement of this modality by real-time imaging.

SPECKLE

The two-dimensional sonogram consists of multiple lines of sight acquired during a finite time interval. The data associated with a particular scan line, however, are not exclusively derived from structures located along that line of sight. Interactions originating outside the main beam path also contribute to the net induced signal. This modulation of scan line data precludes the totally faithful portrayal of anatomical structures.

A scan of a homogeneous object produces an image with variations in brightness. A true representation of the scanned material would exhibit uniform brightness. Brightness non-uniformities, called acoustic speckle, appear throughout a two-dimensional image. Nonspecular reflections within soft tissue, blood, and other fluids scatter ultrasound energy, which ultimately returns toward the transducer along different pathways. Multiple wavefronts from these scattering events strike the transducer simultaneously (Fig. 3-20). The resulting interference pattern is not constant but changes with time. The fluctuating signal causes bright and dark variations in the image, which are responsible for the name "speckle."

Since speckle is a composite of numerous scattering events, the one-to-one correspondence between image brightness and physical structures is lost. Weak echoes from speckle are superimposed on other returning echoes. When echoes from specular reflectors are present, their signals dominate those from speckle and, consequently, speckle is masked in high-echogenic regions. Speckle is usually associated with regions devoid of strong reflectors (e.g., organ parenchyma). A close examination of successive images of the same scan plane shows that brightness variations within the organ parenchyma do occur.

Speckle inhibits the detection of low-contrast structures (i.e., objects with reflective properties similar to the surrounding tissue). Increasing ultrasound intensity does not suppress speckle.

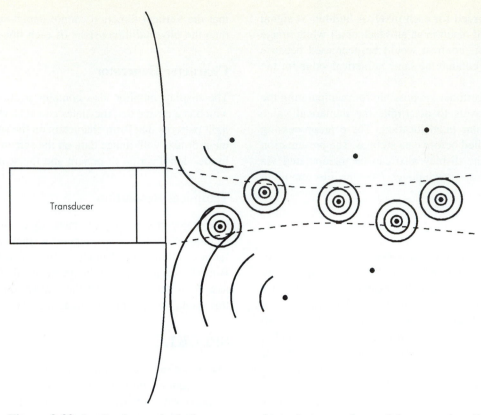

Figure 3-20 Small reflectors in the beam scatter ultrasonic energy. Some of the energy is redirected toward the transducer by additional scatterers located outside the beam. The interference pattern produced by multiple path reflections is called speckle.

GATED-MODE SCANNING

Gated scanning is a type of B-mode imaging that requires the usual B-mode registration arm, transducer, and other associated instrumentation (e.g., an analog or digital scan converter). The only difference is the additional electronics needed for gating purposes. Gating uses a temporal marker or physiological signal to trigger data collection. In static B-mode scanning short (microsecond) pulses of ultrasound are directed into the body, and all the returning echoes along that line of sight are collected before the next pulse is sent out. Occasionally, however, echoes outside the plane of interest will interfere with the desired information or interface motion will cause significant deterioration of the image.

C-Mode Scanning

Interference from overlying and underlying structures in static B-mode scanning is partially eliminated by using constant-depth scanning (C-mode scanning), in which additional gating electronics is incorporated into the standard B-mode unit.

An interface reflects part of the ultrasound beam energy (percentage reflection formula, Chapter 1). All interfaces along a scan line contribute to the normal B-mode image. The gating electronics of C-mode scanning rejects all returning echoes except those received during a specified time interval. Thus only scan data obtained from a specific depth are displayed. Induced signals outside the allowed period are not amplified and thus are not processed and displayed. Detected signals within the specified period are processed and displayed, thereby creating a plane of interest or a slice (tomogram). Ultrasound tomograms are obtained in any orientation. For example, if we were interested in a plane of depth between 5 and 6 cm, this would correspond to a time of flight (transmit and return time) of 65 to 78 μs (5 $\times$ 13 cm μs/cm to 6 cm $\times$ 13 μs/cm). Echoes arriving at the transducer between 65 and 78 μs after the transmitted ultrasound pulse would be amplified and displayed. All other echoes would not be amplified and thus would be lost. Scanning over the region of interest produces a tomogram of the plane of interest (Fig. 3-21). The gate can be adjusted to select both slice location and slice thickness.

■ **Example 3-3**

Determine the thickness of the tomographic slice if the range gates are set for 26 and 52 μs.

The time of travel for 1 cm is 13 μs. The start recording for displaying corresponds to a depth of 26 μs divided by 13 μs/cm, or 2 cm. The end recording for display corresponds to a depth of 52 μs divided by 13 μs/cm, or 4 cm. The slice thickness is equal to the difference between these depths, or 2 cm. This type of gated scanning is not presently practiced for static imaging, but similar principles apply for pulsed Doppler scanning (as discussed in Chapter 6).

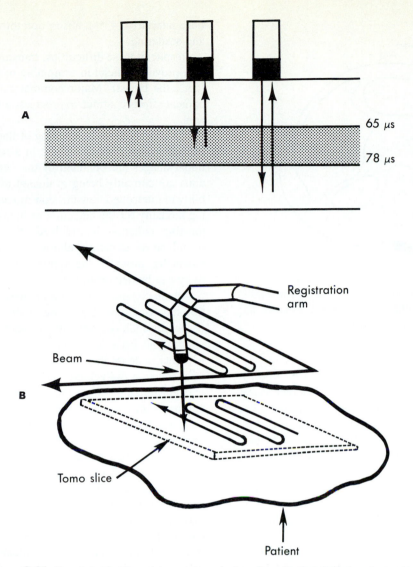

Figure 3-21 Gated-depth (C-mode) scanning. **A,** Interfaces in the *shaded region* are received, processed, and displayed whereas signals generated outside that region are received but not processed or displayed. A change in the gating time allows sampling at different depths. Slice thickness can also be adjusted. **B,** Acquiring a tomographic slice using gated scanning.

Electrocardiograph Gating

Electrocardiograph-gated scanning is designed to reduce motion artifacts obtained from static B-mode scanning of the heart. The motion of the heart creates a blurred image because the positions of the structures are not constant during the time needed to collect the B-mode image. To eliminate the problem, the ECG wave (P-QRS-T complex) acts as a gate to trigger the acquisition of scan data (Fig. 3-22). By selecting the Q part of the wave as the gating point, an image of the heart at the beginning of the ventricular contraction is formed. The assumption is made that the heart walls are in the same spatial configuration during every Q portion of the wave; therefore, if the information is collected, amplified, processed, and displayed only during the time of the Q gate, the heart walls will appear stationary. Repeated short samplings during a well-defined phase of the cardiac cycle prevent blurring of the heart walls in the image. During the remainder of the cardiac cycle the re-

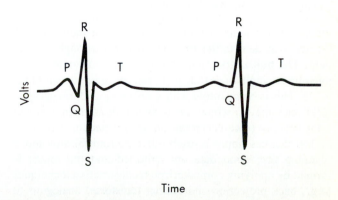

Figure 3-22 The electrocardiographic wave consists of repetitive P-QRS-T complexes. The Q portion of the complex is often used for gating purposes.

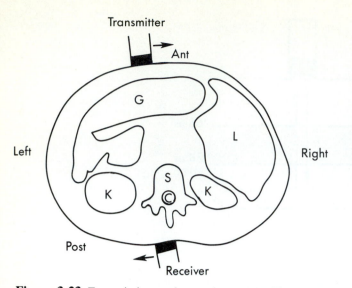

Figure 3-23 Transmission mode scanning system. The transducers are 180 degrees apart and move in concert. *L*, Liver; *K*, kidney; *S*, spine; *G*, bowel gas; *C*, spinal cord.

ceived echoes are not amplified and processed for display. The gate can be changed to acquire data for different phases of the cardiac cycle. Images from systole and diastole are used for measuring the ejection fraction and wall thickness.

With ECG-gating a patient is exposed to the ultrasound beam when no information is being processed for display. A longer scanning time is required to collect the image. Neither C-mode nor ECG-mode scanning has received widespread use. With development and rapid growth of stress echocardiography, however, ECG-gated scanning may become more prevalent.

TRANSMISSION MODE SCANNING

All ultrasound systems discussed thus far have relied on the detection of reflected echoes (echo-ranging principle) to characterize structures along the beam path.

Standard Transmission Mode

Transmission-mode scanning is the only ultrasound scanning method that detects the transmitted beam through the patient. The transmitting and receiving transducers are separated by an angle of 180 degrees and move in concert (Fig. 3-23). This is comparable with x-ray computed tomography (CT) scanning, in which the x-ray source (transmitter) and x-ray detector (receiver) rotate around the patient at an angle of 180 degrees opposite each other. In transmission-mode scanning projection data are collected and the image is formed by applying computerized reconstruction techniques (e.g., back projection and Fourier transform) analogous to those used in x-ray CT.

In most circumstances the transmitted ultrasound wave is of such low intensity that detection is impossible. The intensity of the transmitted ultrasound wave is reduced by reflections at bowel gas-tissue interfaces (99.9%) and tissue-

bone interfaces (43%), absorption through bone, refraction, and scattering.

In spite of these difficulties, transmission-mode scanning may prove beneficial in examining more uniform structures (e.g., the breast). Major commercial research and development efforts continue to progress, although slowly, in this area.

Transmission-mode scanning of the female breast is performed by inserting the breast in a water bath. Cross-sectional images are obtained of the entire breast. Prototype units are currently being evaluated to determine the feasibility of ultrasound transmission-mode scanning as a screening modality for the detection of breast cancer. Because no ionizing radiation is involved, this scanning procedure would be an attractive alternative to conventional mammography, provided the appropriate specificity and sensitivity can be demonstrated.

Attenuation measurements are used to differentiate dense fibrotic masses or less dense cystic masses from normal tissue. In addition, velocity measurements have potential applications because, generally, the velocity of ultrasound is higher in dense than in less dense objects. Combinations of attenuation and velocity measurements may be of benefit in characterizing benign and cancerous lesions from normal tissues. Transmission-mode scanning may be extended to include refracted and scattered ultrasound waves. Because scattering is frequency dependent (f^4 to f^6), scattering may aid in tissue characterization. Dual-frequency examinations with special subtraction techniques are also possible.

The male genitals and the infant head are other possible anatomical sites upon which transmission-mode scanning may have a significant impact. At present, however, the high cost and technical complexities of transmission-mode scanning limit its widespread clinical acceptance.

Reflux Transmission Imaging

An imaging technique called reflux transmission imaging (RTI) has been developed for use in conjunction with ultrasound lithotripsy systems. Reflected ultrasound from a specified depth beyond the focal zone is indicative of the ultrasound transmission through overlying tissues. This technique offers a significant advantage for the identification of gallstones before, during, and after lithotripsy.

SUMMARY

Static imaging techniques, particularly B-mode gray-scale scanners, were the mainstay of ultrasound departments through the mid-1970s. The development of scan converters greatly hastened the acceptance of diagnostic ultrasound in the medical community. B-mode scanners have provided the foundation for extensive applications of ultrasound as a noninvasive diagnostic tool.

Most static imaging systems have now been replaced by real-time and Doppler devices with superior temporal resolution. Many of the same principles of operation, however, still apply.

■■■■ **R E V I E W   Q U E S T I O N S** ■■■■

1. An A-mode scan is a plot of the _____ in one dimension versus _____ in the other dimension.
   a. Amplitude, brightness
   b. Brightness, depth
   c. Amplitude, depth
   d. None of the above

2. The CRT time base sweep rate corresponds to _____ .
   a. 1 m/s
   b. 13 cm/1 μs
   c. 1 cm/13 μs
   d. None of the above

3. In A-mode scanning the amplitude of the signal controls the emission of electrons from the cathode of the CRT to alter the brightness level of the trace.
   a. True
   b. False

4. In A-mode scanning the CRT trace is updated at a rate equal to the PRF.
   a. True
   b. False

5. B-mode stands for _____-mode scanning.
   a. Body
   b. Bridge
   c. Build
   d. Brightness

6. In B-mode scanning increased amplitude of the signal increases the brightness of the dot.
   a. True
   b. False

7. The B-mode signal amplitude controls electron emission from the cathode of the scan converter when operated in the write mode.
   a. True
   b. False

8. The position generator is used to control the location of the dot on the display. The position generator supplies information to the _____ of the scan converter.
   a. X and Y deflection plates
   b. Cathode
   c. Focusing cup
   d. Dielectric matrix

9. Scan converters are analog or _____ .
   a. Prolog
   b. Mechanical
   c. Digital
   d. None of the above

10. The B-mode registration arm is responsible for ensuring that the echo information from a particular interface is displayed at the same location, regardless of the transducer orientation.
    a. True
    b. False

11. The scan converter is so named because this device switches back and forth from the line-by-line acquisition during collection to the raster readout during display.
    a. True
    b. False

12. What are the physical dimensions of a pixel in which a 30 × 30 matrix represents a 10 × 20 cm field of view?
    a. 33 mm × 6.7 mm
    b. 0.67 mm × 0.33 mm
    c. 3.3 mm × 6.7 mm
    d. 0.33 mm × 0.67 mm

13. Static B-mode imaging has good temporal resolution.
    a. True
    b. False

14. C-mode scanning refers to _____ scanning.
    a. Continuous
    b. Constant-depth
    c. Cross-reference
    d. Closed

15. Gated scanning requires the following modifications to the standard B-mode scanner:
    a. Change in transmitter electronics
    b. Change in display
    c. Removal of registration arm
    d. None of the above

16. ECG-gated scanning results in a longer scan time but decreased patient exposure to ultrasound.
    a. True
    b. False

17. Multiple timing points during or following the P-QRS-T complex can be used as a gating trigger for the B-mode receiving electronics.
    a. True
    b. False

18. Transmission mode imaging is the only technique that relies on the echo-ranging principle.
    a. True
    b. False

19. Standard transmission mode imaging can be used for any area of the body without problems.
    a. True
    b. False

20. Gated scanning prevents the _____ of the echoes outside the depth of interest.
    a. Occurrence
    b. Amplification and processing
    c. Detection
    d. None of the above

BIBLIOGRAPHY

Bushong SC: *Radiologic science for technologists: physics, biology, and protection,* ed 5, St Louis, 1993, Mosby.

Curry TS III, Dowdey JE, Murry RC Jr: *Christensen's physics of diagnostic radiology,* ed 4, Philadelphia, 1990, Lea & Febiger.

Hendee WR, Ritenour ER: *Medical imaging physics,* ed 3, St Louis, 1992, Mosby.

Kremkau FW: *Diagnostic ultrasonics: physical principles and exercises,* ed 3, Philadelphia, 1988, WB Saunders.

McDicken WN: *Diagnostic ultrasonics: principles and use of instruments,* ed 3, Edinburgh, 1991, Churchill Livingstone.

Powis RL: *Physics for the fun of it,* Denver, 1978, Unirad Corporation.

Rose JL, Goldberg BB: *Basic physics in diagnostic ultrasound,* New York, 1979, John Wiley & Sons.

Wells PNT: *Physical principles of ultrasonic diagnosis,* New York, 1969, Academic Press.

Wells PNT: *Biomedical ultrasonics,* New York, 1977, Academic Press.

Woodcock JP: *Ultrasonics,* Bristol, 1979, Adam Hilger.

CHAPTER 4

Real-Time Ultrasound Imaging Principles and Instrumentation

Apodization	Frame rate
Beam aperture	Grating lobes
Broadband transducer	Line of sight
Compound linear array	Linear array
Contrast agent	Phased array
Contrast resolution	Pulse repetition frequency
Coprocessing	Scanning range
Curved linear array	Sector scanner
Distortion	Side lobes
Dynamic receive focusing	Slice thickness
Electronic focusing	Subdicing
Endosonography	Three-dimensional imaging
Footprint	

Two-dimensional ultrasound imaging is performed with either static B-mode gray-scale units (as discussed in Chapter 3) or real-time gray-scale scanners. In real-time scanning the displayed image is continuously and rapidly updated with new scan data as the beam is swept repeatedly throughout the field of view. The rate at which new information is displayed can be 30 or more frames per second. Some of the most exciting developments in medical diagnostic ultrasound instrumentation have been in the area of real-time imaging, sometimes referred to as rapid B-scanning (a type of automated B-mode imaging).

Real-time ultrasound imaging techniques have almost totally replaced static B-mode gray-scale imaging. The increased use of real-time imaging is the result of progress in transducer technology, miniaturization of electronics through the development of digital circuitry, advances in computer software, and improved ultrasonic focusing. The final result has been better image quality and higher information content for real-time ultrasound.

The rapid frame rates in real-time imaging eliminate difficulty with motion artifacts, which greatly compromise static imaging. Indeed, the ability to depict motion now makes dynamic studies possible. The total examination time is reduced because the sonographer receives instant feedback with respect to anatomical structures included within the field of view. The scan plane can be changed rapidly to a new orientation.

The major disadvantage is that the limited field of view makes anatomical identification more difficult. Real-time images also appear more nonuniform because the signal to noise ratio (SNR) is reduced compared with static imaging.

PRINCIPLES OF REAL-TIME IMAGING

To understand the basic requirements of a real-time ultrasound imaging system, we must first appreciate some underlying concepts of A-mode and B-mode scanners.

In A-mode scanning a transducer is placed over the area of interest. An ultrasound beam is sent out by exciting the crystal. The pulse lasts approximately 1 μs, and then the transducer is "silent" for 999 μs, waiting for the return echoes before it generates the next pulse. The returning echoes are amplified and displayed as a CRT trace of amplitude versus depth along this single line of sight. To see a different line of sight, we must move the transducer to a different position. Only one line of sight can be observed at any given instant on the display. As long as the transducer is stationary, the trace appears unchanged because the CRT

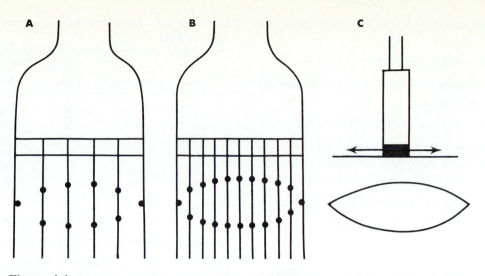

Figure 4-1 An increase in the number of lines of sight improves spatial resolution. **A,** Transducer with few lines of sight. **B,** Transducer with many lines of sight. **C,** Compound B-mode scan with "infinite" lines of sight.

screen is refreshed at the rate of the pulse repetition frequency (PRF).

In static B-mode gray-scale imaging the transducer is placed at the starting position and information is recorded along a single line of sight (similar to a single stop-action photograph or conventional x-ray film). All echoes from a single pulse are assumed to originate from reflections along this line of sight. The amplitude of each signal is represented by the brightness of the dot.

To build up a two-dimensional image, the sonographer moves the transducer manually to a different position or orientation to acquire information along a new line of sight. The previous line of sight data are retained on the display (or in storage). The image, or sonogram, thus is created by obtaining a large number of lines of sight over a 10- or 20-second period. The resolution of the image is improved as the number of lines of sight is increased (Fig. 4-1). Static scanning depends on the object's not moving, because lines of sight are acquired at different times and then combined to form a single image.

Lines of Sight

Real-time gray-scale imaging requires the acquisition of data in a very rapid fashion to give the perception of motion. It can be compared with other dynamic modalities (x-ray fluoroscopy or motion-picture films) in which a series of stop-action shots is taken and then viewed rapidly one after another to depict motion. The ultrasound beam is "swept" or steered through the area of interest (by mechanical or electronic means) in a repetitive automated fashion. Instead of a single sonogram with multiple lines of sight, as in static B-mode scanning, multiple sonograms are formed, each composed of multiple lines of sight. Every line requires one pulse of ultrasound waves to probe interfaces along its path.

The ultrasound beam is first directed along one line of sight, and after the echoes are received it is automatically moved to a new line. A single image is formed by sweeping

through the entire region. This process is repeated to produce successive images of the region. As motion becomes more rapid within the field of view, a faster frame rate is necessary to display the structures without jerkiness (abrupt transitions from one location to another, or blurring). The time for the pulse to travel to the depth of interest and back to the transducer—along with the need for good spatial resolution provided by a large number of lines of sight in each image—imposes a restriction on the frame rate. Frame rates of 5 to 40 images per second are available. The number of scan lines in a frame is usually between 50 and 200 depending on scan conditions. Commonly 120 to 150 scan lines are used.

Frame Rate Limitations

The maximum frame rate (FR) in frames per second (fps) is given by the following equation:

4-1

$$FR = \frac{c}{2\,RN} = \frac{PRF}{N}$$

where c is the velocity of ultrasound in the medium, R the depth of interest, N the number of lines of sight per frame (lpf), and PRF the pulse repetition frequency.

Equation 4-1 indicates that, if the scanning depth and/or number of lines of sight are increased, the maximum frame rate must decrease. The number of frames per second is ultimately limited by the velocity of ultrasound in tissue (1540 m/s). A finite amount of time is required for the ultrasound wave to move away from the transducer, sample the region of interest, and return to the transducer (13 μs for every centimeter of tissue). This sequence must occur for each line of sight.

For instance, assume that the field of view extends to a depth of 10 cm. The data collection time for each line of sight is 130 μs (13 μs/cm × 10 cm). If only one line of sight is desired (as in A-mode), the maximum frame rate would be:

$$(1540 \text{ m/s}) \div ((2) (0.1 \text{ m}) (1 \text{ lpf})) = 7700 \text{ fps}$$

By increasing the number of lines of sight to 100 lines per image the frame rate becomes

$$(1540 \text{ m/s}) \div ((2) (0.1 \text{ m}) (100 \text{ lpf})) = 77 \text{ fps}$$

Extending the depth of interest results in a reduced frame rate. If 100 lines of sight are to be maintained for a change in depth from 10 to 20 cm, the frame rate is decreased:

$$(1540 \text{ m/s}) \div ((2) (0.2 \text{ m}) (100 \text{ lpf})) = 38 \text{ fps}$$

■ Example 4-1

What is the maximum frame rate (FR) if the depth of scanning is 15 cm and 150 lines compose each frame?

Using Equation 4-1

$$FR = \frac{c}{2 \text{ RN}}$$

$$= \frac{1540 \text{ m/s}}{2 (0.15 \text{ m}) (150 \text{ lpf})}$$

$$= 34 \text{ fps}$$

■ Example 4-2

How many scan lines (N) can be acquired for each frame if the range is 10 cm and the frame rate is 24 per second?

Rearranging Equation 4-1

$$N = \frac{c}{2 \text{ R(FR)}}$$

$$= \frac{1540 \text{ m/s}}{2 (0.1 \text{ m}) (24 \text{ fps})}$$

$$= 320 \text{ lpf}$$

■ Example 4-3

If 200 scan lines compose each frame acquired at a rate of 18 frames per second, what is the range of scanning (R)?

Rearranging Equation 4-1,

$$R = \frac{c}{2 \text{ N(FR)}}$$

$$= \frac{1540 \text{ m/s}}{2 (200 \text{ lpf}) (18 \text{ fps})}$$

$$= 0.21 \text{ m or } 21 \text{ cm}$$

To achieve a faster frame rate, the scanning depth and/or number of lines of sight must be reduced. The decreased penetration enables a higher frequency transducer to be used for better axial resolution. Conventional B-mode scanners operate at a PRF of between 200 and 2000 pulses per second. Real-time scanners usually have a much higher PRF (as much as 5000 pulses per second) to preserve lateral resolution while maintaining a high frame rate. Some sacrifice

■ Table 4-1 Frame Rate Versus Depth and the Number of Lines of Sight

Depth (cm)	Frame Rate			
	25 LS*	50 LS	100 LS	200 LS
5	616	308	154	77
10	308	154	77	38
15	205	103	51	26
20	154	77	38	19
25	123	61	30	15
30	103	51	25	12

*Lines of sight.

in scanning depth may be required. Table 4-1 demonstrates the relation between number of lines of sight, depth of scanning, and frame rate.

The manufacturer of real-time equipment sets the frame rate based on the field of view, depth of interest, and number of lines of sight required for the desired image quality. Several approaches are possible to compensate for an increase in scanning depth. The real-time unit may automatically decrease the frame rate but maintain the same number of lines. On the other hand, both frame rate and number of lines may be adjusted downward. The number of lines may be reduced without a loss in resolution by narrowing the field of view. Often, several transducers of different frequencies are available for use with a single ultrasound unit. Each frequency is optimized with respect to the number of lines of sight and frame rate as a function of sampling depth. It is imperative that the sonographer understand these principles when selecting and operating the equipment.

Scan Converter

Multiple lines of sight are the building blocks for each image. As will be discussed shortly, each line of sight represents a particular position of the crystal(s) or activation of a group of crystals in the transducer array, which is established by the scanning mechanism. The ultrasound beam is directed into the patient in a well-defined pattern. Hence, no articulated arm is necessary to determine the position of the line of sight, as in static B-mode imaging. Because the data are collected and displayed in real time, permanent archiving is possible by recording the real-time images on videotape. A storage device (scan converter) is not needed; however, most real-time units incorporate a scan converter to obtain better gray-scale images and provide "freeze frame" capability. The use of digital scan converters also allows for manipulation of the image data to aid interpretation.

MECHANICAL SCANNERS

The most common classification of real-time imaging systems is based on the method by which the ultrasound beam is focused and swept through the region of interest. Mechanical scanners, the first major class, are normally the simplest and least expensive. Mechanical motion of single or multiple crystals sweeps the beam back and forth over the region of interest to collect different lines of sight for images in rapid succession. Focusing is also achieved by fixed mechanical means. The second major class, electronic real-time scanners, is discussed later in this chapter.

Mechanical real-time systems use one or more piezoelectric crystals attached to a stepping motor that moves the crystals to various locations. The changing positions of a crystal allow scan data to be collected from multiple lines of sight. In addition to the previously mentioned limitations on frame rate, the mechanical motion of a crystal restricts the acquisition rate to 30 or 40 frames per second. Mechanical real-time units typically employ one or more of the static B-mode focused crystals and are classified as either contact or liquid path scanners.

Contact Scanners

Contact scanners are those in which the transducer makes physical contact with the patient. Often the crystal is mounted within a liquid medium to eliminate any air interfaces between the moving crystal and the protective front surface of the transducer. The ultrasound path across the liquid medium is narrow (less than 3 mm). Gel is also placed between the transducer face and the patient to remove air-tissue interfaces.

One of the first real-time mechanical systems employed a B-mode crystal (usually focused) attached to a motor (Fig. 4-2). It vibrated or wobbled back and forth during data collection and with a frame rate of 15 per second subtended an arc of 15 to 60 degrees. Some of the early systems vibrated so much, in fact, that they were uncomfortable for both the patient and the sonographer.

When the crystal is at the extreme left position, data collection begins. The crystal is excited and the ultrasound beam moves outward along that line of sight, a fraction of its energy being reflected at various interfaces along its path. After an interval equal to the time needed for the wave to travel to the maximum depth of interest and return to the transducer (13 μs per centimeter), the crystal is moved to the next line of sight by the stepping motor and re-pulsed. This sequence repeats itself until the last line of sight is collected for one image (i.e., the crystal is at the extreme right position). The time required to collect one image depicting information from a depth of 10 cm with 200 lines of sight is 26 ms, and the process is repeated for the next image, which in the present example achieves a frame rate of 38 images per second. The time to collect scan data for each frame establishes the upper limit of the frame rate.

$$FR = \frac{1000 \text{ ms/s}}{26 \text{ ms/frame}} = 38 \text{ fps}$$

Equation 4-1 confirms this analysis:

$$FR = \frac{1540 \text{ m/s}}{(2)(0.1 \text{ m})(200 \text{ lpf})} = 38 \text{ fps}$$

In another version of the mechanical scanner, multiple crystals are mounted on a rotating wheel (Fig. 4-3). The technique for acquiring echo data is very similar to that used

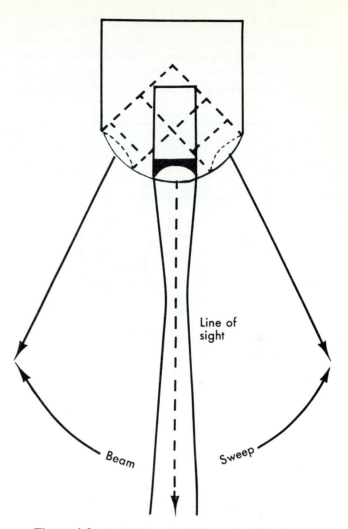

Figure 4-2 Oscillating or wobbling contact transducer.

with the vibrating sector scanner. A crystal is positioned at the extreme left and is excited, and the ultrasound beam probes interfaces along that line of sight. The wheel then moves, and the crystal is excited for the next line of sight. When the crystal moves to the extreme right, the last line of sight is collected for one frame. The neighboring crystal on the rotating wheel is then in position at the extreme left to begin the acquisition for the next frame. This technique may allow for faster frame rates, especially if coprocessing of information is used. In coprocessing, two separate crystals collect data in slightly different areas (nonadjacent lines of sight) simultaneously. The increased rate of sampling allows for more rapid updating of image data. Multiple crystals, each with a different frequency, may also be used to obtain images of the same area with varying spatial detail and contrast.

Characteristics of contact scanners. Oscillating or rotating wheel contact scanners produce an image with a sector or pie-shaped format. Because these sector scanners are physically small, scanning in tight areas between ribs, behind ribs (Fig. 4-4), and elsewhere is possible. Excellent images are produced over a limited range because fixed focused B-mode transducer crystals are used.

Problems with sector transducers do exist, however: Their small size limits the field of view and may make anatomical identification difficult. Their fixed focal length restricts the best lateral resolution to a limited range of depths. The resolution of an image deteriorates with distance

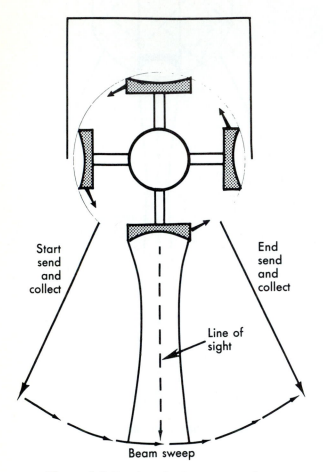

Figure 4-3 Rotating wheel contact transducer.

from the transducer face. There are more lines of sight crossing a given area near the top of the sector than in an equal area near the bottom.

The nonuniform scan-line density is illustrated in Figure 4-5. Streams of water radiating from a shower head demonstrate a similar effect. Near the source they are close together and they become less concentrated as distance from the shower head increases.

In practice, lateral resolution is affected when the distance between two lines is greater than the beam width. Reducing the number of lines to achieve high frame rate sometimes creates this situation (Fig. 4-6). Furthermore, increasing the sector angle to encompass a larger field of view decreases scan-line density (provided the scanning range and frame rate are unchanged) and reduces lateral resolution (Figs. 4-7 and 4-8).

Liquid Path Scanners

Another type of mechanical scanner is the liquid-path scanner, in which the crystals are placed in a liquid bath (usually a water and alcohol mixture). These scanners are further classified as nonreflecting liquid-path or reflecting liquid-path. Single or multiple transducer crystals are incremented in a linear (Fig. 4-9) or a sector (Fig. 4-10) fashion for data collection.

The nonreflecting liquid-path and mechanical contact scanners are said to be in-line transducers. The ultrasound beam travels directly from the transducer into the patient and back to the transducer without striking a mirror. The reflecting liquid-path scanner uses an acoustic mirror to alter the ultrasonic path for purposes of sweeping the beam. Directing or sweeping the beam is accomplished by moving the crystal while reflecting the beam from a stationary mirror (Fig. 4-11) or by reflecting the beam from a moving mirror while the crystal remains stationary (Fig. 4-12). The re-

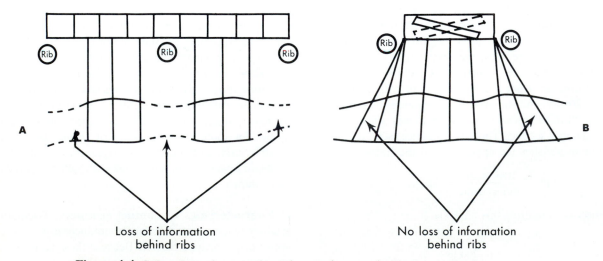

Figure 4-4 Comparison of rectangular and sector formats. **A,** The rectangular format cannot sample the region behind the ribs. **B,** The sector format allows the region between and behind the ribs to be examined.

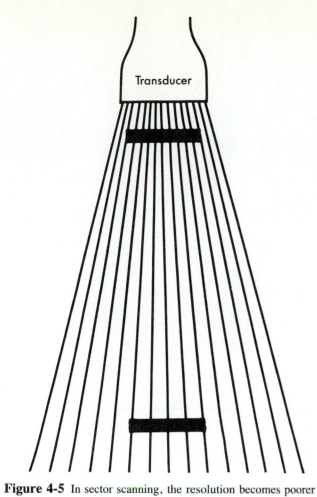

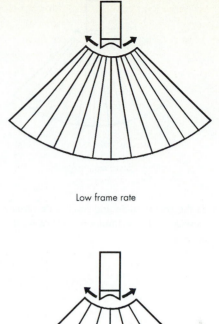

Low frame rate

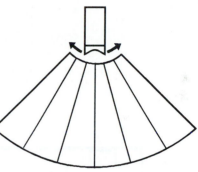

High frame rate

Figure 4-5 In sector scanning, the resolution becomes poorer at increasing depths. Good resolution is obtained in the region near the transducer (large number of lines of sight per unit area). The resolution becomes poorer at greater depths, since the number of lines of sight per unit area decreases. Compare the number of lines of sight through the *rectangular blocks,* which are equal in size.

Figure 4-6 A decease in the number of scan lines allows higher frame rates to be achieved. The sampling range and sector angle remain unchanged.

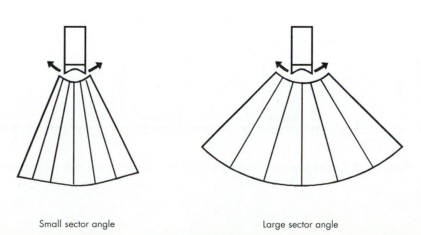

Small sector angle

Large sector angle

Figure 4-7 If the scanning range, frame rate, and number of scan lines remain unchanged, an increase in the sector angle results in a lower line density.

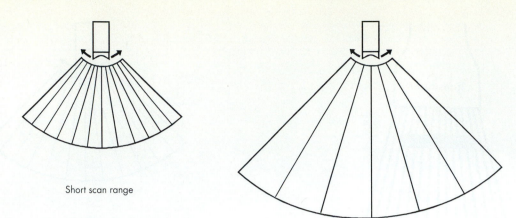

Short scan range

Figure 4-8 If the sector angle and frame rate remain unchanged, an increase in the scanning range lowers the total number of scan lines.

Long scan range

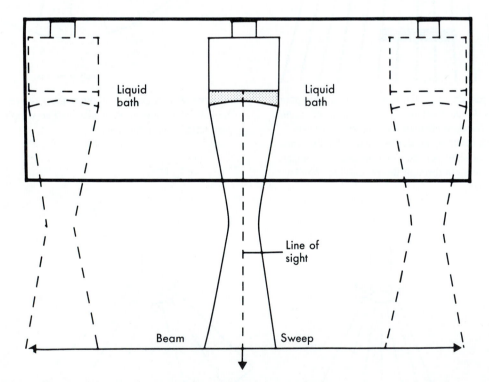

Figure 4-9 Liquid path nonreflecting transducer with one crystal moving linearly.

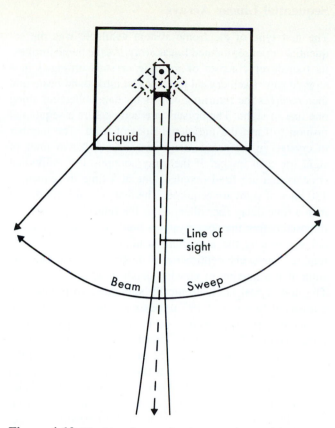

Figure 4-10 Liquid path nonreflecting transducer with an arcing crystal (sector).

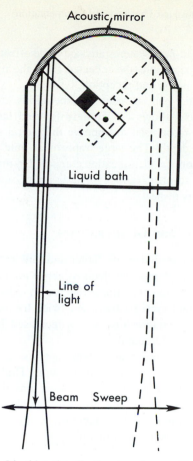

Figure 4-11 Liquid path reflecting transducer with a moving crystal and a stationary mirror.

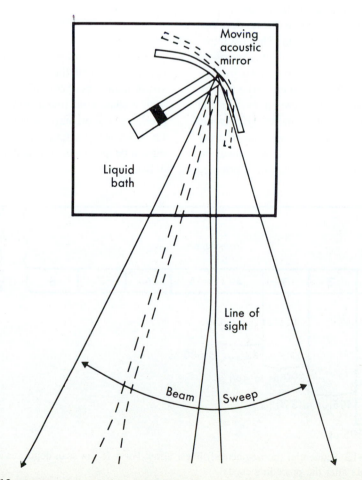

Figure 4-12 Liquid path reflecting transducer with a stationary crystal and a moving mirror.

flecting liquid-path systems are said to be offset because the ultrasound beam must be reflected from the mirror during both transmission and reception.

The liquid path reduces reverberations from shallow structures and allows for strongly focused large-diameter transducers to be used to improve the lateral resolution at the desired depth. The large trapezoidal field of view enhances anatomical identification compared to that obtainable with sector scanners (although static image scanning is superior in this respect).

Advantages and Disadvantages

Liquid-path transducers are larger and bulkier than contact scanners and are more difficult to apply to small or irregularly shaped areas. The frame rate is also reduced, because the liquid path must be traversed twice by the ultrasound beam (the penetration distance is increased by twice the length of the liquid path).

Generally, mechanical systems are less expensive and easier to operate than electronic systems. High-quality images are produced, but mechanical wear may limit the overall lifetime of the transducers. Mechanical wear can be reduced by turning the transducer off when not in use. The mechanical motion also limits the frame rate.

LINEAR ARRAYS

An important advance in medical diagnostic ultrasound instrumentation occurred in the late 1970s with the development of electronic real-time instrumentation. These systems produce high-quality images with high frame rates and many lines of sight without the limited lifetime caused by mechanical wear. The transducer (with one exception) is manipulated electronically to focus as well as to sweep (or steer) the ultrasound beam throughout the region of interest. Electronic real-time units are classified as linear array and phased array systems. Both units are expensive compared with mechanical sectors, although there can be some overlap in pricing.

Sequential Linear Arrays

The first type of electronic system available was the sequential or nonsegmented linear array. As the name implies, its transducer consists of multiple crystals arranged in a straight row. Each crystal produces an ultrasound beam and then receives the returning echoes for data collection along one line of sight. The crystals are activated in a sequential fashion to form the individual lines of sight. The number of crystals in the array determines the number of lines of sight for each image. If the array contains 130 individual crystals that are fired (excited) one at a time in sequence, 130 lines of sight are acquired. The first crystal is fired, and then a time delay for collection of the returning echoes are imposed before the next crystal is fired. The duration of the delay is set by the maximum scanning depth (13 μs are required for every centimeter of depth). For example, assume that a maximum viewing depth of 15 cm is desired. The first crystal is electronically stimulated to produce an ultrasound beam, and 195 μs later (13 μs/cm × 15 cm) the second crystal is excited. After another 195 μs the third crystal is fired. This sequence continues until all 130 crystals are fired to form one image. The process is repeated for the next image. The rate at which this sequence of firing all 130 crystals is repeated determines the frame rate. Figure 4-13 illustrates the timing pattern for a sequential linear array. The 15 cm depth limits the PRF to 5000 pulses per second (pps). With 130 lines per frame (lpf) a maximum frame rate of 38 images per second is obtained:

$$ FR = \frac{5000 \text{ pps}}{130 \text{ lpf}} = 38 \text{ fps} $$

Recall that the physical dimensions of the crystal dictate the width of the ultrasound beam. Linear arrays consist of many small crystals along a row. The major problem with a sequential linear array is that the small crystal size produces a short narrow near field and a rapidly diverging far field. As discussed in Chapter 2, larger crystals produce a deeper near field and a less diverging far field (Fig. 4-14).

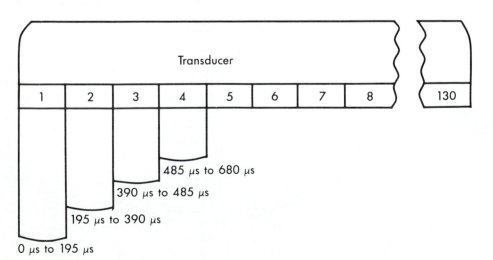

Figure 4-13 Sequential (nonsegmented) linear array. For a 15 cm scan depth, each crystal is fired 195 μs after the preceding crystal.

Segmental Linear Arrays

When a group (segment) of crystals in the linear array is stimulated, it acts in concert to produce a deeper near field and a less divergent far field compared with a single crystal acting alone. This segmental linear array, however, creates fewer lines of sight for the same given area, which causes the spatial mapping to deteriorate although the resultant ultrasonic field provides a more favorable beam pattern. For example, assume that 64 individual crystals are fired in groups of four. The first four crystals are excited simultaneously and then 195 μs (corresponding to the time required to sample 15 cm in depth) elapse before the next four crystals in a group (nos. 5 through 8) are fired. By using adjacent blocks of four crystals, 16 lines of sight that are spaced widely apart can be created (Fig. 4-15). This is less than ideal, although the overall beam pattern for sampling each line of sight at increased depth is improved.

To achieve good lateral resolution at great depths, a combination of large crystal size and high line-of-sight density is required. This is accomplished by using a stepdown segmental crystal array. Figure 4-16 shows the excitation sequence for the first 16 crystals of a 64-crystal linear array. The number of lines of sight is increased by firing crystals 1 through 4, waiting 195 μs, and then firing crystals 2 through 5. After another 195 μs, crystals 3 through 6 are excited. In other words, a set of four crystals is fired as a group or segment to produce the desired beam pattern and, by overlapping groups, the number of lines of sight can be increased. The stepdown segmental array produces 13 lines of sight for the 16 crystals shown, rather than 4 lines of sight obtained by the sequential segmental array. If in an array of 64 crystal elements four crystals are fired at a time

and each group is offset by one crystal, a total of 61 lines of sight will be acquired for each image. Assuming that 15 cm is the desired depth (195 μs between firing each segment), we can see that a maximum of 84 images could be generated each second:

$$FR = \frac{1540 \text{ m/s}}{(2)\,(0.15 \text{ m})\,(61 \text{ lpf})} = 84 \text{ fps}$$

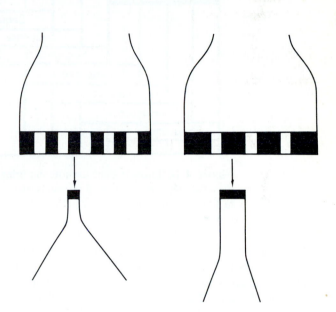

Figure 4-14 Crystal size in the transducer array affects the beam pattern. Small crystals create a short near field and a rapidly diverging far field. Large crystals produce a wider but deeper near field and a less diverging far field.

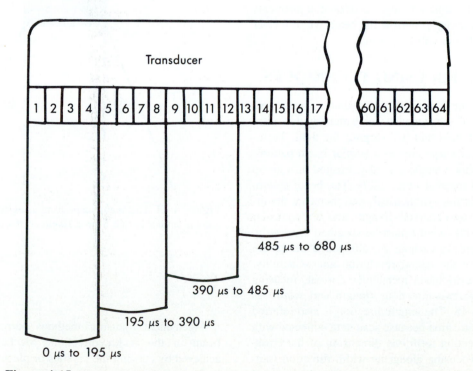

Transducer

| 1 | 2 | 3 | 4 | 5 | 6 | 7 | 8 | 9 | 10 | 11 | 12 | 13 | 14 | 15 | 16 | 17 |

| 60 | 61 | 62 | 63 | 64 |

485 μs to 680 μs

390 μs to 485 μs

195 μs to 390 μs

0 μs to 195 μs

Figure 4-15 Segmental linear array. For a 15 cm scan depth, each group of four crystals is fired 195 μs after the preceding group.

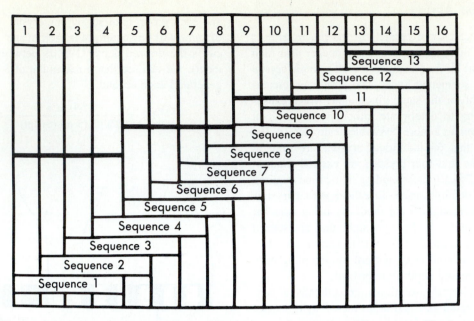

Figure 4-16 Lines of sight for different firing sequences in a segmental linear array. The *large dark lines* represent sequential segments (there are 4). The number of lines of sight is increased to 13 by overlapping segments (referred to by sequence numbers).

The stepdown segmental array with 64 to 200 piezoelectric elements produces good temporal resolution (high frame rate) and good spatial resolution (beam size and number of lines of sight). The field of view is presented in a rectangular format, with the in-plane width equal to the length of the array. The linear array has a flat face, which causes difficulty in maintaining transducer-patient contact when a wide field of view is desired. Nevertheless, this stepdown technique has improved the image quality of real-time scanners dramatically although additional adjustments in focusing are necessary to narrow the beam width further so the spatial resolution will be optimal.

ELECTRONIC FOCUSING TECHNIQUES

As shown in Chapter 2, a circular transducer crystal produces a symmetrical ultrasound beam pattern with a relatively narrow near field and a diverging far field. Fortunately, a rectangular shape creates a similar beam pattern, regardless of whether a single crystal is excited or a group of crystals is fired together (Fig. 4-17). The beam pattern for a linear array is not symmetrical, and therefore the dimension along the row of crystals (length) and perpendicular to the row of crystals (width) must be specified separately. As previously stated (in Chapter 2), ultrasound beams are focused to improve the lateral resolution and sensitivity. Because a linear array has a rectangular format, focusing must be applied in two directions (length and width) as shown in Figure 4-18. The length direction is also referred to as the in-plane direction because scan data collected with respect to this direction form one dimension of the cross-sectional image. Focusing along the width direction (out-of-plane) determines the slice thickness or the thickness of tissue represented by the cross-sectional image (Fig. 4-19).

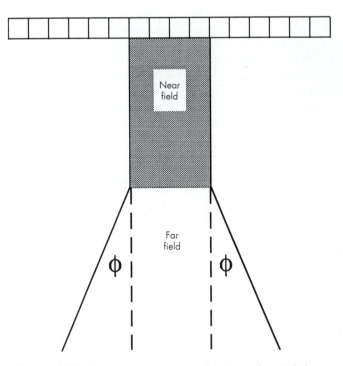

Figure 4-17 The beam shape from a segment of crystals in an array is similar to that from a single crystal circular transducer.

Mechanical focusing methods narrow the ultrasound beam in the width direction. Mechanical focusing is achieved by curving the crystals or placing an acoustic lens in front of the crystals (Fig. 4-20). Focusing in the width direction is applied uniformly to each crystal in the array.

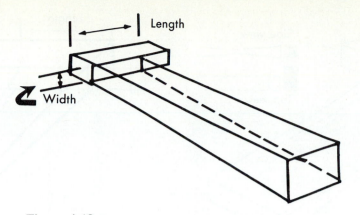

Figure 4-18 Rectangular beam pattern along the length and width directions produced by a segment of crystals illustrating the divergence that occurs in three dimensions.

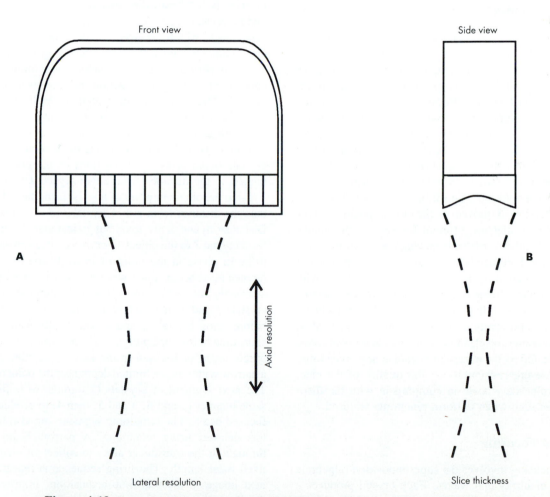

Figure 4-19 Focused beam pattern. **A,** Focusing along the length of the array influences the lateral resolution. For comparative purposes, the direction of axial resolution is also shown. **B,** Mechanical focusing in the width direction determines the slice thickness.

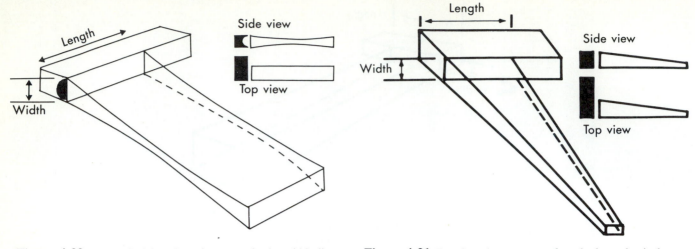

Figure 4-20 Mechanical focusing of an array in the width direction using an acoustic lens or curved crystal elements.

Figure 4-21 Resultant beam pattern from both mechanical width focusing and electronic length focusing.

Focusing Dynamics

The sequence of firing one group of crystals (stepping down) and then firing the next group prohibits mechanical focusing of the ultrasound beam in the length direction. The relative position of a crystal in the group dictates the focusing requirements for that crystal. Because most crystals in the array belong to multiple firing groups, the focusing requirements change and cannot be achieved by static mechanical means. For example, in a stepdown segmented array, crystal 3 is the center of a five-crystal firing sequence involving crystals 1 through 5; when crystals 2 through 6 are fired, crystal 3 occupies the no. 2 position; and when 3 through 7 are fired, crystal 3 moves to the no. 1 position. This changing position dictates different focusing requirements for that crystal and thus prevents mechanical focusing in the length direction. Fortunately, linear arrays are electronically focused in the length direction, which (when combined with mechanical focusing in the width direction) creates a narrow beam (Fig. 4-21). Note that focusing of an ultrasound beam depends on the uniformity of the tissues interrogated. Most scanning of human subjects involves a diverse array of tissue types interrogated by the ultrasound beam at any given time. This places severe restrictions on the quality of the electronically synthesized beam in comparison with the theoretical images seen when uniform phantoms are used.

Principle of Focusing

Electronic focusing involves the superimposition (algebraic summation) of ultrasound waves. Each crystal produces a particular wave pattern, and the overall pattern derived from a group of crystals is the summation of all the wave patterns from the individual crystals (Huygens' principle). Electronic focusing is accomplished by offsetting the firing of various crystals in a group by a small time delay (10^{-9} second). This delay is small compared with the time required for the sound beam to travel to the depth of interest. For a group

of crystals the beam direction is normally centered at the middle crystal. The nanosecond timing is accomplished by delay lines, which are special electronic devices that hold the command signal from the master synchronizer for a specified period. The exact nanosecond timing sequence depends on the crystal position and the focal zone depth desired. The wavefront generated by each crystal in the group is made to arrive at a specific point in the phase, and the result is a focused beam at that point.

Figure 4-22 demonstrates electronic focusing with five crystals of an array. The positions of the crystals are arranged so the distance from either crystal 1 (d_1) or crystal 5 (d_5) to the object or point of interest is the same but greater than the distance from either crystal 2 (d_2) or crystal 4 (d_4). Distances d_2 and d_4 are equal but greater than d_3 (the distance from crystal 3 to the object). For the waves from each crystal to be in phase at the point of interest, constructive interference must occur. Each wavefront must arrive at the point at exactly the same time. This is accomplished by firing crystals 1 and 5 first, delaying a short time (50 to 100 ns) before firing crystals 2 and $4,$ and finally waiting another short time before firing crystal 3. The ultrasound beam thus is reinforced or focused in the length direction, producing a narrow width over a limited depth near the point of interest. The next segment of crystals (2 through 6) is fired in the same manner (2 and 6, 3 and 5, then 4) to produce another focused beam. The remaining segments are also focused by this delayed firing technique. A narrow beam is swept throughout the transducer array to collect an image using a fixed focal length. The firing sequence is repeated for the next image in the real-time acquisition. Improved spatial detail is thus obtained within the focal zone.

Transmit Focusing

Unlike mechanical real-time systems (in which focal depth is fixed), many linear array units allow the operator to select one of several possible focal zones. The depth of the

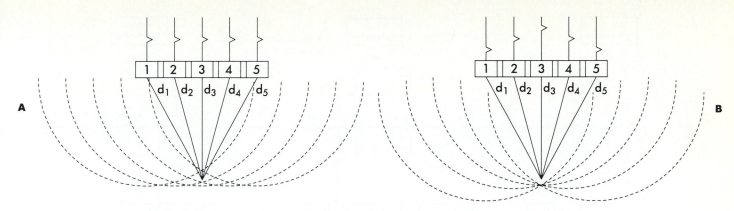

Figure 4-22 Electronic focusing. **A,** If five crystals are stimulated simultaneously, the wavefronts do not arrive simultaneously at the target because the distances d_1, d_2, d_3, d_4, and d_5 are not equal. **B,** Transmit delay lines are used to excite the crystals at slightly different times (nanosecond delays between firings). Then the wavefronts arrive exactly simultaneously at the target point and the result is a focused beam. Crystals *1* and *5* are stimulated first, then *2* and *4*, and then *3*. Changing the time delays allows other points to become the center of focus.

focal zone is altered by varying the delay times between crystal firings. This capability is usually accompanied by increased cost. High-resolution images with several focal zones are obtainable using these variable delay lines. The initial scanning of the region of interest is conducted with a single depth focus. Once the imaging has been completed, the focal zone is changed (by modifying the delay line timing) to rescan the same area with a new focal zone. The beam is focused to a new depth simply by changing the delay times. This technique is called transmit focusing (Fig. 4-23).

In many cases multizone focusing throughout the image is desirable. Multizone transmit focusing slows the frame rate because data must be collected for all the lines of sight across the array with a fixed focal zone depth before the lines of sight are repeated with a different focal zone depth. For example, assume that the unit can be focused to three different depths for the same "image." In reality, three separate images, each focused to a particular depth, must be collected before they are combined into one "final image" for viewing. This reduces the frame rate by a factor of three. For six separate focal zones the frame rate is reduced by a factor of six. Equation 4-1 for maximum frame rate (FR) is modified to read:

4-2

$$FR = \frac{c}{2\,RNn}$$

where n is the number of focal zones used to produce one image, c the velocity of ultrasound, R the depth of interest, and N the number of lines of sight per frame.

Combining multiple zones to form one image may cause a discontinuity at the boundary between the focal zone areas, called the stitch-line artifact. Coprocessing of the echoes restores the frame rate to the original value. The rate of data

collection is increased by simultaneously acquiring multiple lines of sight. Selected portions of each line of sight corresponding to the focal depth are retained for the final image. While the line of sight corresponding to the short focused depth is being collected at one location along the array, other lines of sight with different focal depths are being generated at other locations along the array. Because the data for all three zones have been obtained concurrently, the frame rate is not decreased (Fig. 4-24).

Aperture Focusing

Electronic transmit focusing is also accomplished by switching the number of crystals fired in the segment (Fig. 4-25). For example, two crystals are fired initially as a group to produce a very short narrow near field and a rapidly diverging far field. Then additional crystals in the next group are fired, which extends the depth of the near field and broadens the beam at shallow depths. This method is a quasi-focusing technique based on beam aperture. Large apertures extend the depth of focus.

Aperture focusing is characterized by a quantity known as the f-number, which is defined as the ratio of the focal length (F) to the size of the aperture in the length direction (d):

4-3

$$\text{f-number} = \frac{F}{d}$$

Optimal focusing occurs with an f-number of 2. In reality many manufacturers employ combinations of time-delayed firing and changing beam aperture to optimize focusing at many depths. The normal trade-off is a decrease in frame rate (temporal resolution) unless coprocessing is used.

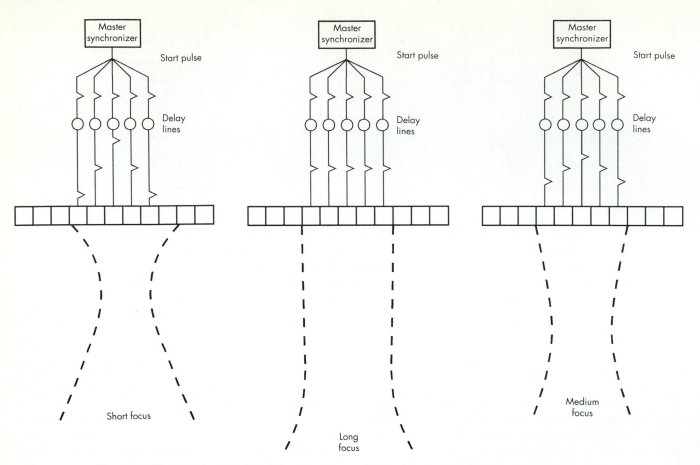

Figure 4-23 Variable delay lines allow focusing at different depths. The delay lines stagger the excitation pulses to the crystals, depending on the degree of focusing desired. **A,** Short focus. **B,** Long focus. **C,** Medium focus.

Dynamic Receive Focusing

Another application is dynamic focusing in the receive mode. The principle of receive focus is difficult to conceptualize. The following analogy may help: Three runners of equal ability begin a race at the same starting point but follow different routes to the finish line. At the finish line an observer is assigned to each runner and must shout the point of origin when the runner crosses the finish line. Because the distance travelled by each runner is not identical, three separate shouts are heard as the race is completed. If an obstacle, such as a wall, is placed in the path of each runner, the sequence of finish can be regulated. The height of the wall is adjusted depending on the distance between the starting point and finish line. To increase the delay before crossing the finish line, the obstacle is made greater. In this case, the shortest route would incorporate the tallest wall. For a certain combination of obstacles, the runners finish the race simultaneously and one loud shout is heard from all the observers identifying the point of origin. The race can be made more complex by varying the starting point. The heights of the obstacles can be adjusted according to the change in distance. Now the observers are given a chart that denotes the starting point based on the elapsed time of the race. This is possible because the participants run at the same speed. The shouts of the observers at the finish line are still synchronized; only the words to identify the starting points vary. Receive focus works in a similar manner.

By means of additional delay circuitry, the returning sound beam is refocused when multiple crystals receive the echo. Dynamic focusing is not limited to one fixed depth, as transmit focusing is, but operates at all depths. In Figure 4-26 five crystals are activated to receive the ultrasound beam reflected toward the transducer from interface P_1. The ultrasound beam diverges during its return to the transducer. The wavefront from P_1 intercepts crystal 3 first, then crystals 2 and 4, and finally crystals 1 and 5. Through the use of receive-time delays the echo-induced signal at crystal 3 is delayed, before being sent for processing to the receiver electronics, until the wavefront reaches crystals 1 and 5. Similarly, the echo-induced signals from crystals 2 and 4 are delayed. The actual time delay is determined for each set of crystals by simple geometry and an assumed constant velocity of ultrasound in soft tissue. The wavefront from P_1 appears to be in phase for all five crystals, resulting in a "focused" beam from that depth of interest. The same prin-

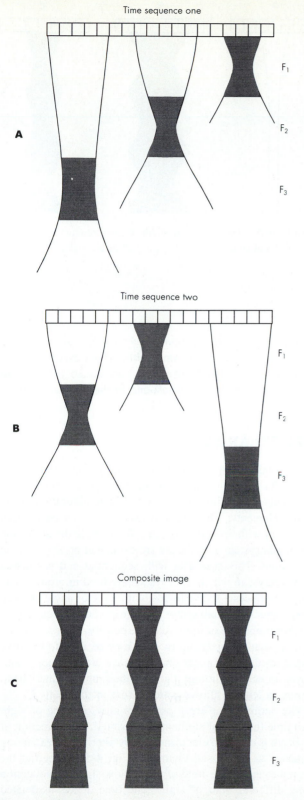

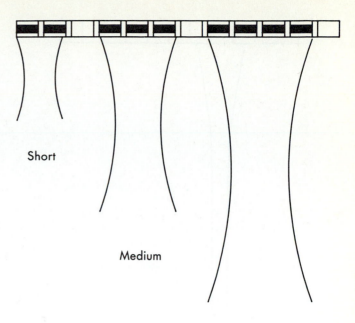

Figure 4-25 Focusing to different depths: two crystals are fired for short focus, three for medium focus, and four for long focus. This is a quasi-focusing technique based on beam aperture.

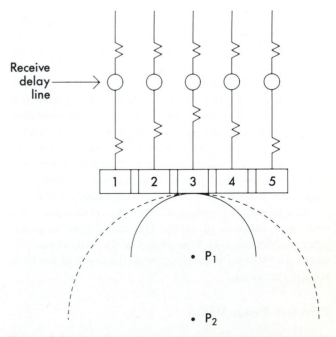

Figure 4-24 Coprocessing. **A** and **B,** Information for three focal zones is collected and processed simultaneously for three nonadjacent lines of sight. **C,** Once all the lines of sight are collected, the data are displayed as one image. The frame rate remains higher than that for multifocal zone units.

Figure 4-26 Dynamic receive focusing. The wavefronts from point 1 (P_1) *(solid semicircle)* and point 2 (P_2) *(dotted semicircle)* arrive at crystal *3* first, then at *2* and *4*, and then at *1* and *5*. By delaying the induced echo signal until the wavefront has arrived at all five crystals, focusing is applied to the received signal (reinforcement or constructive interference).

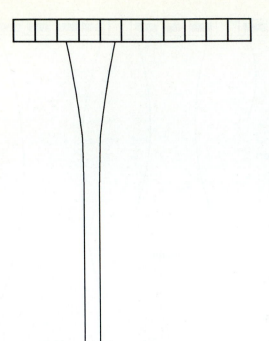

Figure 4-27 Dynamic receive focusing has a narrow echo beam width throughout the scanning range.

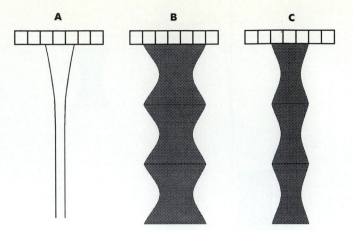

Figure 4-28 Effective beam width, **C,** is a product of the transmit focal zone, **B,** and the received beam width, **A.**

ciple applies to interface P_2 in Figure 4-26, but because of the greater depth the wavefront strikes the crystals with less variability. A shorter receive delay focuses the detected signals from interface P_2. The master synchronizer sends timing messages to the receiver-delay lines to indicate the elapsed time from transmission to reception. The elapsed time determines the delay times (in nanoseconds, just as in transmit focusing) for each crystal. The depth of interest is always known, and thus receive-delay times are constantly changed to yield a continually focused beam at all depths.

The received beam width is uniformly narrow along the line of sight (Fig. 4-27). In essence, therefore, lateral resolution is improved by restricting the tissue volume that contributes to each building block in the image. A dynamic aperture adjusts the number of receiving crystals along the array as a function of depth. This acquisition technique optimizes focusing at a particular depth. Additional elements are included in the aperture as the depth of the focal zone is increased.

Effective Beam Width

Many real-time linear arrays use both fixed transmit focusing and dynamic receive focusing. The effective beam width is the product of the fixed transmit focal zone beam width and the received beam width (Fig. 4-28). As the number of fixed transmit focal zones increases, the composite effective beam width becomes more narrow (Fig. 4-29). Each segment along the line of sight is optimized for a certain focal length. Since the ultrasound beam diverges rapidly beyond

the focal zone, multiple transmit focal zones are necessary to maintain a narrow beam width. The improvement in spatial detail for linear array has contributed to the rapid acceptance of real-time ultrasound in the clinical environment.

PHASED ARRAYS

The second type of electronic real time system is the phased array. Phased arrays are classified as linear, annular, or rectangular according to the geometric configuration of the crystal elements. The linear phased array can be a small transducer with few crystals (16). To generate the ultrasonic beam, all crystals in the array are excited at or nearly at the same time. This contrasts with sequential and segmental linear arrays, in which the crystals are fired in groups. The design produces a sector format with a sector angle as large as 90 degrees. A small sector angle (e.g., 30 degrees) allows a higher frame rate or increased line density. A large number of very small crystals (up to 128) may be used to improve spatial resolution. Linear phased arrays are commonly employed in echocardiology because their smaller size (10 to 30 mm in length) allows better access to the heart.

The entire linear array produces only one line of sight each time the crystal elements are excited. The direction of the beam is changed electronically by altering the excitation sequence to the crystal elements (Fig. 4-30). Steering the beam throughout the field of view allows for data collection along different lines of sight. The time delays associated with beam steering are longer than nanoseconds but shorter than the microseconds needed to acquire data along each line of sight. Electronic steering also relies on the interference of waves for reinforcement within the area of interest—thus the name phased steering or phased array. Small time delays, on the order of nanoseconds, are utilized for fixed transmit focusing purposes as the beam is steered. The linear

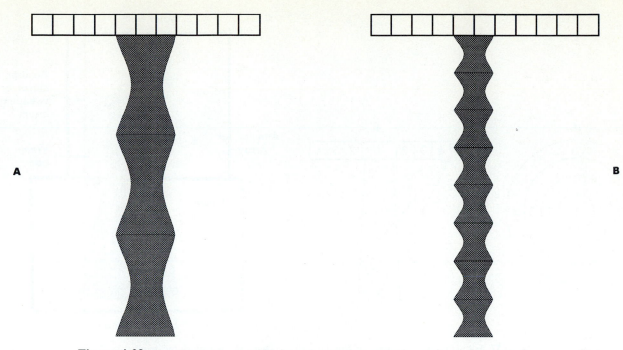

Figure 4-29 The effective beam width is made more narrow by increasing the number of transmit focal zones. **A,** Three zones; **B,** eight zones.

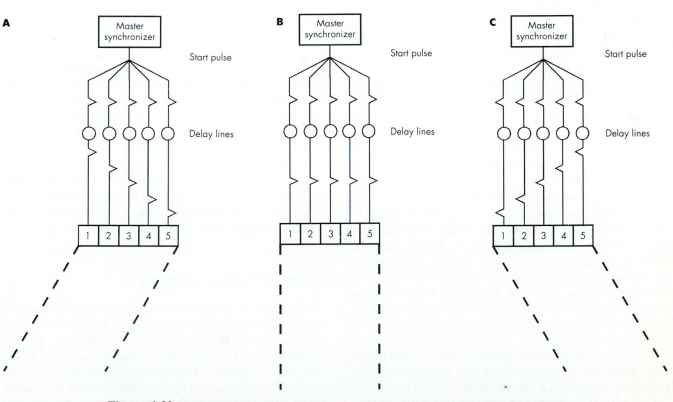

Figure 4-30 Electronic time delays in linear phased arrays steer the beam. The delay lines stagger the excitation pulses to the crystals depending on the direction of sampling. **A,** Sweep left; **B,** no sweep; **C,** sweep right.

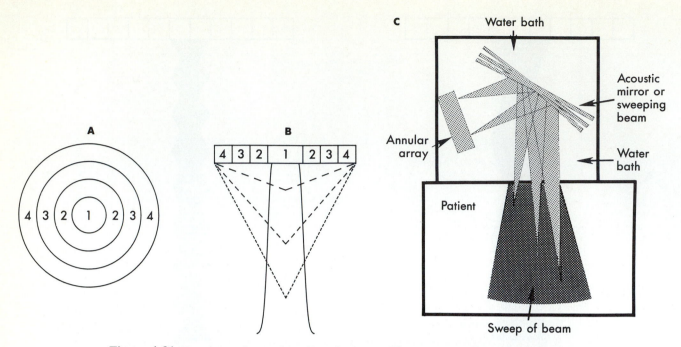

Figure 4-31 Focusing and sweeping of annular arrays. These are normally mechanically swept, but can be liquid path systems. **A,** Top view of an annular array showing four crystal elements. Note that all except the innermost crystal are doughnut shaped. **B,** Side view to show focusing. **C,** Sweeping the beam by a moving acoustic mirror (example of liquid path).

phased array can also be dynamically focused in the receive mode. Outside the central field of view spatial resolution deteriorates because electronic focusing becomes more difficult when large-angle beam steering is performed. Linear phased arrays are mechanically focused in the width (slice thickness) direction.

Annular phased array transducers, when viewed end on (Fig. 4-31), have a central crystal surrounded by concentric rings of additional crystals. Each crystal is pulsed in such a fashion as to permit electronic focusing to a very fine point at all depths along the beam axis. Dynamic receive focusing is also possible, although an annular phased array must be mechanically steered to collect different scan lines. Steering is accomplished by reflecting the beam from a moving mirror or by rotating the transducer mechanically without a mirror. The mirror systems are usually liquid path. The ultrasound beam converges symmetrically to the focal point. The beam width is the same in both the slice-thickness direction and the in-plane direction (similar to a circular transducer). This symmetrical beam should be contrasted with ultrasound beams generated by linear arrays, which have varying dimensions depending on the focusing technique, pulsing sequence, and crystal size.

A rectangular phased array consists of a crystal matrix (e.g., 64 crystals arranged in eight rows and eight columns) embedded in a plastic polymer. Rectangular phased arrays are electronically focused in two dimensions along both directions of the crystal matrix. Mechanical focusing is not needed. Dynamic receive focusing, in conjunction with transmit focusing, defines the depth of focus from any point

in the matrix. Electronic focusing in both dimensions is applied simultaneously, but steering is controlled in only one direction at a time. However, without moving the transducer, the beam can be steered to obtain orthogonal planes (Fig. 4-32).

Compound linear arrays have been developed to incorporate characteristics from both the linear array and the linear phased array. Scan lines for the central field of view are obtained by the stepdown segmental array technique. At the extremes of the field of view the ultrasound beam is steered at wide angles by the phased method. The timed excitation of a large number of crystals is controlled by delay lines. An enlarged effective field of view is created that extends beyond the physical length of the array (Fig. 4-33). Areas of overlapping data are manipulated by the scan converter to form a composite image.

CURVILINEAR ARRAYS

Recently, curvilinear (also called convex, curved linear, or radial) arrays have been developed that produce large sector formats. Crystal elements are arranged along an arc in a linear fashion. The radius of curvature is usually 25 to 100 mm. A large radius of curvature extends the in-plane width of the field of view. As with other types of arrays, the physical dimensions of the crystal elements influence the beam pattern.

As regular linear arrays do, convex arrays sweep the beam by firing multiple crystals in a group, stepping down

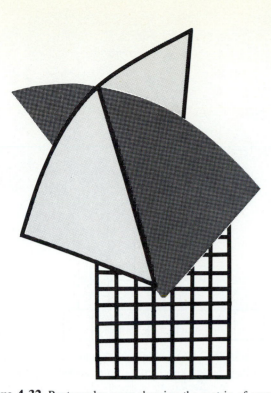

Figure 4-32 Rectangular array showing the matrix of crystals and the orthogonal plane steering of the array.

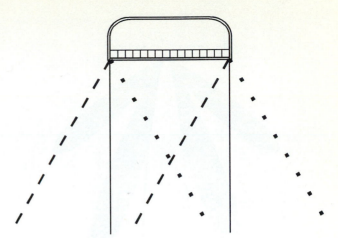

Figure 4-33 Compound linear array illustrating the sweeping and steering of the beam to increase the field of view.

Convex transducer

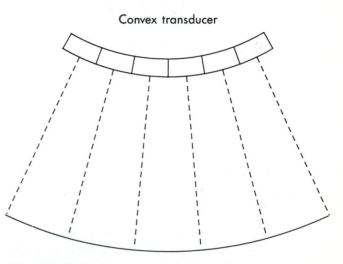

Figure 4-34 Convex or curved linear array. Ultrasonic beams are directed perpendicular to the array surface.

after the appropriate delay, and then firing the next group. The curved crystal arrangement provides lines of sight that are perpendicular to the array surface (Fig. 4-34). No loss of focus occurs at the edges of the field of view; however, beam divergence may limit the useful depth. Analogous to sector scanning, with convex arrays line density is decreased at depth and a loss of lateral resolution can occur. As will be discussed shortly, curved arrays also reduce grating lobes.

PROBLEMS WITH ELECTRONIC ARRAYS

A major problem with electronic arrays is the formation of secondary lobes of ultrasound energy. Secondary lobes originate at the transducer and radiate outward at various angles to the main beam. Artifacts in the image are created by the misregistration of interface position, since all returning echoes are assumed to originate along the main beam axis. Secondary lobes are also responsible for clutter, which inhibits the detection of weak echoes. There are two types of secondary lobes: side lobes and grating lobes.

Side Lobes

Side lobes (Fig. 4-35), which are present with all transducers (single or multiple crystals), result from width and length mode vibrations (radial mode vibrations for circular and annular transducers), immediate reverberations at crystal-tissue interfaces, and interference phenomena. They are

typically of low intensity compared with the main beam (60 to 100 dB). A technique called apodization lowers their intensity for electronic arrays. Apodization employs a variable-strength voltage pulse to the crystals across the aperture during delay line focusing. The excitation voltage to the individual crystals of each segment is maximized at the center and reduced toward the periphery (Fig. 4-36). During reception the contribution to the overall signal from crystals located toward the outer edges of the aperture is also reduced.

Increasing the number of similar elements in the active area of an array (effectively creating a larger generating aperture) reduces the intensity of side lobes. When the side lobes are approximately 60 dB below the main beam intensity, no serious misregistration artifacts in the image are created. Clutter is still present, however, which influences sensitivity. High-frequency transducers reduce the number and intensity of the side lobes.

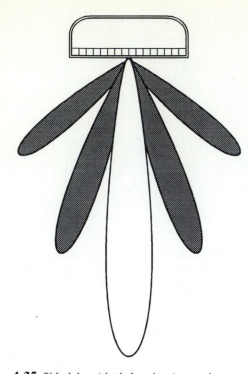

Figure 4-35 Side lobes (shaded regions) at various angles with respect to the main beam.

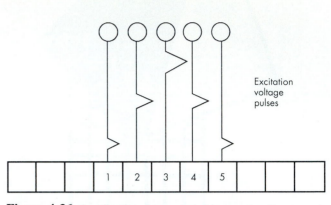

Excitation voltage pulses

Figure 4-36 Apodization demonstrated by varying the strength of the voltage pulse to each crystal (represented by different peak heights in a five-crystal segment). The highest voltage is applied to the center crystal.

Grating Lobes

Another significant secondary lobe problem unique to linear arrays is grating lobes, which are caused by the regular periodic spacing of elements within the array. Grating lobes create artifacts in the image by measuring the time of flight (distance) to an object located outside the main beam and placing the detected echo as if the interface were located along the ultrasound path of the main beam. All scanning units assume that the registered echoes travel in a straight line along the axial line of sight. If grating lobes are present (Fig. 4-37), artifacts appear closer to or farther behind the true position of the object depending on whether the grating lobe strikes the object before or after the main beam (Fig. 4-38). This occurs because the grating lobes are traveling at an angle to the main beam. These artifacts are very prominent at highly reflective interfaces (e.g., the diaphragm behind the liver).

The specific angular location of the grating lobes is given by the following formula:

4-4

$$\sin \phi = \frac{m\lambda}{x}$$

where ϕ is the grating lobe angle from the central axis, m an integer denoting order of the grating lobes (1, 2, 3, etc.), λ the wavelength, and x the center-to-center distance between adjacent array elements.

Equation 4-4 demonstrates that the only way to modify the grating lobes for a given frequency is to change the spacing distance (x). When this distance is decreased to less than one wavelength, the angle of the grating lobes becomes greater than 90 degrees with respect to the main beam and thus the grating lobes are eliminated.

Unfortunately, the elements of the array are always spaced greater than one wavelength from center to center; however, design engineers have found that the grating lobes can be reduced or eliminated by a technique called subdicing. In this technique, the normal element of an array is divided into many smaller subelements with the subelements electronically wired together to form the original-size element. The subdiced elements act in concert as a single crystal. This effectively reduces the center-to-center distance between elements and makes the grating lobes occur at an angle of greater than 90 degrees (Fig. 4-39).

Phased linear array systems have a more severe problem with grating lobes because the steering of an ultrasound beam increases the number and intensity of grating lobes as compared with the nonsteered beam from a stepdown segmental linear array (Fig. 4-40). The grating lobes are a result of the summation of side lobes from the individual crystals. When multiple crystals are pulsed for steering, low-intensity side lobes are added together and create significant secondary lobes of energy. Convex linear arrays partially eliminate grating lobes since the beam is not steered.

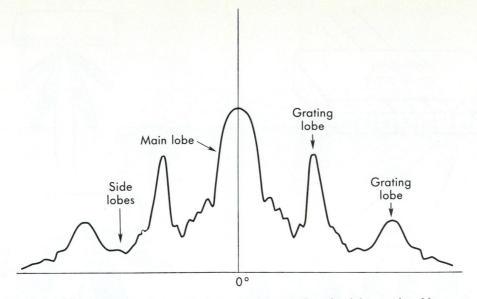

Figure 4-37 Main ultrasonic intensity lobe, side lobes, and grating lobes produced by a segmental linear array.

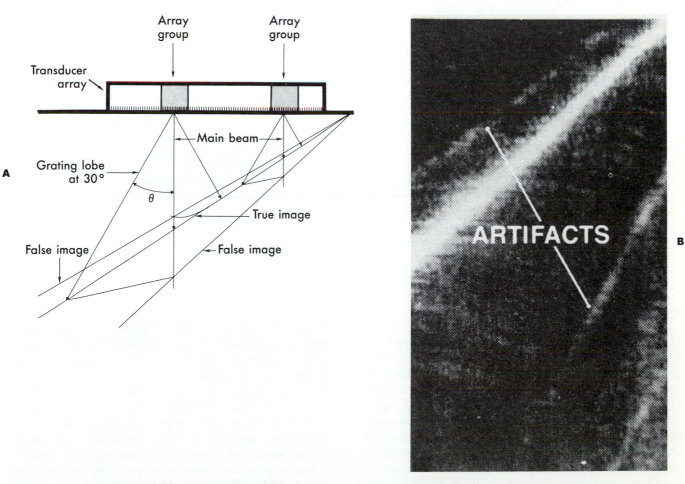

Figure 4-38 Grating lobe artifacts. **A,** Since the interface is at an angle to the main beam, two reflected echoes are produced that correspond to the grating lobes striking the interface before and after the main beam. **B,** The interface in three locations. Artifacts are indicated by *dots* at the ends of the *white line*.

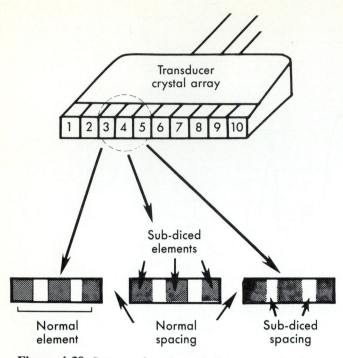

Figure 4-39 Cutaway of an electronic linear array showing the subdiced crystal elements.

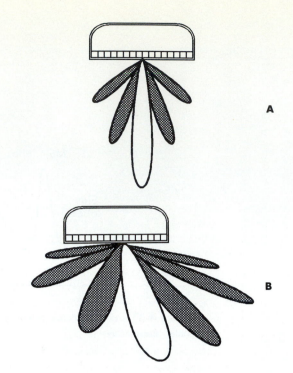

Figure 4-40 Comparison of grating lobes for a stepdown segmental linear array, **A**, and a linear phased array, **B**. The number and intensity of grating lobes are increased for the steered linear phased array.

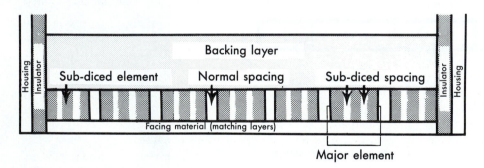

Figure 4-41 The linear array transducer. Note the matching layers, crystal elements, and backing material. When present, the focusing lens is placed between the matching layers and the crystals; or it may form part of the facing material.

Crystal Element Isolation

One additional problem with linear array systems that calls for consideration is interelement isolation, which is a measure of how one element of an array affects adjacent elements. When a voltage pulse excites one element, the other elements should not respond. The same holds true when a crystal receives an echo. No communication (cross-talk) should take place between a supposedly isolated crystal element and neighboring crystals. Electrical and mechanical coupling exists between the array elements and cannot be completely eliminated. The quality of real-time images deteriorates when the crystal elements are not electrically and mechanically isolated from each other. Fortunately, ways to reduce the effects of coupling have been developed.

The array elements are isolated electrically by separate ground wires and separate signal electrodes for each element (including subdiced elements). Nevertheless, the elements are not completely isolated electronically because they act as tiny capacitors (devices that store electrical charge). If the voltage changes in one crystal (due to an excitation or induced radiofrequency [RF] pulse from an echo), the neighboring crystals are affected because of the capacitance of the elements, although this effect can be made quite small.

Mechanical isolation is a much more difficult problem to overcome because the elements are mechanically coupled by the matching layers, focusing lenses, and backing material (Fig. 4-41). Even the housing itself, which is used for electrical and acoustic insulation, serves to couple the elements together. Return echoes pass through the matching layers and focusing lens before striking the crystal element to induce an RF signal. The return echoes are dispersed (similar to light from a cassette screen in radiology) and also strike the adjacent crystals; thus low-amplitude signals are induced in these elements.

Furthermore, crystals must be mechanically isolated to prevent cross-talk (ultrasound transfer between crystals). Air, as a spacing material, partially eliminates this coupling. Any sound produced by a crystal from length mode vibrations is reflected back into the crystal rather than transmitted to the adjacent crystals. An alternative method of isolating crystals is to design the width and length dimensions to be dramatically different from the thickness. If any width or length mode vibration does occur (Fig. 4-42), the vibration is at a different frequency from the center frequency of the transducer (which is caused by thickness mode vibration). The bandwidth of the receiver, normally sensitive to thickness mode frequencies, is adjusted (tuned) to be insensitive to the width and length mode frequencies. An aspect ratio (thickness/length or thickness/width) of 2:1 results in significant cross-talk reduction. As mentioned, total mechanical isolation cannot be achieved because the continuity of matching layers, lenses, and backing material extends over the array.

Other factors that influence the transducer design—the electromechanical coupling coefficient, the Q value, and the acoustic impedance—are discussed in Chapter 2. These factors also affect the performance of electronic real-time transducers.

SMALL-FOOTPRINT TRANSDUCERS

Linear phased arrays with small physical dimensions (miniature probes) are desirable for neonatal applications and small parts scanning. These transducers, however, have, by necessity, a limited area for assembling the piezoelectric elements. The size of their active radiating surface is their footprint.

Electronic focusing becomes suboptimal as scanning range is extended beyond a depth equal to twice the active length of the array. For an aperture of 14 × 8 mm, this corresponds to a depth of 28 mm. Miniature probes, because of their limited range, operate at high frequency (5 to 10 MHz) and have excellent axial resolution. Additional advantages of small-footprint transducers are their reduced weight and relatively wide field of view (90-degree sector format).

BROADBAND TRANSDUCERS

Composite piezoelectric materials have been formulated for lowering the acoustic impedance of the crystal. This design change, in combination with improved matching layer performance, has enabled pulses with higher-frequency components to be generated. The additional frequency components broaden the bandwidth (hence the name, broadband transducers). These transducer modifications result in a shortened pulse length for better axial resolution and higher conversion efficiencies for increased penetration.

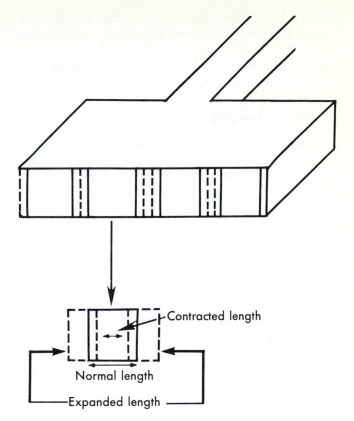

Figure 4-42 Length mode vibrations induce radiofrequency signals in adjacent crystals.

Improved axial resolution is obtained at a cost, however—a loss in lateral resolution. Broad bandwidth pulses contain low-frequency components that increase the focal beam width. A trade-off exists between axial resolution and lateral resolution. The scanning conditions dictate whether the low frequencies should be removed to enhance lateral resolution.

The frequency distribution of the transmitted pulse also affects the beam intensity pattern. High-frequency components tend to increase the intensity maximum in the focal zone and cause a rapid decrease of intensity with depth. The presence of low-frequency components extends the depth of penetration. Thus a trade-off also exists between axial resolution and depth of penetration.

An innovation made possible by broadband transducers is the manipulation of transmit frequency bandwidth and received frequency bandwidth to optimize image data acquisition. The specific adjustments depend on the desired information. High spatial detail at shallow depth can be obtained if the associated increase in beam width and lack of penetration can be tolerated. Improved lateral resolution and increased scanning range are possible if axial resolution is sacrificed.

Real-time units with limited bandwidth are designed by the manufacturer to make the necessary data collection compromises without user input (other than specification of type of examination). Broadband transducers provide flexibility in operation such that image acquisition parameters can be changed during scanning. As the frequency bandwidth becomes wider, the possibility of matching optimal image acquisition parameters with the desired clinical information is improved. Three approaches including multihertz imaging, confocal imaging, and high-definition imaging (HDI) have been implemented.

Multihertz Imaging

In multihertz imaging the available broad bandwidth is subdivided into two or more frequency ranges for transmission and reception of sound waves. The high-frequency portion provides good spatial detail. The low-frequency portion affords maximum tissue penetration. An intermediate-frequency bandwidth between these two extremes is also possible.

The outcome of multihertz imaging is the same as if two independent transducers, each with a different center frequency, were supplied within the same case. The distinct advantage is that one variable-frequency transducer views the patient's anatomy while the center frequency is adjusted. The optimal frequency range can be selected without losing the clinical point of interest in the scan plane.

Confocal Imaging

Confocal imaging is an extension of transmit-zone focusing, except that the focal zone at each depth is formed with a different center frequency. In this imaging scheme the available broad transmit bandwidth is split into multiple frequency ranges. Multiple small transmit bandwidths with different center frequencies are used to collect echo data along each line of sight. This technique provides a very narrow beam width with good spatial detail at all depths.

Since multiple transmit pulses are necessary for each line of sight, frame rate decreases unless additional measures are taken (high PRF, coprocessing). Rapid firing of the crystals causes echoes from different transmit pulses to be incident on the transducer simultaneously. This causes range ambiguity artifacts because each detected echo is assumed to come from the most recent transmit pulse. As described earlier in this chapter, coprocessing of the echo data can reduce range ambiguity artifacts and still allow high frame rates.

High-Definition Imaging

High-definition imaging uses the total transducer bandwidth for the transmitted pulse and then adjusts the receiver bandwidth to lower frequencies as deeper depths are sampled. Since tissue attenuation is frequency dependent (higher frequencies are absorbed more rapidly), a frequency shift occurs as the ultrasound wave propagates through tissue. The center frequency and bandwidth of the echo decrease as the depth increases. By continuously and automatically matching the receiver electronics with the frequency characteristics of the detected echo, HDI provides additional focusing at various depths and improved noise reduction. This technique of adjusting receiver bandwidth during scan line ac-

quisition is called harmonic imaging; it is applied also in multihertz and confocal imaging.

HDI can alter the transmitted bandwidth depending on the scanning range. High-frequency components may be eliminated to extend the depth of penetration. Lateral resolution at shallow depths is improved by removal of the low-frequency components.

Advantages

Broadband transducer technology is still evolving. Each approach offers significant improvement in image quality compared with that from conventional real-time instrumentation. HDI and multihertz methods probably provide superior gray scale contrast when tissue reflectivities are frequency dependent. Confocal imaging enhances spatial detail when tissue reflectivities are relatively independent of frequency.

ENDOSONOGRAPHY (TRANSONOGRAPHY)

The miniaturization of electronics and the refinement of real-time ultrasound transducers have led to the development of a very specialized area of medical diagnostic ultrasound scanning called endosonography or transonography. This type of scanning has also been referred to as PPI (plan-position indicator). Endosonography transducers, such as endovaginal, endorectal, and endoesophageal, are specially designed real-time mechanical, linear, or phased array transducers mounted on probes that can be inserted into various body cavities (even the sinuses).

Beam Steering and Focusing

Several transvaginal (endovaginal) probes are available in which a single, focused crystal (Fig. 4-43) is mounted at the end of the probe. This crystal is mechanically swept up and down to produce a 45- to 110-degree sagittal sector. By rotating and tilting the probe different planes are imaged, although transverse views are not possible. Other transvaginal probes, by mounting the crystal on the top (top-mounted) or side of the probe (side-mounted), are able to acquire transverse planes (Fig. 4-44). The plane of imaging is changed by moving the probe to a different depth. At least one mechanical system allows for collection of sagittal and transverse planes and all planes in between by attaching the crystal to a base that rotates over a 180-degree arc. The sonographer manually turns the base controls while the probe is in place to select the desired plane. The crystal is mechanically swept in an arc through the selected plane (Fig. 4-45). Fetal anatomy is often more clearly presented when transvaginal scanning is used to supplement the more traditional transabdominal scanning (Fig. 4-46).

Linear array and phased array endosonography transducers work in the same manner as the corresponding contact real-time transducers; they are just much smaller. Multiple lines of sight for each image are collected, either by me-

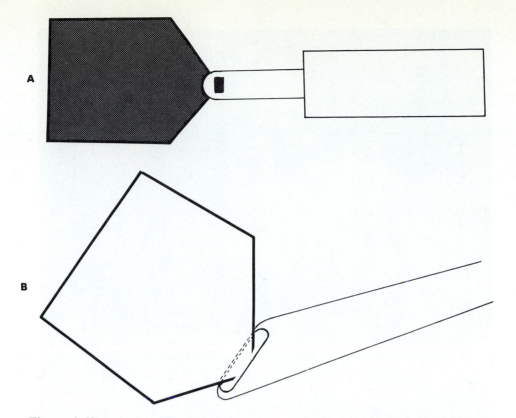

Figure 4-43 A, Endosonography transducer probe showing an end-mounted mechanically sectored crystal. The field of view *(shaded area)* points straight out from the probe that produces a sagittal plane. Other sagittal/coronal planes can be obtained by tilting and rotating the probe. **B,** A 15-degree tilted end-mounted probe.

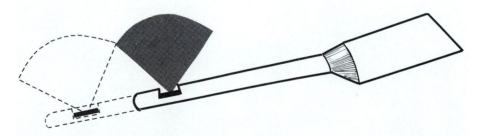

Figure 4-44 Endosonography transducer probe showing a side-mounted mechanically sectored crystal. Scan data are collected in the transverse plane *(shaded region)*. By moving the probe different transverse views are obtained *(dotted region)*.

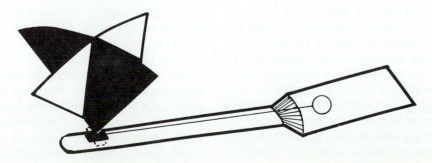

Figure 4-45 Endosonography transducer probe with a top-mounted mechanically sectored crystal. The crystal can be rotated through a 180-degree arc to allow transverse *(shaded)* or sagittal *(white)* planes to be collected.

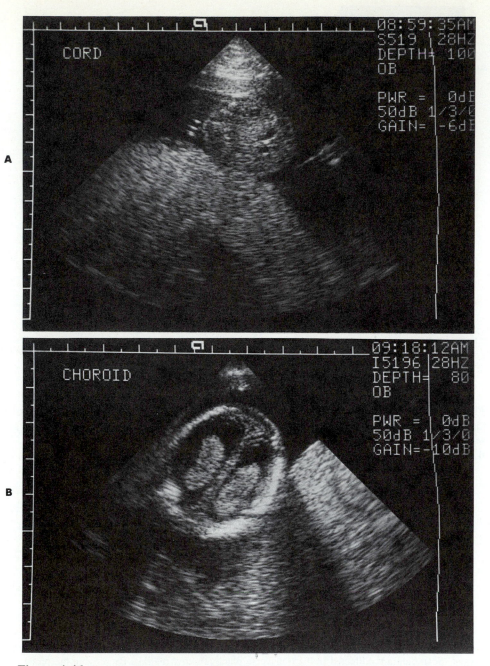

Figure 4-46 Sonogram of a fetus. **A,** Transabdominal scan. **B,** Transvaginal scan. Note the improved tissue contrast compared with sonogram in *A*.

chanically sweeping the beam back and forth or by electronically sweeping or steering the beam over the region of interest. Because the crystals are close to the tissues of interest, and there is thus minimal sampling depth, many lines of sight can be collected to improve the spatial mapping. The obvious necessity of keeping the transducer crystal(s) small creates problems in maintaining a narrow beam, but restricted sampling depth overcomes this difficulty.

Both electronic focusing and dynamic receive focusing are possible. High-frequency transducers are used to optimize axial and lateral resolution. By pulsing at very high PRFs rapid framing rates can be obtained, which is particularly valuable for transesophageal imaging of the heart. Scan data

from multiple planes are acquired throughout the area of interest by rotating or moving the probe within the body cavity. In some cases Doppler flow information is displayed with the real-time image.

Multiple arrays can be incorporated into the same probe so orthogonal planes are visualized without reorienting the probe. The dual-headed probes emit two frequencies for collecting two frequency-dependent images of a single plane. Multiple-frequency acquisitions may be of value for tissue characterization. Phased rectangular arrays steer and focus the ultrasound beam in any orientation for the scan plane desired. Coprocessing of the scan data provides a simultaneous display of multiple planes.

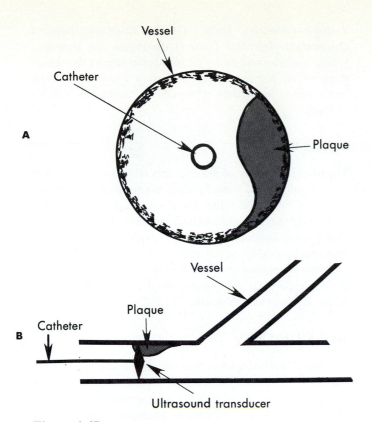

Figure 4-47 Transvascular probe placed in a vessel. **A,** Transverse view; **B,** Longitudinal view.

Scanning Techniques

During transrectal and transvaginal imaging the probe is normally covered with a plastic sheath or condom filled with water to enhance acoustic coupling. These probes have special attachments that are desirable for ultrasound-guided biopsy or amniocentesis. Intraoperative imaging, particularly for brain, liver, pancreas, and gallbladder procedures, is also possible. A special sterilization cover is placed over the probe for intraoperative scanning. Extremely high-detailed images are obtained intraoperatively, and puncture biopsies can be performed with precision using the endoprobes. Operator-controlled angle offsets of the mechanically moved crystal or electronic array are available to define the spatial relations between the anatomic structures of interest more accurately.

Transesophageal probes. Special endosonographic transducers for examination of the heart have been developed. These typically small electronic linear or phased arrays are inserted down the esophagus to acquire two-dimensional images of the heart. Mechanical sector probes are somewhat more difficult to construct with the small dimensions necessary for transesophageal applications. Because the transducer is close to the heart, high frequency, high line density, and high frame rates are achievable. Doppler capabilities can also be included in the probe. Special coupling devices (e.g., water-filled condoms) are not necessary because the esophagus tends to collapse

around the probe. Rectangular phased-array probes are also used to obtain multislice images of the heart in different planes.

Transluminal probes. The miniaturization of electronics and transducer arrays has led to the development of transvascular (transluminal) ultrasound transducers. This is one of the most exciting areas of advancement in instrumentation. Extremely small crystal arrays are mounted on the end of a catheter (Fig. 4-47) to inspect the interior of vessels visually for vascular plaques. These transducers, which operate at 10 to 20 MHz, produce very high-detail images that aid in the placement of balloons for plaque reduction or laser obliteration. Such probes should prove valuable in echocardiology for assessing valves and cardiac vessels, particularly in postinfarction procedures. Placement of catheters through the umbilical cord to the fetal heart may prove invaluable in fetal cardiology. Transluminal probes are also inserted into the fallopian tubes to evaluate the status of a fertilized oocyte.

NONCONVENTIONAL REAL-TIME SYSTEMS

A discussion of real-time instrumentation would not be complete without mentioning quasi—real-time imaging systems. These systems produce images at very low frame rates (typically three to four images per second). Each image is displayed on the output device until updated by the next image. In addition, the systems produce higher-resolution images (more lines of sight) than conventional real-time instruments do. Furthermore, some systems average multiple frames together to improve the image quality by decreasing the variation of detected echoes (signal-to-noise ratio is larger). The temporal solution of these instruments is poor, however.

Ultrafast scanning systems are being developed that acquire and display all scan lines simultaneously in parallel rather than in conventional line-by-line serial fashion. The complex circuitry necessary to parallel-process the scan information is partially eliminated by using optical methods. Several such units are currently being tested.

Ultrasound microscopy is a potential diagnostic tool for surgical biopsies, yielding a very fast response time. The involved tissue preparation required for light microscopy is eliminated. Reflection or transmission ultrasound systems that operate from 30 MHz to 1 gigahertz (GHz) provide high-detail images, similar to light microscopy.

THREE-DIMENSIONAL IMAGING

One major problem associated with 2D real-time imaging is that the small field of view inhibits the presentation of neighboring anatomy. Clinical interpretation of examination results as multiple two-dimensional images is difficult. To solve this problem, three-dimensional ultrasound imaging has been developed that shows tomographic spatial relationships and expands the field of view.

Two-Dimensional Serial Scanning

In one approach the three-dimensional images or multiplanar views are reconstructed from a series of 2D scans through a process similar to the 3D work that has been done in x-ray CT during the past several years. A linear-array transducer is mounted on a mechanical apparatus that translates it in one direction across the imaging volume. Multiple scan planes perpendicular to the plane of motion are collected. Several seconds are required to accumulate the scan data. Real-time imaging is forfeited, and moving interfaces become problematical. Uneven body surfaces also present difficulties.

The pixels in each 2D scan are configured into a 3D data set that can be manipulated for display on a workstation. A workstation is a minicomputer with graphics capability. Data processing is performed off line (separated in time from scan data acquisition). Extensive storage capacity, large computer memory, and fast computer processing are required to display the 3D data in a reasonable response time.

Volume Scanning

A second approach to acquiring tomographic information is to construct a scanning system that sweeps the ultrasound beam throughout the tissue volume by rotating the scanhead. Transducers of this type are called volumetric transducers. Mechanically driven annular-array systems have been developed for this purpose. The imaging volume is conical with an angle of 60 to 70 degrees. Sensors mounted on the transducer register position and orientation and are capable of detecting small positional (0.5 mm) and angular (0.5 degree) changes in movement of the annular array. Scan data can be collected in 5 seconds for one 3D image and updated as rapidly for real-time imaging.

One major drawback of this 3D imaging method, however, is the lack of orthogonal scan planes. Reconstruction of scan data sets into the 3D display is more abstruse than the methods used for CT or MRI. High-speed computer systems are required.

Rectangular Arrays

A third approach is to use a rectangular-array transducer. Ultrasound beam sampling direction is electronically controlled with the appropriate crystal-firing sequence. Coprocessing is necessary to achieve clinically applicable frame rates. Matrix arrays offer the potential for data collection in orthogonal planes. A prototype for 3D color cardiac imaging is currently undergoing testing.

Limitations

Ultrasound and 3D imaging must overcome slow frame rates and relatively long computation times because of large data sets. The latter problem will be solved as the current capabilities of computers are expanded. A more subtle difficulty is that the relationship between the echo-induced signal amplitude and the physical situation is not well defined by a single parameter. Unlike CT, in which one physical characteristic (electron density) determines the measured value, in ultrasound many factors contribute to the reflectivity of an interface. The lack of a common unifying factor makes some data manipulation techniques difficult to apply.

Virtual Reality

The ultimate display of 3D data sets will most likely adopt the methodology of virtual reality, the simulated immersion of an observer within the displayed image. The viewer's point of reference becomes a location within the image rather than a point outside the image as with computer graphic displays. Special headgear with a TV projection system for each eye is required. As the observer's head turns, the TV projection for each eye changes and a different presentation of the 3D image is obtained.

HOLOGRAPHY

Another area of interest is three-dimensional ultrasonic holography. A nonfocused plane ultrasound wave with a frequency between 2 and 5 MHz is transmitted through the region of interest and collected on a holographic plate. When the plate is interrogated with visible light, an image of the transmitted sound beam is formed. Images are displayed in real time. The frequency of the ultrasound wave sets the theoretical limit of resolution. Tubular structures (e.g., tendons and veins of the extremities, which cannot normally be seen in conventional ultrasound) are visualized.

IMAGE QUALITY

Image quality is a combination of interrelated factors. The parameters that describe it include axial resolution, lateral resolution, sharpness, contrast resolution, artifacts, distortion, noise, and temporal resolution. Axial and lateral resolution has been discussed previously. Consistent spatial resolution is desirable throughout the field of view. Individual pixels and scan lines should not be descernible to the viewer. Sharpness describes the ability of the scanner to reproduce tissue boundaries and, consequently, is closely related to spatial resolution. Contrast resolution is the minimum difference in signal strengths from adjacent structures that allows the observer to perceive the structures as separate entities. Artifacts are structures in the image that do not represent the scanned objects (see Chapter 14 for a more complete discussion of image artifacts).

Distortion is a parameter describing the lack of adherence to original geometric relationships. Size, shape, and relative positions of objects within the scan plane should be accurately portrayed by corresponding structures in the image.

The variation in signal level contributed by noise causes brightness fluctuations in the 2D image. Noise originates from both electrical and acoustic sources. Acoustic noise is defined as echo-induced signals that do not correspond to structures along the main beam sampling path. Clutter and speckle are types of acoustic noise. A common example of the effect of noise is snow in the television picture received from a distant station (now virtually nonexistent with the advent of cable transmission). Noise masks the signals from weak echoes and inhibits low contrast resolution. A low noise sonogram is one in which liquid-filled structures exhibit no signal.

Temporal resolution refers to the ability to observe moving tissue along the path of motion. Sampling must occur at frequent intervals during the motion. Thus the frame rate required to visualize a moving object without blurring depends on the speed of the object.

REAL-TIME SYSTEM DESIGN

The following discussion is based on the published work of P.N.T. Wells and his colleagues. The reader is directed to the references at the end of this chapter for a more complete analysis.

Imaging performance is ultimately limited by technical considerations and the manner in which ultrasound is propagated through tissue. Physical properties of the tissue of concern include velocity, attenuation, scattering, inhomogeneity, nonlinearity, and motion. Based on the clinical application system designers attempt to optimize imaging performance within the constraints imposed by these physical properties.

The first consideration is the range of the field of view. The time of travel to the maximum depth of penetration and return imposes a limit on the maximum PRF. The PRF establishes the number of lines of sight per second that can be acquired. Each frame consists of a certain number of lines of sight, which once set imposes a limit on the maximum frame rate. Recall that the PRF is equal to the product of the frame rate and the number of lines per frame.

Detectability of small objects improves as the separation between scan lines decreases. The line density is controlled by the number of lines per frame, the width of the field of view, and the scan format. The useful line density is restricted to what can be accommodated by the display monitor. Typically the trade-off between frame rate and line density is balanced by selecting the lowest frame rate compatible with the clinical application so line density can be maximized. At a minimum, line density should be one line per millimeter in the linear format and one line per degree in the sector format. The velocity of ultrasound limits the lateral resolution and temporal resolution.

Axial resolution improves as frequency is increased. The rate of attenuation, however, increases in direct proportion to the frequency. Once the scanning range is established, the highest frequency compatible with that depth is used. The ability to detect weak echoes from deep-lying structures also depends on noise. As an approximation, modern real-time scanners are capable of a penetration depth equal to 400 wavelengths (corresponding to 4 MHz for 15 cm).

Backscattering is responsible for the fine texture pattern in soft tissue and blood. This interaction is enhanced at high frequencies; but beyond an upper boundary of frequency, attenuation by intervening tissue decreases the returning echo intensity to an unacceptably low level. Again, the highest frequency compatible with the scanning depth should be used.

Physical properties of tissue are often anisotropic. *Inhomogeneity* refers to the dependence of velocity and attenuation on the direction of sound wave propagation in tissue. A different rate of travel during the positive-pressure half cycle from that during the negative-pressure half cycle is classified as nonlinear propagation. The sinusoidal waveform is converted to a sawtooth waveform, which experiences more rapid attenuation. Nonlinear propagation is likely to occur at high intensity levels. Increased acoustic output, neglecting safety considerations, does not have unlimited potential to improve sensitivity. Both inhomogeneity and nonlinearity distort the beam pattern, causing a loss in spatial resolution and contrast resolution.

OPERATOR CONTROLS

Several operator-adjustable controls are available to optimize the two-dimensional image. The most important instrument settings are depth, transmit power, gain, TGC, transmit zone, log compression, and persistence. Preprocessing and postprocessing manipulation of the scan data may also be selected (as discussed in Chapter 10). The type of transducer (linear array, convex array, linear phased array, annular phased array, sector) and the center frequency influence image quality.

The depth control sets the maximum range of the field of view (Fig. 4-48). It also influences the frame rate and line density. These parameters, not typically under direct operator control, are the result of an array of instrument settings.

The power control adjusts the intensity of the ultrasound beam transmitted into the patient. Power levels are commonly expressed in decibels (e.g., 0 dB corresponds to the maximum level, and -9 dB to the minimum). Increased intensity improves the signal to noise ratio (SNR) and enhances sensitivity (weak reflectors can be observed as shown in Figure 4-49). On many scanners a change in the power setting is accompanied by an automatic commensurate adjustment of the gain so the overall image brightness remains constant.

Receiver gain modifies the amplification of signals during signal processing and often is expressed in decibels. TGC is also a type of receiver gain that is varied according to time delay (or depth). TGC must be readjusted when the depth of scanning is changed. The SNR is unchanged by gain. Consequently, gain is used to establish the proper brightness level for echoes of varying strength, but it cannot improve contrast resolution.

The transmit zone selection control adjusts the depth of focusing. Variable transmit zones allow the operator to designate a region within the field of view where enhanced axial resolution is desired. Multiple-transmit focal regions may improve the axial resolution throughout the field of view; however, the frame rate will be reduced unless coprocessing is used (Fig. 4-50).

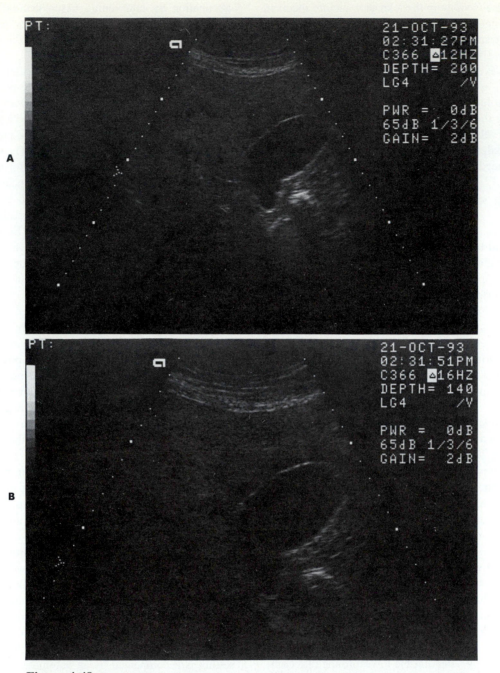

Figure 4-48 Depth control allows adjustment of the scanning range in the acquisition of a sonogram of the gallbladder. **A,** Depth of 20 cm. **B,** Depth of 14 cm.

Log compression is a form of thresholding that alters the dynamic range for the display of signals. Thresholding, by accepting signals greater than a prescribed amplitude, rejects low-amplitude noise. In some circumstances (e.g., a high-reflectivity object located off axis) noise exceeds the threshold value and contributes to the image. Echo strength can vary over several orders of magnitude. Log compression limits the display dynamic range, so the weakest echoes are not depicted in the image. For example, changing log compression to a lower decibel setting removes weak echoes and noise (Fig. 4-51). Improper setting of log compression can prevent visualization of small low-contrast structures.

Persistence is a noise-reduction technique that applies temporal averaging to individual pixels. The operator selects the number of frames during which an average is obtained. Variations in noise at each pixel location tend to offset each another with time, whereas echo-induced signals tend to be reinforced. Fast-moving objects become blurred in the image when persistence is increased.

Real-time imaging depicts motion of moving interfaces, which is lost during freeze-frame display of one real-time image. The cine loop function or video-taping of acquired

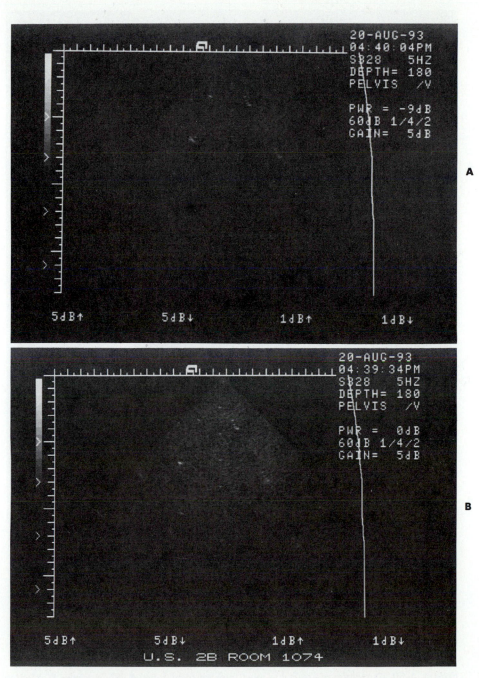

Figure 4-49 Effect of power setting. **A,** Low power. **B,** High power.

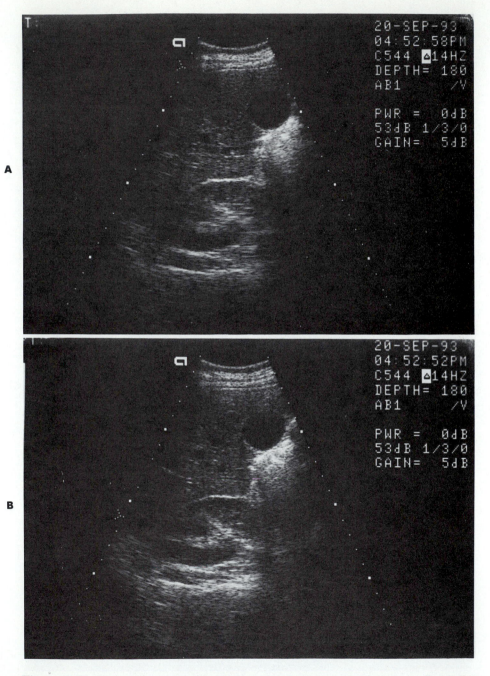

Figure 4-50 Illustration of selectable fixed transmit focal zone. **A,** Short focus. **B,** Medium focus. **C,** Multi-zone focus.

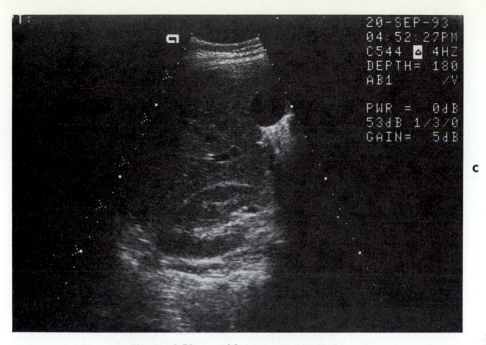

Figure 4-50, cont'd C, Multi-zone focus.

Figure 4-51 Effect of log compression. **A,** Wide dynamic range.

Continued.

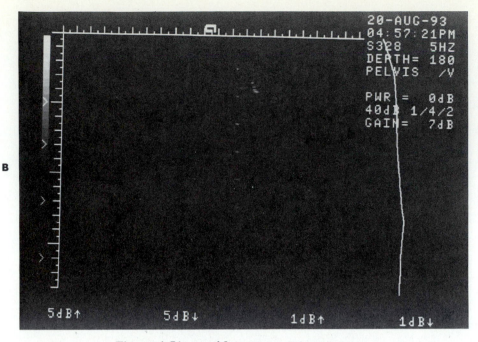

Figure 4-51, cont'd B, Reduced dynamic range.

images allows the operator to review the dynamic relationships. Many frames (150 or more) (corresponding to an acquisition time of several seconds) can be stored in computer memory for immediate playback using the cine loop function. The rate of playback can be adjusted to either coincide with or deviate from the real-time acquisition rate. The slow-motion review capability allows the sonographer to select an appropriate image for study as well as hardcopy recording, if desired.

The reflectivity of small particles is frequency dependent. Thus, transducer frequency can affect contrast in the real-time image. Lesion detectability is sometimes improved by changing transducer frequency.

TISSUE CHARACTERIZATION

Tissue characterization is the identification of tissue type by noninvasive means (e.g., by ultrasonic measurements or imaging). The goal is to obtain a specific pathological diagnosis rather than the more general recognition that an abnormality exists. Five approaches are possible. These include sonogram pattern recognition, signal processing of echoes, specialized measurements of acoustic properties, perfusion pattern recognition, and the introduction of contrast agents.

Certain disease states produce an image with distinctive features. The most important clinical application of pattern recognition is the differentiation between cysts and solid masses. Cystic structures are categorized by having smooth well-defined boundaries, low echogenicity of the liquid contents, no internal echoes, and low attenuation (indicated by signal enhancement distal to the cyst). Distinguishing benign and malignant solid mass lesions is less reliable.

Another method assumes that the returning echoes contain information that if correctly manipulated by signal pro-

cessing would indicate differences in tissue type. High echogenicity of organ parenchyma may be indicative of disease but is nonspecific.

Quantitative methods have been used to evaluate various acoustic properties—including attenuation, speed of sound, acoustic impedance, scattering, tissue motion, and nonlinearity of propagation. None of these properties, however, is sufficiently dissimilar among different tissues to allow tissue characterization.

Vascularization of malignant tumors may have distinctive features. Solid tumors apparently release substances that stimulate new vessel formation. The morphology of the tumor vessels is abnormal: The vessels lack muscular walls and consequently offer low resistance to flow; additionally, vascular pooling occurs in dilated regions. Perfusion detected by Doppler ultrasound may allow features of blood flow in these lesions (high diastolic flow, high velocity, and pooling in areas of dilation) to be characterized. (Doppler instrumentation is discussed in Chapters 6 and 7.)

Contrast agents offer potential for differentiation of tissue types. Applications of contrast agents are discussed in the following section.

CONTRAST AGENTS

The purpose of contrast agents in ultrasound is to improve image quality by introducing a change in the acoustic properties (backscatter, attenuation, or speed of sound) of tissues in which the material resides.

Generally, contrast is enhanced by the increased reflectivity of selected tissues—whether normal tissue, blood pool, or lesion—depending on the biodistribution of the agent. Attenuation effects are subtle, but they can be inferred by observing enhanced or diminished beam penetration distal to the localized material. Speed of sound shifts is not discernible in real-time images. Specialized equipment is required to measure the changes.

Another application of contrast agents is to improve transmission of the ultrasonic beam along the line of sight. Displacement of air from the ultrasound beam path (e.g., in the gastrointestinal tract) increases sound transmission to the underlying structures.

Contrast agents must demonstrate preferential tissue uptake, stability during examination, low toxicity, and safe elimination through a biological or metabolic pathway. Types include free gas bubbles, encapsulated gas bubbles, particulates (colloidal suspensions), emulsions, and aqueous solutions.

1. Free gas bubbles may preexist in a liquid or may be produced by rapid injection of a liquid through a narrow passage. They are excellent scatterers of sound energy, with low toxicity, but are removed by the lungs. Localization in soft tissue following venous injection is not possible with them. Applications are limited to intraarterial injection for imaging parts of the cardiovascular system and to direct injection into the bile ducts.

2. Encapsulated gas bubbles are air-filled microspheres with a thin outer chemical coating. The introduction of an air interface increases the echogenicity of the tissue in which the contrast resides. Backscatter depends on the size and concentration of the microbubbles as well as on the imaging frequency. Bubble size is typically a few microns in diameter; thus the lung capillaries can be safely crossed for systemic distribution following intravenous injection. The composition of the coating is varied to alter the distribution of gas-filled microbubbles (tissue specificity).

   Air-filled albumin microspheres are used as a blood pool agent in echocardiography to increase the reflectivity of the right and left chambers of the heart. Left ventricular border definition and wall motion visualization are improved. The microspheres also improve evaluation of both flow dynamics within the ventricular cavity and valvular regurgitation. As a vascular agent the microbubbles adhere to thrombi, facilitating the diagnosis of venous disease. Infertility in women can be assessed with these agents (i.e., contrast-enhanced sonohysterosalpingography).

   Galactose stabilized by free fatty acids is also used to encapsulate gas bubbles. This contrast agent has vascular applications—including visualization of small vessels in the pancreas, kidney, and liver, evaluation of tumor vascularity, and assessment of peripheral vascular disease.

3. Small particles, approximately 1 μm in diameter, of iodipamide ethyl ester accumulate in the reticuloendothelial system, particularly the Kupffer cells of the liver. Liver metastases, however, do not capture this contrast agent since tumors lack Kupffer cells. The high mass density of iodipamide produces increased backscatter according to the concentration of these particles in the liver. Contrast between liver parenchyma and the lesion can be enhanced. Iodipamide is eliminated within 2 days.

4. Perflubron emulsion is a brominated fluorocarbon in lecithin that persists in the blood for many hours after intravenous injection and is slowly taken up by the liver and spleen. Patients with hepatic metastases have shown increased tumor echogenicity following administration of this agent.

5. Buffered sodium citrate and calcium disodium ethylenediaminetetraacetic acid (EDTA) exhibit higher acoustic impedance as molar concentration is increased. These materials have been proposed to create transiently enhanced tissue backscatter in highly vascularized organs like the kidney. Compared with encapsulated gas bubbles, however, aqueous solutions are poor scatterers and a large target volume is necessary to produce an observable effect.

Imaging of the abdomen is often compromised by shadowing from gas in the adjacent and overlying bowel. The acoustic impedance mismatch, as well as differences in acoustic velocity between soft tissue and gas, causes a loss of ultrasound intensity and various image artifacts. The displacement of bowel gas by an orally administered gastrointestinal contrast agent creates an acoustic window for improved visualization of the stomach and duodenum. Potential gastrointestinal contrast agents must have low toxicity, mild side effects, adequate bulk, and appropriate surface tension (cohesiveness). Studies have reported that cellulose-based suspensions allow distinct bowel wall layers in the body and antrum of the stomach and in the duodenum to be visualized. Cellulose does not induce gallbladder contraction or excessive gas formation.

SUMMARY

In the early and mid-1970s static B-mode gray-scale imaging was the dominant scanning mode used in medical diagnostic ultrasound. Since the late 1970s the development of real-time imaging has progressed so quickly that most institutions currently perform imaging studies with only real-time ultrasound scanners. Contrast resolution (gray-scale mapping of the acoustic properties of individual tissues) has been improved by more precise in-plane and out-of-plane focusing of the ultrasound beam, reduced contributions from side lobes and grating lobes, diminished cross-talk between crystals, more uniform matched performance of crystals in arrays, and greater sensitivity.

Advances in real-time instrumentation (greater variety of transducers, broadband frequency response, reduced transducer size, and increased signal-to-noise ratio) have made ultrasound one of the fastest growing and most exciting areas of diagnostic imaging, and its clinical utility is expanding rapidly. A major advantage of real-time ultrsound, other than the obvious one of improved temporal resolution, has been the ability to combine M-mode and Doppler with imaging. In addition, recently developed specialized transducers for endosonography have created new diagnostic applications.

Contrast agents have improved image quality by altering selected tissue echogenicity. Three-dimensional imaging provides tomographic presentation of the scanned volume.

REVIEW QUESTIONS

1. Real-time imaging provides excellent temporal resolution of motion.
   a. True
   b. False
2. Real-time imaging allows multiple lines of sight for each image and multiple images to be collected each second.
   a. True
   b. False
3. The maximum frame rate in real-time imaging is directly proportional to the depth of interest.
   a. True
   b. False
4. The maximum frame rate is directly proportional to the velocity of sound in the medium.
   a. True
   b. False
5. The maximum frame rate is indirectly proportional to the number of lines of sight for each image.
   a. True
   b. False
6. The maximum frame rate is reduced if the number of fixed transmit focal zones is increased in the absence of coprocessing.
   a. True
   b. False
7. Lateral resolution of the real-time image is not dependent on the number of lines of sight.
   a. True
   b. False
8. Changing the scanning depth from 10 to 15 cm increases the maximum frame rate.
   a. True
   b. False
9. A registration arm is required for real-time imaging systems.
   a. True
   b. False
10. What are the two major classes of real-time imaging systems?
    a. Mechanical, electronic
    b. Electronic, contact
    c. Mechanical, sector
    d. Water path, offset
11. Liquid-path systems allow a higher frame rate compared with nonliquid-path systems.
    a. True
    b. False
12. If the scanning range is reduced by a factor of 2 and the lines of sight is increased by a factor of 2, what is the effect on the maximum frame rate?
    a. Increased
    b. Decreased
    c. Unchanged
13. Electronic linear array real-time systems mechanically focus the beam in the width direction (out-of-plane or slice thickness direction).
    a. True
    b. False
14. The mechanical motion of mechanical real-time units generally prohibits very high-frame rates (i.e., greater than 40 fps).
    a. True
    b. False
15. Electronic linear phased array systems are electronically steered across the region of interest.
    a. True
    b. False
16. The collection time for each line of sight for a real-time transducer, whether mechanical or electronic, depends on the time needed for the ultrasound pulse to travel to the maximum scanning depth and return to the transducer (time of flight).
    a. True
    b. False
17. Multiple crystals are excited simultaneously in a segmental linear array to improve the image quality by producing an effective wider aperture to extend the near field depth.
    a. True
    b. False
18. Effective in-plane (length) focusing of the ultrasound beam for a linear array is accomplished by the use of _____ and _____ .
    a. Mechanical focusing
    b. Delay lines
    c. Changing beam aperture
    d. a and c
    e. b and c
19. Dynamic focusing normally refers to _____ .
    a. Transmit focusing
    b. Receive focusing
    c. Transmit and receive focusing
    d. None of the above
20. Coprocessing uses multiple ultrasound beams with different focal zones to acquire multiple lines of sight simultaneously.
    a. True
    b. False
21. Microsecond time delays are necessary for electronic focusing and phased array steering.
    a. True
    b. False
22. Phased rectangular array transducers are steered and focused in _____ dimension(s).
    a. One
    b. Two
    c. Three
23. Annular arrays are electronically steered to sample along different lines of sight.
    a. True
    b. False
24. Compound linear arrays are steered to expand the field of view.
    a. True
    b. False
25. Convex arrays enlarge the field of view beyond the physical length of the crystal array.
    a. True
    b. False
26. Side lobes and grating lobes do not create artifacts in the image.
    a. True
    b. False
27. Crystals in arrays can be totally mechanically and electronically isolated to prevent cross-talk.
    a. True
    b. False

28. Endosonography probes have small transducers mounted on the probe that can be placed within body cavities.
    a. True
    b. False
29. During echo reception what methods are used to provide focusing?
    a. Delay lines
    b. Changing aperture
    c. Apodization
    d. All of the above
30. Real-time imaging systems have been nearly totally replaced with static imaging systems.
    a. True
    b. False
31. Dynamic receive focusing decreases the frame rate.
    a. True
    b. False
32. What is the maximum frame rate when a single crystal real-time system produces one line of sight per frame? Assume the depth of interest is 15 cm.
    a. 50 fps
    b. 100 fps
    c. 3000 fps
    d. 7000 fps
    e. None of the above
33. Calculate the maximum frame rate if the scanning range is 15 cm and 120 lines compose each frame.
34. Consider a sequential linear array with 100 crystals. How much time is required to form one image if the depth of interest is 10 cm?
    a. 13 μs
    b. 130 μs
    c. 1300 μs
    d. 13 ms
    e. None of the above
35. What is the maximum frame rate for a stepdown segmental curved linear array producing 100 lines of sight with 5 fixed transmit focal zones? Assume the depth of interest to be 10 cm.
    a. 15 fps
    b. 77 fps
    c. 1500 fps
    d. 7700 fps
    e. None of the above
36. Calculate the f-number for a focal length of 5 cm using an aperture 3 cm in length.

BIBLIOGRAPHY

Barnhart J, Levene H, Villapando E, et al: Characteristics of Albunex: air-filled albumin microspheres for echocardiography contrast enhancement, *Invest Radiol* 25:S162, 1990.

Behan M, O'Connell D, Mattrey RF, Carney DN: Perfluorooctylbromide as a contrast agent for CT and sonography: preliminary results, *AJR* 160:399, 1993.

Bom N: Technology of real-time ultrasound. II, *Contrib Gynecol Obstet* 6(2):11, 1979.

Bushong SC: *Radiologic science for technologists: physics, biology, and protection*, ed 5, St Louis, 1993, Mosby.

Curry TS III, Dowdey JE, Murry RC Jr. *Christensen's Introduction to the physics of diagnostic radiology*, ed 4, Philadelphia, 1990, Lea & Febiger.

d'Agincourt L: Transvaginal mode can help detect ovarian cancer. *Diagn Imaging* 9:40, 1987.

d'Agincourt L: Contrast media enhance ultrasound echogenicity, *Diagn Imaging* 15:77, 1993.

Dakins DR: Virtual reality redefines the meaning of real time imaging, *Diagn Imaging* 14:77, 1992.

Fleischer AC: Prostatic endosonography: a potential screening test, *Diagn Imaging* 9:78, 1987.

Goldstein A: Ultrasound devices open new diagnostic avenues, *Diagn Imaging* 11:157, 1989.

Goldstein A: Evaluating image quality in high-res ultrasound, *Diagn Imaging* 13:89, 1991.

Goldstein A: Broadband transducers improve image quality, *Diagn Imaging* 15:89, 1993.

Harris RA, Follett DH, Halliwell M, Wells PNT: Ultimate limits in ultrasonic imaging resolution, *Ultrasound Med Biol* 17:547, 1991.

Hendee WR, Ritenour ER: *Medical imaging physics*, ed 3, St Louis, 1992, Mosby.

Hedrick WR, Hykes DL: A simplified explanation of Fourier analysis, *J Diagn Med Sonog* 8:299, 1992.

Hykes DL, Hedrick WR: Real time ultrasound instrumentation: an update, *J Diagn Med Sonog* 6:257, 1990.

Jones-Bey H: Ultrasound lights path for invasive therapies, *Diagn Imaging* 14:101, 1992.

Kossoff G: Technology of real-time ultrasound. I, *Contrib Gynecol Obstet* 6(2):2, 1979.

Kremkau FW: *Diagnostic ultrasonics: physical principles and exercises*, ed 3, Philadelphia, 1988, WB Saunders.

Kremkau FW: Clinical benefit of higher acoustic output levels, *Ultrasound Med Biol* 15(suppl 1):69, 1989.

Lees WA: 3D ultrasound images optimize fetal review, *Diagn Imaging* 14:69, 1992.

Lund PJ, Fritz TA, Unger EC, et al: Cellulose as a gastrointestinal US contrast agent, *Radiology* 185:783, 1992.

Mattrey RF: Sonographic enhancement of Doppler signals and perfused tissues with perfluorooctylbromide, *Invest Radiol* 25:S158, 1990.

McDicken WN: *Diagnostic ultrasonics: principles and use of instruments*, ed 3, Edinburgh, 1991, Churchill Livingstone.

Mendelson EB, Bohm-Velez M: Transvaginal sonography assesses early pregnancy, *Diagn Imaging* 9:244, 1987.

Ophir J, Parker KJ: Contrast agents in diagnostic ultrasound, *Ultrasound Med Biol* 15:319, 1989.

Powis RL: *Physics for the fun of it*, Denver, 1978, Unirad Corporation.

Stephenson G, Freiherr G: 3D imaging comes to diagnostic ultrasound, *Diagn Imaging* 12:65, 1990.

Taylor KJW, Wells PNT: Tissue characterization, *Ultrasound Med Biol* 15:421, 1989.

Timor-Tritsch IE: High-frequency probes and transvaginal sonography, *Diagn Imaging* 9:98, 1987.

Violante MR, Parker K, Lerner R: Particulate contrast agents for improved ultrasound detection of liver metastases, *Invest Radiol* 25:S165, 1990.

Wells PNT: *Physical principles of ultrasonic diagnosis*, New York, 1969, Academic Press.

Wells PNT: *Biomedical ultrasonic*, New York, 1977, Academic Press.

Wells PNT, Harris RA, Halliwell M: The envelope that tissue imposes on achievable ultrasonic imaging, *J Ultrasound Med* 11:433, 1992.

Wells PNT, Ziskin MC (eds): New techniques and instrumentation in ultrasonography, *Clin Diagn Ultrasound*, vol 5, 1980.

Winsberg F: Real-time scanners: a review, *Med Ultrasonography* 3:99, 1979.

Hemodynamics

Bernoulli's principle
Eddy flow
Hydrostatic pressure
Inertia loss
Laminar flow
Poiseuille's equation

Pressure difference
Stenosis
Turbulence
Velocity profile
Viscosity
Volume flow rate

Doppler ultrasound detects blood flow in vessels. Flow patterns in normal vessels are extremely complex and vary with anatomical location, time within the heart cycle, and exercise. Pathological conditions create more diversity in flow patterns. Before Doppler physics and instrumentation is discussed, basic concepts of hemodynamics will be introduced.

Hemodynamics is the study of the physical principles of blood circulation. Blood is a viscous fluid consisting of cells and plasma. Viscosity is the physical parameter that characterizes a fluid's ability to resist a change in its shape. For a viscous fluid to be deformed, strong intermolecular attractions must be overcome. When pressure is applied to blood in a vessel, the blood is propelled through the vessel by a pressure drop along its path. Resistance to flow depends on the viscosity of the blood and the radius of the vessel lumen. Frictional forces caused by the viscosity of the blood produce variations in velocity across the vessel lumen.

The major cellular component of blood is the erythrocyte or red blood cell (RBC). Normal RBCs are biconcave disks with a diameter of approximately 7 μm and a thickness ranging from 2 μm at the edge to 1 μm in the center. The viscosity of blood at normal hematocrit is 0.03 poise or dynes-s/cm^2, a value approximately four times the viscosity of water. With an increased concentration of RBCs the viscosity becomes greater.

VELOCITY PROFILE

The velocity of blood movement is not uniform across the vessel lumen. When a fluid moves through a long smooth cylindrical tube at a steady rate, concentric layers of fluid flow are formed within the tube. Each layer remains a fixed distance from the tube wall and does not mix with adjacent layers. Friction between the layers alters the velocity. The velocity is not the same in every layer but progressively increases as the distance from the wall increases. The distribution of flow velocities into layers is called laminar flow. Blood often exhibits laminar flow in vessels that are straight and smooth.

Viscous friction between blood and vessel wall causes lowest velocities to occur along the wall. The highest velocities are in the central portion of the vessel. Figure 5-1 depicts the velocity as a function of position through the cross section of a vessel with laminar flow. If the velocity distribution exhibits a wall distance–squared dependence, the velocity profile is described as parabolic. For a parabolic velocity profile the average velocity throughout the lumen is equal to half the maximum velocity.

PRESSURE/FLOW RELATIONSHIP

Poiseuille's Equation

Volume flow rate (Q) is the quantity of blood moving through the vessel per unit of time, usually expressed in cubic centimeters per second. Poiseuille's equation predicts volume flow in a cylindrical vessel:

5-1

$$Q = \frac{\pi p r^4}{8 \, l \eta}$$

where l is the length of the vessel, η the viscosity, p the pressure difference between the ends of the vessel, r the radius of the vessel, and π a constant (value 3.14). Typically the viscosity of blood and the length of vessels in the cardiovascular system do not vary. Flow is regulated by changes in the pressure difference or radius. The dependence of flow on the fourth power of the radius makes small vessels highly resistant to flow. For a small lumen with a radius less than 1 mm, blood no longer acts as a liquid and Poiseuille's equation is not applicable.

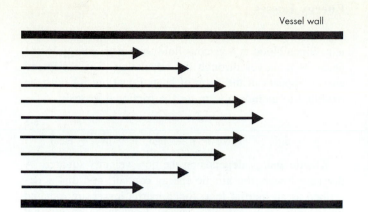

Figure 5-1 Velocity profile of blood exhibiting laminar flow in a vessel.

Blood pressure is usually measured in millimeters of mercury (mm Hg). The units for pressure in the CGS and MKS systems are dynes/cm² and newtons/m², respectively. The conversion factors between these pressure units are

$$1 \text{ mm Hg} = 1333 \text{ dynes/cm}^2$$
$$1 \text{ mm Hg} = 133.3 \text{ newtons/m}^2$$

■ **Example 5-1**

Calculate the volume flow rate through a vessel in which the pressure differential is 20 mm Hg (2.67×10^4 dynes/cm²). The length of the vessel is 10 cm and the radius of the lumen 0.25 cm. The viscosity of blood is 0.03 poise.

Using Equation 5-1

$$Q = \frac{\pi p r^4}{8 \, l \eta}$$
$$= \frac{(3.14) \, (2.67 \times 10^4 \text{ dynes/cm}^2) \, (0.25 \text{ cm})^4}{8 \, (10 \text{ cm}) \, (0.03 \text{ poise})}$$
$$= 136 \text{ cm}^3/\text{s}$$

Intravascular Pressure

Pressure produced by contraction of the heart, static filling pressure, and hydrostatic pressure each contribute to the overall intravascular pressure. Elastic vascular walls allow the lumen to expand and accommodate a higher volume of blood. Filling of the vessel causes additional force, and hence pressure, to be applied to the blood within the vessel by the elastic walls. Just as when a rubber band is stretched it exerts more force in attempting to return to a less distended state, so the elastic walls of a vessel act to exert pressure on the blood. This is called static filling pressure. Static filling pressure is typically much lower (about 7 mm Hg) than hydrostatic pressure and the pressure from heart contractions.

Hydrostatic pressure (p) is generated when a fluid is positioned vertically in a gravitational field. The weight of each overlying layer is transmitted to the bottom layer. More pressure is applied as the height is increased. Hydrostatic pressure is given by

5-2

$$p = -\rho g h$$

where ρ is the density of blood, g the acceleration due to gravity (980 cm/s²), and h the height of the blood. Since the calculation of hydrostatic pressure yields a relative value, height is expressed as the distance from a reference point.

(For the general circulation the right atrium is considered the reference point.) Blood at the same elevation as the right atrium has zero hydrostatic pressure. That below the right atrium experiences a positive hydrostatic pressure, and that above the right atrium a negative pressure. Hydrostatic pressure can be large, comparable to the pressure from heart contractions. In an upright man it causes the intravascular pressure in an artery of the ankle to be approximately 90 mm Hg greater than the hydrostatic pressure in the aortic arch.

■ **Example 5-2**

Calculate the hydrostatic pressure (p) in the ankle when it is located 120 cm below the right atrium. The density of blood is 1.06 g/cm³.

Using Equation 5-2

$$p = -\rho g h$$
$$= -(1.06 \text{ g/cm}^3) \, (980 \text{ cm/s}^2) \, (-120 \text{ cm})$$
$$= 1.25 \times 10^5 \text{ dynes/cm}^2$$

The height has a negative sign to indicate that the ankle is at a lower elevation than the reference point.
Convert the pressure to units of mm Hg

$$= \frac{1.25 \times 10^5 \text{ dynes/cm}^2}{1333 \text{ dynes/cm}^2/\text{mm Hg}}$$
$$= 94 \text{ mm Hg}$$

BERNOULLI'S PRINCIPLE

The movement of blood in the circulation is determined primarily by intravascular pressure. Other factors can influence blood flow, however, even to the extent of causing the blood to move against a pressure gradient. The description of fluid dynamics requires an analysis of fluid energy.

Types of Fluid Energy

Total fluid energy consists of kinetic energy from the blood's moving at a certain velocity, potential energy due to its elevation in a gravitational field, and the work done when pressure (force) is applied to move it. When a nonviscous liquid flows at a steady rate, the total energy content does not change. At any location along the vessel the sum of the work done, the potential energy, and the kinetic energy is the same as that obtained at any other point. The above condition is a statement of Bernoulli's principle. Mathematically, Bernoulli's equation expresses this energy relationship as

$$p + \rho gh + \tfrac{1}{2} \rho v^2 = \text{Constant} \qquad \text{5-3}$$

Some rearrangement of factors has been performed to present this equation in the most common form. It is the fundamental equation of fluid mechanics.

A comparison between any two points can be obtained by rewriting Equation 5-3 as

$$p_1 + \rho gh_1 + \tfrac{1}{2} \rho v_1^2 = p_2 + \rho gh_2 + \tfrac{1}{2} \rho v_2^2 \qquad \text{5-4}$$

where the subscripts denote the respective locations.

Energy Conversion

An important consequence of Bernoulli's principle is the conversion of potential energy to kinetic energy or increased pressure. Water at the top of a waterfall certainly gains momentum as it falls to a lower elevation. Potential energy, by virtue of the water's position in a gravitational field, is changed to kinetic energy.

■ Example 5-3

A fluid flows through a vertical tube at constant pressure and falls a distance of 10 cm. Velocity at the top of the tube is 20 cm/s. Calculate the velocity at the exit. Assume the total fluid energy is unchanged.

Using Equation 5-4

$$p_1 + \rho gh_1 + \tfrac{1}{2} \rho v_1^2 = p_2 + \rho gh_2 + \tfrac{1}{2} \rho v_2^2$$

Since pressure is constant

$$
\begin{aligned}
\tfrac{1}{2} v_2^2 &= \tfrac{1}{2} v_1^2 + g(h_1 - h_2) \\
&= \tfrac{1}{2} (20 \text{ cm/s})^2 + (980 \text{ cm/s}^2)(10 \text{ cm}) \\
&= 10{,}000 \text{ cm}^2/\text{s}^2 \\
v_2 &= 141 \text{ cm/s}
\end{aligned}
$$

■ Example 5-4

A fluid flows through an inclined tube at constant velocity and falls a distance of 10 cm. The pressure at the top of the tube is 50 mm Hg. Calculate the pressure at the bottom. Assume the total fluid energy to be unchanged.

Using Equation 5-4

$$p_1 + \rho gh_1 + \tfrac{1}{2} \rho v_1^2 = p_2 + \rho gh_2 + \tfrac{1}{2} \rho v_2^2$$

Since velocity is constant

$$
\begin{aligned}
p_2 &= p_1 + \rho g(h_1 - h_2) \\
&= 50 \text{ mm Hg} + \frac{(1.06 \text{ g/cm}^3)(980 \text{ cm/s}^2)(10 \text{ cm})}{1333 \text{ dynes/cm}^2/\text{mm Hg}} \\
&= 57.8 \text{ mm Hg}
\end{aligned}
$$

Energy Losses

Equations 5-3 and 5-4 are valid for a frictionless fluid system. Since blood is a viscous fluid, however, energy losses occur as it moves through the circulation. The dissipated energy appears in the form of heat. Equation 5-4 must be modified to include a term for the frictional losses:

$$p_1 + \rho gh_1 + \tfrac{1}{2} \rho v_1^2 = p_2 + \rho gh_2 + \tfrac{1}{2} \rho v_2^2 + \text{Heat} \qquad \text{5-5}$$

Kinetic energy depends on the flow velocity squared. A decrease lowers the kinetic energy content, and this is described as an inertial loss. Since inertia losses are dictated by velocity, they exhibit a strong dependence on luminal size (inversely proportional to the fourth power of the radius). Pulsatile flow, vessel curvature, branching, and vessel dilation can induce a velocity change and cause inertia loss.

The total fluid energy content of blood decreases as it moves through the circulation. Blood ejected into the aorta is at high velocity and high pressure, but on return through the veins it moves more slowly and is at lower pressure. The energy supplied by contractions of the heart is dissipated by frictional losses. An energy gradient is created along the pathway: left ventricle, aorta, arteries, capillaries, veins, and right atrium.

ARTERIAL HEMODYNAMICS

Cardiac Output

The heart rhythmically ejects blood into the aorta. The volume of blood per minute pumped is the cardiac output. The normal cardiac output for a healthy adult man is about 5 liters per minute. Women have, on average, 10% less cardiac output than men of the same body size. Exercise can increase cardiac output 5 to 6 times in a well-conditioned athlete.

Arterial Pressure

High but fluctuating arterial pressure is maintained by the pumping heart. Peak pressure, usually about 120 mm Hg, occurs during systole. Each pressure pulse is transmitted along the aorta to more distant vessels. Pressure progressively decreases from the arterial to venous circulation. Pulsatile pressure fluctuations are damped out by the arteries. Figure 5-2 shows the pressure variations throughout the circulatory system caused by heart contractions.

Large arteries have low frictional losses and provide little resistance to flow. They act as distributors of blood to the remainder of the arterial tree. Flow in them is altered by changes in the peripheral resistance.

Compliance

Arterial vessel walls are strongly elastic, which allows luminal size to increase when additional pressure is applied. As blood is ejected from the heart, the arteries become distended and store large quantities of blood. This property is called compliance. The arteries act as reservoirs that provide continuous flow to peripheral vessels during diastole. The effect of pulsatile action of the heart is diminished by compliant arteries; pressure fluctuations are reduced in magnitude as distance of transmission of the pressure wave is increased.

Pulsatile Flow

Arterial pressure oscillation is a complex combination of several factors, including stroke volume, time course of ventricular ejection, peripheral resistance, and vascular compliance. The pressure fluctuations give rise to pulsatile flow in the arteries. In normal peripheral arteries the flow velocity increases rapidly to a peak during early systole, followed by an end-systolic flow reversal of short duration, and then a resumption of forward flow at lower velocity during diastole (Fig. 5-3).

The changes in velocity within the heart cycle are sometimes characterized by descriptive indices, such as the pulsatility index (PI). Large differences in flow velocity between systole and diastole yield high PI values. Conversely, small differences in flow velocity between systole and diastole yield low PI values.

The velocity pattern is highly variable depending on anatomic location and exercise. Exercise causes vasodilation of lower limb arteries, which decreases the resistance to

flow. Antegrade flow is present during both systole and diastole and produces a low pulsatile flow pattern.

Pathological conditions including obstruction, aneurysm, arteriovenous fistulae, and vasospasm may alter the velocity pattern dramatically. Flow patterns associated with an obstruction are of particular interest and are discussed later in this chapter.

VENOUS HEMODYNAMICS

Venous Function

The major function of veins is to act as a conduit for the flow of blood back to the heart, but the venous system also participates in regulation of the circulation. Veins can constrict or enlarge to change peripheral resistance and alter flow. The walls of veins are not as strongly elastic as those of arteries; for a similar increase in pressure a vein can contain 6 to 10 times the volume of blood as an artery of comparable size. Large quantities of blood can be stored in veins until needed (veins also exhibit compliance).

Venous return tends to increase when blood volume is increased, peripheral venous pressure is increased, or small vessels are dilated. The primary regulatory control on cardiac output is the peripheral resistance. As more vessels dilate in the peripheral circulation, resistance is decreased and cardiac output becomes greater.

Venous Pressure

The pressure pulses in the arteries are damped out before they reach the veins, as illustrated in Figure 5-2. The constant pressure difference along the vessel tends to give rise to continuous flow. Laminar flow is established at low velocities and the velocity flow profile is parabolic.

When distended, large veins have little resistance to flow. Veins are compressed by sharp angulations over bone, however, as well as by outside atmospheric pressure (on superficial vessels) and by the bulk of abdominal organs. With the compression, resistance is increased and flow reduced. Veins inside the thorax are normally distended because the surrounding air pressure is low.

When a person is standing upright, the weight of blood in the vessels creates a hydrostatic pressure that inhibits flow to the heart. Blood tends to accumulate at points of high hydrostatic pressure. The effect is most pronounced the farther it is from the heart, such as in the lower legs

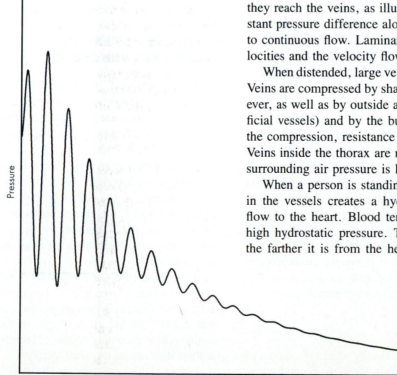

Figure 5-2 Pressure variations throughout the circulation caused by contractions of the heart.

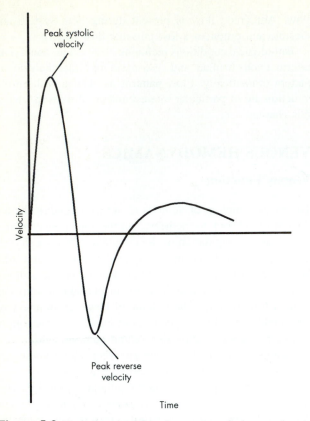

Figure 5-3 Time course of flow in an artery during one heart cycle.

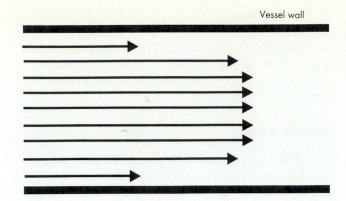

Figure 5-4 Laminar flow is changed to plug flow when blood undergoes acceleration.

■ **Table 5-1** Peak Velocities in Arteries (m/s)

Artery	Systolic	Reverse
Common femoral	0.9 to 1.4	0.3 to 0.5
Superficial femoral	0.7 to 1.1	0.25 to 0.45
Popliteal	0.5 to 0.8	0.2 to 0.4
Internal carotid	0.6 to 1.0	*
External carotid	0.6 to 1.2	*
Common carotid	0.4 to 1.2	*

Modified from Polak JF: *Peripheral vascular sonography: a practical guide*, Baltimore, 1992, Williams & Wilkins. (Also based on our clinical observations.)
*Reverse flow is weak or not commonly present.

and feet. A venous pump counteracts this action of the hydrostatic pressure. Veins contain a series of valves that allow flow only toward the heart. Leg muscular movement compresses the distended veins and propels the blood toward the heart. The valves then block reverse flow as blood accumulates in the next section of the vessel.

Control of Flow

Constriction of the veins increases the peripheral resistance and raises arterial pressure. Also stored blood in the veins is released to increase the blood volume and enhance venous return. Under conditions of extreme cold, the constriction of superficial vessels reduces blood volume flow to conserve body heat.

Severe arterial obstruction can decrease the flow in veins by inhibiting the transport of blood to the capillary bed. Chronic venous obstruction results in edema. Acute venous obstruction is generally associated with the formation of a thrombus, which can lead to pulmonary embolism.

PEAK VELOCITY

Peak velocity is the maximum velocity within the lumen of the vessel. It varies with anatomic location, being highest in vessels near the heart. Peak velocities tend to decrease distal to the heart, because the total cross-sectional area of all vessels increases. Table 5-1 lists the normal range of

peak velocity for various arteries. Exercise and pathological conditions can alter these values.

MODIFICATIONS OF VELOCITY PROFILE

Velocity profile can be affected by accelerated flow, curvature of a vessel, branching to smaller vessels, obstruction in a vessel, and diverging cross section. Velocity components across the lumen also exhibit time-dependent behavior during the heart cycle.

Laminar flow in an artery is converted to a more uniform distribution of flow velocities across the lumen when blood is accelerated or propelled through a narrowed opening (Figs. 5-4 and 5-5). This nonlaminar flow is called blunt or plug flow and commonly occurs in the thoracic aorta, where the blood experiences large accelerations by the pumping heart.

The passageway for blood flow is reduced at an obstruction and when a large artery branches to a small one. The *inlet effect* describes the conversion from laminar flow to a flat velocity profile at the origin of the small artery. The uniform flow gradually reverts to laminar flow after moving a short distance in the small artery.

Laminar flow entering the bend of a tortuous vessel is skewed; thus high velocity components occur at the outer curve of the vessel (Fig. 5-6). *Diverging cross section* refers to a widening of the lumen; it can create regions with mul-

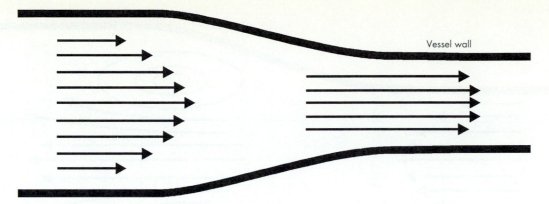

Figure 5-5 A narrowed lumen alters laminar flow to a flat velocity profile.

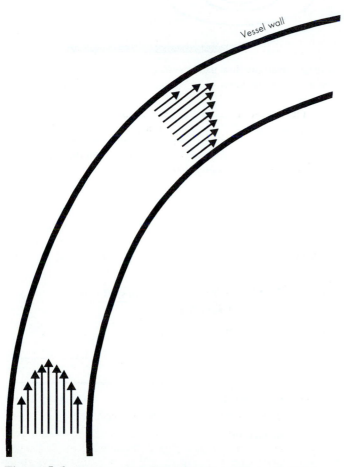

Figure 5-6 Vessel curvature skews the blood flow velocities so higher velocity components are present at the outer edge of the vessel.

tiple flow patterns including uniform high-velocity flow, stagnant flow, and eddy flow (Fig. 5-7).

EDDY FLOW

Eddy flow is the localized slow rotation of concentric blood layers. The rotation creates regions of reversed flow. A zone of stagnant flow, called flow separation, divides the circular motion of eddy flow from the central region of high-velocity

flow. Eddy flow occurs at arterial bifurcations, within vessels undergoing rapid expansion of luminal diameter, and distal to an obstruction.

Regional flow patterns at a bifurcation are extremely complex. The laminar flow incident on the bifurcation is disrupted by the vessel wall. Blood striking the wall is redirected across the vessel lumen, creating flow counter to the prevailing direction. Flow becomes disjointed. Regions of slow and reversed flow are created near the outer vessel wall. Zones of stagnation are also present. A large rock placed in the middle of a gently flowing stream has a similar effect. Water no longer can continue along the projected path but is directed around the rock. Cross currents, flow eddies, and zones of stagnation form as it circumvents the obstacle. The regional flow patterns for the carotid bifurcation are shown in Figure 5-8.

TURBULENCE

Turbulence is chaotic flow in which the coherence of flow velocities across the vessel lumen is lost. Flow is no longer directed along the length of the vessel but occurs crosswise. Velocity components become varied and fluctuate randomly.

Turbulence is more likely to occur at high velocities within large vessels, distal to an obstruction, along a rough surface, and within the sharp turn of a vessel. Vessels typically exhibit laminar flow at normal blood flow velocities. When velocity exceeds a critical threshold, turbulence is induced.

Reynolds Number

The likelihood of turbulence is expressed in terms of the Reynolds number (Re):

5-6

$$Re = \frac{\rho vd}{\eta}$$

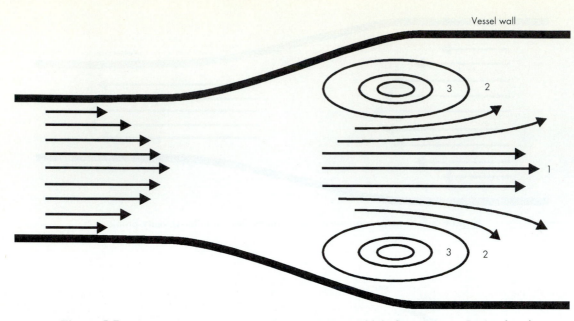

Figure 5-7 A sudden increase in vessel diameter creates multiple flow patterns. *Region 1*, uniform high velocity flow; *Region 2*, stagnant flow; *Region 3*, eddy flow.

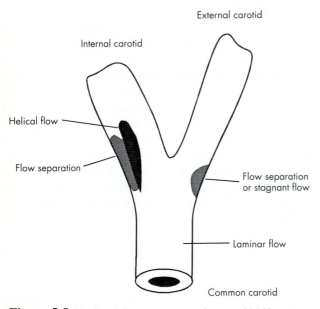

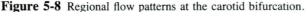

Figure 5-8 Regional flow patterns at the carotid bifurcation.

where v is the velocity (cm/s), ρ is the density of blood (g/cm³), d the diameter of the vessel (cm), and η the viscosity (poise). Vessels with comparable Reynolds numbers exhibit similar flow characteristics. A high Reynolds number (above 2000) in straight smooth vessels indicates turbulent blood flow. If the Reynolds number is less than 2000, blood is constrained to remain in layers by the viscous forces. Local disturbances are suppressed and do not spread through the vessel to disrupt flow in nearby layers. At branches of large arteries a much lower value for the Reynolds number (above 200) may by sufficient to cause turbulent flow. After branching, laminar flow is reestablished in the smooth portion of the vessel.

■ **Example 5-5**

Calculate the Reynolds number (Re) for a 2 cm diameter vessel in which the flow velocity is 80 cm/s.

Using Equation 5-6

$$Re = \frac{\rho v d}{\eta}$$

where ρ is 1.06 g/cm³, v is 80 cm/s, d is 2 cm, and η is 0.03 poise.

$$= \frac{(1.06 \text{ g/cm}^3)\ (80 \text{ cm/s})\ (2 \text{ cm})}{0.03 \text{ poise}}$$

$$= 5653$$

■ **Example 5-6**

Calculate the Reynolds number (Re) for a 0.5 cm diameter vessel in which the flow velocity is 80 cm/s.

Using Equation 5-6

$$Re = \frac{\rho v d}{\eta}$$

where ρ is 1.06 g/cm³, v is 80 cm/s, d is 0.5 cm, and η is 0.03 poise.

$$= \frac{(1.06 \text{ g/cm}^3)\ (80 \text{ cm/s})\ (0.5 \text{ cm})}{0.03 \text{ poise}}$$

$$= 1413$$

The Reynolds number in small vessels is not likely to be high enough to cause turbulent flow.

OBSTRUCTION

Arterial obstruction is usually in the form of a plaque. Plaques are associated with degenerative changes in the

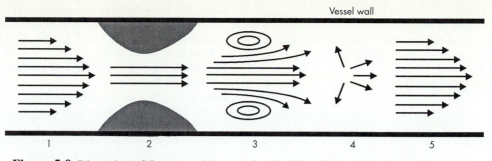

Vessel wall

Figure 5-9 Disruption of flow caused by stenosis (shaded regions). Velocity profiles include *(1)* laminar, *(2)* jet, *(3)* flow reversal, *(4)* turbulence, and *(5)* laminar.

arterial wall accompanied by lipid deposits and, often, calcium deposits as well. When a plaque protrudes into the vessel lumen, flow is disrupted. A high proportion of the artery must be blocked, however, before the flow volume rate is affected.

Certain locations are predisposed to the formation of plaques. Areas of relative stagnation appear more susceptible. A notable site is the carotid bifurcation (in the carotid bulb near the origin of the internal carotid artery).

An obstruction in the flow path reduces the cross sectional area; and thus, if volumetric flow rate is to be maintained, flow velocity must increase across the narrowed lumen. The high-velocity jet at the site of a stenosis has relatively uniform velocity components (flat velocity profile).

As the jet of blood exits the stenotic region, the lumen widens to its normal diameter. The expanded area causes the high-velocity jet to slow and to disperse flow velocities. A zone of flow reversal is formed immediately beyond the narrowed lumen. Distal to the stenosis flow reversal disappears and a region of flow turbulence develops before laminar flow is reestablished (Fig. 5-9). Five distinct velocity profiles are observed in the vicinity of the stenosis. These velocity profiles are summarized in Table 5-2.

If the narrowing of the lumen is severe, pressure and flow distal to the stenosis are reduced. For iliac, femoral, renal, and carotid arteries 70% to 90% of the lumen must be occluded before flow will be significantly impaired. This is classified as critical stenosis. When critical stenosis is reached, small additional narrowing of the lumen causes a rapid decrease in flow and pressure distal to the restriction.

The major consideration is the size of the restricted opening, although many other factors influence the disturbed flow pattern. These include length of the narrowed segment, roughness of the endothelial surface, irregularity of the opening, peripheral resistance, volume flow rate, and pressure differential.

SUMMARY

Arterial and venous flow dynamics is extremely complex. Volume flow rate is regulated primarily by changes in the resistance and pressure differential along the length of a

▣ **Table 5–2**   Velocity Profiles in the Vicinity of a Stenosis

Location	Features
Proximal	Laminar
Coincident	Jet, high velocity, uniform velocity components
Immediately distal	Broadened velocity components, reduced peak velocity from that in jet
Distal	Turbulence
More distal	Laminar

vessel. Friction caused by the viscosity of blood produces velocity variations across the lumen. The velocity profile at a specific location is time dependent and affected by the physical properties of the vessel (curvature, lumen diameter, and branching).

Disease can modify the normal patterns of flow dynamics. For example, severe stenosis creates high-speed jets, eddy currents, and turbulent flow. Volume flow rate may decrease.

An understanding of hemodynamics and a knowledge of normal flow patterns provide the basis for the interpretation of a clinical examination performed with Doppler instrumentation, the topic of the next two chapters.

R E V I E W   Q U E S T I O N S

1. What are the features of laminar flow?
2. Volume flow rate through a vessel is regulated primarily by _____ and _____ .
3. Name the type of pressure produced by the position of blood in a gravitational field.
4. Name the fundamental equation of fluid mechanics. What is the principle of this equation?
5. The total fluid energy content decreases as the blood moves through the circulation. What causes this energy loss? The energy is converted into _____ .
6. A decrease in fluid kinetic energy is called an _____ loss.
7. What factors can modify the velocity profile?
8. Characterize the velocity profile of plug flow.

9. What is eddy flow?
10. What are the features of turbulent flow?
11. Calculate the Reynolds number for a 1.5 cm diameter, straight, smooth vessel in which the flow velocity is 50 cm/s. Is turbulence likely to occur?
12. How is laminar flow altered by a stenosis?

BIBLIOGRAPHY

Burns PN: Hemodynamics. In Taylor KJW, Burns PN, Wells PNT (eds): *Clinical applications of Doppler ultrasound*, New York, 1988, Raven Press.

Carter SA: Hemodynamic considerations in peripheral and cerebrovascular disease. In Zwiebel WJ (ed): *Introduction to vascular ultrasonography*, ed 2, Orlando Fla, 1986, Grune & Stratton.

Guyton AC: *Textbook of medical physiology*, ed 8, Philadelphia, 1991, WB Saunders.

Hatle L, Angelsen B: *Doppler ultrasound in cardiology: physical principles and clinical applications*, ed 2, Philadelphia, 1985, Lea & Febiger.

Polak JF: *Peripheral vascular sonography: a practical guide*, Baltimore, 1992, Williams & Wilkins.

Sumner DS: Hemodynamics and pathophysiology of venous disease. In Rutherford RB (ed): *Vascular surgery*, ed 2, Philadelphia, 1984, WB Saunders.

CHAPTER 6

Doppler Physics and Instrumentation

During the past 10 years Doppler ultrasound has experienced considerable growth in both the number and the diversity of examinations performed. This increase has come about because of the need to evaluate the vascular system noninvasively and the greater sophistication of Doppler instrumentation. Several types of Doppler scanners are available. Although each uses the Doppler principle to detect motion, the manner in which it acquires, processes, and displays signals distinguishes one type of instrument from another. An overview of the various types of Doppler scanners is presented in this chapter, with particular emphasis placed on the explanation of spectral analysis and aliasing.

Doppler instruments often quantify the rate of movement or speed of the moving interfaces within the sound beam. From a physics viewpoint the term *speed* is proper because the magnitude of the movement (a scaler quantity), and not the absolute direction of movement, is of interest. Nevertheless, the term *velocity* has been used tradionally in Doppler ultrasound applications.

DOPPLER EFFECT

The Doppler effect is a phenomenon in which an apparent change in the frequency of sound is observed if there is relative motion between the source of the sound and the receiver. An analogy involving waves striking a boat on the water illustrates the Doppler effect. Assume that the wind is blowing at a constant rate from the west and that the waves all have the same distance between peaks (same wavelength). By remaining stationary in the water, the boat encounters the same number of wave crests each second (constant frequency) as are produced by the source. If it travels westward, the wave crests come more frequently. A person standing on board sees an increase in the wave frequency, although the waves are actually approaching at the same rate. If it reverses its direction and travels eastward (away from the source of the waves), fewer crests are encountered. The observed frequency decreases. As the boat moves faster in either direction, the difference between the actual and observed frequencies *increases*. The only circumstance in which the actual and observed frequencies coincide is when the boat is stationary.

Doppler Shift

A sound source produces a series of concentric pressure spheres moving out and away from it. The same effect (in two dimensions) is seen when a stone is dropped into a pond. Concentric rings form, the most peripheral being the oldest and the most central being the newest. The source determines the frequency of the waves, and the medium determines their speed of propagation. The frequency and speed of propagation together define the wavelength (or space between the spheres radiating from the source).

A stationary receiver views the same number of pressure waves or spheres as are emitted by the stationary source

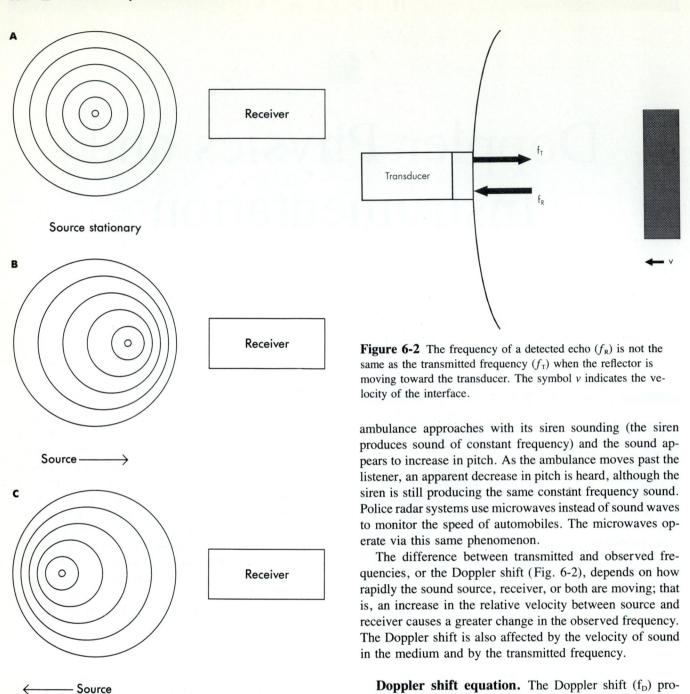

Figure 6-1 The Doppler effect. **A,** Stationary sound source and receiver, showing a constant observed frequency equal to the frequency of the sound source. **B,** Sound source moving toward the receiver, showing an increase in the observed frequency compared with the actual frequency emitted by the sound source. **C,** Sound source moving away from the receiver, showing a decrease in the observed frequency compared with the actual frequency emitted by the sound source.

Figure 6-2 The frequency of a detected echo (f_R) is not the same as the transmitted frequency (f_T) when the reflector is moving toward the transducer. The symbol v indicates the velocity of the interface.

(Fig. 6-1). The observed frequency is influenced by movement of the source or the receiver either toward or away from the other. More or less pressure waves per unit of time strike the receiver and cause a higher or lower pitch to be heard. This is the Doppler shift.

The Doppler shift is experienced in daily life when an ambulance approaches with its siren sounding (the siren produces sound of constant frequency) and the sound appears to increase in pitch. As the ambulance moves past the listener, an apparent decrease in pitch is heard, although the siren is still producing the same constant frequency sound. Police radar systems use microwaves instead of sound waves to monitor the speed of automobiles. The microwaves operate via this same phenomenon.

The difference between transmitted and observed frequencies, or the Doppler shift (Fig. 6-2), depends on how rapidly the sound source, receiver, or both are moving; that is, an increase in the relative velocity between source and receiver causes a greater change in the observed frequency. The Doppler shift is also affected by the velocity of sound in the medium and by the transmitted frequency.

Doppler shift equation. The Doppler shift (f_D) produced by scanning a moving interface in tissue is calculated from the following equation:

6-1

$$f_D = \frac{2\,vf}{c}$$

where c is the velocity of sound in tissue, v the velocity of the interface, and f the frequency of the transducer.

Equation 6-1 is, in reality, an approximation based on the assumption that the speed of the interfaces for biological systems is relatively small (0.5 to 200 cm/s) compared to the velocity of sound in tissue (1540 m/s). As a numerical example, consider an interface moving toward a 5 MHz transducer at a velocity of 15 cm/s. The observed frequency is 974 Hz above the original transmitted frequency of 5 MHz. The calculation of this frequency shift is as follows:

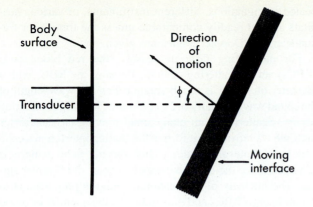

Figure 6-3 Motion of an interface not parallel with the direction of travel of the sound beam. The angle ϕ is used in the Doppler shift equation.

$$f_D = \frac{(2)\,(0.15\ \text{m/s})\,(5 \times 10^6\ \text{c/s})}{1540\ \text{m/s}} = 974\ \text{c/s (or Hz)}$$

If the interface is moving *away* from the transducer at 15 cm/s, the observed frequency will be 974 Hz below the original transmitted frequency.

Remember: The velocity of the sound wave remains constant (it is a function of the medium being scanned). The observed change in frequency occurs because relative motion is present between the source and the detector. The above formula predicts that an increase in velocity of the interface results in a greater Doppler shift. If the frequency shift can be measured, the velocity of the moving interfaces (e.g., red blood cells in vessels) can be determined.

Equation 6-1 is valid only if the direction of motion between the sound source and the moving reflector is parallel to the direction of sound wave propagation. If the sound beam is incident at an angle other than zero degrees with respect to the motion of the reflecting interface (Fig. 6-3), the above equation must be modified by including the cosine of this angle (referred to as the Doppler angle):

6-2

$$f_D = \frac{2\,vf \cos\phi}{c}$$

The combination of v and $\cos\phi$ gives the component of the velocity along the direction of propagation for the ultrasound beam. If the Doppler angle is increased from 0 to 45 degrees, the Doppler shift is found to be 689 Hz instead of the 974 obtained for parallel incidence (974 Hz × cos 45 degrees = 974 Hz × 0.707 = 689 Hz). Doppler shifts as a function of transducer frequency, reflector velocity, and Doppler angle are listed in Table 6-1.

■ **Example 6-1**

Calculate the Doppler shift (f_D) produced by scanning an interface moving at a velocity of 50 cm/s if the angle of insonation is 30 degrees. The center frequency of the transducer is 3.5 MHz. Using equation 6-2

$$f_D = \frac{2\,vf \cos\phi}{c}$$

■ **Table 6-1** Relation Between the Doppler Shift, Transducer Frequency, Velocity of a Moving Reflector, and Doppler Angle

Doppler Shift (kHz)	Transducer Frequency (MHz)	Velocity (cm/s)	Doppler Angle (Degrees)
260	2	10	0
225	2	10	30
184	2	10	45
130	2	10	60
649	2	25	0
562	2	25	30
459	2	25	45
325	2	25	60
2597	2	100	0
2250	2	100	30
1837	2	100	45
1299	2	100	60
649	5	10	0
562	5	10	30
459	5	10	45
325	5	10	60
1623	5	25	0
1406	5	25	30
1148	5	25	45
812	5	25	60
6494	5	100	0
5624	5	100	30
4592	5	100	45
3248	5	100	60
974	7.5	10	0
844	7.5	10	30
689	7.5	10	45
487	7.5	10	60
2435	7.5	25	0
2109	7.5	25	30
1722	7.5	25	45
1218	7.5	25	60
9740	7.5	100	0
8436	7.5	100	30
6888	7.5	100	45
4872	7.5	100	60

$$= \frac{2\,(50\ \text{cm/s})\,(3.5 \times 10^6\ \text{c/s})\cos 30\ \text{degrees}}{154,000\ \text{cm/s}}$$

$$= 1968\ \text{Hz}$$

Actual determination of the Doppler angle may be quite difficult. Minimum shift should occur at a 90-degree angle of incidence because the cosine of 90 degrees is 0. In practice, the signal never goes to zero because there is always some portion of the beam that is not perpendicular to the motion as a result of divergence. Using the position corresponding to the minimum shift as a reference point it is possible to determine the incidence angle by measurement.

Velocity determination. The velocity of a moving interface is calculated from measurements of the Doppler shift and Doppler angle by rearranging Equation 6-2.

6-3

$$v = \frac{f_D c}{2 f \cos \phi}$$

The absolute determination of reflector velocity requires that the Doppler angle be included in this calculation. Ignoring the contribution of the Doppler angle causes an underestimation of the true velocity.

■ **Example 6-2**

Calculate the velocity (v) of a moving reflector if a Doppler shift of 1000 Hz is observed. The angle of insonation is 60 degrees. The center frequency of the transducer is 5 MHz.

Using equation 6-3

$$v = \frac{f_D c}{2 f \cos \phi}$$

$$= \frac{(1000 \text{ c/s}) (154,000 \text{ cm/s})}{2 (5 \times 10^6 \text{ c/s}) \cos 60 \text{ degrees}}$$

$$= 31 \text{ cm/s}$$

Uncertainty in measuring the Doppler angle, particularly at large angles, introduces error in the velocity computation. A 5-degree error for a 70-degree Doppler angle causes the velocity estimation to deviate by 25%. A decrease in the Doppler angle to 40 degrees reduces this deviation to 8% for the same uncertainty of 5 degrees in angle measurement. A greater uncertainty in the Doppler angle further increases the error in velocity computation. As a general guideline, Doppler signals from superficial blood vessels (e.g., the carotids) should be acquired at angles between 30 and 60 degrees. The lower angular limit is recommended because total internal reflection occurs at the vessel wall–blood boundary for small angles and the sound beam does not reach the moving blood. Accurate determination of the Doppler angle is difficult for tortuous vessels that radically change direction. If demonstration of the presence of flow in a vessel is sufficient, however, accurate measurement of the Doppler angle is not required. Some Doppler instruments allow the operator to specify the direction of flow on an image and then automatically calculate the Doppler angle.

Clinical Considerations

Doppler units are designed to extract the Doppler shift(s) from received signals. This change in frequency (as illustrated by the discussion following Equation 6-1) is in the audible range (typically between 200 and 15,000 Hz), which enables audioamplifiers with earphones or loudspeakers to be used as output devices. The display system in this case is very different from the CRT in A-mode scanners or the scan converter in B-mode scanners. A strip chart recorder may be used to generate a hardcopy printout of the Doppler shift(s). The frequency spectrum depicting multiple Doppler shifts may also be presented on a video display. The preferred format is to convert the measured Doppler shift to an absolute velocity, which is independent of instrument parameters. Doppler shifts expressed in kilohertz from repeated examinations, different instruments, or various hospitals are not readily comparable unless the transducer frequencies and Doppler angles are given.

For monitoring flow in vessels, the red blood cells (RBCs) act as scattering centers. Because the RBC, with a diameter of 7 μm, is much smaller than the wavelength of the sound wave (usually 0.2 to 0.5 mm), Rayleigh scattering occurs. Scattering from many small moving targets creates multiple wavefronts that form a fluctuating interference echo pattern in time and space. This varying echo pattern is responsible for the noiselike appearance of the Doppler signal. The intensity of the scattered sound is proportional to the number of RBCs and thus indicates the quantity of blood in the sample volume. The nonspecular reflection from RBCs, however, is small compared to echoes produced by soft tissue interfaces. The echo-free appearance of blood-filled structures on real-time images demonstrates this relatively weak scattering from RBCs. The intensity of the scattered sound is also proportional to the fourth power of the frequency. To produce a strong echo, a high-frequency transducer should be used; but as the frequency is increased, the rate of absorption of the sound beam by the intervening tissues also increases. These two effects must be balanced in Doppler scanning by matching the transducer frequency with the depth of the region of interest. The optimum frequency (f_o) in megahertz for a Doppler examination is given by

6-4

$$f_o = \frac{90}{R}$$

where R is the soft tissue distance to the region of interest in millimeters. In general, the optimal Doppler frequency is lower than the frequency used for imaging. For a depth of 60 mm, imaging is optimized at a transducer frequency of 5 MHz, although Equation 6-4 indicates that a frequency of 1.5 MHz is more appropriate for obtaining Doppler information. Doppler probes usually operate in the frequency range of 2 to 10 MHz because other constraints are placed on the system: a single transducer with dual imaging and Doppler functions, a desired frequency range for Doppler shifts, and the problem of aliasing (discussed later in this chapter). High frequencies, typically 5 to 7 MHz, are employed for peripheral vascular Doppler examinations, whereas examinations of deep-seated vessels are performed at frequencies near 2 MHz.

CONTINUOUS-WAVE DOPPLER

Transducer Design

Continuous-wave (CW) Doppler units use two crystals in the transducer: one to transmit the sound waves of constant frequency continuously and one to receive the reflected echoes continuously (Fig. 6-4). One crystal cannot send and receive at the same time, because an ultrahigh–dynamic range receiver circuit would be required to detect the small echo signals superimposed on the transmitting signal.

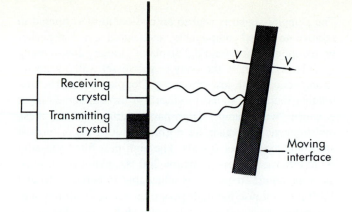

Figure 6-4 Continuous-wave Doppler transducer. One crystal acts as the transmitter, the other as the receiver. The continuous sound wave is reflected from the moving interface.

The sampling region is positioned by geometric arrangement of the crystals. The two elements are angled slightly to allow overlap between their respective lines of sight (transmission and reception). For a moving reflector to be detected, it must be located along the path of the transmitted beam and the resulting echo must strike the receiving crystal. The sensitivity or focal volume is defined by the intersection of the ultrasound field and the reception zone. In essence, each transducer is focused to a particular depth. Depending on the clinical application, the sonographer selects a CW transducer with the appropriate operating frequency and depth of focus.

For an operating frequency below 7 MHz, the transducer consists of two D-shaped elements obtained by cutting a piezoelectric disk in half. The elements are placed as close together as possible within the transducer housing but are electrically and mechanically isolated. They are sometimes angled slightly to maximize the overlap between transmitted beam and reflected echoes. Separate rectangular crystals with dimensions on the order of 1 mm are mounted side by side in a high-frequency CW transducer.

Doppler Shift

The transmitted sound wave interacts with various interfaces, some of which are stationary and others moving. A fraction of the sound wave is reflected at the various interfaces. If the interfaces are stationary, the frequency of the reflected sound wave is the same as the transmitted frequency and consequently no Doppler shift is observed. Moving interfaces initially act as "receivers" of the ultrasound beam and cause the frequency of the reflected beam to shift up or down depending on whether they are moving toward or away from the sound source. The second crystal in the transducer acts as a receiver for the returning echoes. Although the receiving crystal is stationary, another change in frequency occurs because the moving interfaces are now acting as a sound source. These two shifts in frequency are responsible for factor 2 in the Doppler shift equation.

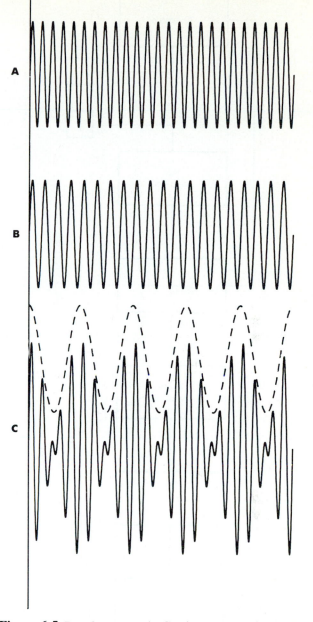

Figure 6-5 Beat frequency. **A,** Continuous transmitted wave of constant frequency (25 cycles are shown). **B,** Continuous reflected wave of constant frequency (20 cycles are shown). **C,** Addition of the transmitted and received sound waves in **A** and **B** produces a complex waveform. The beat frequency (5 cycles are shown) is illustrated as the outer envelope (*dotted line*) of this complex waveform.

Beat Frequency

The method used to measure a Doppler shift is based on the principle of wave interference. The reflected wave received from a moving interface varies slightly in frequency from the original transmitted wave because of the Doppler phenomenon. Waves of different frequencies algebraically add together, giving a resulting frequency called the beat frequency (Fig. 6-5). The beat frequency corresponds to the Doppler shift.

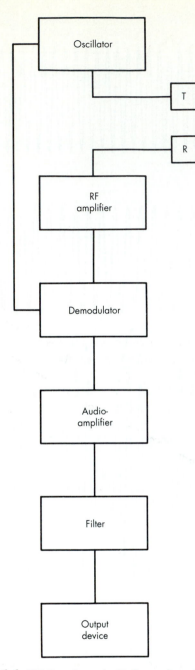

Figure 6-6 CW Doppler unit. *T,* Transmitter; *R,* receiver.

Figure 6-6 illustrates the steps necessary to generate a Doppler signal. An oscillator regulates the transmitter to emit a continuous single-frequency sound wave. The returning echo incident on the receiving crystal is converted to a radiofrequency signal. An RF amplifier increases the RF signal level. The reference signal from the oscillator (mimicking the transmitted wave) is combined with the received signal, which creates a complex resultant wave by wave interference. This wave is demodulated to remove all but the beat frequency. Isolation of the beat frequency forms the Doppler signal, which has a frequency equal to the Doppler shift.

Instrument Design

The Doppler signal is sent to an audioamplifier, filtered to remove unwanted components, and routed to a loudspeaker or earphones for audible "display." Large slow-moving specular reflectors in the body (e.g., vessel walls) generate strong echoes with low-frequency Doppler shifts. The distracting thumping sound produced in the unfiltered output is called "wall thump." High-pass filtering removes these low frequencies, which are normally not of major interest and could mask other signals. The high-pass filter is usually set to remove frequencies below 200 Hz, although on some units the cutoff frequency is adjustable to between 40 and 1000 Hz. Because the high-pass filter removes all frequencies below the cutoff value, Doppler shifts from slow-moving RBCs may be eliminated from the final output. The high-pass filter should be set at the lowest possible value to remove wall thump while not distorting the blood-flow components of the Doppler signal.

A low-pass filter eliminates high-frequency noise, but its application imposes an upper limit for velocity measurement. The pitch of the audio output corresponds to the frequency shift between the transmitted and received sound waves and indicates the speed of flow within the vessel. As the speed of flow becomes greater, a higher pitch is heard.

The CW Doppler unit can detect only speed of movement. It must be modified to determine the actual direction of movement (i.e., whether toward or away from the transducer) such as in blood flow. (The various directional methods will be discussed later.)

Because the Doppler shift corresponding to motion along the direction of sound propagation within a reception zone is detected, no scanning arm is necessary to denote the position of the transducer. The observed Doppler signal can be extremely complex, however, because the sum of Doppler shifts generated by all the moving interfaces within the focal volume is represented. If the focal volume includes multiple vessels, the superposition of resulting Doppler shifts becomes especially problematic.

Furthermore, extensive flow volumes (e.g., those encountered in the left ventricle) cannot be accurately assessed with CW Doppler methods. These units operate at low acoustic power levels but provide no depth information; and since the time between transmitted sound wave and detected echo is unknown, TGC cannot be applied. Consequently, provided they are of similar acoustic properties, superficial moving structures produce stronger signals than deep moving structures do. Depth discrimination is achieved by pulsing the transmitted ultrasound wave.

PULSED-WAVE DOPPLER

Sampling Depth

Pulsed-wave (PW) Doppler units use the echo-ranging principle (Chapter 1) to provide quantitative depth information of the Doppler shift. The transducer is electrically stimulated to produce a short burst of ultrasound and then is silent to listen for echoes before another burst is generated.

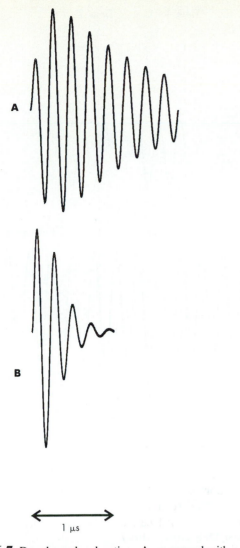

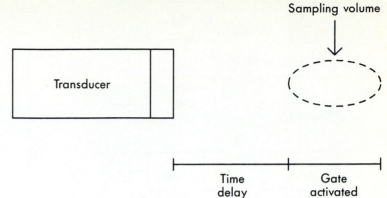

Figure 6-8 In PW Doppler, activation of the gate determines the depth and axial length of the sampling volume.

Figure 6-7 Doppler pulse duration, **A,** compared with real-time pulse duration, **B.**

Beat frequency determination requires a longer pulse duration (minimum of four cycles) than is used in real-time imaging (Fig. 6-7). The received signals are electronically gated for processing so only the echoes detected in a narrow time interval after the pulse, corresponding to a specific depth, contribute to the Doppler signal. Some authors refer to this scanning method as C-mode. The delay time before the gate is turned on determines the axial location of the sensitive volume; the amount of time the gate is activated establishes the axial length of the sample volume (Fig. 6-8). Gate parameters are selectable by the sonographer; thus the depth and length of the sensitive volume can be adjusted. The sample length is usually between 1 and 15 mm. The lateral dimensions of the sampling volume are dictated by the beam width, which is influenced by the transducer frequency and focusing characteristics.

Instrument Design

In PW Doppler the basic CW circuit is modified to accommodate gating and to collect successive processed echoes in a sample-and-hold circuit (Fig. 6-9). The clock functions as a master synchronizer for timing purposes (PRF and gating). Some units allow the sonographer to adjust the pulse repetition frequency manually, whereas others vary the PRF automatically in response to the sampling depth. A single gate limits the interrogation to one depth along the line of sight. Doppler shifts can be acquired simultaneously from multiple separate sample volumes along the direction of propagation by incorporating parallel receiver channels, each with a gate set with a different time delay. Multigate PW systems typically contain 6 to 32 gates, with a minimum axial length of 1 mm for each sample volume. No sacrifice is made with respect to PRF or processing time; the parallel receiver channels act independently during each pulse repetition cycle to process the information from designated sampling regions. Headphones or a spectrum analyzer are typical output devices.

Signal Processing

The received echo must be evaluated to determine whether the reflector is moving. This is accomplished by comparing the phase of the echo with a reference signal for which phase is synchronized with the transmitted pulse. Two waves are described as being in phase if their maximum, minimum, and zero points occur concurrently. The echo from a stationary reflector has the same phase as the reference signal, whereas the echo from a moving structure undergoes a phase shift via the Doppler effect. The phase relation between detected echoes and the reference signal is depicted in Figure 6-10.

The echoes from different reflectors, one moving and the other stationary, are received after different time intervals (time 1 and time 2) following the transmitted pulse. The reference signal has the same frequency and phase as the transmitted pulse but is extended over time so the received signals can be compared with the original transmitted waveform. The dotted lines in Figure 6-10 place the detected echoes on the same time scale as the reference signal. The phase is unchanged for the stationary reflector, whose echo

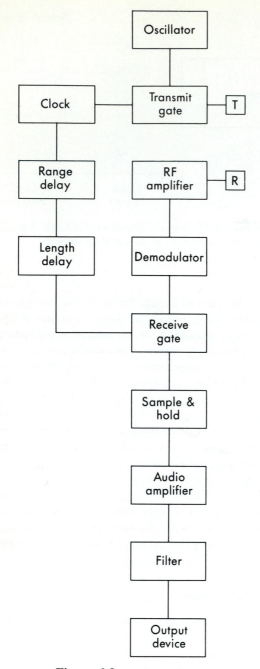

Figure 6-9 PW Doppler unit.

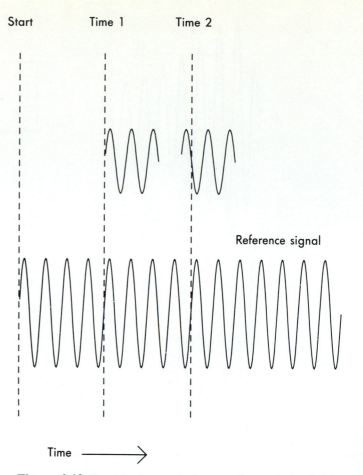

Reference signal

Time ⟶

Figure 6-10 The echo from a stationary reflector received at time *1* is in phase with the reference signal. The echo from a moving reflector received at time *2* is not.

Velocity Detection Limit

At a minimum, two pulses are required per beat cycle to define the beat frequency unambiguously. This creates a very important limitation in PW Doppler scanning. The maximum Doppler shift, $f_D(max)$, that can be detected is related to the PRF:

6-5

$$f_D(max) = \frac{PRF}{2}$$

To measure reflectors moving with high velocity and producing large Doppler shifts, a high PRF is necessary; however, a high PRF limits the depth that can be sampled, because a certain time is required to collect the echoes arising from that depth before the next pulse is sent out. The problem becomes more complex when it is realized that the Doppler shift depends on transducer frequency. Nevertheless, the relation between depth of interest (R), transducer frequency (f), Doppler angle (ϕ), velocity of sound in tissue (c), and maximum reflector velocity (V_{max}) is described by a single equation:

6-6

$$V_{max} = \frac{c^2}{8\ fR\ cos\ \phi}$$

is received at time 1. The shift in phase at time 2 indicates that the reflector at a specific depth is moving.

To obtain the beat frequency, it is necessary that the received signals from multiple pulses be mixed with the reference signal (same frequency as the transmitted pulse). Each transmitted pulse provides one instantaneous value of the Doppler signal. The sample-and-hold circuit assembles the values obtained from multiple transmitted pulses to form the beat frequency. The beat pattern is not as well defined as with CW Doppler because the pulsed echoes are equivalent to sampling the CW signal at discrete intervals (Fig. 6-11). The beat pattern can be more clearly delineated if more pulses are used, which would require an increase in the pulse repetition frequency.

Beat frequency

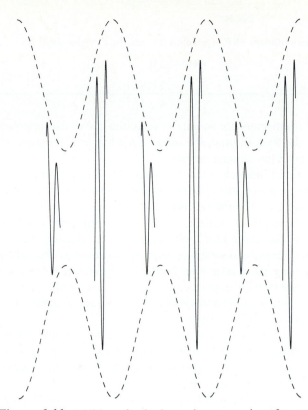

Figure 6-11 Addition of pulsed sound waves to the reference signal yields the interpreted beat frequency (*dotted line*).

	Maximum Velocity Limit* (cm/s)		
Depth (cm)	2 MHz Frequency	5 MHz Frequency	10 MHz Frequency
1	1480	590	295
5	295	120	60
10	150	60	30
15	100	40	20
20	75	30	15

*The Doppler angle is 0 degrees.

possible to increase the maximum velocity detectable to 150 cm/s. Changing the depth of interest to 15 cm, while maintaining the transducer frequency at 2 MHz, lowers the measurable maximum velocity to 100 cm/s. Fortunately, these conditions are such that the physiological velocities of moving structures (except the heart) usually occur within the detectable range of PW Doppler units.

Aliasing

If the sampling rate is not adequate for high-frequency Doppler shifts, artifactual lower-frequency Doppler shifts are displayed. Because beat frequency is sampled intermittently, it must be inferred from the limited data available. When the sampling occurs less than two times during a beat cycle, the data are misinterpreted as being at a lower frequency than the beat frequency. The requirement that the sampling rate must be at least twice the maximum frequency present in the Doppler signal is referred to as the Nyquist criterion. One half of the pulse repetition frequency is the Nyquist limit as defined by Equation 6-5; Doppler shifts above the Nyquist limit are falsely depicted as low-frequency shifts corresponding to slow-moving reflectors. As illustrated in Figure 6-12, imagine that a picture is taken of the amplitude of the beat frequency at various points and that a new waveform is constructed from this collection of amplitude measurements. The actual beat frequency is misinterpreted as a waveform with a lower frequency because sampling occurred only 13 times over 10 cycles. This is called aliasing, and it also is not present in CW units.

The motion picture industry provides a visual example of aliasing. In movies of the old West, a buckboard is often pulled across the prairie by a team of horses. You undoubtedly recall how the wheels on the buckboard appeared to be going backward, which was visually inconsistent with the movement of other objects depicted in the scene. In making the movie, a series of stop-action photographs is taken and shown one after another to give the appearance of motion. There is a time delay between frames, however, which means that the recording system is sampling the motion at discrete intervals. If the motion becomes very rapid, as with the rotating wheel on the buckboard, the sampling cannot properly represent the motion (the wheel moves too

The maximum velocity as a function of depth and transducer frequency for a Doppler angle of 0 degrees is listed in Table 6-2. If the Doppler angle is not 0 degrees, the maximum velocity is increased by the factor $1/\cos \phi$.

The ramifications from Equation 6-6 are twofold. First, if the depth of interest is increased, the maximum reflector velocity that can be measured is decreased. Second, a low-frequency transducer allows greater velocities to be detected. These limitations occur because the motion of the reflector is sampled at discrete intervals and not continuously, as in CW units. Unless low-pass filtering is applied, there is no maximum reflector velocity limit for CW scanners.

The following numerical examples illustrate the maximum velocities measurable in the clinical environment. The maximum PRF for a 10 cm depth is approximately 7700 pulses per second (a 130 μs time delay is required between transmission of the pulse and the reception of the returning echo). With a 3.5 MHz transducer and a Doppler angle of 0 degrees the Doppler shift is limited to 3850 Hz, which corresponds to a maximum velocity for a moving reflector of 85 cm/s.

$$V_{max} = \frac{(1540 \text{ m/s})^2}{(8)(3.5 \times 10^6 \text{ c/s})(0.1 \text{ m})}$$

$$= 0.85 \text{ m/s or } 85 \text{ cm/s}$$

By decreasing the transducer frequency to 2 MHz, it is

True beat frequency

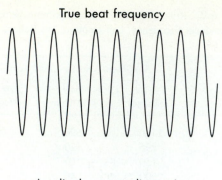

Amplitude at sampling points

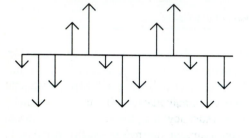

Implied beat frequency

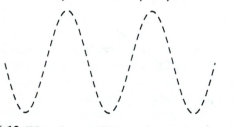

Figure 6-12 When the sampling rate is not adequate, the true beat frequency *(solid line)* tends to be interpreted as a lower frequency *(dotted line)*. The height of an arrow at a particular point represents the amplitude of the sampling at that point. Drawing a line along the tips of the arrows yields the implied beat frequency.

large a distance between successive photographs). To solve this problem the time between frames must be decreased (i.e., more photos taken) so the wheel moves a shorter distance between photographs. More frequent sampling allows the recording system to reproduce the motion accurately. Note that in the movie, only objects moving at high velocity are affected by the sampling rate; the motion of slower-moving objects is correctly reproduced. In ultrasound the boundary for the correct interpretation of object velocity is given by the Nyquist limit, which depends on the PRF.

■ **Example 6-3**

Calculate the minimum PRF necessary to prevent aliasing if the velocity of the moving reflector is 15 cm/s. The angle of insonation is 40 degrees and the transducer frequency is 2 MHz.
Using Equation 6-2

$$f_D = \frac{2 \ vf \cos \phi}{c}$$

$$= \frac{2 \ (15 \ cm/s) \ (2.0 \times 10^6 \ c/s) \cos 40 \ degrees}{154,000 \ cm/s}$$

$$= 298 \ Hz$$

The minimum PRF is equal to 2 times the Doppler shift.

$$PRF = 2 \ f_D$$

$$= 2 \ (298 \ Hz)$$

$$= 596 \ Hz$$

If reflectors are moving at velocities above that imposed by the Nyquist limit, the sonographer has several options to remove the aliasing artifact.

1. An increase in the PRF raises the Nyquist limit, possibly to a level that is sufficient to measure reflector velocity accurately. The PRF is usually set by the pulse transit time to the depth of interest. Nevertheless, adjusting the PRF above the transit time limit can remove the aliasing artifact. An ambiguity in sampling location, however, is created by ignoring the transit time limitation. In effect, echoes are now obtained simultaneously from two sampling volumes. Strategic positioning of one sampling location where no flow is present removes the ambiguity.

2. If reverse flow is not of concern, the baseline can be adjusted to devote the entire range of velocity detection to forward flow. This technique doubles the maximum velocity that can be measured without aliasing.

3. Examination of Equation 6-6 reveals that the Doppler angle and transducer frequency also affect the Nyquist limit. By increasing the Doppler angle or lowering the transducer frequency, the sonographer can eliminate aliasing.

4. Finally, switching from PW to CW modes enables the fastest motion to be observed without an aliasing artifact (although depth information is then sacrificed in the CW mode).

PW Bandwidth

The transducer in a PW Doppler unit does not produce a single-frequency sound wave. Because the ultrasound beam is on for only a short time, each sound pulse consists of a range of frequencies characterized by the bandwidth. As with imaging transducers, a very short pulse creates a spectral distribution of frequencies with a wide bandwidth. The multiple frequency components cause frequency variations in the observed Doppler shifts and a reduction in the signal-to-noise ratio. Decreasing the bandwidth by lengthening the pulse improves the system's ability to detect weak Doppler shifts but degrades the spatial resolution. PW Doppler units require pulses that consist of at least four to five cycles. Manufacturers compensate for the poor signal-to-noise ratio (compared with CW units) by increasing the acoustic power.

The spectral distribution of frequencies poses two additional problems. First, the preferential attenuation of high-frequency components as the beam traverses tissue causes a downward distortion in the frequency distribution, which is interpreted incorrectly as a Doppler shift. This attenuation effect varies with the depth of the moving reflectors. Second, the frequency dependence of scattering enhances the high-

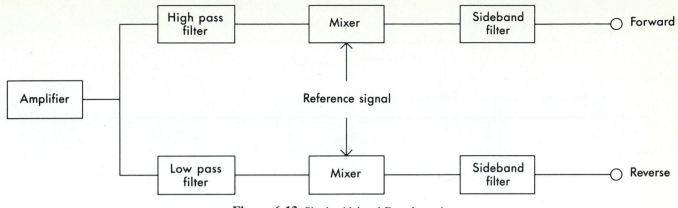

Figure 6-13 Single sideband Doppler unit.

frequency components in the echo and thus tends to counteract the effect of attenuation.

DIRECTIONAL METHODS

The received echo from a moving reflector is shifted in frequency above or below the reference signal depending on whether the motion is toward or away from the transducer. This process of demodulating the signal indicates that a shift has occurred but it cannot identify whether the shift is positive or negative. Three processing methods—including single sideband, heterodyne, and quadrature phase detection—have been developed to distinguish between motion toward and motion away from the transducer.

Single-Sideband Detector

The operation of a single-sideband detector system is shown in Figure 6-13. The received signal consists of reflected echoes from both stationary and moving structures. The reflections from stationary structures are equal in frequency to the transmitted beam, whereas those from moving structures are offset in frequency.

The signal from the radiofrequency amplifier is split into two components and then filtered. One filter is designed to pass all frequencies above the reference signal (forward motion) and the other all frequencies below the reference signal (reverse motion). The output of each filter is mixed with the reference signal and then filtered by a sideband filter in which all components except the shifted signals are removed. This results in two separate signals corresponding to the forward and reverse motions.

Heterodyne Detector

In a heterodyne detector the offset signal combines with the reference signal before being added to the received signal to obtain the Doppler shift. This technique displaces the Doppler shift to a new frequency range. Forward and reverse motions are differentiated by the magnitude of the Doppler shift compared with the offset frequency. For example, if the offset frequency is 5 kHz, the Doppler shift (f_D) is given as

$$f_D = f_R - (f - 5 \text{ kHz})$$

6-7

where f_R is the frequency of the received signal and f the transmitted frequency.

Note that Equation 6-7 reduces to the usual definition of Doppler shift (the difference in frequency between received and transmitted signals) if the offset signal is set to zero. The offset signal, however, allows reverse motion ($f_R < f$) to be displayed as frequencies below 5 kHz and forward motion ($f_R > f$) to be displayed as frequencies above 5 kHz (usually up to 15 kHz).

Quadrature Phase Detector

Figure 6-14 illustrates quadrature phase detection, the most commonly used directional technique. The signal from the radiofrequency (RF) amplifier is split into two components, and each is mixed with the reference signal (one channel 90 degrees out of phase with the other). After filtering, the output from each channel contains a mixture of forward and reverse flow signals. In time domain processing the presence of flow in one direction only causes each channel to exhibit the same voltage variation as a function of time, although the pattern is shifted in time. If flow is in the forward direction, the output from channel A shows the leading edge of the pattern first. Flow in the opposite direction causes the output from channel B to precede the output from channel A. The outputs from both channels are analyzed simultaneously by comparing their relative phase to determine whether flow is in the forward or reverse directions. This detection system does not work properly, however, if forward and reverse flow signals occur concurrently. The method also is susceptible to switching flow artifacts if high noise levels or strong low-frequency signals are present.

A technique called frequency domain processing is applied after quadrature phase detection to generate two output signals, each associated with a particular direction of flow. These signals can be routed to headphones in which the sounds in one ear represent motion toward the transducer and those in the other ear correspond to motion away from the transducer. Figure 6-15 demonstrates the operation of the frequency domain detector. A pilot signal within the

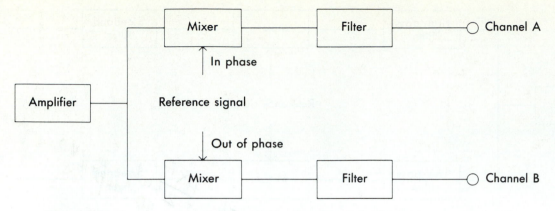

Figure 6-14 Quadrature phase detection divides the received signal into two components and then mixes these with a varying phase reference signal.

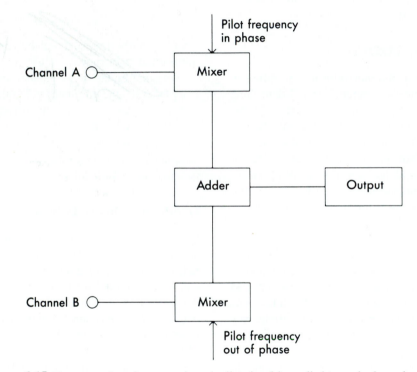

Figure 6-15 Frequency domain processing. A pilot signal is applied to each channel output from a quadrature phase detector. The two signals are added and the frequency components of the output are analyzed to separate the forward and reverse flow signals.

audible frequency range is mixed with the channel output signals from the quadrature phase detector. A 90-degree phase difference in the pilot signal is maintained between the two channels. The resulting signals from each channel are then added together and sent to an output device where the frequency components are analyzed and displayed. Forward flow is represented by output frequencies above the pilot frequency, and reverse flow by frequencies below the pilot frequency.

COLOR-FLOW IMAGING (STATIC MODE)

A two-dimensional image of the flow is constructed by displaying the detected Doppler shifts as the transducer is moved across the scanning area (Fig. 6-16). Each point in the image corresponds to a particular location of the transducer. The transducer is mounted on a scanning arm (similar to the static B-mode scanner), which enables its position to be known. A collection time of 2 to 3 minutes is necessary for acquiring the scan data in an image. Some devices display the detected Doppler signals as different colors depending on the magnitude of the frequency shift. This imaging technique was originally called color Doppler, but the terminology is now antiquated by real-time color Dopper imaging. Static color-flow imaging systems may operate in either the CW or the PW mode.

CW systems produce flat-plate images of blood flow across a vessel, but no depth information is given (Fig. 6-17). Each point in the image is a composite of all the Doppler signals along a single line of sight. Several lines of sight

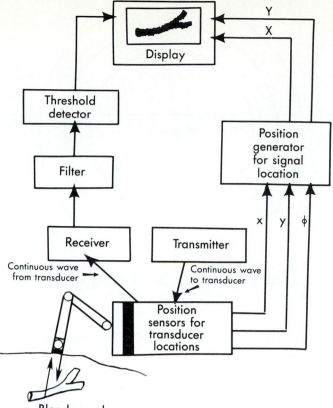

Figure 6-16 CW flow imager with scanning arm to denote position of the transducer.

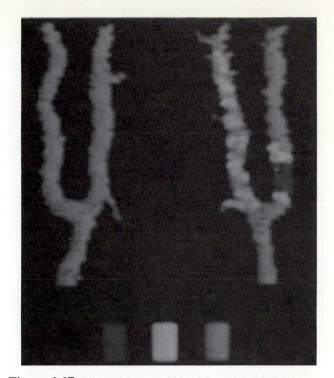

Figure 6-17 Bilateral image of blood flow through the carotids produced by a CW Doppler imaging system. The arteries are color coded according to the velocity of flow at each point across their lumina. The left internal carotid demonstrates stenosis. Compensatory increased velocity is exhibited by the left external carotid. (Courtesy Diagnostic Electronics Corporation, Lexington, Mass.)

are combined to form a two-dimensional mapping of the flow.

PW systems (sometimes called range-gated Doppler) provide depth information and, consequently, depict flow in three dimensions. The depth range along the line of sight is divided into many sections (usually about 30) of 1 mm each. Multiple processing gates are employed to select the Doppler signals according to depth. These units can also detect the direction of flow.

DUPLEX SCANNERS

Duplex Doppler units combine real-time imaging with CW or PW Doppler detection. The real-time image depicts stationary reflectors (e.g., plaques inside the vessel and other anatomical structures) whereas the Doppler mode provides flow information for a selected region. The display of anatomical structures aids in selecting the line of sight for CW Doppler or the sample volume for PW Doppler. Markers for the sampling region are superimposed on the real-time image. Visualization of the physical size and shape of plaque with real-time scanning is an important factor in the diagnosis of vascular disease. Duplex scanners were developed to overcome two major disadvantages of static color flow imaging: (1) the neighboring stationary structures are not displayed and (2) the scanning time for two-dimensional flow mapping is long.

The duplex scanner must perform both imaging and Doppler functions. Because the optimal design specifications for each of these functions are not the same, a variety of transducer configurations have been developed. Mechanical sector, annular phased array, linear phased array, and linear array transducers are used for real-time imaging and then switched to operate in the Doppler mode (Fig. 6-18). Real-time imaging is interrupted while the flow information is acquired, usually over a period of several milliseconds. The ultrasound beam must be repeatedly directed along one line of sight in the Doppler mode. Multiple echoes from the same reflector are necessary for determining the beat frequency. The rotational inertia of mechanical sector transducers prohibits rapid switching between imaging and Doppler modes. The electronic interleaving of Doppler pulses between imaging pulses in simultaneous duplex scanning permits real-time imaging, though at a reduced frame rate. Some systems use a separate transducer operating at a different frequency for the Doppler mode. A linear array with an offset Doppler transducer is one example. The offset transducer also provides a more appropriate Doppler angle, but good coupling between the probe and skin is difficult.

A single broadband transducer operating at low frequency in the Doppler mode and high frequency in the imaging mode is also feasible. An annular phased array has been developed that obtains the image data at 5 MHz and then

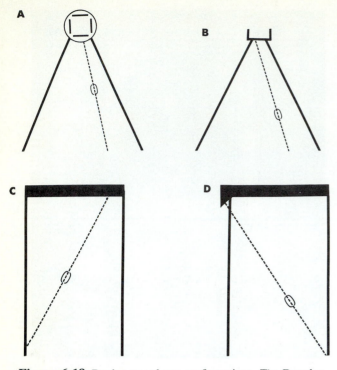

Figure 6-18 Duplex transducer configurations. The Doppler lines of sight are denoted by a *dotted line*. **A,** Mechanical sector; **B,** linear phased array; **C,** linear array; **D,** linear array with an offset transducer.

activates the central disk only for Doppler detection at 3 MHz.

In duplex scanning, the flow information is acquired for a highly restricted region and displayed in real time. The pattern of flow must be ascertained by sampling multiple regions one after the other. Isolated flow disturbances may go undetected.

SPECTRAL ANALYSIS

In the cross section of a vessel, RBCs at various radii from the center are moving at different velocities, resulting in a Doppler signal that is a combination of all the frequency shifts. The process of determining the individual frequency shifts from this complex Doppler signal is called spectral analysis.

The analysis of complex Doppler signals is usually accomplished with a mathematical algorithm called the Fast Fourier Transform (FFT). Fourier analysis is the process of separating a waveform into a series of single-frequency sine-wave components. When algebraically combined, these components yield the original waveform. A more complete description of Fourier analysis is presented in Appendix B. Other methods (e.g., the parallel filter bank and time compression) have also been used to quantify individual frequency components in the Doppler signal. Parallel filter bank and time compression are discussed later. Several examples follow to illustrate the principle of spectral analysis.

Figure 6-19 is a cross-sectional view of a vessel lumen. In regions *1, 2,* and *3* RBCs move at different velocities

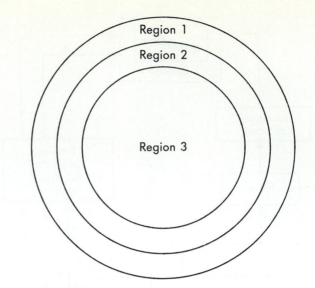

Figure 6-19 Regions of red blood cell velocity across a vessel lumen.

($v_3 > v_2 > v_1$) through the vessel. For simplicity, the same total number of RBCs is assumed to pass through each region and to flow at a continuous (nonpulsatile) rate. If the ultrasound beam is made very small so each of these regions is sampled individually, a characteristic Doppler shift is obtained for each region (Fig. 6-20). Three frequency shifts are observed (f_1, f_2, and f_3). The frequency shift is largest for region 3, because RBCs in this region are moving at the greatest velocity. Because an equal number of RBCs is present in each region, the amplitude of the individual frequency shifts is the same. This is represented by the heights of the waveforms in Figure 6-20, which are identical.

If all three regions are sampled by the ultrasound beam at the same time, a very complex Doppler signal will be obtained, as shown in Figure 6-21, that is an algebraic sum of the three waveforms in Figure 6-20. This detected signal must be simplified to associate groups of RBCs with individual frequency shifts and thus with rates of movement. Spectral analysis separates the complex signal into its individual frequency components and determines the relative importance of each; that is, the waveform in Figure 6-21, the detected signal, is mathematically converted into the various individual frequency shifts shown in Figure 6-20.

Power Spectrum

An alternative way to display the spectral analysis is in the form of a power spectrum in which the magnitude of individual frequency components is plotted against the frequency (Fig. 6-22). This converts the complex Doppler signal from the time domain into the frequency domain. The power spectrum is an extremely useful analysis technique because it displays the desired flow information, the distribution of Doppler shifts, directly. The magnitude is determined by the amplitude of the respective waveform corresponding to a particular frequency and represents the relative importance of each frequency (i.e., the number of

Region 1

Region 2

Region 3

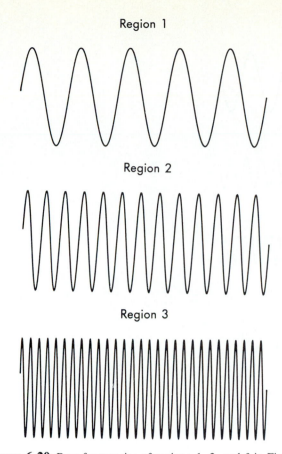

Figure 6-20 Beat frequencies of regions *1*, *2*, and *3* in Figure 6-19. Note that they increase with increasing velocity of the RBCs.

Complex

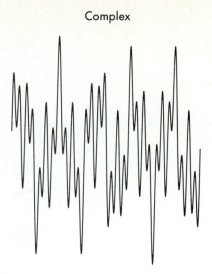

Figure 6-21 This complex Doppler signal is the sum of the waves in Figure 6-20.

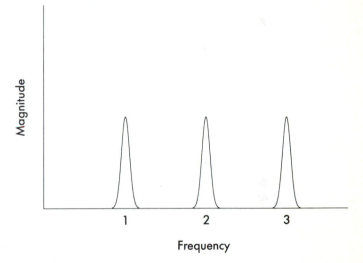

Figure 6-22 Power spectrum of the complex Doppler signal in Figure 6-21. The peaks corresponding to the regions are the same height.

RBCs moving at the velocity given by the frequency shift). Suppose, for example, that the number of RBCs moving through region *1* is doubled. The amplitude of the beat frequency corresponding to this region also doubles and results in an altered complex Doppler signal, as shown in Figure 6-23. The frequency of the Doppler shift for region *1* remains the same, because the velocity of the RBCs has not changed. The spectral analysis presented by the power spectrum in Figure 6-24 depicts the increased importance of the lowest frequency by the increased height of the peak corresponding to this frequency. The display of the complex Doppler signal as a function of time does not allow the sonographer readily to ascertain this increase in flow through region 1, but it can be easily interpreted from the power spectrum.

The relationship between the frequency domain display and the velocity of RBCs is further illustrated by the power spectrum associated with plug flow. Plug flow is blood moving at a single velocity. Suppose that all the RBCs throughout the vessel are moving slowly at a constant velocity; the power spectrum contains a single peak at low frequency (Fig. 6-25, *A*). If the velocity of the RBCs increases, the power spectrum once again shows a single peak but at a higher frequency (Fig. 6-25, *B*).

In reality, blood does not typically flow in discrete ve-

locities; rather, it exhibits a wide range of velocities. A sample velocity distribution of RBCs is depicted in Figure 6-26. The fullness of each bin indicates the number of RBCs within the corresponding velocity range. Note that all velocity ranges are not equally represented. Laminar flow consisting of many components is often encountered in the vascular system. Laminar flow with a velocity profile ranging from zero near the vessel wall to a maximum in the central portion of the vessel yields a continuous power spectrum, as shown in Figure 6-27. The power spectra associated with other velocity profiles are presented in Figures 6-28 and 6-29.

Stenosis creates disturbed flow, which is characterized by fast jets, slowly moving elements, and circulating eddies. The power spectrum demonstrates a broad range of frequency components, including negative values (which indicate reverse flow) (Fig. 6-30).

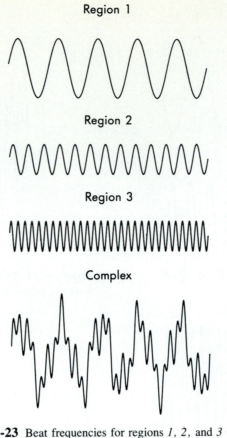

Region 1

Region 2

Region 3

Complex

Figure 6-23 Beat frequencies for regions *1*, *2*, and *3* (Fig. 6-19). Region *1* contains twice as many RBCs as the other regions, and changes in the complex Doppler signal arise from doubling the number of RBCs in that region.

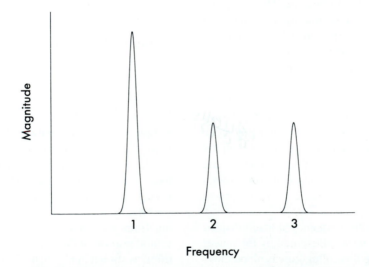

Figure 6-24 Power spectrum of the complex Doppler signal in Figure 6-23.

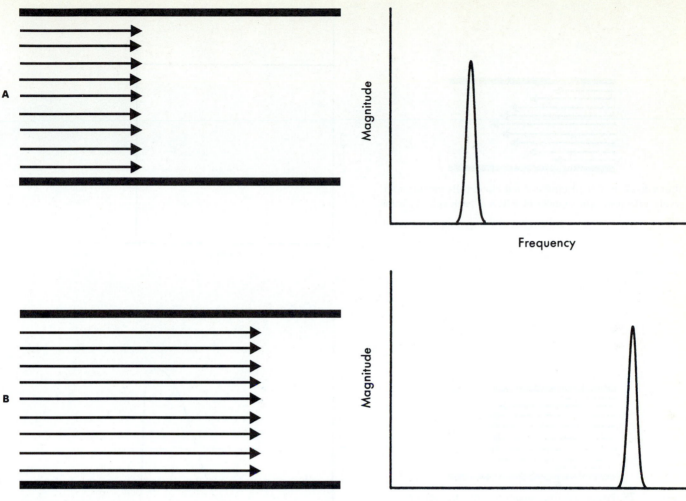

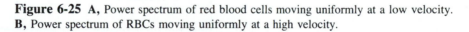

Figure 6-25 A, Power spectrum of red blood cells moving uniformly at a low velocity. **B,** Power spectrum of RBCs moving uniformly at a high velocity.

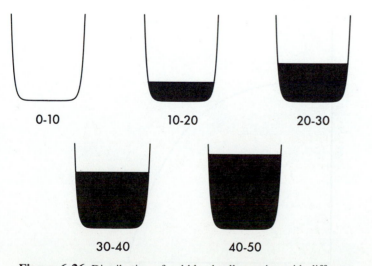

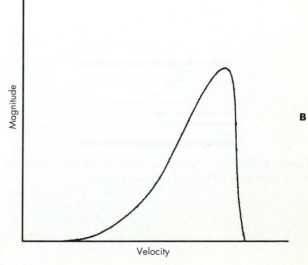

Figure 6-26 Distribution of red blood cells moving with different velocities across the vessel lumen. **A,** The fullness of each bin indicates the number of RBCs within that velocity range. All velocities are not equally represented. **B,** Power spectrum of the different velocity components represented.

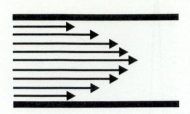

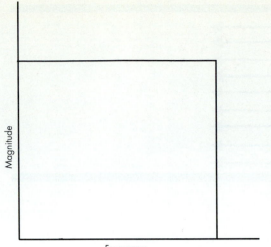

Figure 6-27 Power spectrum of red blood cells moving with varying velocities. The number of RBCs at each velocity is the same.

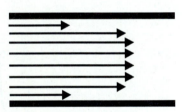

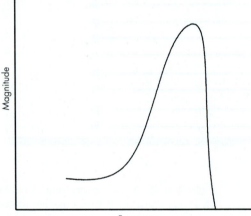

Figure 6-28 Power spectrum obtained when the velocity profile is dominated by high-velocity components.

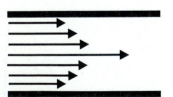

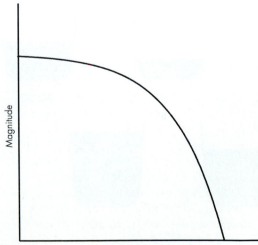

Figure 6-29 Power spectrum obtained when the velocity profile is dominated by low-velocity components.

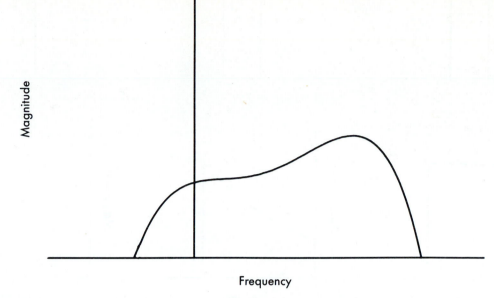

Figure 6-30 Power spectrum produced by turbulent flow.

Influence of Beam Shape

In the previous examples of power spectra associated with different velocity distributions, the magnitude of the frequency component indicated the volume of blood moving at the velocity given by that particular frequency. The ultrasound beam is assumed to be large enough to insonate all RBCs within the vessel uniformly. PW Doppler scanners are designed to generate highly directional beams that restrict sampling to small volumes. Beam shape, as characterized by cross-sectional uniformity and sample axial length, has a major effect on the detected Doppler signal. This beam-shape dependence becomes particularly problematical in the quantitative measurement of blood volume flow rate.

Consider once more the situation of laminar flow in which the velocity profile varies from zero near the vessel wall to a maximum in the central portion of the vessel. The effect of ultrasound beam shape on the power spectrum is shown in Figure 6-31 for three different sampling volumes. If the ultrasound beam encompasses the entire vessel uniformly, an accurate power spectrum depicting the various velocities is obtained. When the vessel is insonated nonuniformly, the contribution to the power spectrum by the slowly flowing RBCs near the wall is diminished. If the beam were restricted to the central portion of the vessel, only the most rapidly moving RBCs would contribute to the Doppler signal and the power spectrum would then become distorted. In each case the conditions of blood flow would not change but the measurement process would yield very different results depending on the relative dimensions of the vessel and the ultrasound beam.

The actual Doppler sampling volume may not correspond to the region selected by the sonographer. Refraction by soft tissue interfaces sometimes causes the sound beam to deviate from the anticipated straight-line path. If the ultrasound beam partially intercepts the vessel, the Doppler spectrum will not accurately portray flow velocities throughout the vessel.

Time Display of the Power Spectrum

In vessels the velocity distribution is not constant with time; rather, cyclic pressure changes give rise to pulsatile flow. Consequently, it is desirous to display the changing flow patterns depicted by the power spectrum as a function of time (called Doppler waveform). Three variables (frequency, magnitude, and time) must be included in this display. The magnitude in the power spectrum is now represented by varying the brightness level to indicate the relative importance of each frequency. Consider the power spectrum in Figure 6-32, *A*, in which the high-velocity group of RBCs produces twice the signal as the middle-velocity group, which in turn produces twice the signal as the low-velocity group. This information is converted to points of varying brightness along a straight line, representing the frequency axis (Fig. 6-32, *B*). Increased distance along the axis corresponds to higher frequency. Note that, in this example, the high frequency is brighter than the middle frequency, which is brighter than the low frequency.

Flow hemodynamics is not constant throughout the cardiac cycle. Peak flow velocities typically occur at peak systole. Good temporal resolution is necessary for the interpretation of flow patterns. The dimension of time is obtained by sampling the Doppler signal repeatedly in small increments of a few milliseconds. A fast Fourier transform (FFT) frequency analysis is then applied to each short time

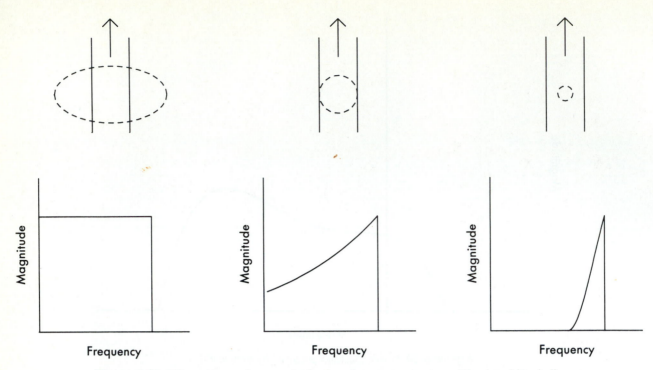

Figure 6-31 Effect of beam shape on the laminar flow power spectrum. The *dotted line* indicates the sampled region in each case. On the *left*, sampling of the entire vessel lumen with uniform intensity. In the *middle*, sampling with decreased intensity at the vessel wall. On the *right*, sampling restricted to the central portion of the lumen.

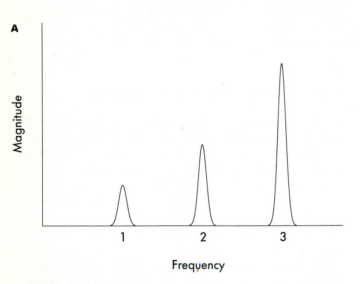

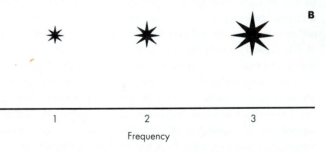

Figure 6-32 A, Power spectrum of three discrete groups of red blood cells in which the signal decreases in importance from high frequency to low frequency. **B,** Gray-level representation of the power spectrum.

segment of the Doppler signal. High-speed digital integrated circuits perform the necessary calculations on the most recently collected data while the Doppler signal for the following time segment is being acquired. The FFT processing allows a series of power spectra to be analyzed in real time. The display of these multiple analyses consists of a vertical axis corresponding to frequency, a horizontal axis corresponding to time, and varying brightness levels representing magnitude. Each analysis of a short time segment of the Doppler signal is presented as a single vertical line. By placing succeeding frequency analyses side by side, a fixed distance apart, the vertical lines scroll left to right with time to build up a pattern. The ability to display quickly changing velocities within the vessel is thereby achieved (Figs. 6-33

and 6-34). Time-varying physiological signals (e.g., an electrocardiogram) can be displayed in conjunction with the brightness-modulated power spectra.

The frequency or velocity scale of the spectrum analyzer is adjusted by changing the PRF. Aliasing is characterized by wraparound, whereby the high-velocity components above the Nyquist limit appear below the baseline (Fig. 6-35, *A*). The aliasing artifact is removed by adjusting the baseline (Fig. 6-35, *B*) or increasing the PRF (Fig. 6-35, *C*).

A high-pass filter, applied to the Doppler signal to eliminate the distracting low-frequency wall thump, may remove low-velocity blood flow components in the power spectrum. Under these conditions the velocity distribution becomes distorted by the application of a filter. Operator-controlled amplifier gain may also influence the Doppler waveform.

A

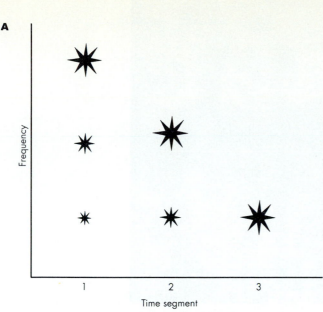

B

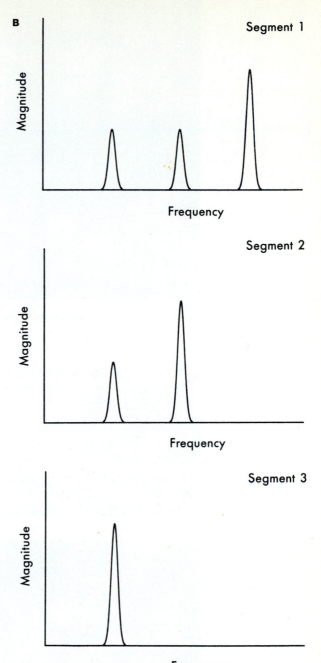

Figure 6-33 **A,** Time sequence of the gray-level representations of varying power spectra shown in **B. B,** Power spectra corresponding to the three time segments in **A.**

High gain broadens the velocity components that are displayed. Flow information can be lost at low gain settings, however.

Another improper presentation of the power spectra, called the mirror image artifact, occurs when weak Doppler signals are detected with high gain settings (Fig. 6-36). The large amount of clutter from stationary scatterers prevents the receiver from processing all incoming Doppler signals. The quadrature phase detector becomes saturated, resulting in a loss of directional discrimination.

Limitations of FFT Analysis

The FFT (fast Fourier transform) is applied to a block of data that have been collected previously. For the spectral display to respond to rapid changes in the velocity distribution, short sampling times are desirable. The duration of the analyzed segment, however, determines the frequency resolution. Each brightness-modulated dot in the power spectrum represents a range of shift frequencies equal to the inverse of the sampling time. A time segment of 5 ms yields a frequency resolution of 200 Hz; a longer time segment, 10 ms, improves the frequency resolution to 100 Hz.

Because the Doppler signal is a changing entity, statistical variations are introduced into the FFT analysis. To reduce these inaccuracies, several FFTs are performed within each time segment and the results averaged to generate the final spectrum. For example, an FFT calculated every 5 ms within a sampling time of 20 ms provides a redundancy of four analyses.

The observation of a single-frequency Doppler shift for a reflector moving at constant velocity is attained only for a very large-plane target insonated by a large acoustic field. As the reflector moves across a finite-width beam, the strength of the echo varies. The rise and fall of the detected signal causes the beat frequency to vary in amplitude, which is interpreted as additional frequency components above and below the idealized Doppler shift (Fig. 6-37). The broadening of the spectrum is called transit time broadening and creates difficulties in spectral interpretation. The spectrum produced by scatterers moving at different velocities is the same as that observed when scatterers are moving at constant velocity with transit time broadening. The overall effect of transit time broadening is to smear the magnitude of a frequency component over a wider range of frequencies.

Narrowing the beam width and shortening the receiver gate in PW mode accentuate the broadening effect. The simultaneous measurement of reflector position and velocity in PW Doppler limits the ability of these systems to deter-

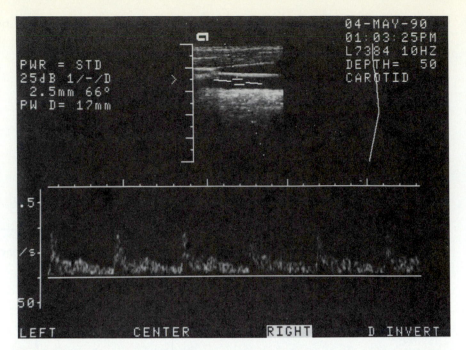

Figure 6-34 Brightness-modulated power spectra obtained for the internal carotid artery.

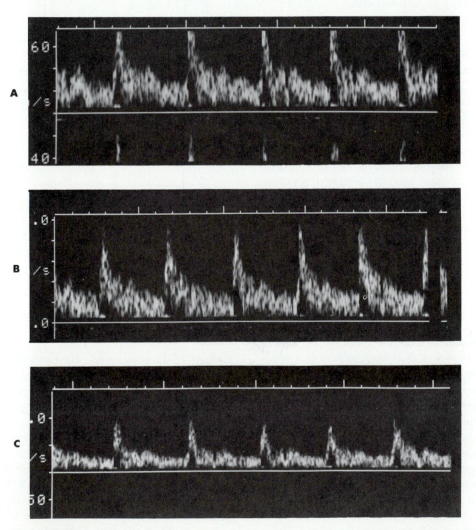

Figure 6-35 A, Aliasing artifact in which high velocity components demonstrate wraparound. The velocity range on the vertical scale is −0.4 to 0.6 m/s. **B,** Adjusting the baseline to remove the aliasing artifact. The velocity range is 0 to 1.0 m/s. **C,** Increasing the PRF to remove the aliasing artifact. The velocity range is −0.5 to 1.0 m/s.

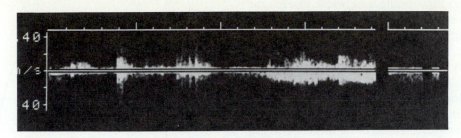

Figure 6-36 Mirror image artifact.

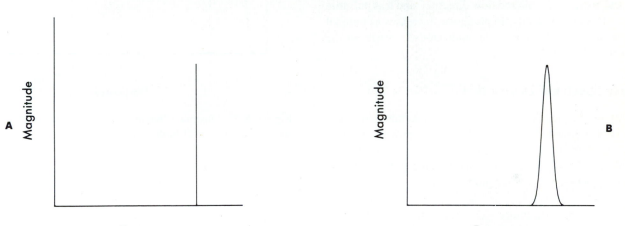

Figure 6-37 A, Idealized power spectrum for a constant-velocity reflector. **B,** The effect of transit-time broadening on this power spectrum.

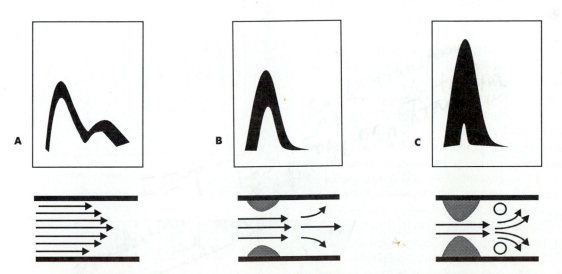

Figure 6-38 Brightness-modulated power spectra. **A,** Normal. **B,** Partially blocked lumen. **C,** Severe stenosis.

mine high-velocity flow in small localized regions. Longer pulse lengths with a corresponding loss in positional information are necessary to assess high-velocity jets accurately.

The transmitted pulse consists of multiple frequencies, which introduces variations into the received frequency and contributes to spectral broadening.

Disturbed Flow Power Spectra

For a vessel with a nearly uniform velocity distribution the spectral display, particularly during systole, shows a characteristic window appearance (Fig. 6-38, *A*). The window is an area between the high-velocity components and the baseline that is relatively signal free. Doppler shifts are confined to a relatively narrow velocity range. Partial blockage of a vessel causes flow disturbance, which extends the velocity distribution over a wider range. The increased variation in Doppler shifts is evidenced by a broadening of the spectral display (Fig. 6-38, *B*). The window is reduced and is not as distinct. A nearly blocked lumen creates high-speed jets with rotating flow elements (Fig 6-38, *C*). Arterial regions with eddy flow exhibit time-dependent behavior in which the velocity distribution reverts to laminar flow during periods of reduced pressure. The spectral display changes shape to reflect a loss in pulsatility. In summary: the four features of disturbed flow include increased peak velocity, spectral broadening, altered flow direction, and less pulsatile shape. The peak velocity, in particular, increases as luminal size decreases and is used as an indicator of severity of the stenosis.

Power Spectrum Descriptors

Maximum frequency, mean frequency, median frequency, and mode frequency are descriptors of the power spectrum that help characterize vascular Doppler signals. Various signal-processing techniques are incorporated within the PW unit to generate these descriptors.

Maximum frequency. The maximum Doppler shift (f_{max}) corresponds to the fastest-moving RBCs within the sample volume at the time of measurement. Each FFT segment is analyzed for the maximum frequency shift, which then is presented as a time-varying trace on the display.

Often the maximum Doppler shift in each time segment is converted to velocity using transducer frequency and Doppler angle. This trace is referred to as the maximum velocity waveform. An ECG tracing may be included in the display to associate events with the cardiac cycle. Many units are designed to provide an automatic derivation of the velocity waveform. Usually a 1% to 5% upper cutoff limit is applied to prevent the maximum Doppler shift from being associated with high-frequency noise. The cutoff limit indicates the portion of the power spectrum that is above the calculated maximum frequency. Perhaps the alternative description is easier to conceptualize: 100 minus the cutoff limit gives the percentage of total Doppler signal that lies below the calculated maximum frequency. Figure 6-39 illustrates the relation between FFT analysis and maximum frequency. If the power spectrum demonstrates a relatively steep falloff in magnitude for the high-frequency components, f_{max} is a good approximation of the true maximum frequency.

Mean, median, and mode frequencies. The mean frequency (f_{mean}) is calculated from the weighted sum of all frequencies in the power spectrum, in a manner similar to finding the statistical mean for a set of measurements. It can also be presented as a time-varying trace on the display. If insonation is uniform throughout the vessel, the average Doppler shift will correspond to the average velocity within the sample volume. Estimation of volume flow rate is commonly based on measurement of the average velocity. The

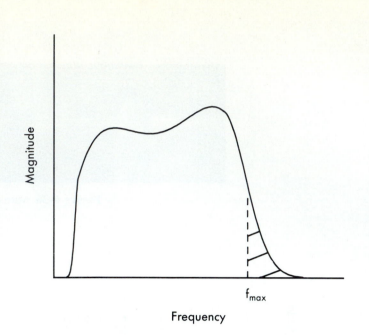

Figure 6-39 Maximum frequency derived from the power spectrum with a cutoff limit of 5%.

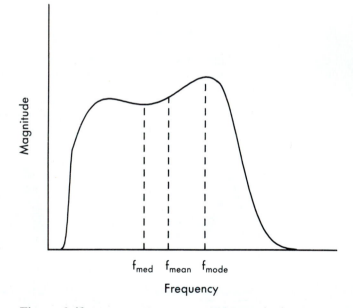

Figure 6-40 Mean, median, and mode frequencies in a power spectrum.

preferential absorption of high-frequency components by tissue causes a downward shift of the mean frequency, which is dependent on ultrasound path length. The application of a filter can also alter f_{mean} by removing low-frequency components.

The Doppler shifts of all reflectors are equally divided above and below the median frequency. The mode frequency indicates the prevalent Doppler shift in the power spectrum (the frequency at which the peak occurs). The relation of these three descriptors is illustrated in Figure 6-40.

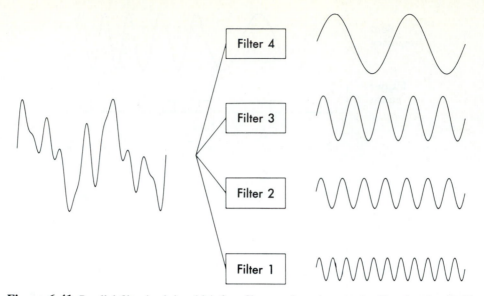

Figure 6-41 Parallel filter bank in which four filters analyze the complex Doppler signal with respect to four frequencies.

ALTERNATIVE METHODS OF SPECTRAL ANALYSIS

With advances in the speed of computer systems, the fast Fourier transform technique has rapidly become the method of choice for analyzing the Doppler signal; however, the methods of parallel filter bank and time compression have also been employed for frequency analysis.

The parallel filter bank analyzer contains a large number of filters each of which passes signals within a narrow frequency range. The analysis is performed in real time by simultaneously introducing the complex Doppler signal to each of the filters (Fig. 6-41). A disadvantage is that the large number of filters required for simultaneous analysis of multiple frequency ranges is very expensive.

In time compression the complex Doppler signal is sampled for a short time (8 ms) and then stored in digital memory. Once stored, it can be played back at an accelerated rate (250 times normal speed). The time compressed signal is analyzed during the time that the next Doppler signal is being collected for analysis. A filter with a bandwidth of 150 Hz is swept through a wide frequency range (200 Hz to 15 kHz). In other words, the filter is initially set at a baseline of 200 Hz with a window of 150 Hz, and the Doppler signal is examined for frequency components in this range. The baseline is then incremented by 150 Hz and the Doppler signal is reexamined for frequency components in this new range. The process is repeated several times until the Doppler signal is analyzed throughout its entire frequency range. The accelerated rate of playback is necessary to complete the analysis of multiple frequency windows in real time.

ZERO CROSSING DETECTORS

Zero crossing detectors are designed to monitor how rapidly the complex Doppler signal is oscillating between maximum and minimum. This provides an indicator of the frequency shifts that make up the Doppler signal.

Each time the Doppler signal crosses zero in one direction (e.g., moving from below zero to above zero), a trigger pulse is generated (Fig. 6-42). To reduce the influence of electronic noise, the signal must exceed a threshold value above zero for a trigger pulse to be produced. The number of pulses per second gives rise to the zero crossing frequency, which represents an averaging of all the frequencies in the Doppler signal. This spectral average is described as the root mean square of the instantaneous frequency distribution, which approximates the mean frequency waveform. The zero crossing frequency is similarly dependent on the velocity components of the flowing blood; that is, it increases if the velocity of flow becomes faster. It is susceptible to error when broad frequency spectra are encountered, however, and consequently FFT methods are generally preferred for the evaluation of flow.

The output of a zero crossing detector can be modified so each pulse appears as a dot on the display. The time-interval histogram (or TIH) is generated by positioning the dot vertically according to the reciprocal of the elapsed time from the previous pulse (Fig. 6-42). If two zero crossings occur rapidly, one immediately after the other, the dot corresponding to the second will be located high on the vertical scale. Thus the time dependence of the rate of zero crossings is visualized, and this yields a pattern similar to that obtained by spectral analysis. The TIH does not provide quantitative analysis of flow; only the pattern from plug flow is readily interpreted. This method also is not applicable when turbulent flow is present.

DOPPLER CONTRAST AGENTS

Encapsulated microbubbles injected intravenously are used as vascular contrast agents to depict small vessels, detect

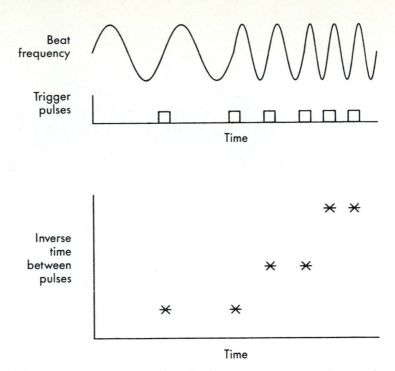

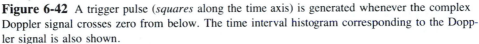

Figure 6-42 A trigger pulse (*squares* along the time axis) is generated whenever the complex Doppler signal crosses zero from below. The time interval histogram corresponding to the Doppler signal is also shown.

small tumors in low-sensitivity areas, evaluate tumor vascularity, and distinguish tumors from pseudotumors. Flow signal enhancement is usually observed in vessels near the site of injection, although normal and tumor tissue reflectivity is unchanged by the introduction of contrast agent.

The technique known as harmonic imaging minimizes echogenic contributions from tissue by detecting reflected sound waves at twice the transmitted frequency. The small microbubbles resonate and emit sound waves at the harmonic frequencies. By tuning the receiver to a harmonic frequency it is possible to enhance contrast because tissue does not produce reflected waves at this frequency.

SUMMARY

Doppler instrumentation detects the presence, direction, and velocity of motion. The Doppler shift is extracted by combining the detected echoes with the reference signal followed by demodulation to produce the beat frequency. PW Doppler allows the depth of the moving reflector to be determined, but a maximum velocity detection limit is imposed. Aliasing occurs if reflector velocity exceeds this limit. CW Doppler eliminates aliasing artifacts, although spatial information is also lost.

The Doppler signal obtained from RBCs is analyzed for frequency (and hence, velocity) components using the fast Fourier transform (FFT). The power spectrum shows the relative contribution of each velocity component. Velocity profile across the vessel lumen and sampling conditions affect the power spectrum. Time-dependent flow velocities within a vessel are depicted by brightness-modulated power spectra acquired successively in short time segments.

The information content of the brightness-modulated power spectra is simplified by displaying the maximum velocity waveform. This time-varying trace corresponds to the maximum Doppler shift and thus the fastest-moving RBCs within each FFT segment.

■ **REVIEW QUESTIONS** ■

1. Which of the following statements is true regarding the Doppler effect?
   a. The Doppler shift is the difference between the transmitted frequency and the observed frequency.
   b. The amount of the Doppler shift does not depend on the relative velocity between the source and receiver.
   c. The maximum Doppler shift will occur when the direction of ultrasound wave propagation is perpendicular to the motion.
   d. All of the above.
2. Assuming that an 8 MHz transducer is aimed at an interface moving toward the transducer with a velocity of 15 cm/s, what is the Doppler shift? The angle of incidence is 0 degrees.
   a. 779 Hz
   b. 1558 Hz
   c. 155,800 Hz
   d. None of the above
3. For Question 2, what is the frequency of the echo incident on the transducer?
   a. 1558 Hz
   b. 7,998,442 Hz
   c. 8,001,558 Hz
   d. None of the above

4. For Question 2, what is the Doppler shift if the Doppler angle is increased to 60 degrees?
   a. 390 Hz
   b. 779 Hz
   c. 900 Hz
   d. 77,900 Hz

5. Calculate the velocity of the moving reflector if a Doppler shift of 800 Hz is observed. The angle of insonation is 45 degrees. The center frequency of the transducer is 3 MHz.
   a. 9 cm/s
   b. 29 cm/s
   c. 58 cm/s
   d. 87 cm/s

6. Calculate the minimum PRF in pulses per second to prevent aliasing if the velocity of the moving reflector is 25 cm/s. The angle of insonation is 60 degrees, and the transducer frequency is 5 MHz.
   a. 410
   b. 812
   c. 1624
   d. 2100

7. Which of the following statements is true regarding the beat frequency?
   a. It is derived from the algebraic addition of transmitted and received waveforms.
   b. It is equal to the difference between the transmitted frequency and the received frequency.
   c. It corresponds to the Doppler shift.
   d. All of the above.

8. What is the purpose of the high-pass filter in a CW Doppler scanner?
   a. Remove echoes from stationary reflectors.
   b. Remove wall thump.
   c. Remove components from fast-moving reflectors.
   d. All of the above.

9. The CW Doppler unit
   a. Provides depth discrimination.
   b. Requires a scanning arm.
   c. Produces aliasing artifacts.
   d. None of the above.

10. In PW Doppler the sampling volume is defined by
    a. Gating the received signals.
    b. Changing the PRF.
    c. Increasing the gain and power.
    d. Mixing the received signal with the reference signal.

11. Which of the following statements is true regarding aliasing?
    a. It is an artifactual display of low-frequency components caused by an inadequate sampling rate of high-frequency Doppler shifts.
    b. It may be prevented by increasing either the PRF, the transducer frequency, or the depth of interrogation.
    c. It can occur in CW Doppler if the Doppler shift approaches 25% of the transducer frequency.
    d. It has no threshold in PW Doppler.

12. The power spectrum
    a. Places the Doppler shifts in the frequency domain (or equivalently, velocity).
    b. Shows the relative importance of each frequency component in the Doppler signal.
    c. Is usually obtained via the FFT technique.
    d. All of the above.

13. The brightness-modulated power spectrum combines _____, _____ , and _____ in a two-dimensional display.
    a. Frequency, depth, time
    b. Depth, signal strength, time
    c. Frequency, magnitude, time
    d. None of the above

14. What are the features of disturbed flow as presented on a spectral display?
    a. Higher frequency shifts
    b. Spectral broadening
    c. Presence of negative frequency components
    d. All of the above

15. The maximum frequency in the power spectrum:
    a. Correlates with the fastest moving reflectors.
    b. Is determined by the most prevalent frequency component.
    c. Represents an average of all reflector velocities.
    d. Is time independent.

16. Which of the following statements is true regarding zero crossing detectors?
    a. Zero crossing frequency depends on flow changes.
    b. FFT analysis is performed.
    c. Zero crossing frequency represents the maximum frequency in the Doppler signal.
    d. All of the above.

BIBLIOGRAPHY

Burns PN: The physical principles of Doppler and spectral analysis, *J Clin Ultrasound* 15:567, 1987.

Burns PN, Jaffe CC: Quantitative flow measurements with Doppler ultrasound: techniques, accuracy, and limitations, *Radiol Clin North Am* 23:641, 1985.

Hedrick WR, Hykes DL: Doppler physics and instrumentation: a review, *J Diagn Med Sonogr* 4:109, 1988.

Merritt CRB: Doppler US: the basics, *Radiographics* 11:109, 1991.

Nelson TR, Pretorius DH: The Doppler signal: where does it come from and what does it mean? *AJR* 151:439, 1988.

Smith H, Zagzebski J: *Basic Doppler physics*, Madison Wisc, 1991, Medical Physics Publishing.

Taylor KJW, Burns PN, Wells PNT: *Clinical applications of Doppler ultrasound*, New York, 1988, Raven Press.

Taylor KJW, Holland S: Doppler ultrasound, I, Basic principles, instrumentation, and pitfalls, *Radiology* 174:297, 1990.

Wells PNT: Ultrasonic Doppler equipment. In Fullerton GD, Zagzebski JA (eds): *Medical physics of CT and ultrasound-tissue imaging and characterization*, New York, 1980, American Institute of Physics.

Zagzebski JA: Physics and instrumentation in Doppler and B-mode ultrasonography. In Zweibel WJ (ed): *Introduction to vascular ultrasonography*, ed 2, Orlando, Fla, 1986, Grune & Stratton.

Color-Flow Imaging

K E Y   T E R M S

Asynchronous scanner

Autocorrelation

Baseline control

Capture function

Color aliasing

Color gain

Color gate

Color reject

Color threshold

Combined Doppler mode

Dwell time

Echo wavetrain

Mean frequency estimation

Motion discrimination

Packet size

Power map

Quadrature detection

Speckle tracking

Synchronous scanner

Time domain correlation

Variance map

Velocity map

Velocity scale

Velocity tag

Color-flow imaging is a relatively new scanning mode that combines gray-scale imaging with two-dimensional mapping of flow information in real time. Frame rates are slower than those achieved by real-time scanning (considerably more computational analysis is required), although speeds of 4 to 32 frames per second (fps) are possible. The gray-scale component of the color-flow image is designated as real-time, gray-scale, 2D, or B-mode. Motion is depicted throughout the field of view by superimposing different colors on the two-dimensional gray-scale image. A single representative velocity (usually the mean) at each sampling site is color encoded by hue or intensity. Typically, red indicates motion in one direction and blue motion in the opposite direction. Regions with high-velocity flow are displayed by decreased color saturation (increased whiteness). Flow turbulence may be color-coded in green.

CLASSIFICATION OF INSTRUMENTS

The first type of color-flow instrument developed processed Doppler signals to obtain velocity information and, hence, was called a color Doppler (CD) imager. A time domain correlation method to measure reflector velocity directly has recently been developed as an alternative to Doppler signal processing, and the term *color Doppler* has been retained to describe this imaging technique.

Both stationary and moving structures are detected by analyzing the received echoes with respect to amplitude, phase, and frequency in the Doppler-signal method or time shift in the direct velocity–measurement method (Fig. 7-1). Stationary structures are assigned a gray-scale level based on signal strength as previously shown for real-time scanners. Moving reflectors cause a phase shift or time shift that indicates the presence and direction of motion. For Doppler signal processing the magnitude of the frequency shift gives the relative velocity of the moving reflector via the Doppler-shift equation (not corrected for Doppler angle). When flow determination is made by time domain correlation, reflector velocity is directly proportional to the measured time shift in the received echoes from the moving reflector. Fast-moving reflectors are represented in light shades of red or blue, and slow-moving reflectors in dark shades (Fig. 7-2). Other color schemes are also used.

VELOCITY DISPLAY

The range of displayed velocities is set by the sonographer. For arterial work a high velocity range is appropriate, but for venous flow a low velocity range is necessary. If the phase shift is positive, the reflector is moving toward the transducer and is depicted in red. If the phase shift is negative, the reflector is moving away from the transducer and is depicted in blue. The association of color with a particular direction of flow is interchangeable, however. The importance of the two-color scheme is not to code for arterial and venous flow but rather to depict simultaneous flow in opposite directions on the real-time image. The highest priority in color-flow imaging is the observation of motion. If certain criteria are met, the display of motion in color always takes precedence over the gray-scale image of stationary reflectors.

The major disadvantage of duplex scanning is that flow is not evaluated simultaneously throughout the field of view but rather is sampled at a particular location as selected by

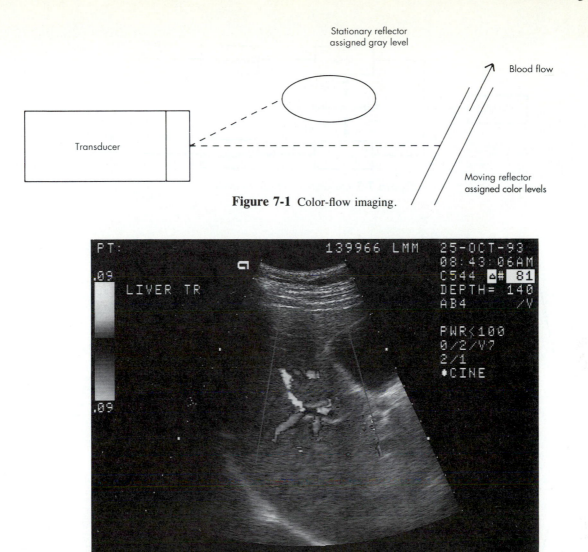

Figure 7-1 Color-flow imaging.

Figure 7-2 Color-flow imaging of the portal vein. Flow in the anterior right portal vein and the posterior right portal vein is shown. (See Color Plate 1A.)

the sonographer. To establish the regional flow pattern, the fast Fourier transform (FFT) analysis must be performed at multiple sites throughout the vessel, which requires precise positioning of the sampling volume. Focal regions of abnormal flow are sometimes overlooked. The repetition of sampling is also a time-consuming process. By displaying the two-dimensional spatial distribution of the velocities and the temporal changes in these velocity patterns, real-time CD imaging overcomes these difficulties and enables regions of flow disturbance to be more easily visualized.

VELOCITY DETECTION

To assess motion, multiple echoes from the same reflector must be collected using a series of transmitted pulses. As an analogy, a series of stop-action photographs of a moving car allows its velocity to be determined but a single photograph in the series does not indicate whether it is moving or not. Color-flow imaging requires positional information

as well as velocity of the moving reflector. Spatial origin of the echoes is obtained by gating the detected echoes.

PW Doppler FFT

Velocity information must be obtained for a large number of sample volumes throughout the field of view in a very limited amount of time. Range-gated PW Doppler spectral analysis requires a relatively long sampling time for each line of sight (typically about 10 ms). The sampling time or dwell time is the product of the PRP and the number of pulses used to interrogate the moving reflectors along one line of sight. Parallel processing of a multigated system allows several locations along the line of sight to be examined with no increase in sampling time. The gates are activated sequentially following the excitation pulse. Each gate corresponds to one pixel. Hundreds of gates, to acquire the Doppler signals from the entire scan line simultaneously, are necessary. The most important consideration is the time

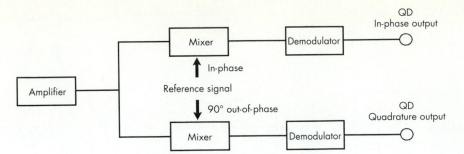

Figure 7-3 Quadrature detection circuit.

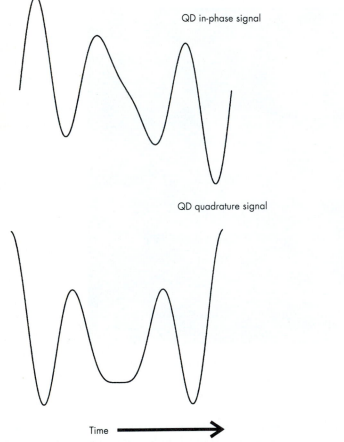

Figure 7-4 Output signals from the quadrature detection circuit. The in-phase signal and quadrature signal are not the same but are mathematically related.

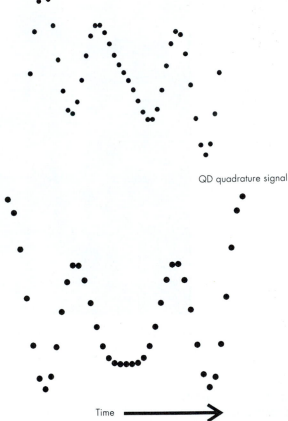

Figure 7-5 A PW Doppler sampling depicts the in-phase and quadrature signals in Figure 7-4 as a series of points.

constraint imposed by the requirement that the image must be updated every 0.05 to 0.1 second (corresponding to a frame rate of 10 to 20 images per second). Range-gated PW Doppler spectral detection does not satisfy this condition, because the time necessary to form an image of the Doppler signals is on the order of seconds. Each image consists of multiple scan lines and each scan line requires a dwell time of 10 ms. A faster method to detect Doppler signals is needed.

Quadrature Detection

Spectral analysis has a high informational content in that the individual frequency components of the Doppler signal

are identified. By characterizing the Doppler signal with a single parameter (usually the mean frequency) informational content is sacrificed but the sampling time can be shortened considerably. The rapid acquisition and analysis of flow data are achieved with multigate PW Doppler by zero crossing detection, time derivative of Doppler signals, autocorrelation, and autoregression.

Doppler signal processing is initiated with a quadrature detection (QD) circuit (Fig. 7-3). Two output signals labeled in-phase and out-of-phase (or quadrature) are generated (Fig. 7-4). For reflectors interrogated with a CW sound beam as illustrated in Figure 7-4, the QD signals are continuous waveforms. The pulsed wave technique is necessary to ob-

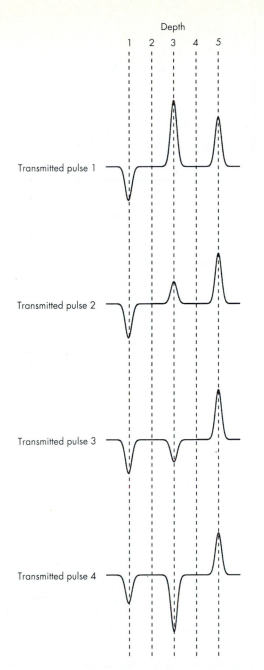

Figure 7-6 Quadrature channel output from four successive pulses along the line of sight. Motion is detected by changes in the signal level at a particular time (depth). The reflectors at depth segments *1* and *5* are stationary; that at depth segment *3* is moving.

signals to be generated from many depth segments during the dwell time for the line of sight. The depth sampling interval can be made 0.5 mm or smaller.

Zero Crossing Detection

Zero crossing detection evaluates the density of oscillations in one channel and the polarity in the other. It provides both the mean frequency and the phase. However, it underestimates high-frequency Doppler signals and is subject to error when signal-to-noise is poor.

Time Derivative of Quadrature Signals

An estimate of the mean frequency can be calculated by taking the time derivative of the phase, which is the arctangent of the ratio of the QD signals. Accurate mean velocity estimates are possible over a wide signal-to-noise range. Because of the superior performance and hardware simplicity of autocorrelation, however, that technique has become the standard for mean frequency estimation of the Doppler signal.

Autocorrelation

In quadrature detection the time-varying output from each channel is a complex function of amplitude and phase of the echo signals. Both stationary and moving reflectors contribute to this waveform, called the echo wavetrain. The phase of the received signal from a stationary reflector is constant, whereas the phase of the received signal from a moving reflector fluctuates with time. Consequently, sampling with another pulsed sound wave at a later time introduces a change in the signal level at the point in the echo wavetrain corresponding to the depth of a moving reflector (Fig. 7-6). Each echo wavetrain is partitioned according to depth by sequentially clocked gates (Fig. 7-7). A plot of QD output from successive transmitted pulses, segmented according to depth, indicates that moving reflectors produce signals with varying magnitude (Fig. 7-8). Note that two time measurements are required to obtain the information in Figure 7-8. First, the time following the transmitted pulse assigns depth; each transmitted pulse contributes one data point to the Doppler signal at every depth segment. Second, intermittent sampling of the Doppler signal at a particular depth is achieved by a succession of transmitted pulses. Data points are separated by a time interval equal to the PRP.

Autocorrelation is a comparison of measurements acquired from the same reflector. Processing of the echoes received from multiple depths is done concurrently. The stream of echoes along the entire scan line is examined by delaying the previous echo wavetrain obtained from the immediately preceding pulse by a time equal to the pulse repetition period (PRP). This places the stream of echoes on the same time scale, and thus reflector location is designated by the time interval following the transmitted pulse. Each echo wavetrain is divided into segments by depth. At every location the individual echoes from consecutive

tain positional information, which necessitates discrete sampling of these signals (Fig. 7-5). A succession of echoes from the same reflector is collected by sequential transmitted pulses, processed through the QD circuit, and placed in a hold circuit. In the time following a transmitted pulse the output from each QD channel is segmented into different depths by means of sequentially clocked gates. Each PRP contributes one data point to the composite in-phase signal and the composite quadrature signal at each depth. Multiple transmitted pulses allow the buildup of time-dependent QD signals (Fig. 7-6). The time between data points is equal to the pulse repetition period. This scheme allows Doppler

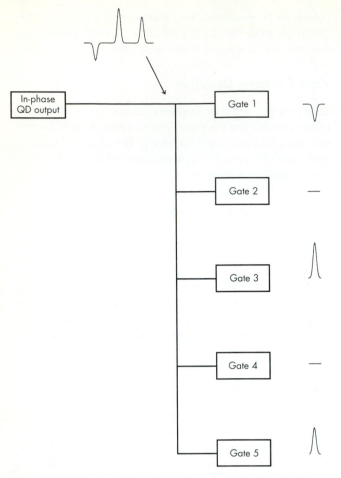

Figure 7-7 Gating of the QD output allows the signal to be segmented according to depth. One channel output is shown.

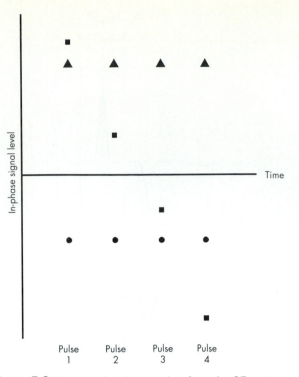

Figure 7-8 Doppler signal generation from the QD output. Each data point for a depth segment requires one transmitted pulse. Reflectors in depth segment *1 (triangles);* reflectors in depth segment *3 (squares);* reflectors in depth segment *5 (circles).*

samplings are multiplied together and the product is added in the integrator to the values from other samplings (Fig. 7-9). Registers store the computational results while the data are accumulated for one line of sight.

Both channels of the QD circuit provide input to the autocorrelation detector. For each depth two separate registers hold the output from the autocorrelation detector. At the conclusion of sampling along the line of sight, velocity and phase are computed at each depth from the values stored in registers corresponding to that depth. The phase is equal to the arc tangent of the ratio of the output values, and the velocity is equal to the phase divided by the sampling time interval, the pulse repetition period. Variance can also be determined.

Dwell time. A minimum of three observations is required to determine the Doppler shift. Generally, each scan line is sampled 4 to 10 times, although it may be as many as 32 times. *Packet size* or *ensemble length* describes the number of pulses used to interrogate a single color line of sight. Large packet size (long integration time) provides the highest color definition (most accurate frequency estimates), but a long dwell time lowers the frame rate.

The dwell time for each color line using autocorrela-

tion will now be examined. The frame rate (FR) is determined by

$$\text{7-1}$$

$$\text{FR} = \frac{1}{(\text{PRP}) \, Nn}$$

where N is the number of lines per frame (lpf) and n is the packet size. For a scanning range of 8 cm (PRP of 104 μs) under the conditions of 15 fps and 64 lpf, 10 pulses are used to sample each line of sight. The dwell time is 1.04 ms. At a PRF of 5 kHz or higher, autocorrelation provides rapid acquisition of the Doppler data to allow real-time imaging of the flow.

Fixed echo canceller. To lower the dynamic range of the QD input to the autocorrelation detector, strong echoes from stationary structures are often eliminated. Echoes from stationary reflectors remain unchanged in successive wavetrains; otherwise, varying echoes would be attributed to moving reflectors. Echoes from stationary reflectors are removed by subtracting identical echoes in consecutive pulses through the introduction of a fixed echo canceller (Figs. 7-10 and 7-11). The inability of mechanical transducers to generate an extremely stable beam path inhibits their use in CD imaging.

Velocity estimation. The autocorrelation detector does not depict spectral analysis of the Doppler signal from each sample volume. An average, not maximum, Doppler shift

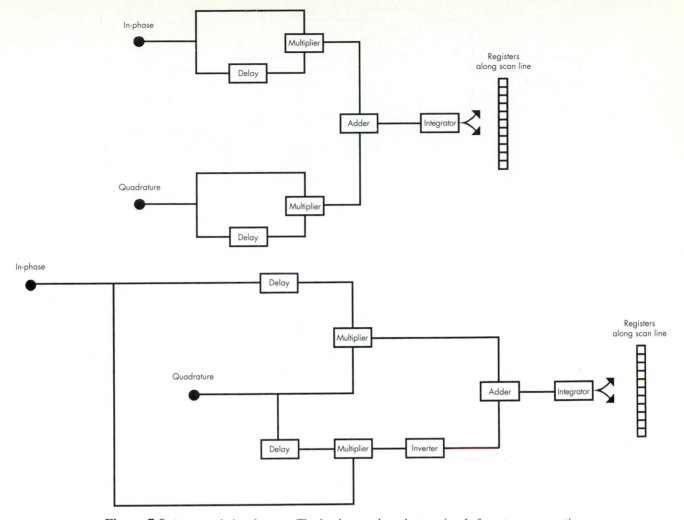

Figure 7-9 Autocorrelation detector. The in-phase and quadrature signals from two consecutive transmitted pulses are segmented by depth and then manipulated in a series of multiplication and addition steps. An integrator sums the computational results at each depth from repeated samplings and stores them in registers.

is determined. Although this is not ideal, a region with high mean velocity is likely to be a region with maximum velocity as well. The maximum Doppler shift could be presented, but this parameter is more sensitive to noise and spectral broadening.

CD imaging with autocorrelation is a PW Doppler technique that uses a relatively long pulse duration with a narrow bandwidth. Variance in the mean frequency estimate is increased when the pulse is shortened to improve axial resolution. Attenuation and diffraction of the ultrasound beam affect the velocity estimation, and the measured mean frequency of reflectors moving with the same velocity is depth dependent.

Autocorrelation is based on a pulsed sampling technique and, as such, is subject to aliasing. If flow exceeds the velocity range set by the sonographer (Doppler shift greater than half the PRF), color aliasing occurs. A high-frequency shift above the Nyquist limit is interpreted as a low-frequency shift in the opposite direction. Aliasing causes the

motion to be represented by a color level corresponding to reverse flow. For example, lighter and lighter reds progress to light blue where aliasing is present; also at a very high velocity (i.e., greater than twice the Nyquist limit) flow is depicted incorrectly, with a low-velocity color level in the correct direction.

Autoregression

An alternative to the Fourier method of frequency analysis has been introduced recently. The autoregressive technique uses a linear difference equation of past values of a measured variable to predict the current value. For Doppler signal analysis the QD outputs from each transmitted pulse compose the time-dependent data sequence. Regression coefficients used to estimate the mean frequency and maximum frequency are obtained by solving a set of recursive formulas. The mean frequency is identical to the frequency determined by the autocorrelation technique.

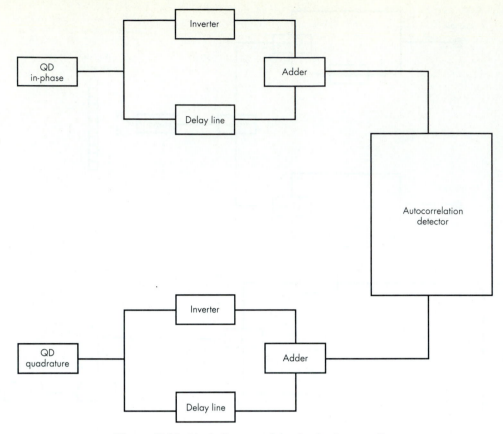

Figure 7-10 Block diagram of the fixed echo canceller.

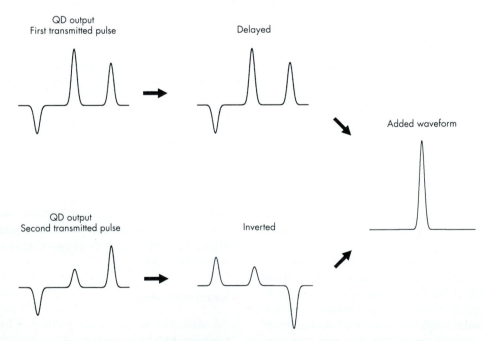

Figure 7-11 Manipulation of echo wavetrains by the fixed echo canceller.

Time Domain Correlation

A recently developed method, called time domain correlation, determines the velocity of a moving reflector by measuring the change in spatial location during a known time interval. Successive echo wavetrains along a fixed line of sight reveal that the echo associated with a moving reflector is displaced in time (Fig. 7-12). Using the echo-ranging principle, time (δt) is converted into distance (x) by assuming a value for the velocity of sound in the medium (c):

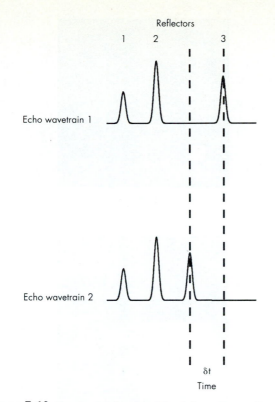

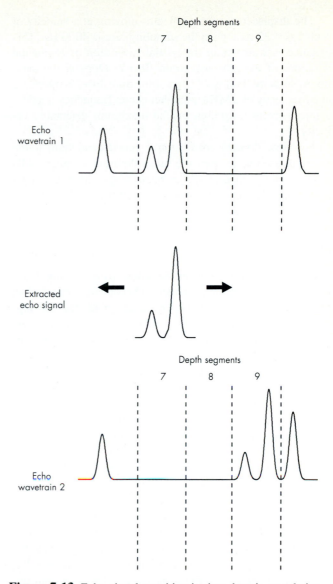

Figure 7-12 Received echo signal level from three reflectors at different depths. Reflectors *1* and *2* are stationary. Reflector *3* moves during the time between transmitted pulses. The shift in time indicates the distance of movement.

7-2

$$x = \tfrac{1}{2} c \, (\delta t)$$

Since the time between transmitted pulses is known (equal to the PRP), the velocity of the reflector (v_1) is calculated by

7-3

$$v_1 = \frac{x}{PRP}$$

Because sampling occurs along one direction only, Equation 7-3 yields the velocity component along the beam axis. The total reflector velocity (v) can be determined if the angle (ϕ) between the beam axis and the direction of motion is known:

7-4

$$v = \frac{v_1}{\cos \phi}$$

Echo pattern matching. The unique feature of time domain correlation is the ability to (1) identify a particular echo signal waveform in multiple echo wavetrains consisting of many echoes and (2) track the individual echo signals in time. Echo pattern matching is achieved by searching for a time position with maximum correlation. The echo wavetrain is segmented by depth, and the echo signal in each segment is extracted. A second echo wavetrain is acquired. Extracted echo signals in the first echo wavetrain are compared with echo signals at the corresponding depth and with

Figure 7-13 Echo signal matching in time domain correlation. The extracted signal from segment *7* in the first echo wavetrain is compared with various segments of the second echo wavetrain. The best match occurs at segment *9*.

signals at the neighboring segments in the second echo wavetrain until a match is found (Fig. 7-13). Moving reflectors are identified by a different depth assignment in the successive echo wavetrains. The time shift (δt) between the two segments provides the measurement by which the reflector velocity can be determined.

Velocity detection limit. The time correlation function has one maximum; no ambiguity is present as occurs in PW Doppler when the phase shift exceeds one cycle (aliasing). Time shifts greater than the period of the RF signal can be measured. Consequently, the velocity limits imposed by time-domain correlation are less restrictive than those with PW Doppler techniques. A velocity limit does arise, however, because the reflector must remain within the beam on successive pulses.

The displacement for a reflector moving at a velocity of 1 m/s is 0.25 mm when the sampling rate is 4000 Hz. This distance is well within the spatial resolution of segmental divisions of the echo wavetrain. In PW Doppler the maximum velocity limit is 77 cm/s if the transducer is operating at a frequency of 2 MHz. A higher center frequency imposes a more severe restriction on the maximum detectable velocity.

For time domain correlation a broad-bandwidth transducer is used to shorten the pulse duration (similar to B-mode). The decreased spatial pulse length improves axial resolution of the color display. Pixels in gray scale and color are comparable in size.

Speckle Tracking

The speckle pattern produced by echoes from moving RBCs is tracked in successive images. The distance traveled in the acquisition interval between frames yields the velocity. Both axial and lateral components of the motion are determined. A two-dimensional image of blood flow is constructed by tracking multiple regions within the field of view. The velocity for each region is color encoded and superimposed on the gray scale image.

Tracking of the speckle pattern is accomplished by identifying a small region (called a kernel) in the first image and then searching the subsequent image for the matching region (Fig. 7-14). The search area in the second image is limited to a small region surrounding the kernel. The location of the match for the kernel indicates the distance moved by the RBCs in the time between frames.

Recent developments in computer technology have enabled speckle tracking to be performed in real time at a frame rate of 30 fps. Spatial resolution of the color-encoded velocity display is inferior to that in gray-scale images because the pixel size is twice as large. The maximum detectable velocity is 1 to 2 m/s but, in theory, could be as high as 8 m/s.

The major advantage of speckle tracking is that an angle-independent color map of flow is produced. Conventional color-flow imaging, in which sampling is performed along one line of sight, provides mapping of only the axial component of motion. Consequently, quantitative assessment of flow velocity is compromised because the Doppler angle is not accurately known.

Doppler Spectral Analysis

Regardless of the velocity-detection method, a two-dimensional mapping of flow within the field of view is produced. To obtain information regarding the individual velocity components, range-gated PW Doppler with FFT analysis is performed for selected regions of interest. Since areas with abnormal flow pattern are rapidly identified, CD imaging has the potential to reduce examination time greatly by facilitating placement of the sampling volume for FFT analysis.

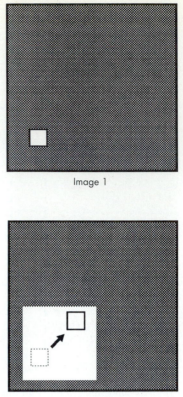

Image 1

Image 2

Figure 7-14 Speckle tracking. The reflectors producing the signal from a pixel in image *1* move from the original location *(dotted line)* to a new location *(solid line)* in image *2*. The search area is denoted in *white*.

ASYNCHRONOUS VERSUS SYNCHRONOUS IMAGING DEVICES

CD imaging devices are classified as asynchronous or synchronous based on how the scanner acquires the two-dimensional gray-scale and velocity information. Asynchronous systems collect imaging and flow data at different times, whereas synchronous systems collect the two data sets simultaneously.

We can use a linear array to see how the two-dimensional gray-scale and flow data are acquired separately and later superimposed to form the asynchronous image. The gray-scale image is obtained by generating sequential dynamically focused beams along the length of the array. Parallel lines of sight compose the two-dimensional gray-scale image, which allows for sampling perpendicular to the blood movement (the vessel is assumed to be parallel to the skin surface). This geometry is ideal for imaging but not for assessing flow (for which the interrogation angle would be 90 degrees). To place the beam at a more appropriate Doppler angle for measuring flow, it is steered at an angle to the array (Fig. 7-15). The beam angle is adjustable by the operator.

Separate complete field-of-view sweeps for two-dimensional gray-scale and flow imaging displace tissue position and flow in time. Consequently, small groups of steered and

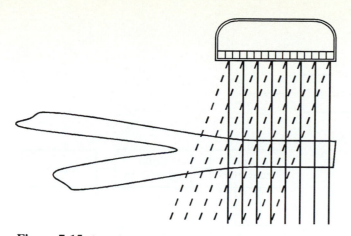

Figure 7-15 Asynchronous linear array with two-dimensional lines of sight *(solid)* and steered lines of sight *(dotted)*.

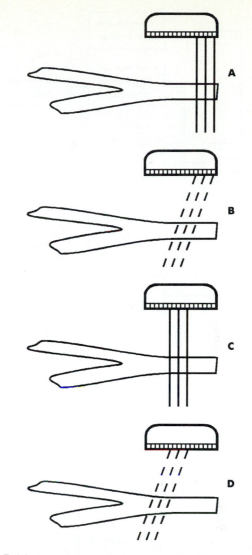

Figure 7-16 Asynchronous linear array with time sharing. A small portion of the field of view is sampled with gray scale, **A,** and then color, **B,** lines of sight before the next section of the field of view is probed, **C** and **D.**

unsteered lines of sight are alternated in a time-sharing scheme. These scan lines are interwoven in a digital scan converter to compose the final image (Fig. 7-16).

Figure 7-17 diagrams an asynchronous autocorrelation system. Separate transmitters form either the steered or the unsteered beam. If the beam is steered, the induced signal is directed to the Doppler channel. Otherwise, the gray-scale channel is active. The image data are processed and sent to the scan converter. In the Doppler channel a quadrature detector coupled with autocorrelation quantifies forward and reverse flow signals, which are numerically encoded and placed in the scan converter. The numerical values in the scan converter are translated into gray and color levels before being displayed on the monitor.

The basic CRT design is modified to display color-flow images. The uniform phosphor layer is replaced by an array of small dots consisting of red, green, and blue phosphors. Three electron beams scan the phosphor array simultaneously, each striking one type of phosphor. Different colors are formed by altering the mix of red, green, and blue light (primary colors) contributed by the respective phosphor types. Primary-color light intensity is varied by controlling the electron beam current.

The asynchronous autocorrelation scanner allows the transmitted beam to be optimized for both Doppler and two-dimensional gray scale because each component is collected independently of the other. The transducer frequency and transmit power may be adjusted for each component. Transmitted pulses can be switched between a gray-scale frequency of 5 MHz and a Doppler frequency of 3 MHz. The dual-frequency transducer entails some compromises: sensitivity is reduced, and beam manipulation becomes more difficult as the frequency is offset from the center frequency. Although a narrow beam width is desirable for good lateral resolution in the two-dimensional gray-scale mode, it causes spectral broadening in the Doppler mode. Transmitted power in the Doppler mode can be increased to improve detection of weak-flow signals.

Because the field of view is scanned twice for each frame, the frame rate is reduced. Most of the acquisition time is devoted to collecting the flow image. Only one pulse per scan line is required for the two-dimensional gray-scale mode although multiple pulses are necessary to compose a color line. To compensate partially for the longer acquisition time, fewer lines of sight, a smaller field of view, a higher-frequency threshold for the minimum displayed velocity, or a combination of these is used in the color mode (Figs. 7-18 and 7-19). Interpolating between lines fills in the gaps (spatial persistence). The axial sampling interval for Doppler is usually greater (as much as several millimeters), which means that the Doppler and two-dimensional gray-scale spatial resolution are not the same.

In a synchronous autocorrelation scanner (Fig. 7-20) am-

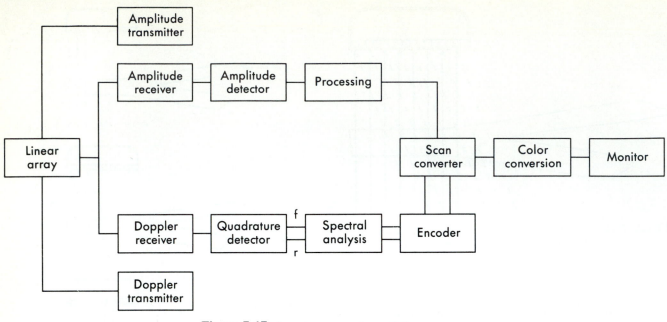

Figure 7-17 Asynchronous autocorrelation scanner.

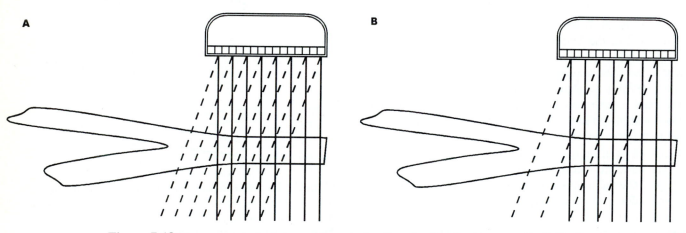

Figure 7-18 Frame rate can be increased by reducing the color line density across the field of view. Color lines of sight are shown as dotted lines. **A,** High-density. **B,** Low-density.

plitude, phase, and frequency of the detected echo are analyzed simultaneously. After reception, the induced signal is divided into two parts and then processed separately for two-dimensional gray-scale and flow information. Image manipulation and color encoding are similar to those described for the asynchronous scanner, the major distinctions being generation of the ultrasound beam and initial routing of the induced signals in the receiver circuit.

Each sampling site throughout the field of view, on a pixel-by-pixel basis, is evaluated for gray scale and color. The field of view and spatial resolution are the same for both gray scale and Doppler.

A suitable Doppler angle is necessary for the detection of flow. If the direction of flow is perpendicular to the transducer line of sight, flow will not be visualized. A stand-off wedge can be used with linear arrays to change the

relative orientation of the moving reflectors so an adequate Doppler angle is achieved. The fluid-filled wedge attenuates the ultrasound beam and lowers the PRF because the path length is increased. Current systems alter beam steering by permitting the operator to select the insonation angle.

Because the transmitted beam is used for both the two-dimensional gray-scale and Doppler modes, the optimum pulse length and other beam characteristics are sacrificed. High-frame rates are possible, however, because two-dimensional gray-scale and flow information is collected concurrently.

CD PARAMETERS

Commercially available CD instruments have multiple controls that affect the color image. These operator-adjustable

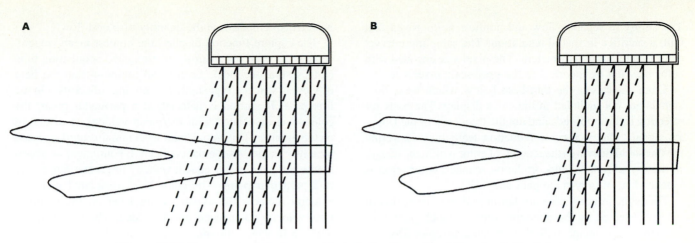

Figure 7-19 Frame rate can be increased by reducing the width of the color field of view. Color lines of sight are shown as dotted lines. **A,** Wide field of view. **B,** Narrow field of view.

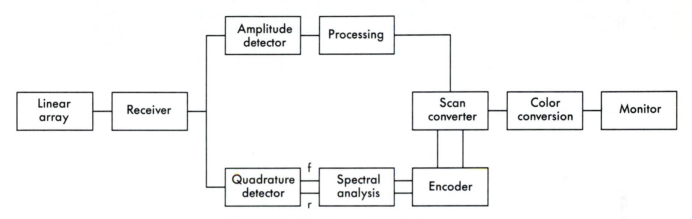

Figure 7-20 Synchronous autocorrelation scanner.

parameters contribute markedly to the overall complexity of CD imaging. Fortunately, many of the controls have a function similar to that described for CW and PW Doppler. The terminology used to label the controls has not become standardized, however, and each manufacturer has adopted its own set of descriptors.

Autocorrelation

Echoes from blood are weak compared with echoes from tissue. This property (in the form of signal amplitude) is evaluated using an echo-versus-color threshold to differentiate flow from moving tissue. Strong reflections that exceed the threshold value are assigned a gray level. Weak echoes from tissue are sometimes depicted in color at low gain settings. Proper gray-scale gain creates an image in which tissue is free of color. Excessive gray-scale gain can suppress color within the vessel and mask the flow.

The velocity scale specifies the range of velocities that are presented in the color display. The PRF is set by the velocity scale and the depth of scanning. For applications in peripheral vascular imaging in which a low-velocity flow is encountered, decreasing the PRF lowers the maximum detectable velocity and improves the velocity resolution. Some manufacturers alter the transducer frequency in response to a shift in velocity scale.

The center of the velocity scale is initially set at zero so the magnitude limits for forward and reverse flow are equal. The baseline control shifts the center of the velocity scale up or down to display a greater range of velocities in one direction. The total velocity range is unchanged. For example, if the initial velocity range was -0.5 to 0.5 m/s, an adjustment in baseline could establish a new velocity range as -0.2 to 0.8 m/s (higher velocities in the forward direction are displayed without aliasing).

Color gain is the amplification applied to the Doppler component during signal processing. High-color gain increases the system's sensitivity for color and expands the number of pixels encoded with color.

The axial length of the Doppler sampling volume is adjusted by the color gate. Increasing the color gate enlarges the region from which PW Doppler signals are examined.

The ability to separate flow and nonflow is improved, but with a sacrifice in spatial resolution. The sampling interval can extend several millimeters. The pixel size encoded with color may not be identical to the gray-scale pixel size.

Color reject sets the threshold below which weak flow signals are not included in the color display. The basis for rejection is the amplitude and not the frequency of the Doppler signal. This is a noise-reduction technique. Lowering the threshold increases the amount of color within the image. In the asynchronous autocorrelation scanner, color reject is independent of gray-scale gain and TGC.

For asynchronous autocorrelation scanners the region of interest selected by the operator controls which portion of the gray-scale image will be subjected to color Doppler analysis. The width of the color region has a considerable impact on frame rate. The dwell time for a color line is long because multiple pulse repetitions are required for the Doppler analysis (denoted by packet size). In general, as the color field of view is expanded, more lines of sight are necessary and the frame rate is reduced. Many scanners, however, automatically adjust packet size and line density as a function of field width to optimize the frame rate for a particular application.

Color persistence is a temporal smoothing technique to reduce noise. Images are displayed at a rapid rate (e.g., 30 fps). By combining previous frames with the most recently acquired frame, the color in the displayed image is averaged. The time interval of the averaging is controlled by the number of frames added together. Color persistence may enhance regions with a low-velocity flow. (A more complete discussion of persistence is presented in Chapter 10.)

A velocity map, similar to a gray-scale map in real-time imaging, assigns flow velocities to various color shades. The "blue away, red toward" (BART) and "red away, blue toward" (RABT) formats use color saturation to code for velocity. Deep shades represent low velocities, and light shades high velocities. Maps consisting of rainbow-colored hues also encode flow information. Red progressing to yellow allows rapid flow in opposite directions to be more easily differentiated.

The velocity tag function emphasizes a selected range of velocities by highlighting regions of flow within this range with a contrasting color (usually green or white). The color bar adjacent to the displayed image indicates (with the same contrasting color) that portion of the velocity scale selected for tagging.

The color image is not limited to a display of mean velocity, however. Additional information (e.g., the spread of velocities within a sampled region) can also be depicted. The variance is a statistical measure of the velocity distribution within each sampled volume. Regions with plug flow demonstrate little spread, whereas those with laminar flow exhibit more variation. The turbulence or variance map provides a means of displaying a two-dimensional color image of the variance.

Another possible display mode is the power map. The power image presents the intensity of the Doppler signal without an indication of the velocity. The intensity depends on the number of RBCs within the sampled volume. The power map emphasizes the quantity of blood flow.

The capture function displays the highest mean velocity detected at each pixel during an elongated acquisition time (1 to several seconds). Each small region within the field of view is scanned repeatedly for moving reflectors. On the first pass, if motion is detected at a particular point, the color level associated with the mean velocity is displayed on the monitor. This initial color level remains until replaced by a new value. As the data collection continues, measurements may yield a subsequent velocity of greater magnitude at a particular point. The color level associated with this velocity replaces the existing color level on the monitor. Low-velocity color levels are discarded. Thus an image is built up in which the maximum mean velocity detected at each pixel is displayed. For vessels with intermittent Doppler signals the capture function is useful in defining whether flow extends to the wall of the vessel.

As the angle of insonation relative to the vessel segment approaches 90 degrees, low-frequency Doppler shifts are generated that may not be depicted in the image. When a steered beam collects the Doppler signal, the angle of insonation can be selected to provide a more favorable geometry between the direction of flow and the ultrasound beam.

Time Domain Correlation

Color-flow imagers based on the time domain correlation principle use many of the same controls as described for autocorrelation scanners. These include transmit power, color map, velocity scale, baseline adjustment, velocity tag, color persistence (enhance), capture function (quantify), restrictive color field of view, and beam insonation angle.

A flow-angle marker establishes the direction of flow relative to the beam axis. By correcting for insonation angle, the velocity scale indicates the absolute velocity of reflectors. If multiple vessels are present within the field of view or the vessel is tortuous, the color-coded velocity may not be correct. The magnitude of the velocity scale is adjusted by altering the PRF. Operation in slow flow mode is susceptible to color flash since sensitivity for motion is maximized.

Frame rate is adjusted by changing the width of the color field of view and by selecting the appropriate resolution versus speed setting. The latter control increases the frame rate by reducing the line density. Decreasing the depth of the color field of view typically does not alter the frame rate.

Thresholding designates the low velocity cutoff. Measured velocities below the threshold value are not displayed. Color noise, in which weak stationary reflectors are depicted with color, occurs if the threshold is set too low.

COMBINED DOPPLER MODE

In the CD image a single parameter, usually the mean velocity, is represented by a variation in color. A more detailed presentation of the velocity profile requires an FFT time-dependent power spectrum. The combined Doppler mode or duplex mode displays the CD image and the Doppler spectral analysis.

A specific sampling volume for spectral analysis is identified on the CD image. Because the beam must be shared among two-dimensional gray-scale, color-flow, and PW Doppler modes, the refresh rate of the color image is slowed to a new frame every 1 to 5 seconds.

Spectral invert displays the negative velocity components in the power spectrum above the baseline. Spectral smoothing averages information along the velocity or time axis. Smoothing is a technique to reduce rapid fluctuations in the displayed spectrum. Smoothing in time is accomplished by combining the results of the most recent FFT analysis with the preceding power spectra. The smoothing effect is enhanced by increasing the number of power spectra added together. Smoothing in velocity averages the magnitudes of adjacent Doppler shifts.

CLINICAL APPLICATIONS OF COLOR-FLOW IMAGING

The presence of flow, direction of flow, characteristics of flow, and existence of focal differences in velocity within the vessel are all assessed by CD imaging. Specific clinical applications are listed in the box. For cardiac applications temporal resolution is essential. To achieve high frame rates, the sonographer needs to minimize the field-of-view width, scanning depth, and line density. Often, when a larger field of view is selected, line density is adjusted automatically to maintain a high frame rate. Slow flow in peripheral vessels is analyzed by a low PRF, long dwell time, and low wall-filter setting. The Doppler transmit frequency influences the limit for the lowest velocity that can be detected. High frequency reduces the low-velocity limit. Under the same conditions the low-velocity limit is 15 cm/s and 6 cm/s for 3 MHz and 7.5 MHz, respectively. Deep slow flow in the abdomen requires a low frequency to penetrate tissue and a narrow field of view to counteract the effect of a long dwell time and low PRF on the frame rate.

The major advantage of CD imaging is that the pattern of flow throughout the vessel within the field of view is visualized instantaneously as the hemodynamics changes during the cardiac cycle. Vessels too small to be discerned with real-time gray-scale imaging are located with CD imaging. Improved ease of vessel identification allows for examination of large vascular territories. In addition, vascular and nonvascular structures are more readily differentiated. Determination of the presence or absence of flow in peripheral vessels is also enhanced.

CD IMAGE QUALITY

CD image quality is characterized by four factors. These are (motion discrimination, temporal resolution, spatial resolution, and uniformity.) The term *color sensitivity* has also been applied to describe this collection of factors.

Color is associated with movement, but it does not necessarily indicate flow. Movement of the transducer, peristaltic motion, and cardiac motion all may contribute spu-

■ **Clinical applications of color flow imaging**

Diagnosis of vascular stenosis
Visualization of organ perfusion
Tumor vascularity
Evaluation of aneurysm, pseudoaneurysm, and dissection
Examination of large vascular territories
Imaging of the heart

rious color to the image and give an artifactual impression of flow. The ability to distinguish moving blood from moving tissue and at the same time depict subtle flow patterns is the ultimate goal. Low-frequency shifts from slowly moving tissue are selectively removed with a wall filter. A variety of filters is used depending on the application. Often the PRF is adjusted automatically to be as high as possible for the depth of interrogation. The wall filter is altered in conjunction with this change in PRF. Unfortunately, this technique is not completely effective in eliminating high-amplitude low-frequency Doppler shifts associated with vessel wall movement. Also low-velocity flow components are excluded by this high-pass filter. To better differentiate flowing blood from stationary fluid and moving soft tissue, the amplitude and the Doppler shift are examined. Weak reflections are associated with blood and other fluids. Gray-scale values are assigned to strong echoes. An alternative method, called multivariate motion discrimination, has been introduced recently by one manufacturer. Several parameters of the motion (not only velocity and amplitude) are evaluated to ascertain whether the motion is characteristic of tissue or flowing blood.

Flow hemodynamics varies throughout the cardiac cycle. The ability to detect changing flow patterns depends on the frame rate. Temporal resolution is improved as the frame rate is increased. A high frame rate is achieved by reducing the number of scan lines, the field of view, the dwell time, or a combination of these.

Spatial resolution characterizes a scanner's ability to depict small structures at the proper location. The axial dimension of the Doppler sampling volume is defined by the sampling time interval (color gate). The out-of-plane dimension (slice thickness) is determined by the beam size along that direction. The beam width and scan line density affect the lateral resolution. As the interrogated volume is reduced in size, weaker-amplitude signals are generated (lower signal-to-noise ratio), which are less likely to be encoded in color. The precision of the Doppler shift measurement also deteriorates. Spatial filtering is a technique to diminish random color variations throughout the image. Pixels are encoded in color only if they neighbor other pixels previously encoded in color. Small vessels with weak flow must be visualized with the spatial filter off. Another type of spatial filtering (sharp/smooth processing) manipulates the presentation of the boundary between color and gray scale pixels.

Generally, real-time imaging provides superior gray-scale spatial and temporal resolution compared with CD imaging. The CD temporal and frequency resolution of the Doppler shifts is less than that obtained by spectral analysis in which the sampling time is typically 10 to 20 ms with 50 to 100 Hz frequency resolution.

(*Uniformity* implies that vessels with identical properties are depicted in a similar manner regardless of their respective locations within the field of view; that is, vessel size and color pattern should not be altered by a change in position.) Dynamic focusing enables pixels of constant size to be portrayed throughout the field of view. Pixel size for color Doppler and two-dimensional gray scale modes may not be the same, however.

COLOR FLOW LIMITATIONS

The rapid acceptance of CD imaging indicates that this scanning technique has unique applicability in the clinical environment. Nevertheless, CD imaging is not without limitations, many of which have been discussed previously.

Color coding is based on the average, rather than the peak, Doppler shift. Measurement of peak velocity from the CD image is not appropriate. Velocity estimates do not include the correction for Doppler angle. A sector transducer interrogates a linear segment of a vessel oriented parallel to the skin surface with a variable angle of insonation. The angle is greatest in the center of the field of view and decreases toward the periphery. Progressing across the field of view, a vessel with constant flow is depicted first as red, then with no color, and finally as blue. Comparatively, a linear array with a constant angle of insonation demonstrates uniform color throughout the field of view. Presentation of an apparent velocity deviation at the bend of the vessel may be attributed to a change in Doppler angle (Fig. 7-21).

Short pulses optimized for gray-scale imaging are interspersed with longer pulses that provide Doppler informa-

tion. The pulsing sequence and extensive computations limit the frame rate. A wide dynamic range of 110 dB is necessary in the receiver circuit to accommodate both the echoes and the Doppler signals.

The shades of red and blue are not sensitive indicators of velocity variation. Color assignment is based on the direction of flow but can be reversed. The direction of flow in the vessel of interest should be established by the orientation of the vessel with respect to the transducer or by reference to another vessel of known origin.

The presence of gas also produces color artifacts because the velocity of sound in air is not the same as in tissue. The highly focused beam is readily attenuated by a calcified plaque. Shadowing obscures the lumen of the artery and gives the impression of an absence of flow. Vessel tortuosity, poor scanning technique, and weak Doppler signal may also cause flow not to be visualized in an image.

SUMMARY

Color-flow imaging combines gray-scale imaging with two-dimensional mapping of flow velocity in real time. Motion is depicted throughout the field of view by color encoding the flow information. The mean velocity at each sampling site is depicted by hue or intensity of color. Regional flow patterns within the color field of view are portrayed.

CD imaging has limitations and depends on operator-selected imaging parameters. The shades of red and blue are not sensitive indicators of velocity variation. Color assignment, based on the direction of flow, can be reversed. The direction of flow in a vessel of interest can be established by the vessel's orientation with respect to the transducer or by reference to another vessel of known origin.

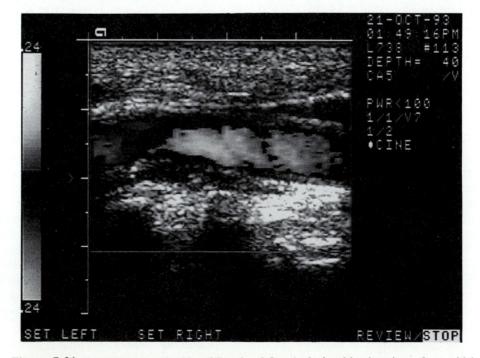

Figure 7-21 A tortuous vessel with unidirectional flow is depicted in changing colors, which suggests a reversal of flow. (See Color Plate 1B.)

Motion discrimination, temporal resolution, spatial resolution, and uniformity all contribute to overall image quality. Numerous controls including gray-scale gain, packet size, color gate, color gain, color reject, velocity map, velocity tag, and capture function are available to manipulate the collection and processing of the CD data.

REVIEW QUESTIONS

1. In processing scan data for color flow imaging,
   a. A phase shift or time shift indicates the presence and direction of motion.
   b. A stationary reflector is assigned a gray level based on amplitude of the detected echo.
   c. Magnitude of the frequency shift or time shift provides velocity information.
   d. All of the above.
2. The number of transmitted pulses along one color line of sight required to determine the velocity of the moving reflector is _____ .
   a. One
   b. Two
   c. Three or more
3. To acquire the Dopple frequency information rapidly, color flow imaging uses a _____ .
   a. CW transducer
   b. Range-gated PW detector with spectral analysis
   c. Autocorrelation detector
   d. Mechanical sector transducer
4. The method used to measure velocity by detecting a time shift in the echo signal is _____ .
   a. Autocorrelation
   b. PW Doppler spectral analysis
   c. Time domain correlation
   d. Time derivative of the quadrature signal
5. What is a characteristic of the asynchronous scanner?
   a. Separate lines of sight collect flow and gray-scale information.
   b. It operates in real-time and static color-flow imaging modes.
   c. Color field of view and gray-scale field of view are always the same.
   d. It allows more rapid framing than is possible with a synchronous scanner.
6. The number of pulses along one line of sight to acquire the velocity information is called the _____ .
   a. Packet size
   b. Dwell time
   c. PRF
   d. Pulse duration
7. Aliasing does not occur in color flow imaging.
   a. True
   b. False
8. What flow information is typically encoded by the color scale?
   a. Median velocity
   b. Maximum velocity
   c. Mean velocity
   d. All velocity components at each pixel
9. The axial length of the Doppler sampling volume is set by which control?
   a. Baseline
   b. Velocity scale
   c. Color gate
   d. Packet size
10. What control shifts the center of the velocity scale to display a greater range of velocities in one direction?
    a. Baseline
    b. Color reject
    c. Color gain
    d. Packet size
11. What adjustment is made to improve the velocity estimates of the moving reflectors?
    a. Increase the line density.
    b. Increase the packet size.
    c. Increase the color gate.
    d. Increase the frame rate.
12. What adjustment is made to increase the frame rate?
    a. Decrease the line density.
    b. Decrease the packet size.
    c. Decrease the width of the color field of view.
    d. All of the above.

BIBLIOGRAPHY

Barber WD, Eberhard JW, Karr SG: A new time domain technique for velocity measurements using Doppler ultrasound, *IEEE Trans Biomed Engin* 32:213, 1985.

Bohs LN, Friemel BH, McDermott BA, Trahey GE: Real-time system for angle-independent ultrasound of blood flow in two dimensions: initial results, *Radiology* 186:259, 1993.

Bonnefous O, Pesque P: Time domain formulation of pulse-Doppler ultrasound and blood velocity estimation by cross correlation, *Ultrason Imaging* 8:73, 1986.

Foley WD, Erickson SJ: Color Doppler flow imaging, *AJR* 156:3, 1991.

Hoeks APG, Peeters HHPM, Ruissen CJ, Reneman RS: A novel frequency estimator for sampled Doppler signals, *IEEE Trans Biomed Engin* 31:212, 1984.

Kasai C, Namekawa K, Koyano A, Omoto R: Real time two-dimensional blood flow imaging using an autocorrelation technique, *IEEE Trans Son Ultrason* 32:458, 1985.

Loupas T, McDicken WN: Low-order complex AR models for mean and maximum frequency estimation in the context of Doppler color flow mapping, *IEEE Trans Ultrason Ferroelectr Frequency Control* 37:590, 1990.

Merritt CRB: Doppler color flow imaging, *J Clin Ultrasound* 15:591, 1987.

Mitchell DG: Color Doppler imaging: principles, limitations, artifacts, *Radiology* 177:1, 1990.

O'Leary DH, Polak JF: Interrogating the carotids with color Doppler imaging, *Diagn Imaging* 10:204, 1988.

Powis RL: Angiodynography: a new look at the vascular system, *Appl Radiol* 15:55, 1986.

Powis RL: Color flow imaging: understanding its science and technology, *J Diagn Med Sonogr* 4:236, 1988.

Smith H, Zagzebski J: Basic Doppler physics, Madison, Wisc, 1991, Medical Physics Publishing.

Taylor KJW, Burns PN, Wells PNT: *Clinical applications of Doppler ultrasound*, New York, 1988, Raven Press.

Wells PNT: Doppler ultrasound in medical diagnosis, *Br J Radiol* 62:399, 1989.

Zweibel WJ: Color-encoded blood flow imaging, *Semin Ultrasound CT MR* 9:320, 1988.

Zweibel WJ: Color duplex imaging and Doppler spectrum analysis: principle, capabilities, and limitations, *Semin Ultrasound CT MR* 11:84, 1990.

CHAPTER 8

Vascular Ultrasound

KEY TERMS

Compression technique
Deep venous thrombosis
Doppler spectral analysis
Doppler waveform
High-velocity jets
Intravascular imaging
Maximum velocity
   waveform

Plaque
Pulsatility index
Resistive index
Spectral broadening
Stenosis
Triphasic waveform
Turbulence
Volume flow rate

The third leading cause of death in the United States (after cancer and heart disease) is stroke. Stroke is caused primarily by atherosclerosis, the accumulation of lipid deposits on arterial walls. A history of TIA (transient ischemic attack) increases the risk of stroke by a factor of 3. Pulmonary emboli caused by venous thrombosis also contribute to the mortality rate attributable to vascular disease. Disruption of blood flow in the peripheral vascular system may lead to the loss of an extremity.

With the development of high-resolution x-ray imaging chains, digital subtraction angiography (DSA), computed tomography (CT), and magnetic resonance imaging (MRI), imaging of the vascular system has become very sophisticated and highly effective. These techniques, however, often involve the introduction of contrast agents whereas ultrasonic imaging is usually noninvasive. Ultrasonography provides flow dynamics, vessel wall anatomy, and tissue characteristics that cannot be obtained by other means. In addition, ultrasound equipment costs are lower than the costs associated with alternative imaging modalities.

Instrumentation with both real-time and Doppler capabilities (e.g., Duplex and color Doppler scanners) are used extensively in vascular work. Real-time imaging provides anatomical information regarding the vessel and surrounding tissues. Vessel size is depicted. Perivascular masses and luminal thrombi are usually well visualized. Because the echoes from RBCs are weak, however, real-time imaging does not depict blood flow. Flowing blood appears as a signal void. Doppler methods are necessary for the investigation of blood flow dynamics. The presence of flow, its direction, and other physiological aspects of flow (pulsatility, resistivity, high-velocity jets, and turbulence) are assessed with Doppler techniques.

MAXIMUM VELOCITY WAVEFORM DESCRIPTORS

Frequently the Doppler spectral waveform is simplified by displaying the time dependence of a single parameter, the maximum velocity. The maximum velocity is determined for each Doppler sampling time segment and then plotted as a function of time. This display format readily shows the fastest-moving reflectors within the cardiac cycle. In addition, the maximum velocity waveform is analyzed to evaluate other aspects of flow.

Several Doppler indices have been formulated to characterize the maximum velocity waveform. Pulsatility index (PI) is commonly used to quantify impedance or resistance to flow. This index is calculated from the systolic peak velocity (A), the end-diastolic peak velocity (B), and the mean velocity throughout one cycle as illustrated in Figure 8-1:

8-1

$$PI = \frac{(A - B)}{Mean}$$

High values of the PI describe pulsatile waveforms. Advantages of this index include the following: (1) the Doppler angle and vessel size do not need to be known; (2) abnormal waveforms are identified with high sensitivity; and (3) vessels too small or too tortuous to image can be evaluated. The PI should be calculated for each of several cardiac cycles and the values averaged to obtain the final result.

Two other parameters, the resistive index and the systolic/diastolic ratio, are commonly used clinically:

8-2

$$Resistive\ index = \frac{(A - B)}{A}$$

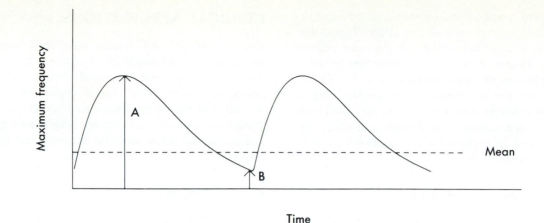

Figure 8-1 Parameters of the maximum velocity waveform used to calculate the pulsatility index and resistive index.

8-3

$$\text{Systolic diastolic ratio} = \frac{A}{B}$$

where A and B are defined as for Equation 8-1.

With these indices computation is easier because the mean velocity does not need to be determined. The resistive index has been used to assess vascular rejection of renal transplants. In obstetric sonography, waveforms from the umbilical cord and uteroplacental arteries have been characterized with the systolic/diastolic ratio. Intrauterine growth retardation is evaluated by measuring placental impedance.

Pressure gradients are sometimes estimated using peak values in the maximum velocity waveform. The derivative of this waveform yields flow acceleration. To depict acceleration with reasonable precision, time segments must be short. Mean or median velocity, when normalized to maximum velocity, tends to decrease as spectral broadening occurs.

VOLUME FLOW RATE MEASUREMENTS

Volume flow rate delineates the amount of blood moving through the vessel per unit of time. Its estimation is commonly derived from measurements of the velocity distribution and the cross-sectional area of the vessel. The velocity distribution is analyzed to obtain the mean velocity. The product of the mean velocity and the cross-sectional area yields the volume flow rate (Q):

8-4

$$Q \ (\text{cm}^3/\text{s}) = \text{Mean velocity (cm/s)} \times \text{Area (cm}^2)$$

For an accurate assessment of volume flow rate to be obtained, all velocity components must be included in the calculation of mean velocity. Several methods have been developed to quantify volume flow rate.

Velocity Profile Method

A PW Doppler system with a small sample volume is used to evaluate the mean velocity at multiple locations across the vessel lumen. At each measurement point the mean velocity is followed throughout the cardiac cycle to obtain a time average. A profile of velocities across the lumen is thus generated. Provided the lumen is circular, total flow is determined by adding the product of the velocity and the corresponding semiannular area at each point in the profile. A multigate Doppler system containing 16 or 32 gates (each approximately 1 mm in axial length) provides instantaneous presentation of the velocity profile. Volume flow rate can be assessed during a single cardiac cycle, which is less susceptible to beat-to-beat variations. This method is most suitable for large and easily accessible vessels (e.g., the aorta and common carotid arteries), which allow a high-frequency transducer to be placed directly on the vessel.

Even Insonation Method

The mean velocity is determined for the entire vessel, which is insonated with a uniform beam. This is multiplied by the cross-sectional area of the lumen to yield the instantaneous volume flow rate. Averaging the instantaneous value over the cardiac cycle results in the time-averaged flow rate. The cross-sectional area fluctuates during the cardiac cycle. Therefore the instantaneous mean velocity and cross-sectional area should be determined simultaneously. In practice, this cannot be achieved because imaging of the luminal diameter should be conducted with the beam positioned perpendicular to the direction of flow and the Doppler signal should be obtained with the beam oriented along the direction of flow. As an alternative, the mean velocity and cross-sectional area are measured separately, individually averaged over time, and combined to estimate the volume flow rate.

The even insonation method is subject to a wide variety of additional problems. The cross-sectional area is often calculated from the luminal diameter. The dependence of the area on the square of the diameter necessitates that the diameter be determined accurately. A nonuniform intensity throughout the vessel deemphasizes the low-velocity components near the vessel wall, causing an upward shift in the spectral distribution and an overestimation of the mean velocity. A high-pass filter has a similar effect. Transit-time broadening, clutter, and noise all distort the mean velocity measurement. Frequency-dependent attenuation by intervening tissue lowers the observed mean velocity. The response of the receiver is not time and frequency independent. The flow is assumed to be parallel to the vessel wall. The intensity of the scattered sound beam is altered if turbulence is present. Consequently, this method cannot be used to assess turbulent flow.

Assumed Velocity Profile Method

The velocity profile is determined at one segment of a vessel, and this profile is assumed to exist at different locations in the vessel. For vessels exhibiting plug flow (in which the velocity profile is nearly uniform) the mean velocity is equated to the maximum velocity, an easily measured parameter. This method has limited validity because velocity profiles are known to change during the cardiac cycle and along various segments of a vessel.

Attenuation-Compensated Flow Volume Ratemeter

A device called an attenuation-compensated flow volume ratemeter has been developed to overcome the difficulty of path-dependent attenuation on velocity measurements. An annular array transducer alternately generates a wide, then narrow, beam. The wide beam encompasses the entire vessel with a uniform ultrasonic intensity. The narrow beam samples the central portion of the vessel only. Because both beams traverse the same ultrasonic path, the effect of attenuation is identical and any difference in received signal strengths is attributed to the increased amount of blood in the large sample volume. The spectral distribution from the broad beam is also analyzed for mean frequency. A calibration factor is required to convert the measured parameters of mean frequency, broad-beam signal strength, and narrow-beam signal strength into volume flow rate. However, the Doppler angle and luminal cross-sectional area need not be known for this estimation of volume flow rate.

Time Domain Velocity Profile Method

The time domain Doppler detection technique measures displacement of the acoustic speckle pattern associated with a group of RBCs. Since the time interval between measurements is known, the velocity of the RBCs can be determined. Time domain processing uses a wide bandwidth, which allows accurate presentation of spatial information.

The velocity profile is measured along a single line of sight. Good temporal resolution is achieved by sampling at high PRFs. The spatial extent of the velocity profile indicates the size of the lumen. By assuming circular symmetry of the lumen, it is possible to calculate the volume flow rate. The angle of incidence with respect to the direction of flow must be known, however.

CLINICAL APPLICATIONS

Real-time images and Doppler waveforms must be interpreted based on a knowledge of anatomy, hemodynamics, disease processes, and ultrasound physics and instrumentation. This overview of clinical applications is arranged according to the topics discussed—carotid arteries, intracranial arteries, peripheral arteries, deep venous thrombosis, abdominal and pelvic vascular anatomy, and intraluminal imaging.

Carotid Arteries

Ultrasound has proved to be an effective method of screening patients for carotid occlusive disease. Patients with a history of transient ischemic attack, stroke, or vascular disease elsewhere, with a carotid bruit or vertebrobasilar symptoms, are usually candidates. Ultrasound is of value for monitoring the progression of atherosclerotic stenosis and for determining the effectiveness of endarterectomy.

Real-time imaging and PW Doppler are both essential for evaluating the carotid arteries. Although not required, color Doppler can enhance the data collection process and shorten the examination time.

A 5 or 7 MHz linear array is used to image the common carotid (CCA), internal carotid (ICA), and external carotid (ECA) arteries in the longitudinal and transverse planes. Gray-scale images can depict the location and size of plaques.

A Doppler spectrum using a small gate (e.g., 2 mm) is acquired throughout the arteries. A Doppler angle between 30 and 60 degrees must be maintained at each sampling point. Doppler measurements should be expressed in units of velocity rather than frequency. This removes the dependence of the Doppler measurement on transducer frequency and Doppler angle, which facilitates comparisons of the results obtained with different equipment from subsequent examinations. All segments of these arteries must be interrogated, because normal flow patterns can be reestablished within a short distance of stenosis.

Color Doppler depicts global hemodynamics within the field of view. Turbulent flow and high-velocity jets associated with focal stenosis are usually readily identified. Placement of the Doppler sampling volume is eased when flow within the vessel is visualized. Color Doppler also depicts tortuous vessels and vessels with low volume flow. One limitation of color Doppler is that flow information is obtained at a single angle, which must be set at 60 degrees or less. Inaccurate measurement of velocity will occur if the vessel changes direction with respect to the transducer.

Doppler spectral analysis yields waveforms that are characteristic of flow within the respective arteries. The normal ICA waveform (Fig. 8-2) demonstrates a maximum peak velocity during systole with a narrow distribution of velocities. This provides the window appearance of the waveform during systole. The low resistance of downstream vessels in the brain allows antegrade flow during diastole. The normal ECA waveform (Fig. 8-3) demonstrates a relatively

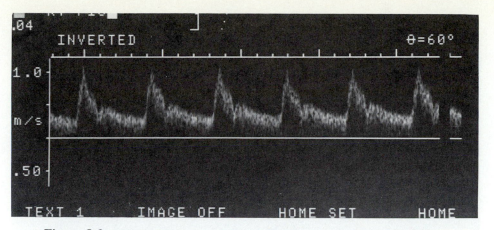

Figure 8-2 Normal Doppler waveform obtained from the internal carotid artery.

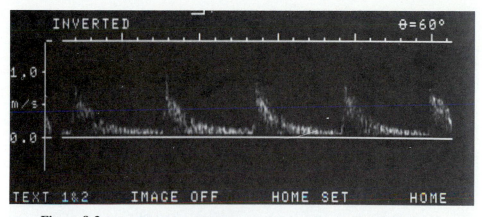

Figure 8-3 Normal Doppler waveform obtained from the external carotid artery.

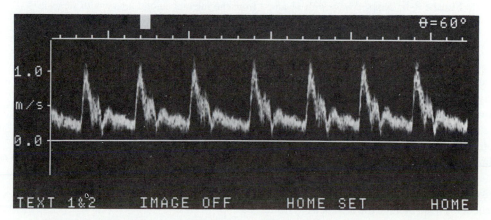

Figure 8-4 Normal Doppler waveform obtained from the common carotid artery.

sharp maximum velocity peak during systole with possible flow reversal in early diastole. The high resistance of downstream vessels in muscle hinders antegrade flow during diastole. The normal CCA waveform (Fig. 8-4) is a composite of the ICA and ECA waveforms. In the carotid bulb multiple velocity components, including reverse flow, are expected (Fig. 8-5). Typically, peak velocities in the carotid arteries

are between 60 and 100 cm/s. The ECA may have slightly lower peak velocity than the ICA and CCA. Flow is symmetrical on the left and right.

Stenosis, which causes a 75% reduction in cross-sectional area (or, equivalently, a 50% reduction in luminal diameter), disrupts the normal flow patterns. High-velocity jets are formed at the stenosis. A broadening of flow velocities and

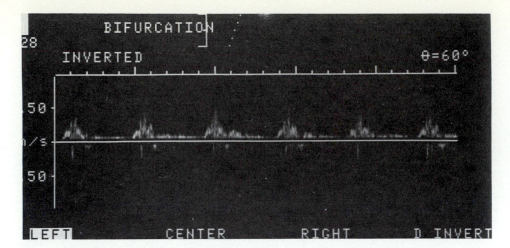

Figure 8-5 Normal Doppler waveform obtained from the carotid bulb.

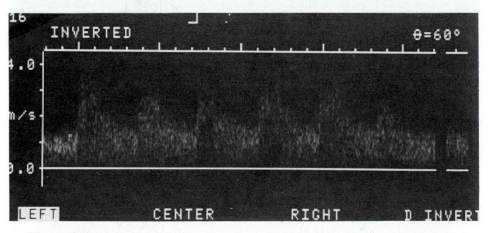

Figure 8-6 Doppler waveform obtained from the internal carotid artery with stenosis.

turbulence occur distal to the stenosis. Spectral analysis detects these changes as an increased velocity peak and a fill-in of the window (Fig. 8-6). Color Doppler depicts high-velocity jets with a single hue, elevated on the velocity color scale (e.g., saturated color on the blue or red scales). Post-stenotic velocity broadening is represented by multiple hues (Fig. 8-7).

Multiple velocity measurements or ratios have been used as predictors of stenosis. These include the ICA peak systolic velocity, ICA/CCA systolic velocity ratio, ICA end-diastolic velocity, ICA peak diastolic velocity, and ICA/CCA diastolic velocity ratio. The ICA peak systolic velocity, as a single index, appears to be a good predictor of stenotic disease and is easy to measure. Its criteria are presented in Table 8-1. Stenosis classification is not improved by the use of additional velocity parameters. The sonographic appearance of the plaque does not predict progression of disease.

Examination of the ICA to differentiate between occlusion and high-grade stenosis with slow flow is extremely important. The highest sensitivity settings must be used.

■ **Table 8-1** Diagnostic Criteria for ICA Stenosis

	Reduction in Luminal Area (%)			
	<75	75% to 90%	90% to 98%	>98%
Peak systolic velocity (cm/s)	<150	150 to 250	250 to 615	Low

Special ultrasound equipment with low flow detection capability may be required. If the ICA is occluded, the CCA spectral waveform resembles that obtained from the ECA.

Although ultrasonographic examination of the carotids has become a well-accepted clinical diagnostic procedure, limitations do exist. Improper Doppler angle or incorrect placement of cursor (not parallel to the direction of flow) introduces error in the Doppler measurements. Attenuation artifacts from calcifications may obscure a segment of the vessel (Fig. 8-8). Stenosis at the origin of the CCA or within the intracranial ICA is difficult to detect.

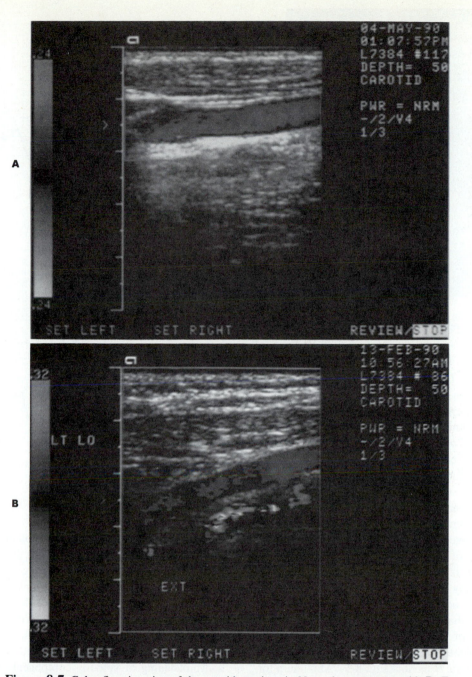

Figure 8-7 Color-flow imaging of the carotid arteries. **A,** Normal common carotid. **B,** External carotid with moderately severe focal stenosis. (See Color Plates 1C and 1D.)

Intracranial Arteries

Attentuation by bone inhibits examination of the intracranial circulation. Transcranial scanning of the anterior cerebral, middle cerebral, anterior communicating, and posterior communicating arteries has recently been introduced. A low-frequency transducer operating at relatively high power levels is positioned over the thin portion of the temporal bone. Although the field of view is limited by the small acoustic window available through the temporal bone, stenosis of the middle cerebral artery is detectable by trans-

cranial scanning. Transcranial scanning, however, has not achieved widespread clinical use.

Peripheral Arteries

Peripheral arterial ultrasonography is most often concerned with possible stenosis in the femoral and popliteal arteries. Applications also include assessment of arterial graft patency after surgery, monitoring the effectiveness of peripheral vascular angioplasty, evaluation of dialysis shunt pa-

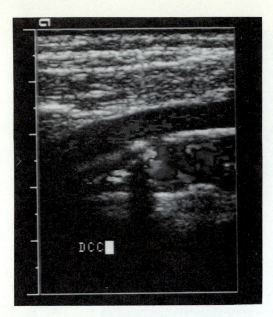

Figure 8-8 Shadowing by calcified plaque obscures flow in the vessel. (See Color Plate 1E.)

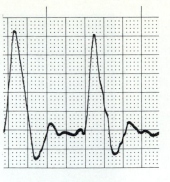

Figure 8-9 Normal Doppler maximum velocity waveform obtained from the common femoral artery.

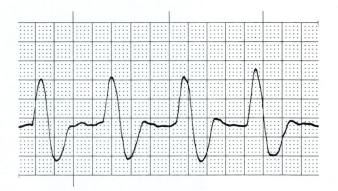

Figure 8-10 Normal Doppler maximum velocity waveform obtained from the popliteal artery.

tency, and detection of aneurysm, pseudoaneurysm, and vascular malformation.

An arteriovenous fistula is a congenital malformation in which abnormal shunting between an artery and a vein causes high-velocity, possibly pulsatile, flow in the vein. It may also be induced by trauma.

Pseudoaneurysm usually presents as a hypoechoic mass in which blood flows into the cavity during systole and exhibits a swirling pattern. These features allow differentiation between the pseudoaneurysm and a post-angiographic hematoma or arteriovenous fistula.

Ultrasonography of the peripheral arteries provides anatomical location of the plaque and the degree of stenosis. A 5 MHz linear array is used to image arteries in the leg, but the operator may adjust frequency upward or downward depending on body habitus. Doppler spectra are acquired with a narrow gate of 2 to 3 mm.

The normal maximum velocity waveform of the femoral artery exhibits triphasic behavior (Fig. 8-9). Maximum forward flow occurs during systole, followed by reverse flow in early diastole, and then slow forward flow in late diastole. Flow reversal is caused by arterial pressure wave reflection from the distal muscle arterioles, which have high resistance. Arterial compliance is responsible for reestablishing the forward flow in late diastole. This late phase may be lost or greatly reduced in elderly patients. The normal maximum velocity waveform of the popliteal artery is also triphasic and similar to that from the femoral artery (Fig. 8-10), the major difference being that forward flow in late diastole is low or nonexistent.

A gradual reduction in peak systolic velocity is observed in arteries more distal to the heart. For example, maximum velocity in the common femoral and popliteal arteries is 90 cm/s and 59 cm/s respectively.

Color Doppler is beneficial in identifying the plaque and

showing vessel tortuosity. Flow around the plaque is depicted in color, which contrasts with the gray-scale presentation of the plaque. Doppler sampling volume is more easily defined when flow within a curved vessel is shown. Detection of slow flow is facilitated by color Doppler. Occlusion is demonstrated by the absence of color within the vessel and by the observation of collaterals.

Monophasic waveform, increased maximum velocity, and broadening of velocity components are characteristics of the Doppler spectrum when significant stenosis is present (i.e., greater than 75% reduction). The maximum velocity may change by a factor of 4 to 7 above the normal value. The peak velocity provides an indirect measure of the pressure gradient in a vessel segment.

Many of the ultrasonographic limitations described for the carotid arteries (calcifications, tortuosity, and slow flow) are also present in the peripheral arteries. Body habitus is a factor as well. The superficial femoral artery at the adductor canal is a prime site for stenosis, but because of its depth in tissue this segment is difficult to interrogate.

Deep Venous Thrombosis

Ultrasonography has become the primary screening method for deep venous thrombosis (DVT) of the lower extremity.

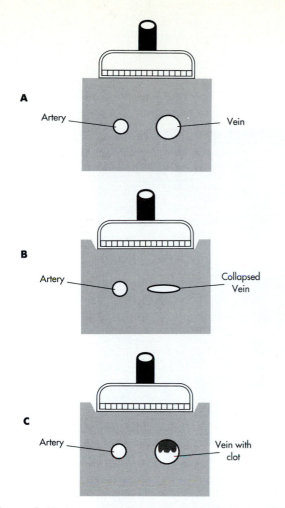

Figure 8-11 Compression technqiue to detect deep venous thrombosis. **A,** No compression. Both the artery and the vein are visualized. **B,** The normal vein collapses when compression is applied. **C,** The vein with a clot does not collapse when compression is applied.

Acute DVT can lead to an expansion of the clot and to pulmonary emboli if a portion of the clot is released into the arterial system. Most pulmonary emboli are attributed to thrombic disease in veins of the lower extremities and pelvis. Chronic venous insufficiency can damage valves and induce venous wall changes that result in pain, swelling, and edema.

Although the femoral and popliteal veins are routinely examined, the efficacy of including calf veins in the examination is subject to debate. Their small size, slow flow, and complex anatomy hinder evaluation. The lack of clear evidence showing adverse effects from clots localized to the calf veins also contributes to the controversy.

The echogenicity of a clot is variable and erratic. The gray scale presentation depends on transducer frequency, age of the clot, and extent of the thrombotic process. Fresh clots are often not visualized.

A compression technique is used to diagnose DVT. The image of a vein is obtained in the transverse plane as pressure is applied with the transducer. For a normal vein such compression causes the lumen to collapse completely. If a clot is present, coaptation does not occur and the lumen remains (Figs. 8-11 and 8-12). For an artery, compression should not alter the lumen. The compression technique may not be effective in obese individuals or in patients with swollen extremities.

Augmentation and valvular competency are evaluated with Doppler spectral analysis. Augmentation is the increase in flow induced in a normal vein by massaging the thigh or leg below the point of interest. Valvular incompetency is demonstrated by retrograde flow in the vein when compression is applied above the point of interest. Properly functioning valves prohibit flow away from the heart.

Color Doppler supplements real-time imaging and PW Doppler. Color extends throughout the lumen of a normal vein but is displaced by nonocclusive thrombi in a diseased vein (Fig. 8-13). Color Doppler is also helpful in establishing the presence of venous collaterals.

The differentiation of acute and chronic clots is based on the size of the vein and the presence of venous collaterals and wall thickening. The latter two characteristics are indicative of chronic disease. Large vein size (as much as two times the diameter of the associated artery) is consistent with an acute clot.

Abdominal and Pelvic Vascular Ultrasonography

Vascular ultrasonographic applications in the abdomen and pelvis include determination of vessel patency, detection of aortic aneurysms, pseudoaneurysms, arteriovenous fistulas, and other vascular malformations, visualization of large vessels supplying neoplastic tumors, and evaluation of suspected thrombosis. Complex vascular systems can be examined by means of color Doppler scanning (Figs. 8-14 and 8-15).

The demonstration of flow within the testis eliminates testicular torsion as a possible diagnosis. Preoperative and postoperative assessment of the patency of hepatic vessels is essential in the management of liver transplant patients. The Doppler spectrum of arteriovenous fistulas is distinguished by high-velocity diastolic flow attributable to the low resistance created by shunting.

The renal hilum, splenic hilum, and porta hepatis can be evaluated for thrombosis. Cirrhosis and portal hypertension may affect the patency of the portal vein, and these are detectable by ultrasonography. The bile ducts are readily distinguished from the hepatic artery and portal vein by means of Doppler techniques. Obesity, massive ascites, bowel gas, high attenuation rate of a diseased liver, and the inability to achieve an appropriate Doppler angle may all compromise examination of the liver. Overlying bowel gas obstructs insonation of the inferior vena cava and the iliac and pelvic veins.

In renal transplant patients obstruction, peritransplant fluid collections, and thrombosis of the transplant artery and vein are assessed with ultrasonography. Renal transplant

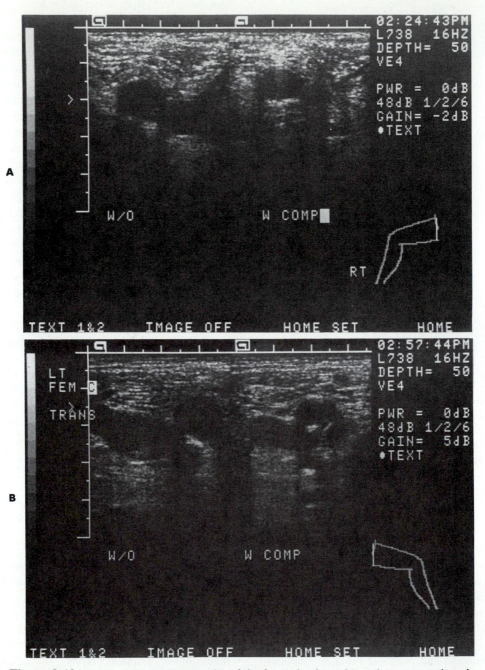

Figure 8-12 Compression ultrasonography of the femoral vein to detect deep venous thrombosis. **A,** Sonograms of the normal vein with and without compression. **B,** Sonograms with and without compression showing a clot.

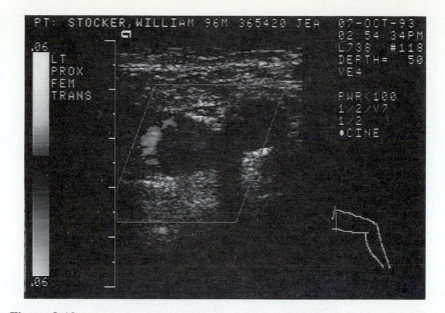

Figure 8-13 Color-flow image of the femoral vein with a clot. (See Color Plate 1F.)

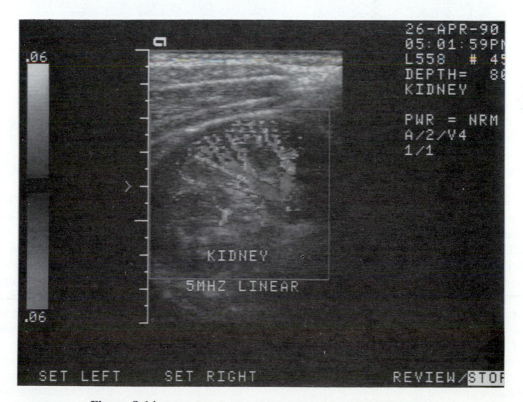

Figure 8-14 Color-flow image of the kidney. (See Color Plate 1G.)

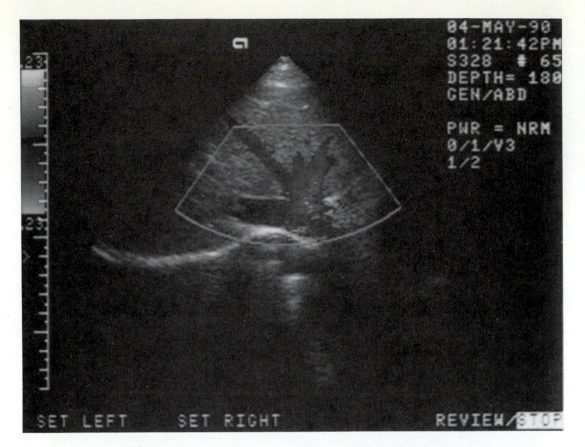

Figure 8-15 Color-flow image of the liver. (See Color Plate 1H.)

biopsies are conducted under ultrasound guidance. Although the specificity is low, elevated pulsativity and resistivity indices may denote vascular allograft rejection.

Intravascular Imaging

A phased array or mechanical transducer is mounted at the catheter tip. The catheter is placed in the artery, and a two-dimensional image of the vessel wall is obtained at each point of interest. The scanning range is 1 to 2 cm. A very high frequency extending from 20 to 40 MHz is used. The axial images are often reconstructed in three-dimensional format to aid in the presentation of scan data.

This technique allows examination of the vessel wall not immediately adjacent to the lumen. Information concerning the histological layers is now available that cannot be obtained by angiography. The severity of disease may be more accurately assessed with intravascular scanning.

Other information provided by intraluminal ultrasonography includes the extent of plaque formation, the measurement of luminal area and percent stenosis, the elasticity of vessel walls, and the tissue characterization of plaques. Fibrous and calcific plaques have been differentiated based on sonographic appearance. Lipid-containing plaques are more difficult to identify.

Intravascular imaging may provide a means to evaluate therapeutic interventions. Luminal size and percent stenosis are measured before and after atherectomy. An intraluminal transducer may be mounted with balloons or lasers to monitor plaque removal during the procedure.

SUMMARY

Real-time imaging and PW Doppler spectral analysis are both necessary for evaluations of the vascular system. Vessel size and surrounding anatomy are shown in the gray-scale image, and clots and plaques when present are often visualized. Hemodynamic information is acquired via Doppler techniques. The time-dependent spectral Doppler waveform indicates the velocity components in a small segment of the vessel. However, multiple samplings must be obtained before a composite representation of regional flow can be formed.

Color Doppler presents the global hemodynamics within real-time images. The collection of sonographic data is enhanced by shortening of the examination time, easing the placement of Doppler sampling volumes, visualizing tortuous vessels, and the prompt detection of high-velocity jets.

Clinical applications of vascular ultrasonography include the evaluation of stenosis, the detection of aneurysms, pseudoaneurysms, and vascular malformations, and the screening of patients for deep venous thrombosis. For these applications vascular ultrasonography has become a well-accepted clinical diagnostic modality.

▰ R E V I E W   Q U E S T I O N S ▰

1. Why is the vessel lumen depicted as a signal void in real-time imaging?
2. What is the maximum velocity waveform?
3. Name three methods used to measure volume flow rate.
4. How is focal stenosis in the carotid arteries identified by duplex scanning?
5. State the importance of insonation at the proper Doppler angle.
6. What changes occur in the Doppler spectrum when stenosis is present in the femoral artery?
7. What technique is used to diagnose deep venous thrombosis?
8. What are the advantages of vascular imaging with color Doppler?

BIBLIOGRAPHY

Cronan JJ: Ultrasound evaluation of deep venous thrombosis, *Semin Roentgenol* 27:39, 1992.

Cronan JJ: Venous thromboembolic disease: the role of US, *Radiology* 27:39, 1992.

Dorfman GS, Cronan JJ: Venous ultrasonography, *Radiol Clin North Am* 30:879, 1992.

Grant EG, White EM (eds): *Duplex sonography*, New York, 1988, Springer-Verlag.

Hertzberg BS, Carroll BA: Ultrasonography of the vascular system. In Taveras JM, Ferrucci JT (eds): *Radiology: diagnosis, imaging, intervention*, Philadelphia, 1993, JB Lippincott.

Katzen BT: Current status of intravascular ultrasonography, *Radiol Clin North Am* 30:895, 1992.

Robinson ML: Duplex sonography of the carotid arteries, *Semin Roentgenol* 27:17, 1992.

Sacks D: Peripheral arterial duplex ultrasonography, *Semin Roentgenol* 27:28, 1992.

Taylor KJW: Arterial vascular ultrasonography, *Radiol Clin North Am* 30:865, 1992.

Zwiebel WJ (ed): *Introduction to vascular ultrasonography*, ed 2, Orlando, Fla, 1986, Grune & Stratton.

CHAPTER 9

M-Mode and Two-Dimensional Echocardiography

Color M-mode
Ejection fraction
M-mode scanning
Stress echocardiography

Strip chart recorder
Transesophagel
    echocardiography

The practice of diagnostic cardiology has changed dramatically over the past decade as new techniques and sophisticated equipment including single photon emission computed tomography (SPECT), positron emission tomography (PET), computed tomography (CT), and magnetic resonance imaging (MRI) have been incorporated. Developments in ultrasound instrumentation have also played a significant role in noninvasive evaluations of the heart. M-mode scanning, the mainstay of cardiac ultrasound, has been supplemented by advances in color M-mode scanning, real-time two-dimensional imaging with improved transmit and receive focusing, CW and PW Doppler ultrasound, and two-dimensional color Doppler imaging.

IMAGING CONSIDERATIONS

The temporal and spatial imaging properties and lack of demonstrated adverse effects make ultrasound attractive for cardiac imaging. Temporal resolution is the ability of an imaging system to interrogate the structures of interest repeatedly in a very short time. Ultrasound travels through tissues at an average speed of 1540 m/s or 1 cm every 6.5 μs. The time required for passage to a depth of 15 cm (the most distal cardiac structures) and back is 195 μs. Conse-

quently, an ultrasound system can interrogate the heart at least 5000 times each second for one line of sight. This provides the ability to sample numerous times during one cardiac cycle. Two dimensional imaging with many lines of sight requires longer collection times and therefore is achieved at slower frame rates.

Spatial resolution refers to the ability of an imaging system to detect and display, as separate entities, anatomical structures that are close together. Axial resolution and lateral resolution must both be considered. Axial resolution depends on the spatial pulse length and is typically between 0.5 and 2 mm. The development of specialized electronic transmit and receive focusing techniques has resulted in newer transducers with lateral resolutions of 1 to 3 mm. Transesophageal and transluminal transducers achieve even better axial and lateral resolution over a limited depth because high frequency and small crystals are used. Compared with fluoroscopy, angiography and especially radioisotope techniques, ultrasound provides superiorly detailed studies of cardiac anatomy in real time.

To date the lack of observed deleterious effects from diagnostic ultrasound ensures patient and personnel safety. The ultrasonic exposure received by a patient depends on the pulse duration, intensity of the ultrasound pulse, and volume of the tissue interrogated. Typically, less than 1% of the actual examination time is spent transmitting pulses into the patient. Most of the time the transducer is in a passive mode, receiving the echoes. The maximum intensity for each pulse is limited by the manufacturer. Sonographers are trained to conduct the examination with exposure controls (e.g., dB, output, and transmit) as low as possible to acquire the necessary clinical images and complete the examination quickly. In addition, new focusing techniques have led to the need for smaller sampling volumes, which reduces the ultrasonic exposure to neighboring tissues while improving the spatial detail.

PHYSICAL PRINCIPLES

The physical principles of ultrasound remain unchanged regardless of the application; that is, ultrasound physics that applies to general pelvic and abdominal examinations also applies to cardiac studies. Although a short consideration of ultrasound physics is included in this chapter, the echocardiographer should consult Chapter 1 for a more detailed discussion.

The ultrasound wave, a form of mechanical energy that is propagated through a medium, consists of alternating regions of molecular compression and rarefaction. The number of times a compression or rarefaction occurs at a point each second is called the frequency (f). For cardiac imaging the transducer operates at a frequency between 1.5 and 7.5 MHz. The frequency remains constant when progressing from one tissue type to another, but the velocity (c) changes. A shift in the wavelength (λ) of the ultrasound wave also occurs because the previous three parameters are related by the following equation:

9-1

$$c = f\lambda$$

Small changes in wavelength may have an effect on the spatial resolution of the image (as discussed later).

Ultrasound waves undergo various interactions with cardiac tissues, the most notable being reflection, in which a portion of the incident ultrasound beam is returned toward the transducer when a structure is encountered. The amount of reflection at an interface is determined by the difference in acoustic impedance (Z):

9-2

$$Z = \rho c$$

where ρ is the density and c the velocity. Large acoustic impedance differences produce strong echoes.

The orientation of the structure also contributes to the strength of its detected echo. An interface located perpendicular to the beam produces higher-amplitude reflections than one that is oriented at some other angle to the beam. The heart, a highly complex and variably shaped moving organ, produces interfaces that change in their orientation to the stationary ultrasound beam throughout the cardiac cycle. Except for the large structures (specular reflectors) such as the heart walls, a perpendicular interface geometry is difficult to maintain.

The physical size of the reflector can also have a profound effect on the strength of the echo. Interfaces greater in width than the ultrasound beam are very strong directional reflectors. Structures smaller in width scatter ultrasound energy independent of the incident beam angle. For strong reflective surfaces the quality of an echocardiac scan depends on the angle of the transducer.

The ultrasound beam can undergo various other interactions as it is transmitted through the cardiac structures. When it strikes an interface at an angle other than 90 degrees to the surface, it is bent from the expected stright-line path if the two media forming the interface have different acoustic velocities. This is called refraction (see Chapter 1 for a description) and is not normally a problem in echocardiography.

Ultrasound energy is absorbed in the medium by the back-and-forth movement of molecules during the compression and rarefaction phases (i.e., frictional losses). As the frequency increases, this oscillating motion occurs more often and results in a more rapid decrease of energy. A lower-frequency transducer may be necessary to probe deep-lying structures.

Reflection, scattering, and absorption all act to decrease or attenuate the intensity of the ultrasound beam. The transmitted pulse and returning echo both undergo attenuation. Thus a very small fraction of the original pulse intensity ultimately reaches the transducer for detection. The loss of intensity with depth makes deep-lying structures difficult to visualize. Most echocardiographic units are equipped with controls (e.g., time gain compensation, depth gain compensation, and sensitivity) that allow the operator to compensate, at least partially, for attenuation with depth.

BASIC ECHOCARDIOGRAPHIC INSTRUMENTATION

The main requirements of an echocardiographic unit include instrumentation that can generate an ultrasound beam to be directed toward the heart and that can detect the returning echoes for display in a format understandable to the observer. The echocardiographic scanner is similar to the basic unit described in Chapter 2 (Fig. 2-1).

Pulse Repetition Frequency

The transducer is excited by a short voltage pulse from the transmitter that causes the crystal to expand (compressing molecules in the adjacent tissue) and then contract (decreasing the molecular concentration). The progression of these pressure differences through the cardiac tissues constitutes the ultrasound beam.

The number of times the transmitter excites the crystal each second is the pulse repetition frequency (PRF). Typically the PRF ranges from 200 to 5000 per second and is set by the manufacturer. For some scanners the operator can adjust the PRF in relation to the transducer, type of study, and greatest depth of interest (R). The maximum PRF is given by

9-3

$$PRF_{(max)} = \frac{c}{2R}$$

where c is the velocity of ultrasound in tissue. The depth control on some units automatically reduces the PRF as the depth of penetration increases.

Data Acquisition

Once the ultrasound beam enters the patient, the various interactions decribed in Chapter 1 take place. Reflection redirects some of the ultrasonic energy back toward the transducer in the form of an echo. The returning pressure wave induces an electrical signal in the transducer crystal that is amplified from a microvolt or millivolt range to a few volts. One component of this amplification process is time gain compensation (TGC), sometimes referred to as depth gain compensation (DGC). Log compression converts the echo dynamic range of $10^6:1$ to a usable storage and display dynamic range of $60:1$. After further processing, the scan data are presented on a display device, normally in different shades of gray, that shows the relative amplitudes of the echoes.

Operator Controls

Each manufacturer has its own set of "knobs" or machine controls, which are manipulated by the operator to optimize the informational content of the examination. One type is the output, transmit, dB, power, or course gain control, which varies the excitation voltage to the piezoelectric crystal to increase or decrease the intensity of the transmitted pulse. Weak echoes that go undetected may be subsequently visualized by raising the output to increase the intensity of returning echoes. Manufacturers set a limit for the transmitted intensity depending on the application.

Most echocardiographic units have a series of gain controls that amplify the received signals but do not increase patient exposure because the transmitted pulse intensity is not changed. TGC, DGC, and sensitivity controls vary the amplification as a function of elapsed time (depth) to counteract the progressive weakening of the ultrasound signal due to attenuation.

Ancillary controls may be associated with TGC. The near gain, near depth, or fine gain modifies the amplification of induced signals from echoes originating close to the transducer. Normally, in the near depths, little amplification is necessary because attenuation of the beam is minimal. The delay determines the depth at which the TGC slope or true TGC actually begins. Beyond a certain depth (denoted as the end of TGC slope) the maximum amplification is set by the far gain. In the far gain region, signal strength exhibits exponentially decreasing behavior because the amplification is constant. Most echocardiographic units have adjustable slide controls to change the amplification at about every 1 cm of depth. This provides a great deal of flexibility in regulating the acquired scan data.

The overall gain, also called fine gain, control amplifies all signals by a constant factor regardless of the depth of origin. Patient exposure is not affected because only the received signal is manipulated.

The reject or compress control permits the elimination of weak signals from extraneous sources (e.g., electrical noise, clutter, and low-level scattering). The reject control may also be set to exclude extremely high-level signals. Often TGC, by altering signal amplification, is used as a reject control.

Automatic Controls

Some cardiac units have a switched gain, or oscillator, control that electronically switches the receiver gain between a high setting optimized for the endocardium and a low setting optimized for the epicardium. Measurements of ventricular wall thickness are easier to perform and more accurate when this technique is used.

Some echocardiographic units contain a pulse power or damping control to shorten the voltage excitation pulse to the crystal electronically. The reduced duration of the crystal vibration shortens the ultrasound pulse and provides better axial resolution. Pulse damping decreases the ultrasonic energy available, which may result in poor or no visualization of distant structures.

Display Device

Each cardiac unit has brightness and contrast controls on the display device, whether a cathode ray tube (as in early M-mode units) or a television (black and white or color). The brightness or intensity control determines the light output. Too high an intensity broadens the dots and deteriorates the spatial detail. Contrast establishes how the range of signal levels is displayed as different shades of gray. If it is not correct, either the full range of signals or all shades of gray will not be exhibited. Improper contrast and brightness settings may distort measurements of distance, area, or volume when cardiac structures are being assessed.

Normally a computer keyboard is used to write information on the display. Each manufacturer incorporates additional controls for preprocessing and postprocessing of the echo data, particularly for real-time, Doppler, and color Doppler scanners.

Data Analysis

Most cardiac units have preassigned analysis packages that require specific measurements to be performed in a predetermined order. The echocardiographer must understand the sequence of events for the examination and must know the calculation algorithms—for example, whether the Bullet model, Simpson's rule, or some other model is being used for determination of left ventricular volume and what measurements are needed from the two-dimensional gray-scale images to determine the volume.

M-MODE SCANNING

The first motion-detection device used in diagnostic ultrasound was the M-mode (or motion-mode) scanner. It emphasized the movement of interfaces, including rate, amplitude, and pattern of motion. Also called TM (time-motion) or PM (position-motion) mode, it was first used to interrogate the mitral valve in cardiac ultrasonography.

Summary of A-mode and B-mode

A review of the basic principles of A-mode and B-mode instrumentation aids in the understanding of M-mode. A-mode scanning uses the echo-ranging principle. A short burst of ultrasound is transmitted into the body, and at various interfaces some of the energy is reflected toward the transducer. When the echo strikes the crystal, a radiofrequency (RF) signal is induced, amplified, and sent to the processing unit. The amplitude of the signal is converted to a spike on the CRT display. The height of the spike is proportional to the reflectivity of the interface. The time delay between transmission and reception denotes the depth of the interface. The coordination of timing pulses is extremely important for the correct placement of a spike at the proper depth. As long as the transducer is pointed along a particular direction (line of sight), the same one-dimensional "image" is repeatedly portrayed at the rate of the pulse repetition frequency, which is usually at least 1000 per second. To the observer the image appears unchanging, although the scan data are being replaced 1000 times per second.

B-mode scanning converts the A-mode spike into a brightness-modulated dot, which is varied in response to the amplitude of the echo-induced signal. The position of the dot is derived from the time-of-flight information. Two-dimensional static B-mode imaging requires the collection of dots from individual lines of sight, one at a time, and the storing of the scan data until all lines of sight that form the image are collected.

Effect of Motion

For nonstationary interfaces the A-mode spike moves back and forth on the display, showing the changing position of the interface (Fig. 9-1). The fidelity of the motion depicted depends on the pulse repetition frequency. Because most A-mode scanners are pulsed at least 1000 times per second, the motion appears continuous. The display can be recorded on videotape for viewing. Hardcopy-film imaging (Polaroid or multiformat camera), however, is not practical because the moving spike is frozen in one position and the effect of motion is lost. This limits the usefulness of one-dimensional A-mode imaging for detecting motion.

Motion of interfaces during two-dimensional B-mode scanning poses similar problems (Fig. 9-1). Blurred borders around the moving interface are produced in the image. Each line of sight freezes the interface at a particular position, but the interrogation of the interface from multiple lines of sight separated in time places the interface at different locations. Static imaging is not useful for detecting motion because of the poor temporal resolution, particularly for cardiac studies.

Data Acquisition

The moving B-mode dots are combined with the dimension of time to form a two-dimensional recording called an M-mode scan (Fig. 9-1). In this particular scanning technique, data are collected along one line of sight only (similar to A-mode) and therefore no registration arm is required (Fig. 9-2). The transducer is moved to view another line of sight. A time-trace signal from the master synchronizer

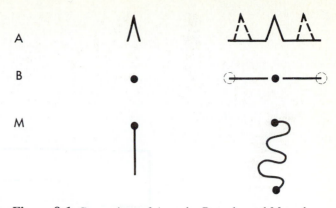

Figure 9-1 Comparison of A-mode, B-mode, and M-mode displays of a stationary and a moving interface.

causes one set of deflection plates to sweep the electron beam across the screen at 25 to 100 cm/s. Other sweep rates are also possible. In the other dimension, B-mode dots that represent the depths of various interfaces along the line of sight are displayed. The brightness of the dots corresponds to the reflection properties of the interface. Stationary interfaces are recorded as straight lines on the display, whereas moving interfaces produce oscillating waveforms. The M-mode traces in Figure 9-3 illustrate strong specular reflection from the ventricular wall and the low-amplitude nonspecular reflection (scatterers). The sweep rate can distort the pattern of the M-mode trace, depending on the speed of the moving interface (Fig. 9-4).

Recording

M-mode traces can be recorded on Polaroid film from a persistence CRT or on continuous-roll 35 mm film. Film development is time consuming and expensive. The most common archiving method uses the strip chart recorder, which provides a continuous reproduction of the trace.

The M-mode trace is recorded in a line-by-line sequence as the recording paper moves past a specialized CRT. The CRT has a narrow band of phosphor deposited on the glass plate. An electron beam sweeps horizontally across the phosphor and is modulated in response to the echoes detected along the path. To prevent diffusion of the light and subsequent blurring of the trace, light from the phosphor strip is transferred to the recording paper via fiber-optic light guides (Fig. 9-5). Thousands of optic fibers are placed parallel to each other across the phosphor plate to provide continuity. The speed of the recording paper can be varied. Some paper is sensitive to ultraviolet light; other paper requires development by a thermal or film processor. The latter two methods improve the gray-level reproduction.

M-mode is a two-dimensional data-presentation technique that provides a plot of distance (i.e., the depth of the interfaces relative to the face of the transducer along one line of sight) versus time. The M-mode trace is descriptive of the speed of the interface, the distance traveled by the interface, and the direction and type of motion of the interface. The speed of the interface is obtained by the slope of the trace. M-mode scanning gives an excellent evaluation

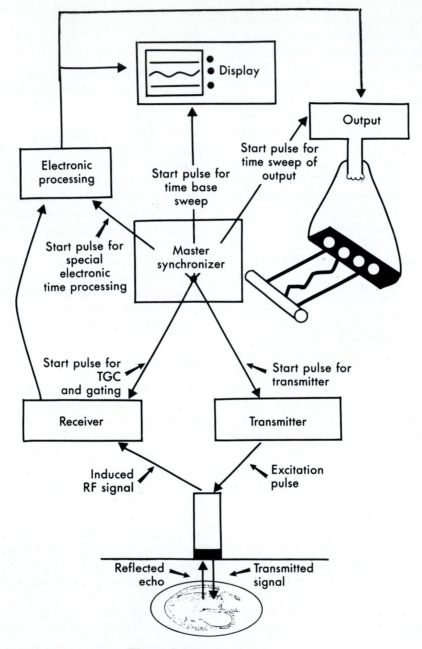

Figure 9-2 The M-mode scanner.

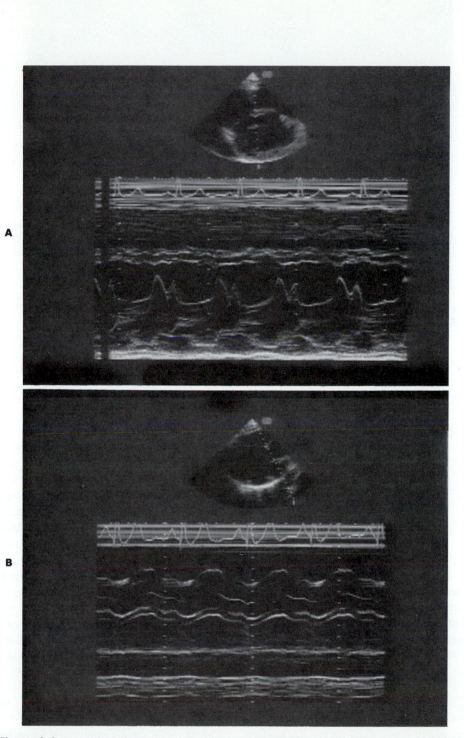

Figure 9-3 Two-dimensional gray-scale images with M-mode line-of-sight delineation at 50 cm/s. The strong reflectors show up white. **A,** Normal mitral valve. **B,** Normal aorta and aortic valve cusps.

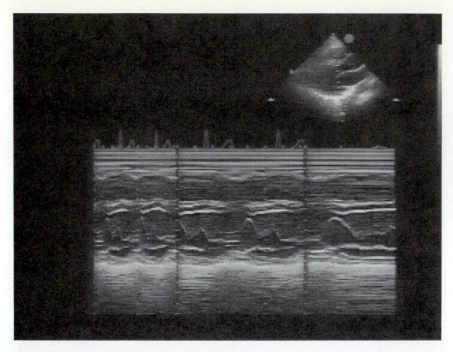

Figure 9-4 M-mode traces of normal mitral valve at 25 cm/s, 50 cm/s, and 100 cm/s. The pattern is changed as the trace speed is increased.

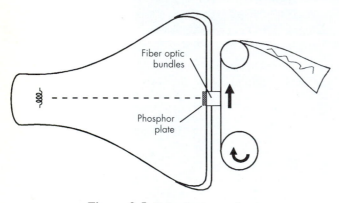

Figure 9-5 Strip chart recorder.

of the object's size and motion in the axial direction. The scroll feature allows viewing of information stored in the memory. The length of viewing depends on the sweep rate. A stored M-mode trace may be recorded on videotape or a strip chart.

Applications

An M-mode trace can be acquired by using dedicated units with either a circular, pencil-type, fixed-focus, single-element transducer or a two-dimensional real-time scanner. The scan is obtained from the left parasternal, suprasternal, subcostal, or apical approach. Measurements are usually made at end diastole and end systole, as denoted by a simultaneously recorded ECG. Recommendations for performance measurements using M-mode techniques have been published.

The parameters assessed by M-mode scanning include dimensions and a cross-sectional area of the left ventricle,

dimensions of the ventricular septum, left ventricular wall thickness at end systole and end diastole, and left ventricular volume. Various indices derived from these parameters (e.g., fractional shortening, fractional area change, and ejection fraction) are used as indicators of cardiac function. Measurements of the aorta, left atrium, right ventricle, and the mitral, tricuspid, and pulmonic valves during systole and diastole are also performed. Special analysis packages are available for making necessary calculations after the appropriate scans have been collected.

Color M-mode imaging combines M-mode with Doppler information encoded in color. As a truly duplex scanning system, data along one line of sight are evaluated for both interface motion and blood flow. The flow data and M-mode pattern are displayed in conjunction with the corresponding segment of the cardiac cycle given by the ECG. Color M-mode thus provides important information about timing of flow across the valve. A color M-mode scan obtained from a patient with mitral regurgitation and aortic insufficiency is shown in Figure 9-6.

Advantages and Disadvantages

The M-mode scan is interpreted by pattern recognition, but it does not correlate with the usual two-dimensional structural anatomy as depicted in real-time imaging. Although the axial and temporal resolution is excellent, motion in the lateral direction (perpendicular to the beam axis) is not portrayed because of the limited field of view (sampling is along one line of sight only).

Another limitation of M-mode scanning is based on assumptions of geometric shapes when measurements along one dimension are extrapolated to calculate two-dimensional

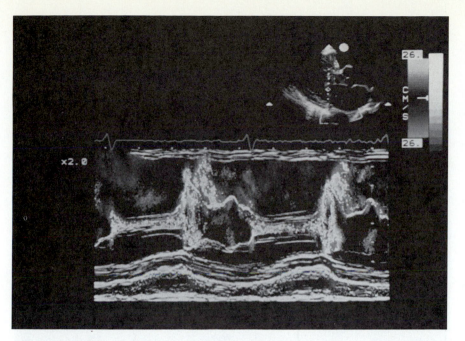

Figure 9-6 Color M-mode trace of aortic insufficiency and mitral valve regurgitation. (See Color Plate 2A.)
(Courtesy Hewlett-Packard Imaging Systems.)

areas and three-dimensional volumes. Only real-time two-dimensional imaging techniques can portray lateral motion and depict shape.

Because of its simplicity, high axial resolution, and superior temporal resolution, M-mode scanning will continue to play an important role in echocardiology. Recent advances in two-dimensional instrumentation, however, have created new opportunities for invasive and noninvasive imaging of the heart.

TWO-DIMENSIONAL ECHOCARDIOGRAPHY INSTRUMENTATION

Because the interfaces of the heart are blurred, two-dimensional static cardiac imaging is not practical in echocardiography. ECG-gated scanning (as discussed in Chapter 3 [image data acquired during part of the P-QRS-T complex so the heart motion is frozen]) relies on the premise that cardiac structures are always in the same location during the ECG-triggered gate. Image definition is improved but at the price of both increased examination time and increased patient exposure.

Real-Time Imaging

Real-time sector scanners, both mechanical and electronic, have been used to acquire two-dimensional images of the heart. They are small enough to be positioned within the intercostal space. Phased array systems have been especially valuable, not only for their small size and superb image quality but also for the rapid frame rates that are obtainable. Typically, these transducers operate at a frequency of 1.5

to 7.5 MHz. The small probes can be oriented in any direction to collect different two-dimensional views of the heart. Each image (frame) consists of multiple lines of sight. The frame rate (FR) is limited by the velocity of ultrasound (c), the depth of penetration (R), and the number of lines of sight (N) in each image:

9-4

$$FR = \frac{c}{2\ RN}$$

Note that the frame rate is equal to the PRF divided by the number of lines of sight. Gray-scale images of the heart are shown in Figure 9-7.

The miniaturization of electronics and the formulation of better focusing and steering techniques have led to the development of small probes that are inserted into the esophagus to obtain high-detail images of the heart. Because these transesophageal probes are close to the heart, several advantages are gained—high-frequency transducers, many lines of sight, and rapid frame rates are all possible. Despite the fact that it is somewhat invasive, transesophageal scanning has become a valuable tool in cardiac imaging. Figure 9-8 presents two-dimensional gray-scale images of the heart obtained with a transesophageal probe.

Extremely small transluminal probes (transducers attached to the end of a catheter) have been introduced in the study of vascular disease. They provide highly detailed images of the cardiac chambers and valves.

Real-time imaging with multiple lines of sight per frame delineates structures in both the beam axis and the lateral directions. This improves the accuracy of area and volume determinations. Sampling rates, however, are reduced, which results in poorer temporal resolution.

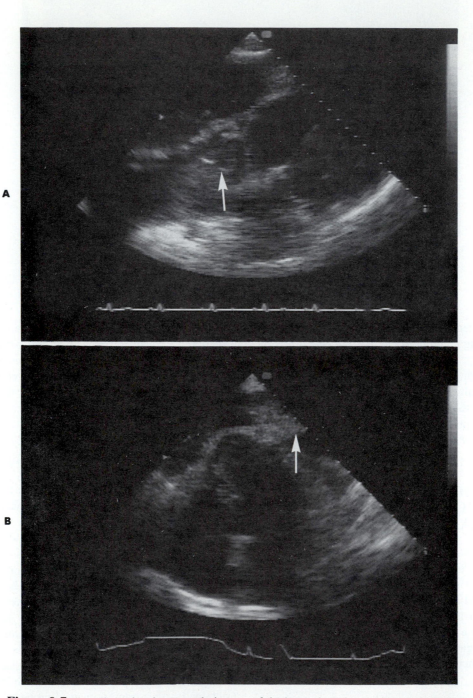

Figure 9-7 Two-dimensional gray-scale images of the heart. **A,** Subcostal four-chamber view demonstrating a tumor *(arrow)* in the right atrium. **B,** Apical four-chamber view demonstrating a tumor *(arrow)* adjacent to the left ventricle.

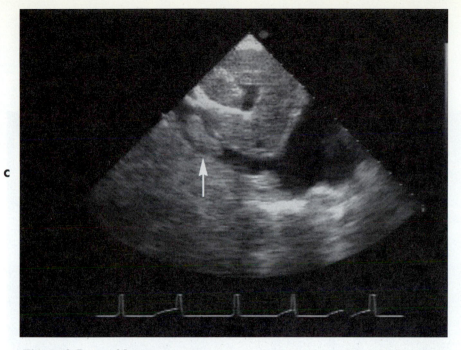

Figure 9-7, cont'd C, Subcostal view demonstrating a mass *(arrow)* in the inferior vena cava.

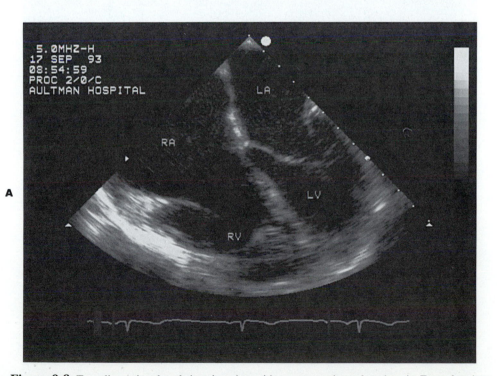

Figure 9-8 Two-dimensional real-time imaging with a transesophageal probe. **A,** Four-chamber view, long axis. *LA,* Left atrium; *RA,* right atrium; *LV,* left ventricle; *RV,* right ventricle.

Continued.

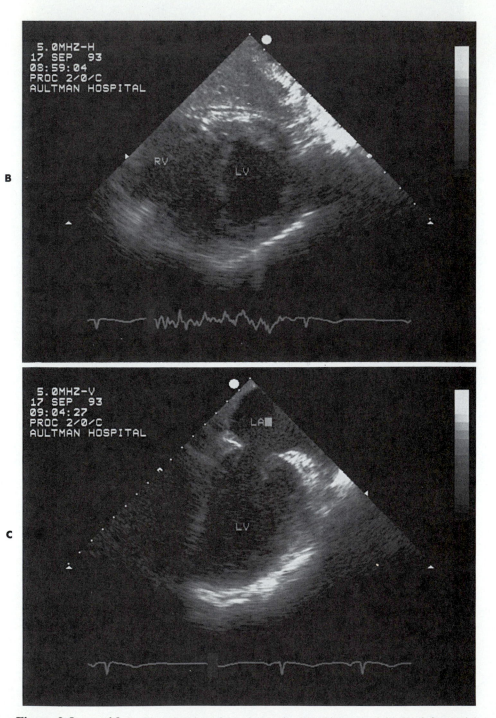

Figure 9-8, cont'd B, Two-chamber view, short axis. *RV,* Right ventricle; *LV,* left ventricle. **C,** Two-chamber view, long axis. *LA,* Left atrium; *LV,* left ventricle.

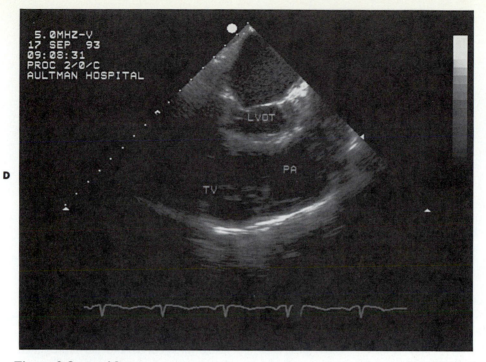

Figure 9-8, cont'd D, Long axis view showing the left ventricle outflow track *(LVOT)*, pulmonary artery *(PA)*, and tricuspid valve *(TV)*.

Stress Echocardiography

Stress echocardiography examines regional systolic function under conditions of increased oxygen demand in patients with suspected coronary artery disease. Systolic function is evaluated by the extent of endocardial motion and myocardial thickening. Stress is achieved by physical exercise or by pharmacological agents (dipyridamole, adenosine, dobutamine). Myocardial segments at rest and during stress are compared by means of side-by-side image displays on the monitor. The cineloop function facilitates assessment of abnormal wall motion. Quantitation of the ejection fraction (i.e., the fractional change in left ventricular volume between diastole and systole) during stress may identify global dysfunction. The diagnostic accuracy of stress echocardiography appears comparable to that obtainable with radionuclide imaging (thallium-201). Examination of patients 2 to 3 weeks after an acute myocardial infarction has provided prognostic information. Patients with detectable ischemia are at higher risk of a future myocardial infarction.

DUPLEX INSTRUMENTATION IN ECHOCARDIOGRAPHY

Duplex scanning incorporates the simultaneous or near-simultaneous acquisition of M-mode or Doppler information with two-dimensional gray-scale images on one monitor. The echocardiographer can view the two-dimensional image while directing the M-mode or Doppler acquisition to a particular region of interest. Imaging in conjunction with M-mode or Doppler is accomplished in a time-sharing fashion. Mechanical sector scanners generally contain a separate crystal dedicated for the collection of M-mode or Doppler data. Electronic phased arrays direct ultrasound pulses along the appropriate paths as required for each mode.

Early Scanners

Early duplex systems divided the real-time and M-mode or Doppler functions into two distinct pathways. The two-dimensional gray-scale image was collected by means of a mechanical or electronic transducer. A separate crystal (housed in the transducer) and independent signal-processing circuitry acquired the M-mode or Doppler data. The real-time image had to be frozen so the M-mode or Doppler sampling indicator (line of sight or region) could be moved to the position of interest. The active mode was switched back and forth between gray-scale imaging and M-mode or Doppler waveform. The real-time image, once frozen, could not be updated until the M-mode or Doppler data were collected. This lack of simultaneous acquisition created a lag in the real-time image, reducing the temporal resolution and inhibiting placement of the M-mode or Doppler sampling site.

Phased Arrays

Electronic linear phased arrays provide greater flexibility by allowing a scan line to be used for either imaging or Doppler sampling. The beam electronically sweeps throughout the field of view, and, the received signal is directed through separate real-time and Doppler processing pathways. A specific scan line is repeated for ascertaining the Doppler shifts while other scan lines are collected for imaging. This allows a continuous update of the real-

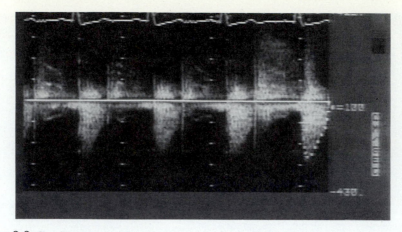

Figure 9-9 Continuous-wave Doppler spectrum of the aortic valve. The positive component above the baseline indicates aortic insufficiency.

time images for accurate placement of the Doppler sampling volumes. To measure high velocity, the Doppler mode requires higher PRFs than the imaging mode. A longer dwell time for a given Doppler line of sight reduces the real-time frame rate but improves the accuracy of the Doppler shifts.

Figure 9-9 demonstrates aortic valve motion as depicted by the Doppler waveform. Valvular stenosis is characterized by high pressure gradients across the opening. The pressure gradient (P) in millimeters of mercury is estimated by

$$P = 4 \, v^2 \qquad \text{9-5}$$

where v is the peak velocity (in meters per second) of flow at the narrowing. For the mitral valve the severity of stenosis is indicated by the pressure half-time (i.e., the time required for the peak pressure in early diastole to decrease to half its value).

The desire for a simultaneous presentation of regional flow with the two-dimensional real-time image led to the development of a new field of cardiology called cardioangiodynography or cardiac CD (color Doppler) imaging.

CARDIAC COLOR DOPPLER IMAGING

Beam formation and steering by electronic phased array, well-defined beam position relative to the scan head, near synchronous signal processing, and rapid data collection have all led to the development of CD imaging of the heart. Cardiac CD imaging combines two-dimensional mapping of flow with real-time imaging. M-mode scanning, including color M-mode, can be incorporated with CD to form a complex scanning system. This multiple-mode instrument is a powerful diagnostic tool for evaluating cardiac flow and function. The first CD image obtained was of blood flow through the heart. It has since been extended to color flow vascular imaging.

Data Collection

The returning echo is examined with respect to amplitude, phase, and frequency. Strong reflections correspond to soft tissue interactions and are represented in shades of gray. The two-dimensional gray-scale image is created by dividing the field of view into a discrete set of sampling sites, which are stored in the digital scan converter. The time to collect the information along each line of sight depends on the depth of the field of view. A single pulse-listen cycle is sufficient to sample one line of sight. The image is composed of multiple lines of sight, which are updated periodically to achieve real-time frame rates.

Doppler detection, by contrast, requires a longer sampling time along the color line of sight. The echo data must be collected over several pulse-listen cycles (4 to 32) for a determination of the speed of flow to be made.

A compromise between frame rate and the estimation of Doppler frequency (velocity flow determination) is thus necessary. A rapid frame rate requires a short dwell time and consequently leads to poorer Doppler estimates. The reverse is also true. A longer dwell time provides improved assessment of flow though at a lower frame rate.

Two types of signal-generation processing (synchronous and asynchronous) are employed to extract two-dimensional gray-scale and color flow data. As discussed earlier, synchronous processing examines the returning echo concurrently for two-dimensional gray-scale and flow information. Asynchronous processing uses echoes generated at different times to collect data separately from each mode. Often the frequency is varied between the two-dimensional gray-scale and Doppler modes. The two-dimensional gray-scale lines of sight are interwoven with the color lines of sight in a time-sharing fashion.

The colors (red and blue) show regions of flow relative to cardiac anatomy (gray scale) and cardiac cycle (Fig. 9-10). The direction of flow relative to the transducer is depicted in red (toward) and blue (away). The color assignment can be reversed. Higher Doppler shift frequencies cause color saturation (more whiteness) or a change in hue.

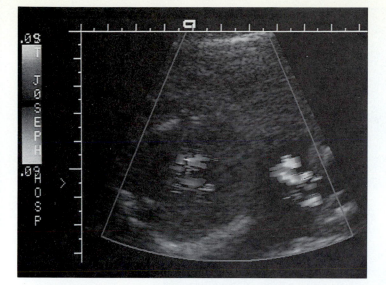

Figure 9-10 Color Doppler image of a fetus. Flow is demonstrated in the fetal heart and the umbilical cord. (See Color Plate 2B.)

Turbulence appears as a third color (green) or as a mosaic pattern.

CD Controls

In addition to the usual transmit (dB, output, course gain) and TGC controls, a variety of CD parameters is available to optimize the imaging process. As with any ultrasound system, a higher output increases the transmitted beam intensity and influences sensitivity.

The color-on-and-off control switch selects two-dimensional gray-scale images only or two-dimensional images with color and gray scale (see Fig. 9-11 for comparative images; an M-mode scan of the patient is also included). The beam-sharing requirements when color is present reduce the real-time frame rate. Color lag in the real-time image can be improved by switching to a synchronous scanner.

The color gain control adjusts the system's sensitivity to the received Doppler signals. A higher gain increases the amount of color displayed. The color depth control specifies the depth of the color field of view, which is set separately from the two-dimensional gray-scale mode. Increased color depth reduces the frame rate.

The color map assigns color levels to various flow velocities. Turbulent flow may be depicted as a mosaic pattern (Fig. 9-12). Special maps emphasize high-amplitude low-velocity Doppler shifts associated with heart walls or valves. This has applicability in assessing damage following an infarct. When blood flow is of interest, the clutter filter removes wall movements from the color display.

The map invert reverses the conventional color coding of blue (away) and red (toward the transducer) to red (away) and blue (toward). Persistence is a frame-averaging technique used to reduce color fluctuations, with some sacrifice in temporal resolution. Spatial filtering averages scan lines

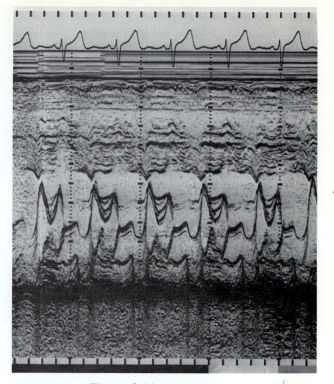

A

Figure 9-11 A, M-mode trace.

Continued.

to allow for higher frame rates, but with a loss of spatial detail.

The accuracy of the velocity estimates is improved by increasing the packet size (the number of pulses sampling the Doppler line of sight). A large packet size translates to a longer dwell time for each color line of sight and a reduction in frame rate.

The width of the color field of view overlaid on the two-dimensional gray-scale image can be changed. A small portion of the two-dimensional gray-scale image is sampled for flow, thus increasing the frame rate or improving the flow estimates. The position of the color field of view can be varied within the two-dimensional gray-scale image to obtain flow information from a particular area of interest.

Most units also allow for adjustments of the color intensity (brightness) and tint (hue) on the monitor. Cine loops enable stored image data to be reviewed at variable frame speeds for better visualization of flow data.

Applications

Clinical applications of CD imaging include the visualization of structural changes altering flow patterns (congenital heart disease, intracardiac mass, cardiomyopathy) and the presentation of flow velocity changes (regurgitation and high pressure gradients). Regurgitation is identified by flow reversal or turbulence in the region of the valve during diastole. Increased flow velocity is associated with high pressure gradients.

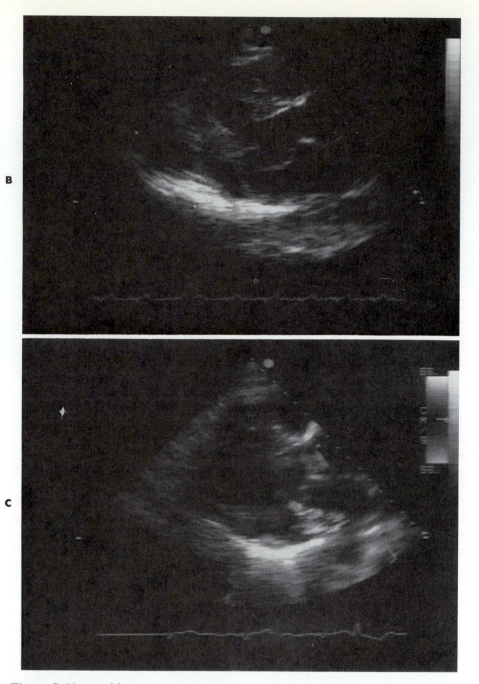

Figure 9-11, cont'd **B,** Two-dimensional gray-scale (parasternal long-axis view) of mitral valve prolapse. **C,** Color Doppler image of mitral valve regurgitation. (See Color Plate 2C.)

TRANSDUCER SELECTION FOR ECHOCARDIOGRAPHY

The selection of an appropriate transducer depends on several factors. The characteristics of short wavelength, broad bandwidth, and extended near-field depth make a high-frequency transducer desirable. The short spatial pulse length allows for early detection of echoes (decreased dead zone) to evaluate objects located near the transducer face (i.e., the right ventricle). In addition, high-frequency transducers can be made to fit easily between the ribs. The problem, however, is that high-frequency ultrasound beams are less

penetrating because the attenuation by tissue is enhanced. For some patients, lower-frequency transducers are needed. Improved focusing techniques have been developed to enable these transducers to be used.

M-mode scanning, based on the time trace of the B-mode dots along a single line of sight, uses medium-focused low- to medium-frequency transducers that were developed for A-mode and B-mode scanning. A fixed-focused single crystal (under certain conditions) provides adequate resolution for M-mode scanning.

ECG-gated scanning also uses a fixed-focused trans-

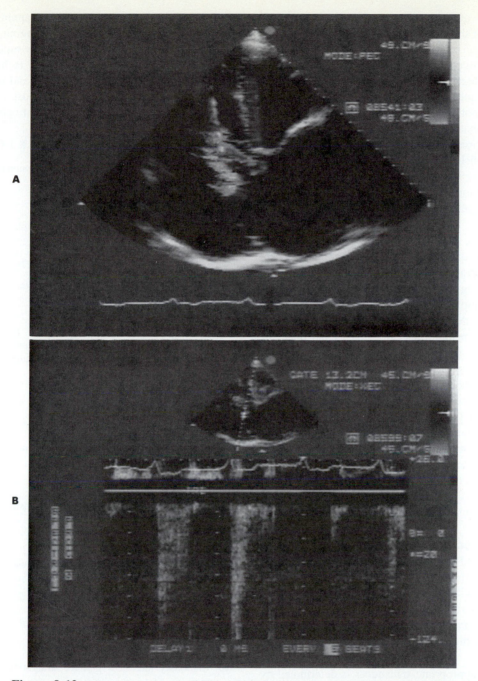

Figure 9-12 Tricuspid valve regurgitation. **A,** Color Doppler (apical four-chamber view). A mosaic pattern denotes the regurgitation. **B,** Pulsed-wave Doppler demonstrating reverse flow. (See Color Plates 2D and 2E.)

ducer. Two-dimensional real-time mechanical cardiac imaging systems employ a fixed-focus B-mode crystal driven across the field of view. These transducers are small in size and provide a sector view of the heart between the ribs. Frame rates, however, are relatively slow for cardiac studies. The fixed focal zone creates problems when different views of that heart are needed because the changing depth of the cardiac structures compromises spatial resolution.

Electronic arrays have improved image quality by allowing for changeable focal zones, faster frame rates, smaller sizes, and more sophisticated processing techniques. The stepdown segmented array is usually too long to be placed between the ribs, as is necessary for cardiac imaging.

A linear phased array, by contrast, produces a sector format and is small. High frame rates and narrow beam widths are possible. A disadvantage is the increased production of side lobes and grating lobes from beam steering; however, the advantages far outweigh these, particularly for CD imaging.

Transmit and receive focusing depends on the type and uniformity of tissues encountered by the ultrasound beam. Cardiac structures are extremely variable in content (i.e., walls, valves, and blood), which makes focusing unreliable. In addition, further degradation of lateral resolution occurs as a result of the frequency response of the transducer and the depth-dependent shift in the echo frequency distribution.

Annular phased array transducers are concentric rings with four or five circular elements. The are 1 to 4 cm in diameter with the degree of focusing enhanced by a larger aperture. Proper sequencing of the annuli produces a symmetrical beam in both the in-plane and the out-of-plane directions. Unfortunately, the beam must be mechanically steered, which requires a fluid standoff or liquid path. Beam focusing is accomplished in uniform liquid rather than nonuniform tissue. The ability to combine modalities for simultaneous acquisition of color-flow and two-dimensional gray-scale information is difficult.

The curved linear array enlarges the beam aperture for deeper focusing while decreasing the skin contact area. Grating lobes are reduced because the beam formation is perpendicular to the array and beam steering is not applied. Out-of-plane focusing is accomplished by means of a mechanical lens, and in-plane focusing is achieved by the transmit and receive time delays. The disadvantage of the curved array is that lateral resolution is reduced as the depth of penetration becomes greater, although this is also true with any sector format (Fig. 4-5).

The compound linear array couples the segmental and phased array format to create a field of view that extends beyond the physical length of the array. Parallel lines of sight generated perpendicular to the array are acquired and stored in the digital scan converter. Multiple lines of sight are then collected at an angle to the array. These data also are stored in the scan converter. Corrections are applied for areas in which scan lines overlap (Fig. 4-33). The frame rate is reduced because data collection is achieved over a wider area.

Rectangular phased arrays are electronically focused in both the in-plane and the out-of-plane directions simultaneously. A very narrow symmetrical beam is steered in different directions without moving the transducer. Specific lines of sight can be reserved for M-mode or Doppler data collection. CD imaging also can be completed. The major disadvantage is the high cost associated with the complex electronics.

Selection of an appropriate transducer is determined by the clinical needs of the institution. The applications must be identified and the transducer selected accordingly. Electronic formation and focusing and steering of the ultrasound beam allow near-simultaneous collection of data from several modes—including M-mode, two-dimensional gray scale, and Doppler—which can be combined into one image. Serious consideration must be given to the flexibility of the transducer and the processing options available.

SUMMARY

M-mode scanning evaluates the motion of an interface. Both reflector position and velocity are depicted by the M-mode trace. Highly detailed two-dimensional real-time gray-scale imaging of the heart is possible with small probes introduced near or into the heart. Duplex scanning combines real-time imaging with M-mode and Doppler scanning. The extension of duplex scanning has led to CD imaging, which provides a two-dimensional presentation of flow superimposed on the real-time image. All these scanning techniques are optimized by specific transducer designs and signal-processing techniques. The echocardiographer must understand the instrumentation necessary to produce an optimal image.

■ REVIEW QUESTIONS ■

1. Cardiac real-time imaging with ultrasound provides good temporal and spatial resolution.
   a. True
   b. False
2. Ultrasound physics for echocardiography is dramatically different from other ultrasound physics.
   a. True
   b. False
3. Reflector size, shape, and composition affect ultrasound reflectivity.
   a. True
   b. False
4. Real-time imaging of the heart is usually accomplished with a higher PRF than used to image abdominal organs.
   a. True
   b. False
5. M-mode scanning is a static imaging technique.
   a. True
   b. False
6. The M-mode scan is a two-dimensional plot of depth versus time.
   a. True
   b. False
7. M-mode scanning forms a two-dimensional spatial image by collecting multiple lines of sight.
   a. True
   b. False
8. The most common recording device used for M-mode scanning is the strip chart recorder.
   a. True
   b. False
9. M-mode is useful for the evaluation of heart valves.
   a. True
   b. False
10. Stationary interfaces produce straight lines on the M-mode trace.
    a. True
    b. False
11. Static B-mode imaging provides superb images of the heart with well-defined edges.
    a. True
    b. False
12. Duplex scanners incorporate both M-mode and real-time capabilities.
    a. True
    b. False
13. Color M-mode scanning combines Doppler and M-mode data collection along one line of sight.
    a. True
    b. False
14. Color M-mode portrays detailed anatomical information of the heart.
    a. True
    b. False

15. High frame rates are important for two-dimensional real-time cardiac imaging.
    a. True
    b. False
16. Simultaneous display of the ECG with the real-time image or M-mode trace is valuable in cardiac imaging.
    a. True
    b. False
17. Duplex imaging allows simultaneous or near-simultaneous collection of Doppler data and the real-time image.
    a. True
    b. False
18. Long dwell times during Doppler data collection increase the real-time frame rate in duplex scanning.
    a. True
    b. False
19. In CD imaging, the frame rate depends on the depth of interest and the dwell time for the color line of sight.
    a. True
    b. False
20. Multiple pulses for each line of sight are required for two-dimensional gray-scale in CD imaging.
    a. True
    b. False
21. In CD imaging, blue normally indicates flow toward the transducer.
    a. True
    b. False
22. Persistence is a frame-averaging technique.
    a. True
    b. False
23. Electronic linear phased array is used in cardiac imaging because of its small size, sector field of view, changeable focal zone, and high frame rate.
    a. True
    b. False

24. An annular phased array produces a symmetric beam pattern.
    a. True
    b. False
25. Transducer selection is dictated by the clinical application.
    a. True
    b. False

BIBLIOGRAPHY

American Institute of Ultrasound in Medicine: Syllabus: advanced small animal ultrasound imaging seminar, Bethesda, MD; 1990, The Institute.

Feigenbaum H: *Echocardiography,* ed 4, Philadelphia, 1986, Lea & Febiger.

Goldberg SJ, Allen HD, Sahn DJ: *Pediatric and adolescent echocardiology: a handbook,* ed 2, Chicago, 1980, Year Book Medical Publishers.

Lee RM, Riesen BE: Diagnostic cardiology: noninvasive imaging techniques. In Come PC (ed): *Diagnostic cardiology: non-invasive imaging techniques,* Philadelphia, 1985, JB Lippincott.

McDicken WN: *Diagnostic ultrasonics: principles and use of instruments,* ed 3, New York, 1991, Churchill Livingstone.

Silverman NH, Snider AR: *Two-dimensional echocardiography in congenital heart disease,* New York, 1982, Appleton-Century-Crofts.

Talano JV, Gardin JM: *Textbook of two-dimensional echocardiography,* New York, 1983, Grune & Stratton.

Woodcock JP: *Ultrasonics,* Bristol, 1979, Adam Hilger.

▲

CHAPTER 10

Digital Signal and Image Processing

During the past 15 years the scan converter used in ultrasound imaging hardware has undergone a transition from analog to digital. The newer devices are essentially solid-state computer memories. Long-term stability of the displayed image is achieved, and day-to-day variations in electronic drift can be reduced compared to analog storage tubes. Digital scan converters also provide superior accuracy and longer life compared with their analog counterparts. Incorporation of the digital scan converter in real-time instruments has facilitated the rapid development and acceptance of real-time scanning. The digitization of scan data provides an additional advantage: quantitative manipulation and analysis of the received echoes are possible in an expeditious fashion using current computer technology. Time gain compensation (TGC), edge enhancement, logarithmic compression, frame averaging, and gray-scale mapping are all examples of techniques available for processing the scan data.

In this chapter the binary number system, computer hardware, computer operation, analog-to-digital conversion, and matrix representation of digital images are reviewed before incorporation into the presentation of real-time scanners.

An overview of the signal-processing techniques used in acquisition and display of scan data is then presented. Computer programming and database management as practical tools in the clinical environment are introduced. Finally, computer requirements for an integrated all-digital imaging department are discussed.

BINARY REPRESENTATION

Digital computers are based on the binary system, in which two symbols or states are used to encode information (numbers, characters, and instructions). Similar to Morse code, in which a series of dots and dashes represents numbers and characters, the binary system employs combinations of 0s and 1s. The on-off operation of switches in the computer is ideally suited to representing these two possible states (the "off" position corresponding to 0 and the "on" position to 1).

The relative ease of representing 2 symbols in the binary system instead of the 10 symbols necessary in the decimal notation dictates that computers operate in binary. Furthermore, electrical circuits designed according to the Boolean principles (a mathematical treatment of logic developed by George Boole in the middle of the 19th century) could perform logic comparisons as well as execute complex calculations.

Bit and Byte

A single binary digit (called a "bit") can be either 0 or 1 and thus is limited to two configurations. To increase the number of possible configurations, several bits are combined and treated as a single entity called a "word" (Fig. 10-1). *Word length* denotes the number of bits that are moved as a group in and out of a location in computer memory and also dictates the maximum number of bits used in computation. The design of a specific computer fixes the word length.

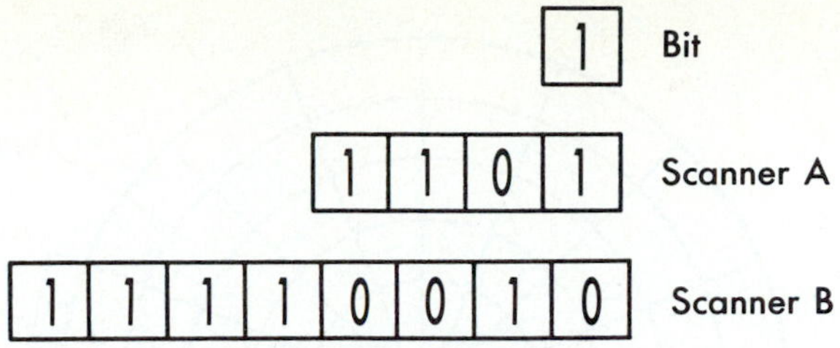

Figure 10-1 Relationship between bit and word. *Scanner A* has a 4-bit word, and *Scanner B* an 8-bit word. *Scanner B* is able to represent the received echo with many more combinations of 0s and 1s.

Another term that describes a collection of bits is *byte*. A byte is a group of 8 bits and is required to code a single character, such as one letter of the alphabet. The capacity of data storage units (e.g., floppy disk drives and magnetic tapes) is expressed in bytes or megabytes (millions of bytes). The total number of bytes indicates the total number of characters that the storage device can hold.

Binary Notation

The problem of how to represent the usual decimal numbers in this binary notation is solved as follows: In the binary system the base is 2. Each position in a multidigit binary number is denoted by the base raised to a particular exponent, which increases right to left. The number 1 in a column signifies that the value of the power of 2 represented by that position contributes to the overall sum. For example:

Column value	2^3	2^2	2^1	2^0
Binary number	0	1	0	1

This means that the sum of 0×8, 1×4, 0×2, and 1×1 is five (the corresponding decimal equivalent of the number 0101 in binary notation).

■ Example 10-1

Calculate the decimal equivalent of the binary number 1101.

Assign the value to each position.

2^3	2^2	2^1	2^0
1	1	0	1

Sum the contribution from each column.

$$1 \times 8 + 1 \times 4 + 0 \times 2 + 1 \times 1 = 13$$

The decimal equivalent of 1101 thus is 13.

Several binary numbers and the associated decimal numbers are listed in Table 10-1.

Mathematically the number of combinations that could be denoted by a collection of bits is given by 2^n, where n is the number of bits in the word. A 4-bit word can represent 16 different combinations of 0s and 1s because the base 2 raised to the fourth power equals 16. Obviously, a word with more bits can be configured in more combinations and can represent varying echoes with greater magnitude or with

■ **Table 10-1** Translation of Binary Numbers to Decimal Equivalents

Binary System	Decimal System
0000	0
0001	1
0010	2
0011	3
0100	4
0101	5
0110	6
0111	7
1000	8
1001	9

greater precision. As illustrated in Figure 10-1, scanner *B*, with a bit depth of eight, corresponding to 256 combinations, is superior to scanner *A*, which has a bit depth of four.

COMPUTER SYSTEMS

The computer system is classified into three major components: hardware, software, and documentation. Hardware is the physical equipment such as the central processing unit (CPU), disk drive, printer, cathode ray tube (CRT), keyboard, light pen, and joystick. Software is the set of programs (or instructions) that tell the computer what to do. The collection of programs to perform specialized tasks is called an application package. Documentation consists of the manuals that instruct the operator how to use the computer hardware and the application package.

HARDWARE

A computer accepts information from an input device, applies some prescribed process (dictated by the software), and communicates the results to the outside world. The input device acquires data and/or conveys operator instructions. For example, the transducer is used to input scan data to the CPU.

Central Processing Unit

The CPU manipulates the scan data by sequentially executing programmed instructions. All mathematical manipulations and logic functions are performed in the CPU. The CPU coordinates all operations, including data transfers from one device to another in the system.

Memory

The read only memory (ROM) contains permanent instructions to be implemented by the CPU to configure the system. Usually the ROM is accessed during the startup procedure, called booting. Its contents are changed by replacing the integrated circuit chip. Random access memory (RAM) is accessible by the CPU for temporary storage of scan data or instructions. It is erasable and can be updated with new information as required.

Input/Output Devices

Numerous input/output (I/O) devices are available that can be interfaced to the computer system. Sometimes these devices are called peripherals because they are controlled by the CPU. A device may be designed for input only, output only, or both input and output. The output devices are used to display, list, or store the results of manipulations performed by the CPU.

The transducer is representative of many detector systems in medicine that supply image information to the computer. Since the computer can handle only binary data, however, the signals coming from the transducer must be translated into a digital form. This occurs at the interface, which contains an analog-to-digital converter (ADC).

Information in the form of alphanumerics (letters, numbers, and symbols), images, and graphs is provided to the operator. Within the computer system data communication assumes a form (e.g., magnetic fields, polarized laser light, and voltage pulse height) that is efficiently handled by the hardware devices. For example, most scanners contain a keyboard. The depressed key is translated into binary code as a series of voltage pulses before being communicated to other devices. A modem allows information to be transferred over telephone lines by converting digital data to audible tones. For analog devices such as the modem the rate of data transmission is designated in bauds, 1 baud equaling 1 bit per second.

Storage Devices

Memory is expensive and limited in capacity. Therefore information (both program and data) is stored as files outside the memory until needed. The most common storage devices are magnetic disks (e.g., Winchester disks, removable magnetic cartridges, or floppy disks). The magnetic disk consists of a base material coated with a thin layer of magnetic material, usually ferrous oxide. Data in the form of 0s and 1s are represented by small regions of magnetizations in the ferrous oxide (the magnetic field in one direction corresponding to 0 and in the opposite direction to 1).

The disk is divided into tracks and sectors, which allows a directory of the location of data on it to be generated (Fig. 10-2). Each track in a sector corresponds to one block. A block is the smallest data group that can be transferred to and from the disk. A block is usually equal to 256 or 512 words. If a file is 300 words large in memory, it requires 2 blocks on disk for storage (assuming 1 block contains 256 words).

The information is transferred to and from the disk via read/write heads. One read/write head is associated with each disk surface. The disk is spinning rapidly, and the read/write head moves in and out above the sensitive layer. By positioning the read/write head directly on a particular

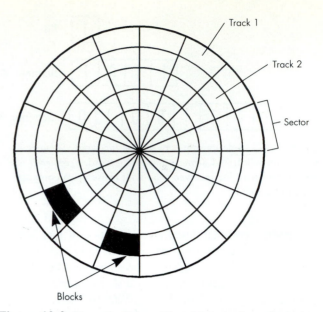

Figure 10-2 Magnetic disk partitioned into tracks and sectors. One block of data is contained on the track through one sector. The designation of track and sector of a file indicates the storage location on the disk.

■ **Table 10-2** Disk Characteristics

Type	Storage Capacity (megabytes)	Transfer Rate
Floppy	0.3 to 4	Slow
Optical disk	100 to 1000	Medium
Disk cartridge	2.5 to 80	Fast
Winchester	10 to 1000	Fastest

track and sector, it is possible to read or write the desired file. This is an example of random access, since the information can be transferred without examining other blocks. A particular track may contain several files, but all the data making up a single file are contiguous on the disk.

Optical disks may be written on only once or may be erased and rewritten with new information. The first type is called WORM, which means write once read many. Erasable optical disks are designated MOD (magneto-optical disk). A small laser light beam (less than 1 μm in diameter) scans across the reflective surface of the optical disk. At each location on the reflective surface, a value of 0 or 1 is encoded by manipulating the properties of the surface. In the WORM format a pit is etched into the surface to alter the amount of light reflected by the readout laser beam. The presence or absence of the pit codes for a 0 or a 1. The erasable format uses the polarization of reflected light to code for the two binary states. In the write mode the polarizing properties of the reflective surface are switched by heating the sensitive layer while laser light is incident. The small physical dimensions of the laser beam allow high recording density, and thus a large storage capacity is achieved.

Disks are characterized by data capacity and rate of transfer of data (Table 10-2). Each device has advantages and disadvantages (capacity, transfer rate, cost, size). The primary disadvantages of the floppy disk are its slow rate of data transfer and its limited capacity. Many institutions use the floppy disk as a portable storage device for the transfer of patient studies between computers.

SOFTWARE

Software is the set of programs that are used to control the computer. These may be permanently stored in ROM, which can be only read, or they may be stored on magnetic disk and transferred to RAM when needed. The advantage of this storage method is that the programs can easily be rewritten with newer versions (software updates).

Software supplied by the manufacturer is designed primarily to transform the hardware into usable tools. In addition, a set of programs is provided that allow users to create and run programs of their own design. These user-generated programs are usually written in the high level programming languages of Fortran or Basic, but they can also be written in assembly language.

Operating System

The operating system is a collection of programs that direct all the activities of the computer, including control of hardware devices and execution of application programs. Communication between the computer system and the user is essential. The computer system must offer clear and direct methods to acquire data and to select processing options. The responses of the user must be converted by the operating system to forms understood by the computer. The operating system must select programs that can fulfill the request of the user. The basic approach is to separate the many functions into discrete modules, which are retrieved from the storage device and placed in memory as necessary. Each module is a program designed to do a certain task. The operating system must also maintain records of stored programs and data.

Programming Languages

Selection of a particular language to write programs depends on the application (business or scientific) and the specific hardware devices available. In all cases the program language must eventually be translated into machine code (the instruction set in 0s and 1s for the computer). Machine code is not universal but rather is computer specific.

Assembly language programming requires every execution step by the CPU to be defined. The assembly language is converted to machine code by translation programs called assemblers. Assembly language is machine dependent. This low level language provides for greatest programming flexibility and speed; however, such programs often become large and complex for the general user. Operating systems are usually written in assembly language.

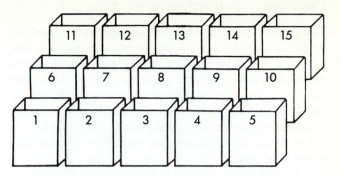

Figure 10-3 A collection of wastepaper baskets can be used to represent computer memory. Each wastepaper basket (location in memory) has a numerical label (address) to distinguish it from the others. One instruction or multidigit binary number is held at each memory location.

■ **Table 10-3** Computer Memory Example

Wastepaper Basket	Contents*
1	Erase pad (i.e., put number 0 on pad)
2	Add number at location 12 to contents of pad
3	Add number at location 11 to contents of pad
4	Place value on pad in wastepaper basket 10
5	Stop
6,7,8,9	0 (0000 0000)
10	8 (0000 1000)
11	5 (0000 0101)
12	3 (0000 0011)

*Can contain either an instruction or an item of data (number).

High-level languages are constructed so they are machine independent. Language interpreters and translators are required to translate the program written in a high-level language to specific machine code.

COMPUTER OPERATION

Suppose memory is represented by a group of wastepaper baskets numbered 1 through 15, as shown in Figure 10-3. The numerical label is used to identify a particular basket. Each basket is limited—that is, it can hold only one piece of paper on which an instruction or number may be written. You are now given a pen and a scratch pad and told to go to basket number 1, retrieve the piece of paper, and perform the instructed task. When you have completed the first assignment, move on to the next basket to retrieve your next instruction. You proceed and find the scenario outlined in Table 10-3. The result of your work is that the number 8 in binary notation with a word length of 8 (0000 1000) is stored in basket 10.

Execution of Instructions

This example illustrates how a computer works. Each location (or address) in memory, corresponding to a basket, holds one instruction or one multidigit binary number. The person represents the central processing unit (CPU) and the pad acts as the accumulator, which is a working area for calculations. A set of instructions is carried out in a carefully planned sequence (which is designated by the program). In this program the instructions are performed in order from basket 1 to basket 5. In a different program the user may be told to jump to a nonconsecutive location for the next instruction. The execution would then proceed in sequence from that point.

Although, in the example you had to go to basket 12 to get some numerical information, you still came back to the next basket in sequence for the next instruction. (After completing the instruction at location 2, you went to location 3 for the next instruction). Note that you had to be told where to start (which location in memory contained the first instruction in the program to be executed).

The program must be placed in memory before instructions are executed. This program, for example, could have been stored on a floppy disk and then transferred to computer memory before being run. The process is called "loading." Before the program was stored on the floppy, it would have to have been entered as a set of instructions line by line via the keyboard by the software developer. The data in locations 11 and 12 would also have to have been entered before the program was run.

Memory Capacity

The total number of baskets dictates the size of the computer memory. As the number of baskets increases, more instructions and data can be held in memory, and this results in faster execution times. The memory capacity is usually designated by the number of locations, expressed as K. The symbol K (for kilo) denotes the numerical value of 2^{10}, or 1024. For example, a 32K computer would have 32×1024 or 32,768 locations available in its memory. Each storage location contains one word. The length of the computer word is dictated by the computer system (most computers have a word length of 32 bits). Therefore the memory with 32K locations would be described as a 32K word memory. Sometimes the memory size is denoted by the number of bytes. For a 32-bit computer word in which each word contained 4 bytes, a 32K word memory would also be described as having 128K bytes or 128 kilobytes. Memory capacity has been greatly expanded in recent years and is often specified in the unit of megabytes (MB). One megabyte is equal to 2^{20} or 1,048,576 bytes.

Each wastepaper basket has a numerical label to distinguish it from neighboring wastepaper baskets. This label is the unique memory address of that particular basket. The address and binary information placed in the word are separate entities (just as the writing on the piece of paper is not the same as the numerical label of the wastepaper basket). For a 32-bit word the information held at any memory location is coded in the form of some 32-digit combination of 0s and 1s.[10]

Computer Speed

The speed of a computer is measured by the number (in millions) of instructions it can execute in 1 second (MIPS). Another, more complex, means of gauging computer speed is to note the number of floating point operations it can perform in 1 second (MFLOPS). These parameters establish the computer's speed on a relative scale, but other factors influence the execution time necessary for a particular program. Test programs have been used to determine the speed of different systems designed for the same application.

ANALOG-TO-DIGITAL CONVERSION

Some accuracy is sacrificed when the echo signal is digitized, as occurs in the translation of information from the detection system (signal amplitude and location of the reflecting structure) to a form that is understood by the computer. The translation process is called analog-to-digital conversion and is limited by the number of bits available in the digitization process. The analog signal is a continuously variable entity, whereas the digital signal is expressed in discrete steps.

Height Conversion

Imagine that there are two ways (via a staircase or via a ramp) of ascending to the second floor from the first floor in a building. By using the stairs, a description of your position (height above the first floor) consists of the number of the step you are standing on multiplied by the height of a single step. You are constrained to standing on one of the steps; a position between steps is not possible. If you stand on step no. 2 and each step is 2 feet high, your location is designated as 4 feet above the first floor. At step no. 3 you move to a height 6 feet above the first floor. The description is limited to discrete intervals of distance established by the size of the step (in this case increments of 2 feet). However, by taking the ramp, you would reach *any* height above the first floor.

If we replace each step in the staircase with two smaller steps, we can now describe the height as increments of 1 foot. In Figure 10-4 , a height 5.75 feet above the first floor can be represented precisely by the ramp but it would be approximated by step no. 2 in staircase A (at a height of 4 feet) or by step no. 5 in staircase B (at a height of 5 feet). An error is introduced in the quantitative description of the variable (in this case position) because discrete units are used. If we divide the discrete units into smaller and smaller steps, however, the accuracy of the conversion process is improved. In general, staircase B provides a more accurate assessment of position than does staircase A because many more steps are used in the conversion process. The same effect is achieved by employing more bits in the digitization of analog signals.

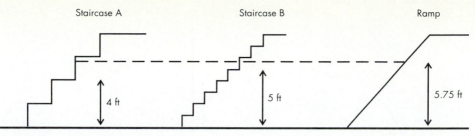

Figure 10-4 Comparison of analog and digital representations. The 5.75-foot height above the floor *(dotted line)* can be represented exactly by the ramp but is only approximated by the stair-cases. *Staircase A* (with large steps) is less accurate in its representation than *Staircase B*. The fifth step in *Staircase B* is closer to the actual height than the second step of *Staircase A* is.

Voltage Conversion

In ultrasound scanning the analog signal is a voltage wave-form generated by the returning echo that strikes the trans-ducer. Increased intensity of the received echo is represented by an increased value of the voltage. The transformation of this analog signal to a digital format is limited to discrete steps, the size of each step being dictated by the bit depth of the analog-to-digital converter (ADC). Suppose the ADC for each of two scanners is configured to digitize the received signals over a range of 0 to 5 V. Scanner A has a 2-bit ADC (or four discrete steps) and scanner B a 3-bit ADC (or eight discrete steps). The corresponding step size, which is cal-culated by dividing the range (5 volts) by the total number of discrete steps available (either 4 or 8), is 1.25 and 0.625 V. The 2-volt peak in Figure 10-5 is interpreted as digital step 01 (or 1×1.25 V $= 1.25$ V) by scanner A and as digital step 011 (or 3×0.625 V $= 1.875$ V) by scanner B. Once more, the accuracy of the conversion process is improved by increasing the bit depth because each step corresponds to a smaller physical quantity.

Serial Sampling

In the previous examples one digital value was assigned to the analog signal. Other applications may require that the time-dependence of the analog signal be preserved. The analog signal is repeatedly sampled during the time interval and the instantaneous value at each sampled point is digi-tized. Figure 10-6 illustrates the digitization of a voltage waveform varying in time. Once more, the analog-to-digital conversion process yields discrete steps (in this case, with respect to both voltage and time).

Bit Depth

Word length sets the upper limit for the number of bits that can be used in the digitization of a signal. The actual bit depth of the ADC does not necessarily correspond to the word size. Some manufacturers use ADCs with fewer bits than the number available in a word. The prospective pur-chaser of ultrasound equipment should ascertain the bit depth maintained throughout the imaging chain, for it ul-timately will affect both contrast and dynamic range.

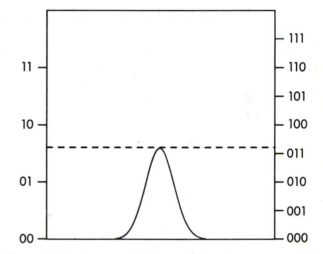

Figure 10-5 Analog-to-digital conversion of a voltage peak. With a 2-bit scanner the voltage peak is represented as 01, but with a 3-bit scanner as 011. The smaller divisions between digi-tizer steps allow greater accuracy.

SPATIAL REPRESENTATION

The information obtained from a scanned area is divided into small square picture elements called "pixels," which are combined to form the image. Each pixel corresponds to a particular region, designated by spatial coordinates, and is associated with the echo amplitude reflected from that region. The amplitude of the received signal is converted to a digital number (1s and 0s) by the ADC before storage in computer memory. The number of pixels available de-pends on the matrix size, which denotes the number of rows and columns in the pictorial representation. For example, a 512×512 matrix has 512 rows and 512 columns. The image is composed of a total of 262,144 individual pixels (the number of rows multiplied by the number of columns).

During data collection the digitized signal is stored in a particular location of memory specified by its address. Each pixel has one location reserved in memory for holding the amplitude of the signal associated with that pixel. The ad-dress is determined from the X and Y coordinates, which are generated from the transducer's position-sensing elec-tronics and the time between the transmitted pulse and the received echo (Fig. 10-7).

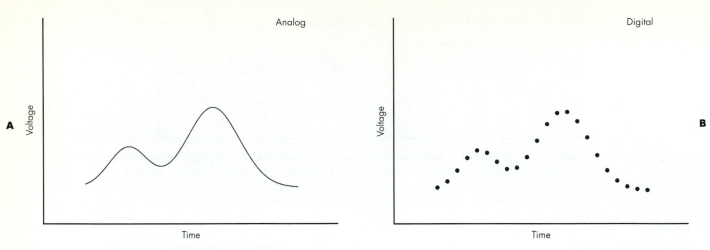

Figure 10-6 Analog-to-digital conversion of a time-varying voltage waveform. **A,** Analog signal; **B,** Digital signal.

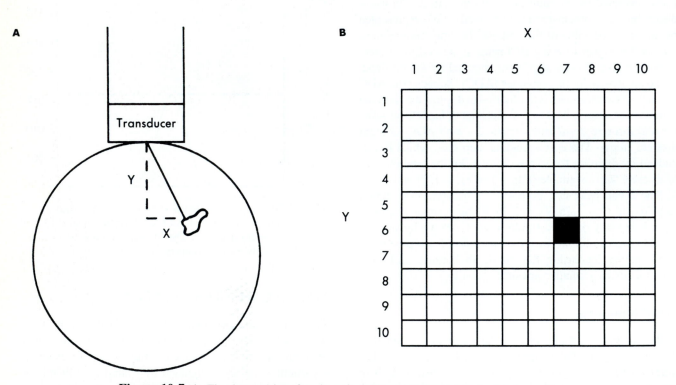

Figure 10-7 A, The detected interface is assigned *X* and *Y* coordinates to denote position. **B,** The coordinates are then used to place the signal amplitude of the received echo in the proper pixel location within the matrix.

The digitized amplitudes for all pixels contained in computer memory must be recombined to form the image. The image is constructed in such a manner that X and Y coordinates in the image correspond to X and Y coordinates in the area scanned. The address in memory designates the position of the pixel in the image, and the value stored at that address represents the signal amplitude of that pixel in the image. This is analogous to a jigsaw puzzle. Each piece of the puzzle is imprinted with a portion of a scene (signal amplitude) and must fit into the puzzle in a specified manner (address) to reproduce the scene. In the digital format each piece of the puzzle is restricted to a square (which is a

uniform shade of gray). Each pixel has its own shade, but only one value is stored in memory for that pixel. The same value is assumed to exist throughout the pixel. This assumption is most appropriate for pixels with small physical dimensions. Once more, some accuracy is sacrificed by the digital representation of spatial location. As the matrix size increases, the system has the potential of presenting more spatial detail, which is demonstrated by the digitized pictures of Abraham Lincoln in varying matrix sizes (Fig. 10-8). However, computer memories with a larger capacity are then necessary to store the information. Currently, most real-time scanners use the 512 × 512 matrix, which is

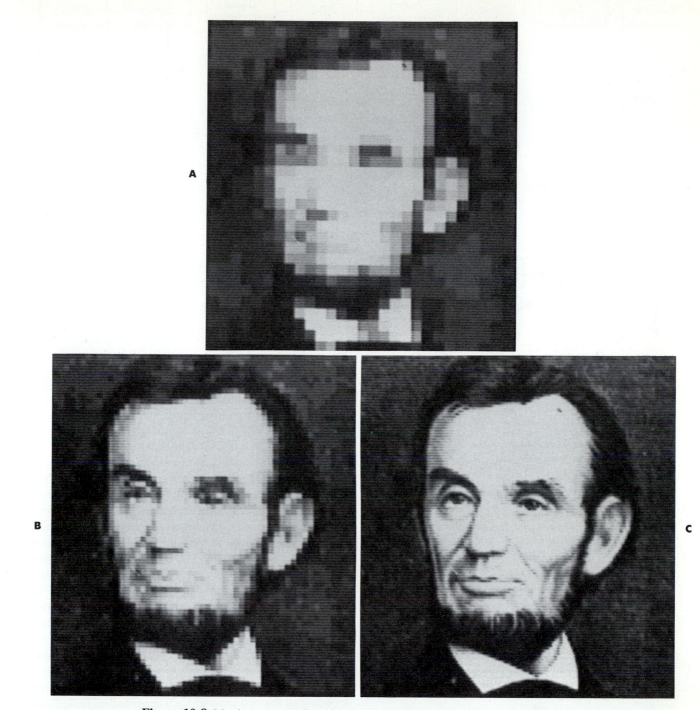

Figure 10-8 Matrix representation of a portrait of Abraham Lincoln. **A**, 32×32 matrix; **B**, 64×64; **C**, 128×128.

adequate for representing the spatial resolution achievable by the rest of the imaging chain.

IMAGE ACQUISITION

Figure 10-9 is a block diagram of the image acquisition components of a scanner. On command, the transmitter generates an ultrasound pulse of short duration and sends it into the body. The beam interacts with various interfaces,

and a fraction is reflected to the transducer. The transducer/ receiver converts the returning echo to an electronic pulse that can be subsequently processed and displayed. The amplifier increases the relatively weak received signals (a few millivolts) to the range of 1 V for analog-to-digital conversion. In the preprocessing section the received signal is modified by applying time gain compensation (TGC), edge enhancement, logarithmic compression, or a combination of these.

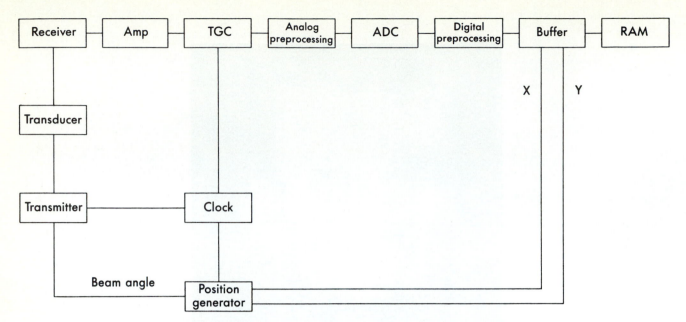

Figure 10-9 Image-acquisition components of a real-time scanner.

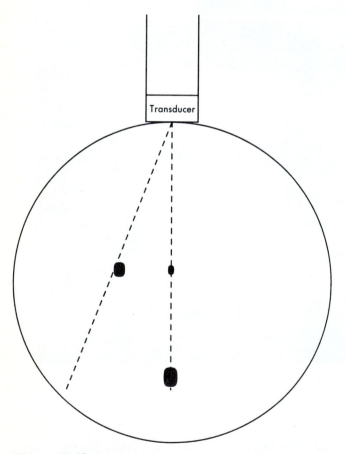

Figure 10-10 Sampling of a patient along two lines of sight. Note that the two interfaces are detected along the central line of sight. The size of the *black dot* is directly proportional to the intensity of the reflected echo.

Image Matrix

The ADC converts the amplified signal to digital format. Processing of the scan data may also occur in digital format. For the digitized representation of the echo to be placed at the correct location in the image matrix, the X and Y coordinates must be specified. This is accomplished by a position generator, which uses the time of travel for the ultrasound pulse and position sensors for beam direction. The beam sweeps through the region of interest either electronically or mechanically in a repetitive fashion. The signal amplitude and position coordinates for multiple lines of sight are placed temporarily in the buffer before final storage in random access memory (RAM). The format is changed from signal levels along successive lines of sight to the matrix notation, which represents a composite of all scan data. The buffer also serves to hold the scan data acquired at a very rapid rate until the computer is able to store the information in memory.[4,13]

Figure 10-10 shows two successive line-of-sight samplings of an object. Three reflecting structures of varying amplitude are detected. The contents of the buffer corresponding to the two lines of sight are listed in Table 10-4, where the signal amplitude is recorded as a function of the X and Y coordinates. Alternatively, the beam angle and elapsed time could be placed in the buffer to indicate position (with the X and Y coordinates calculated from these two parameters).

The signal amplitudes are assigned to the appropriate pixels in a 10 × 10 matrix (Fig. 10-11). The X and Y coordinates dictate the location within the matrix (also the address in memory), and the signal amplitude dictates the numerical value of the pixel. In this example the pixel locations corresponding to the various interfaces are assigned different values based on the intensity of the reflected echoes.

■ **Table 10-4** Contents of the Buffer for Successive Scan Lines

Signal Amplitude	X Position	Y Position
000	5	1
000	5	2
000	5	3
000	5	4
001	5	5
000	5	6
000	5	7
000	5	8
000	5	9
111	5	10
000	5	1
000	4	2
000	4	3
000	3	4
010	3	5
000	2	6
000	2	7
000	2	8

0	0	0	0	0	0	0	0	0	0
0	0	0	0	0	0	0	0	0	0
0	0	0	0	0	0	0	0	0	0
0	0	0	0	0	0	0	0	0	0
0	0	2	0	1	0	0	0	0	0
0	0	0	0	0	0	0	0	0	0
0	0	0	0	0	0	0	0	0	0
0	0	0	0	0	0	0	0	0	0
0	0	0	0	0	0	0	0	0	0
0	0	0	0	7	0	0	0	0	0

Figure 10-11 A 10×10 matrix depicting the three structures observed in Fig. 10-10. Note that the pixels corresponding to the various interfaces are assigned different values based on the intensity of the reflected echoes.

Data Manipulation

The incorporation of a digital scan converter in real-time instruments has dictated that images be manipulated in the matrix format. The digitization of scan data provides additional advantages of quantitative manipulation and analysis of echo data in rapid fashion. A wide variety of digital signal-processing techniques is available for this purpose. A large amount of information can be presented in a compact and more easily recognized form. Received echoes configured in a pictorial format as light and dark regions on a video monitor are more readily comprehended than a series of voltage spikes on an A-mode CRT display. Changing the shade of gray associated with a particular received echo in accordance with well-defined processing techniques may enhance the observer's ability to interpret the scan data. TGC, edge enhancement, logarithmic compression, frame averaging, and gray-scale mapping are some of the techniques used in the clinical environment.

Signal-processing techniques in ultrasound imaging are classified according to when they occur with respect to the computer storage of scan data. *Preprocessing* refers to the manipulations that take place during data collection before the scan data are stored in computer memory. *Postprocessing* denotes the operations applied after storage. Changing the manner in which the stored information is displayed constitutes a postprocessing technique.[11]

PREPROCESSING

Preprocessing is the manipulation of scan data during collection before their storage in computer memory. The data may be in an analog or digital format. The most common types of preprocessing include TGC, selective enhancement, logarithmic compression, fill-in interpolation, edge enhancement, image updating, and write zoom.

Time Gain Compensation

The attenuation of an ultrasound beam with depth causes equally reflective interfaces to produce different signal levels depending on their relative distances from the transducer. It is often advantageous to display reflectors of similar size, shape, and reflection coefficients with equal amplitude (see Fig. 2-51). Exponential amplification as a function of elapsed time from the transmitted pulse is used to correct the received signals for attenuation; that is, the reduction in signal level caused by the increased depth at which echoes are generated is compensated by applying time-dependent amplification to the received signal. This processing technique is called time gain compensation (TGC) (see Chapter 2).

Selective Enhancement

Amplification of the received signal (in addition to TGC) may be applied in a nonuniform manner to highlight echoes generated within a particular region of interest. In this technique, referred to as selective enhancement, the amplification is applied as a function of depth. The operator uses a series of slide control keys to set the depth, each key corresponding to a certain depth; the displacement of a key denotes the amount of amplification.

Logarithmic Compression

In general, the digitized signal amplitudes are stored in RAM as 6 to 8 bits. With 8 bits a total of 256 values is available

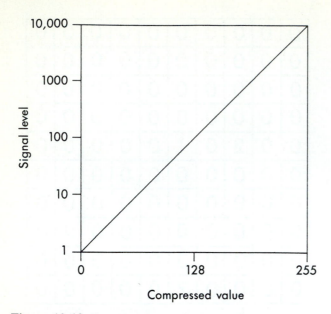

Figure 10-12 Signal levels over four orders of magnitude are assigned values between 0 and 255 for an 8-bit scanner. The vertical scale is logarithmic.

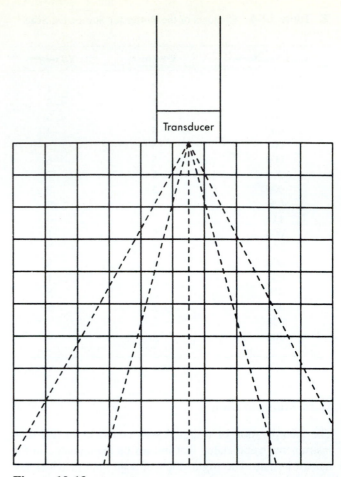

Figure 10-13 Lines of sight *(dotted)* superimposed on the matrix to demonstrate that not all pixels are sampled by the sound beam. The value assigned to the unsampled pixels is calculated by averaging signal amplitudes in the neighboring pixels.

to quantify the signal amplitude. If a linear representation is used, the maximum signal can be only 256 times the weakest signal. The range of values of the received signals after TGC and amplification, however, may extend over four or more orders of magnitude. A logarithmic transformation of the signal levels (1 to 10^4) is employed to compress the signal level to a narrower range (0 to 255). Figure 10-12 illustrates the relationship between signal level and the stored pixel value.

Because the display device is unable to process an extremely wide range of signal levels, compression is necessary. Increasing the depth beyond 8 bits allows a greater range of values to be stored, but the increased signal levels are ultimately compressed by the display device.

Fill-In Interpolation

The scanned area is probed by a series of ultrasound pulses directed along various lines of sight. By superimposing all the lines of sight on the image matrix, it can be demonstrated that several pixels are not sampled by the ultrasound beam (Fig. 10-13). If these blank pixels were each displayed with a 0 signal level, a disconcerting checkerboard image would result. Manufacturers avoid this by averaging the signals from nearby pixels that are sampled to generate a fill-in value for the blank pixel. A value for the blank pixel can thus be inferred by examining the surrounding region.

Edge Enhancement

Ultrasound imaging is ideally suited to the detection of interfaces or boundaries between structures. Edge enhancement is a filtering technique that can be applied to the line-of-sight data (or in some applications to the matrix image

data) to emphasize further a change in signal levels across an interface. Suppose eight pixels along one line of sight have the initial values shown in Table 10-5. The filtering process uses a kernel (i.e., a collection of weighting factors or convolution coefficients) applied to the original values. In this example the kernel is applied to three sequential pixels with weighting factors of -1, 3, and -1. To calculate the edge-enhanced value for pixel no. 4, the kernel is centered on pixel number 4. The sum of each weighting factor times its respective original value in the three-pixel sequence is calculated. This yields a new value of 300 for pixel 4. The numerical operations are

$$(-1 \times 200) + (3 \times 200) + (-1 \times 100) = 300$$

The edge-enhanced values for the remaining pixels are determined in a similar manner, by moving the center of the kernel to each pixel along the line of sight. Centering the kernel at pixel 5, for example, yields an edge-enhanced value of 0:

$$(-1 \times 200) + (3 \times 100) + (-1 \times 100) = 0$$

Note that the original value and not the new value for pixel 4 was used in this calculation. The kernel always operates

■ **Table 10-5** Numerical Example of Edge Enhancement

Pixel No.	1	2	3	4	5	6	7	8
Original value	200	200	200	200	100	100	100	100
Kernel			−1	3	−1			
Edge-enhanced value	200	200	200	300	0	100	100	100

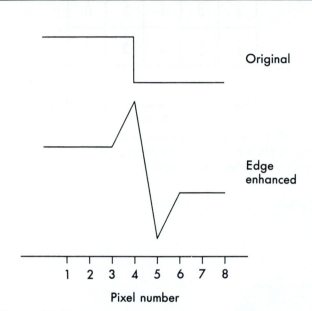

Figure 10-14 Edge enhancement. The original change in signal level detected along a particular line of sight is manipulated mathematically to produce a more dramatic difference at the boundary.

on the original data; the edge-enhanced results must be maintained separately from the initial values. Figure 10-14 is a graphical representation of edge enhancement. The amount of edge enhancement can be modified by changing the magnitude or number of weighting factors used in the filtering process.

Image Updating

Because the ultrasound beam sweeps repeatedly through the patient, new information is constantly becoming available. The most recent scan data are held in the buffer for updating the image data in memory. Several techniques by various manufacturers are employed for this purpose. Most simply, the old value at a particular location stored in memory is replaced by the current value for that pixel location. This is referred to as last-value mode. The image data are updated continuously and rapidly with the newest echo data (Fig. 10-15). The average of the old value and current value may also be used to replace the stored scan data.

A

0	0	5	0	0
0	0	4	0	0
0	0	3	0	0
0	0	2	0	0
0	0	1	0	0

B

0	0	5	0	0
0	0	4	0	0
0	0	7	0	0
0	0	2	0	0
0	0	1	0	0

C

0	0	5	0	0
0	0	4	0	0
0	0	5	0	0
0	0	2	0	0
0	0	1	0	0

Figure 10-15 Image updating. **A,** Old matrix data. **B,** Last-value mode or most recent matrix data. **C,** Pixel-by-pixel average of these two matrices.

Write Zoom

Write zoom (also called regional expansion, reduced field of view, and zooming) is a magnification technique applied during data collection. The operator designates a region

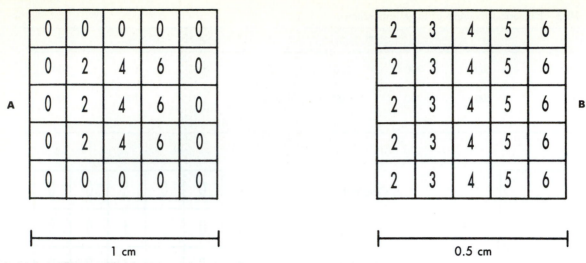

0	0	0	0	0
0	2	4	6	0
0	2	4	6	0
0	2	4	6	0
0	0	0	0	0

A

├──────── 1 cm ────────┤

2	3	4	5	6
2	3	4	5	6
2	3	4	5	6
2	3	4	5	6
2	3	4	5	6

B

├──────── 0.5 cm ────────┤

Figure 10-16 Write zoom. **A,** Original sampled region. **B,** Central portion of the original region scanned in write-zoom mode. Although the number of pixels is constant, a smaller region is sampled in write zoom and thus each pixel corresponds to a smaller physical size.

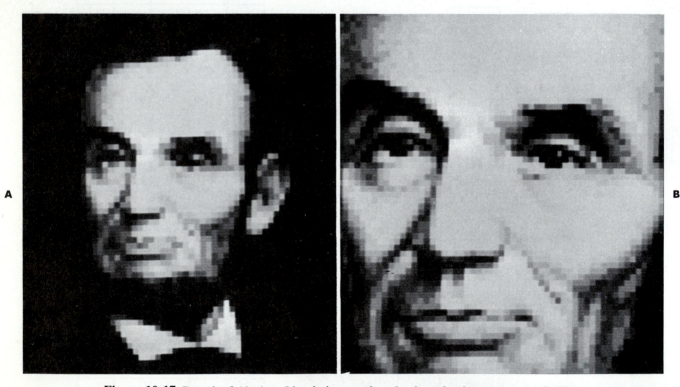

Figure 10-17 Portrait of Abraham Lincoln in normal mode, **A,** and write-zoom mode, **B.** The number of pixels in each matrix is identical but in write-zoom mode spatial detail is improved.

within the field of view to be magnified. The signals received from echoes within this expanded region are placed in pixels to generate the image matrix. Because the physical dimensions of the expanded region are much smaller than the original field of view, however, more pixels are available to represent the signal amplitudes within the expanded region. This may lead to increased spatial resolution.

For example, in Figure 10-16, a 5 × 5 matrix is used to store an image of an object that has physical dimensions of 1 × 1 cm. By designating the central region for expansion, the same 5 × 5 matrix can be made to represent a 0.5 × 0.5 cm portion of the object. The same number of pixels is available in each case, but in the magnified mode the pixels are distributed over a smaller fraction of the original. In the magnified mode the physical size of the object represented by a single pixel decreases from 0.2 × 0.2 to 0.1 × 0.1 cm. Improved spatial detail is thus possible with the application of regional expansion. The disadvantage of write zoom is that the field of view is limited. The portrait of Abraham Lincoln displayed with the same number of pixels in normal and magnified modes illustrates the effect of write zoom (Fig. 10-17). The normal and magnified

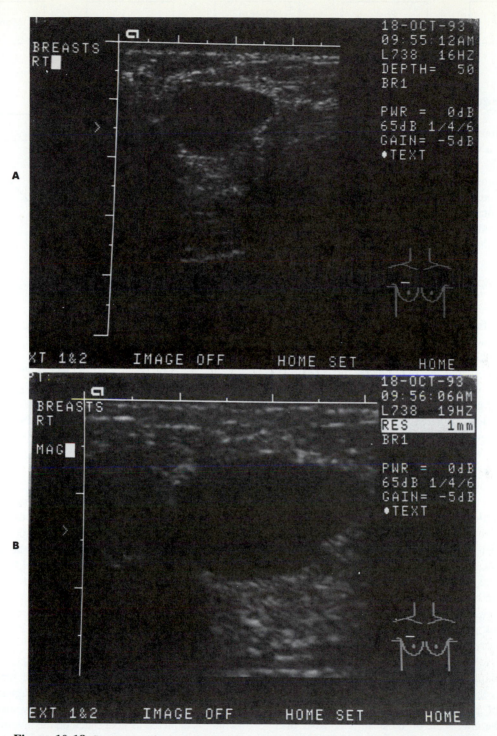

Figure 10-18 Sonogram of a breast containing a cyst. **A,** Normal mode; **B,** Write-zoom mode.

views of a breast containing a cyst (Fig. 10-18) demonstrate write zoom. In practice, the gain in resolution is usually limited by the beam width and spatial pulse length.

Panning

Panning is an image-acquisition technique that allows the operator to shift the expanded region to a new anatomical location during scanning. The maximum field of view for a particular transducer is well defined. During panning, a portion of this field of view is displayed and the sonographer can move the expanded region to a new position within the field of view of the transducer. In essence, panning provides a write-zoom image that can be translated vertically and horizontally under operator control to sample different regions.

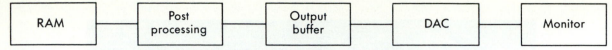

Figure 10-19 Image output components of a real-time scanner.

POSTPROCESSING (DISPLAY)

The image data stored in memory are converted into a video signal and sent to a video monitor for display. The standard video signal implies a specific format for information transmittal. A frame consists of 525 raster lines subdivided into two fields. Alternate raster lines are assigned to each field; thus half of the total raster lines are placed in a field. At the monitor the fields are interlaced to re-form the original frame. The transmission rate is 30 frames per second.

Gray-Scale Mapping

The image data are transferred to an output buffer, which is read in a raster fashion. The signal amplitudes are converted back into analog signals via a digital-to-analog converter (DAC) and fed into the monitor (Fig. 10-19). Postprocessing options enable the operator to manipulate the image data before viewing. Each pixel is displayed as a particular shade of gray depending on the signal amplitude versus brightness level relationship (gray-scale map) selected by the operator.

The number of values that can be stored at any one location in computer memory is determined by the number of bits. If each memory location could store 1 bit of information, each pixel would be "on" or "off" (0 or 1) and a bistable image would be created. A system that was 2 bits deep could represent four different values (four combinations of 1s and 0s—00, 01, 10, 11—equivalent to the decimal numbers 0, 1, 2, and 3). Most units are 5 to 8 bits deep, creating up to 2^8 or 256 numerical representations in memory, and these stored values can be translated into various shades of gray on the display screen. A 2-bit system displays 0 as black, 1 as dark gray, 2 as light gray, and 3 as white. Systems with more bits can exhibit more shades of gray.

At this point, it is important to differentiate between the number of values that can be stored in computer memory and the number of gray levels that can be displayed on the output device. The gray scale on most units consists of 32 or 64 levels. If the computer word is 8 bits (with 256 numerical configurations possible), obviously each value cannot be represented as a separate and distinct shade of gray. A range of numerical values must be associated with each gray level. The translation of the range of pixel values (stored values in RAM) to brightness levels is called gray-scale mapping. Figure 10-20 is a gray-scale map in which eight brightness levels are available. Pixels with values between 191 and 223 are all displayed as brightness level 7. Several methods, including linear, logarithmic, and enhancement algorithms, can be selected by the operator as postprocessing options for converting the digitized ampli-

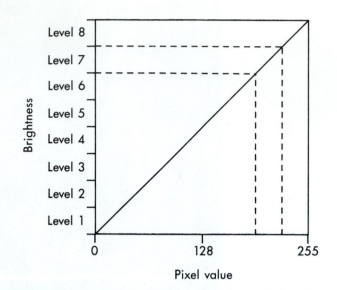

Figure 10-20 A gray-scale map provides the translation of stored pixel values to different brightness levels. For this system, eight brightness levels are possible. Usually level 1 is black and level 8 is white. Pixels with values from 191 to 223 are all displayed with brightness level 7.

tudes into various shades of gray. Pixels with similar values are displayed with either the same or different brightness levels depending on the gray-scale mapping. Altering the gray-scale mapping does not change the stored value in RAM; rather, it modifies how that pixel is displayed based on its stored value. (This is discussed in more detail on page 224.)

Black and White Inversion

In black and white inversion the brightness levels on a gray-scale map are inverted to extend from white (at the low signal amplitude) to black (at the high signal amplitude). A pixel value of 240, which is normally displayed as near white, is depicted as near black on the inverted image (Figs. 10-21 and 10-22). Note the reversal of brightness levels on the vertical scale in Figure 10-21.

Freeze Frame

The freeze-frame option allows the operator to select an image of interest for prolonged viewing. A single frame is held in the output buffer, and updating is discontinued while the freeze-frame option is activated. The output buffer is repeatedly read in raster fashion, which allows the monitor to be constantly refreshed with the same information. The framing rate for the display is 30 per second; but because the same frame is shown over and over, the image appears unchanging to the observer.

Frame Averaging or Persistence

Noise is the variation in signal level introduced by the interactions of ultrasound with tissue and by limitations in the detection system. In other words, multiple measurements of the reflected echo from a particular interface yield not the same but slightly different values. Thus a uniform object would be depicted by nonuniform pixel values throughout the image. Real-time scanners acquire images at a rate of several frames per second. Frame averaging (also called persistence) allows successive frames (as many as four or more) to be added together to increase the signal-to-noise ratio. Image quality is improved because the variations in signal level from regions of comparable-strength echoes are reduced. However, because, in effect, the sampling occurs over a longer time interval, temporal resolution is poorer. The rate of movement of the interfaces must be small; otherwise, motion will induce lag or blurring. During imaging of the heart, high persistence levels are not appropriate because the small rapid motions of the valves cannot be perceived when several frames are added together. The technique of frame averaging does allow high-quality abdominal scans to be obtained.

A series of temporary storage areas (sometimes called banks) is created that sequentially accept the most recent frame. The displayed image is the average of all accepted frames in the storage areas (Fig. 10-23). Note that the mem-

ory requirements for four frames, each with a 512 × 512 matrix, are 4 × 256K bytes.

Read Zoom

Read zoom is a display magnification technique applied to the scan data after collection. The pixels that compose the image are shown in a larger format on the monitor; that is,

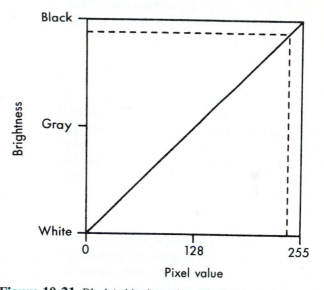

Figure 10-21 Black/white inversion. The brightness levels on the gray scale map are inverted. High pixel values such as 240 are displayed as near black.

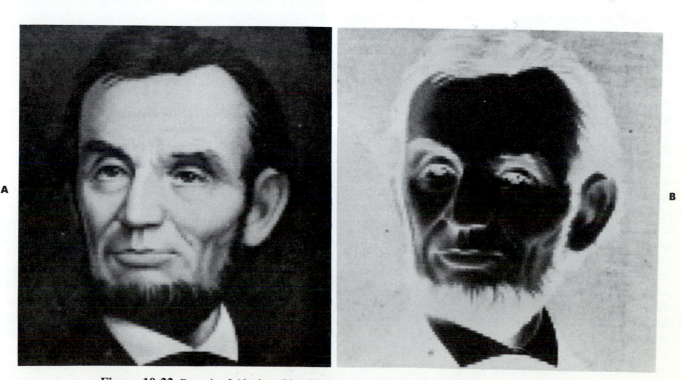

Figure 10-22 Portrait of Abraham Lincoln displayed with the original gray-scale map, **A**, and with black/white inversion, **B**.

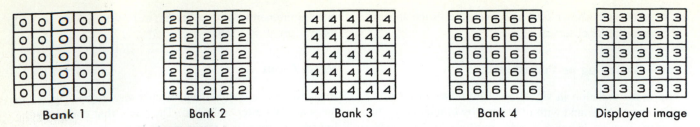

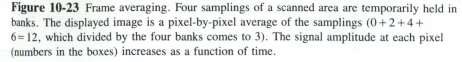

Figure 10-23 Frame averaging. Four samplings of a scanned area are temporarily held in banks. The displayed image is a pixel-by-pixel average of the samplings $(0 + 2 + 4 + 6 = 12$, which divided by the four banks comes to 3). The signal amplitude at each pixel (numbers in the boxes) increases as a function of time.

the portion of the monitor screen associated with each pixel is enlarged. The number of pixels throughout the scanned area remains constant, and the area of tissue represented by each pixel does not change. Unlike write zoom, this technique fails to improve spatial detail. Figures 10-24 and 10-25 illustrate the change in display format when read zoom is selected. Read zoom is called display zoom or magnification by some manufacturers.

To increase the number of pixels in the displayed matrix during read zoom, a technique known as bilinear interpolation is applied. The original image data are unaltered. Every pixel in the read zoom matrix is replaced by four smaller pixels. One pixel is set equal to the value of the original large-size pixel. The remaining three are each assigned a value by averaging the values of the nearby pixels (Fig. 10-26). The most frequently used method creates a linear variation between original pixels. Bilinear interpolation provides a more pleasing image since the individual pixels are less discernible. Spatial resolution, however, is not improved by increasing the displayed matrix size. Figure 10-27 illustrates the effect of bilinear interpolation on the matrix data.

POSTPROCESSING (DATA MANIPULATION AND ANALYSIS)

Additional manipulation and analysis of the echo data are possible because the image information has been digitized and stored in computer memory. The postprocessing techniques of thresholding, contrast enhancement, filtering, and region-of-interest definition can be performed. Thresholding is a technique whereby values less or greater than a reference value are not displayed. This allows weak signals to be acquired and manipulated for display purposes. Pixels with similar values over a narrow range can be displayed with differing brightness levels via contrast enhancement. Thus these pixels can be distinguished from each other on the displayed image. Digital filtering is used extensively in other imaging modalities. *Filtering* refers to the modification of a pixel value based on the values of surrounding pixels. Smoothing and edge enhancement are forms of digital filtering. Region-of-interest definition enables the operator to specify a portion of the image for special consideration.

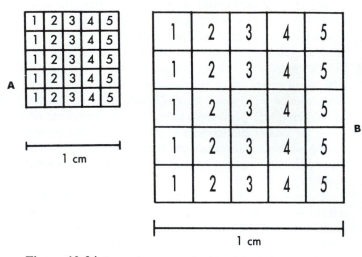

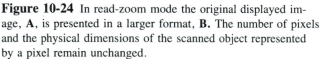

Figure 10-24 In read-zoom mode the original displayed image, **A**, is presented in a larger format, **B**. The number of pixels and the physical dimensions of the scanned object represented by a pixel remain unchanged.

Contrast Enhancement

Contrast enhancement is an especially powerful technique. For example, if the echo data in computer memory range from 0 to 210 and the pixel values are to be visualized in eight shades of gray, every pixel with a value of 0 will be depicted as black and the remaining pixels will be linearly distributed over seven levels of gray. Each gray level is associated with a specific spread of values. Thus pixels with values between 61 and 90 are all displayed in the same shade of gray (level 3). Suppose values less than 56 (weak echo signals) are not of interest and can be eliminated for viewing purposes. By depicting these pixels as black and redistributing the gray scale over a new range of values (57 to 210), image contrast is enhanced. The range of pixel values associated with each gray level is then decreased from 30 to 22 following contrast enhancement and pixels with similar values are more likely to be separated by being displayed at different gray levels. Whereas pixels with relative signal amplitudes of 65 and 85 were displayed as gray level 3 initially, after contrast enhancement they are pre-

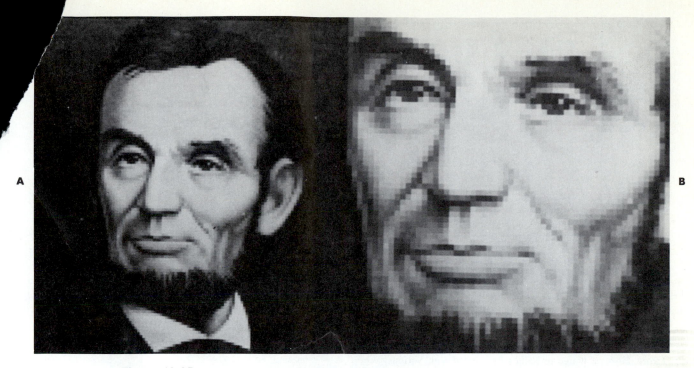

Figure 10-25 Portrait of Abraham Lincoln in normal-size mode, **A,** and in read-zoom mode, **B.** In read-zoom mode the central portion of the image has been magnified by a factor of two.

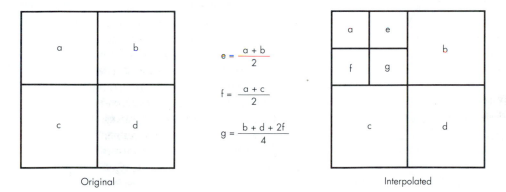

$$e = \frac{a + b}{2}$$

$$f = \frac{a + c}{2}$$

$$g = \frac{b + d + 2f}{4}$$

Original

Interpolated

Figure 10-26 Bilinear interpolation. Each original pixel is replaced by four smaller pixels. The values assigned to the originals are calculated from values in the surrounding pixels.

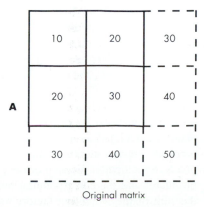

Figure 10-27 A 2 × 2 portion of the original data matrix, **A,** is expanded to contain more pixels (16) by bilinear interpolation, **B.** Values for neighboring pixels in the original matrix required for the bilinear calculation are shown by the *dotted lines*.

Read zoom matrix with bilinear interpolation

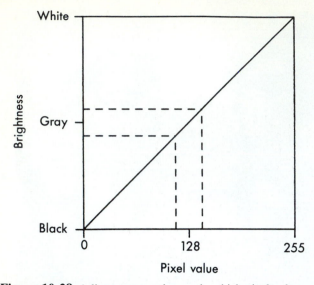

Figure 10-28 A linear gray-scale map in which pixel values near 128 are displayed as intermediate shades of gray.

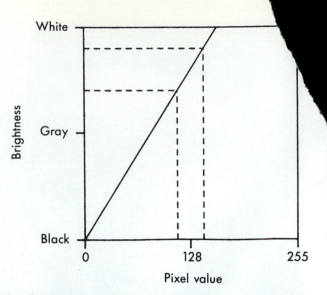

Figure 10-29 An enhanced gray-scale map in which pixel values near 128 are displayed as near white. The range of brightness levels for pixel values near 128 is wider than in Figure 10-28.

■ **Table 10-6** Change in Values Associated with Various Gray-Scale Levels Using Contrast Enhancement

Original Values	Gray Level	New Values
181 to 210	7 white	189 to 210
151 to 180	6	167 to 188
121 to 150	5	145 to 166
91 to 120	4	123 to 144
61 to 90	3	101 to 122
31 to 60	2	79 to 100
1 to 30	1	57 to 78
0	0 black	0 to 56

sented as gray level 1 and gray level 2 (Table 10-6).

Contrast enhancement can also be illustrated with the aid of gray-scale mapping. Figure 10-28 is a linear gray-scale map used to translate pixel values from 0 to 255 to the different brightness levels in a linear fashion. Pixels with values near 128 are displayed with intermediate shades of gray. If the gray-scale map is changed so pixel values from 0 to 160 are distributed linearly over the various brightness levels and if values above 160 are displayed as white, pixels with values near 128 will be displayed with very light shades of gray (Fig. 10-29). There are more brightness levels available to display a fixed range of values for the contrast-enhanced gray-scale map (e.g., Fig. 10-29) than for the original gray-scale map (Fig. 10-28). In other words, the distance along the vertical axis corresponding to a particular range of pixel values is greater for the enhanced gray-scale map (Fig. 10-29) than for the initial map (Fig. 10-28).

Figure 10-30 is a sonogram of the liver displayed with different gray-scale maps. The stored pixel values remain unchanged. The presentation of data is manipulated by the operator-selected gray-scale maps. In many scanners, gray-scale assignment is available as a preprocessing function.

Smoothing

Smoothing is an image-processing technique for the reduction of noise. Noise is the variation in signal level associated with a particular interface. It has no well-defined spatial pattern, which prohibits using a mathematical correction to eliminate its contribution in the image. Noise can be reduced, however, by averaging the values in nearby pixels if the pixels are representative of the same physical entity. This assumption fails at sharp boundaries, where a rapid change in pixel value occurs.

The digital portion (i.e., conversion to the digital format with subsequent digital processing) of the scanner does not introduce random noise to the image.

Smoothing is a two-dimensional averaging technique whereby values in the surrounding pixels are used to calculate a new value for the pixel of interest. The most common smoothing operation employs a nine-point spread function, or kernel. A set of weighting factors is arranged in a 3×3 minimatrix as shown:

$$\begin{matrix} 1 & 2 & 1 \\ 2 & 4 & 2 \\ 1 & 2 & 1 \end{matrix}$$

The center of the kernel is superimposed on the pixel of interest in the raw data matrix. The smoothed value for that pixel is calculated as a weighted sum of the value of the pixel of interest and the values of the neighboring eight pixels. Specifically, the sum of the product of each weighting factor and the corresponding pixel value is divided by the sum of the weighting factors to generate a new value for the pixel of interest. The kernel is subsequently placed over every pixel (except those along the edge) to produce the smoothed values. Each application of the kernel on the raw data matrix creates one new pixel value for the new

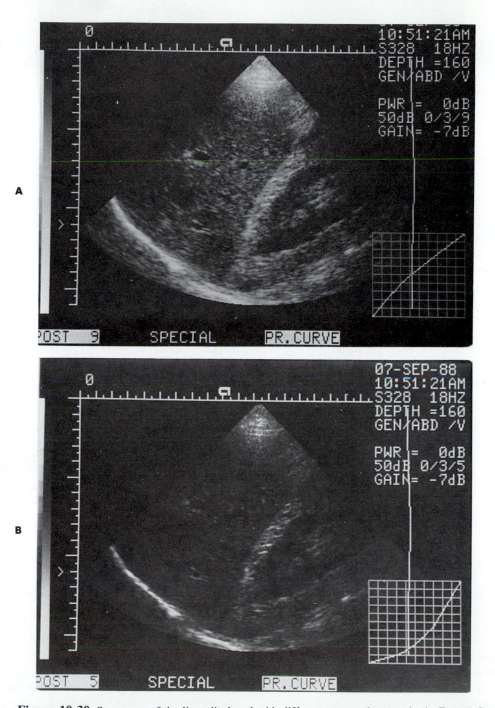

Figure 10-30 Sonogram of the liver displayed with different gray-scale maps in **A, B,** and **C.** The gray-scale map for each image is presented in the lower right. The data in RAM are unchanged, but the translation of pixel values to brightness levels is altered to produce radically different images.

Continued.

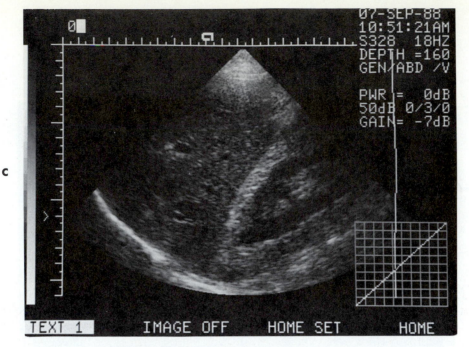

Figure 10-30, cont'd. For legend see page 227.

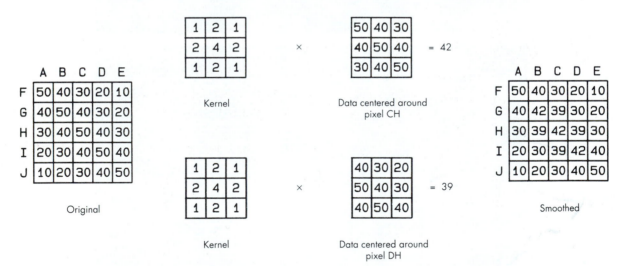

Figure 10-31 A kernel (collection of weighting factors) is applied to the original matrix data to generate the smoothed matrix data.

matrix of smoothed values. All calculations are applied to the raw data, which requires that the smoothed matrix be generated separately from the raw data matrix.

Figure 10-31 illustrates the nine-point smoothing operation applied to a 5 × 5 image matrix. Calculations for pixel CH (column C, row H) and pixel DH (column D, row H) are shown. The new value for pixel CH is found by

$$(1 \times 50) + (2 \times 40) + (1 \times 30) + \\ (2 \times 40) + (4 \times 50) + (2 \times 40) + \\ (1 \times 30) + (2 \times 40) + (1 \times 50)/16$$

The factor 16 is the sum of the weighting factors. To complete the smoothing operation on this 5 × 5 matrix, the

kernel must be applied a total of nine times (the pixels along the border are not included). For each calculation the same weighting factors are used to modulate the contribution of the surrounding pixels to the pixel of interest. For a larger-sized matrix the kernel would be applied many more times.

The degree of smoothing is modified by changing the weighting factors or by increasing the size of the kernel (e.g., a 5 × 5 instead of a 3 × 3 minimatrix). Weighting factors of equal magnitude or those averaging a greater number of surrounding pixels produce a stronger smoothing effect.

The disadvantage of smoothing is that some spatial detail is lost because the smoothed value represents the averaging

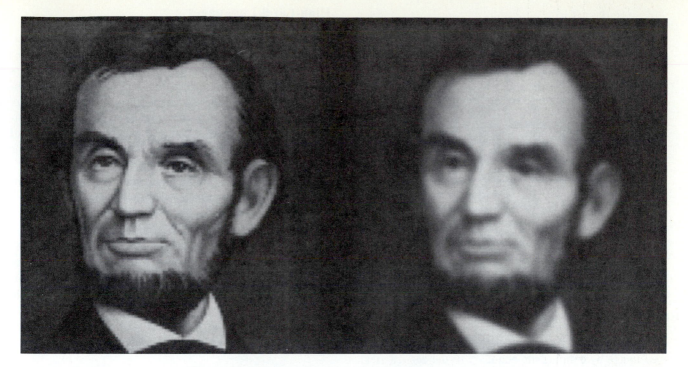

Figure 10-32 Smoothing. The smoothed image is on the right.

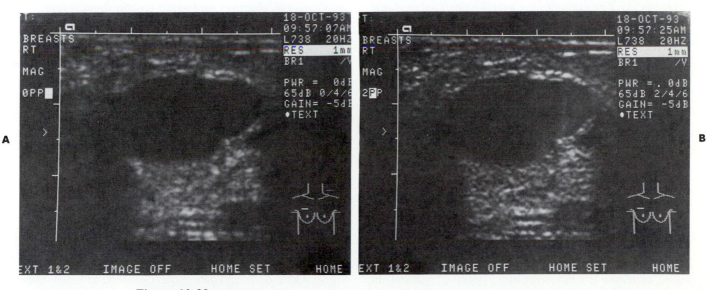

Figure 10-33 Edge enhancement applied to the sonogram of a breast containing a cyst. **A,** Smooth; **B,** Sharp.

over the nearby region. Compare the portrait of Abraham Lincoln after undergoing the smoothing operation with the original (Fig. 10-32).

Edge Enhancement

Edge enhancement (also called sharpness) is a filtering technique that can be applied to the matrix image data to increase the visibility of small high-contrast structures. The filtering process uses a kernel applied to the original values in the same manner as described for smoothing. The set of weight-

ing factors, however, arranged in a 3 × 3 minimatrix assumes different values:

$$\begin{matrix} 0 & -1 & 0 \\ -1 & 5 & -1 \\ 0 & -1 & 0 \end{matrix}$$

Figure 10-33 shows the effect on a sonogram of the breast processed with edge enhancement. The amount of edge enhancement can be modified by changing the magnitude or number of the weighting factors used in the convolution.

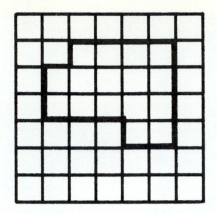

Figure 10-34 Region of interest. The *darkened line* denotes the boundary of the region of interest. Pixels within this boundary are included in the region of interest.

Region of Interest

The operator may denote the region of interest on the displayed image by defining the boundary of the desired area. This is accomplished by moving a visible cursor on the screen via a joystick, light pen, or track ball. Pixels within the boundary are now designated for special consideration (Fig. 10-34). For example, the average pixel value within a particular area of the liver can be determined.

Distance Calculation

The image matrix is calibrated in terms of physical size. The side of one pixel corresponds to a known length (e.g., 1 pixel equals 0.2 mm), which is dictated by the transducer and the collection parameters (matrix size and field of view). The distance between any two points of interest on the displayed image therefore is readily calculated by the computer. The operator must identify the two locations, which is usually accomplished by moving a visible cursor on the screen via a joystick. Once the separation in number of pixels is determined, the actual distance is calculated by the computer using the product of the number of pixels and the calibration factor (0.2 mm per pixel). Distance measurements of femur length, crown-rump length, biparietal diameter, and many other structures are routinely performed in the clinical environment. Accuracy of distance measurements is compromised when a matrix with few pixels is used for imaging.

PROGRAMMING LANGUAGES

Programming languages provide the individual user with the ability to solve problems by directing the computer to execute a series of instructions. The solution to a particular problem requires a precise and unambiguous statement of the exact sequence of tasks to be performed. This description of the necessary steps in the solution process is called an algorithm, and it must be translated into the terminology of a specific programming language.

High-Level Languages

Several high-level programming languages—including Basic, Pascal, Forth, COBOL, C, and Fortran—are available. Each has a unique vocabulary of symbols, words, and letters that code for particular operations. In addition, for the computer to interpret each instruction correctly, rules of syntax must be followed exactly. Interpreters, translators, or compilers are present in the operating system so the high-level language can be converted to a machine code (instructions in binary) that is understood by the computer.

No single programming language is best for all circumstances; rather, each offers certain advantages depending on the application. For example, Fortran provides a more elaborate set of mathematical operations and a faster execution time than Basic; however, Basic has been adopted by personal computer manufacturers because it is relatively easy to learn and the difference in execution times for short simple programs is insignificant. The ease by which a Basic program can be altered, updated, and debugged also has contributed substantially to Basic's acceptance in the personal computer marketplace.

Clinical Applications

A personal computer can be very effective in the clinical environment.[6] Various parameters (crown-rump length, femur length, head circumference, abdominal circumference, and biparietal diameter) have been shown[7-9,16] to be excellent predictors of fetal age. The computer can be programmed to calculate fetal age based on the measurements of a particular structure. The equation relating fetal age and the measured parameter is assimilated into an algorithm that is then translated into program code.

A simple Basic program designed to calculate menstrual age (MA), given measurements for biparietal diameter (BPD), femur length (FL), head circumference (HC), and abdominal circumference (AC) is listed in the box on p. 231. For readers wishing to learn Basic, Marateck[14] has written an excellent textbook providing practical instruction on programming techniques. For readers already familiar with Basic, the program is divided into four sections: initialization (lines 10 to 60), data input (lines 70 to 460), calculation (lines 470 to 640), and data output (lines 650 to 1310). Data input allows for both patient demographics (lines 70 to 260) and measurements of the various parameters (lines 270 to 460). If a particular parameter is not of interest, a zero entered will cause the program to ignore the menstrual age calculation using that parameter. A sample report generated by this program is shown in the box on p. 232.

Although the sample program in the box does accomplish the designed purpose of calculating fetal age based on ultrasonically measured parameters, its usefulness in the clinical environment would be enhanced if it were modified. Changes would include the ability to edit the input data, identify the hospital on the printed report, and select calculation alternatives (e.g., fetal weight and multiple variable analyses for fetal age). In addition, storage of the information (examination date, patient demographics, and measured parameters) for subsequent retrieval and analysis is very desirable.

Real-time scanners are becoming microprocessor based, which means that most of their functions are computer controlled. Many units allow for direct calculation of fetal age by incorporating equations relating the age of the fetus with measured parameters into the scanner. Some units even allow the operator to modify these equations. Because several equations are available based on the work of different researchers, the operator should know which ones are used by his or her scanner.

DATABASE MANAGEMENT

The database is a collection of data pertaining to a particular project that are stored in files. These data are maintained as a source of reference and often include identification, statistical and historical information, physical measurements, and images. The files must be updated when new data become available. Data extracted from the files can be used to compare results and produce a report.[5]

Database management will become increasingly important during the next few years in ultrasound imaging. Although the computers used to manage a database will be separate from the imaging devices, quick retrieval of the results from previous examinations saves personnel time and aids the diagnostic process. Personal computers could easily be employed to accomplish this task by using Basic programs or database application packages to manipulate the information contained in the data files.[12,15]

Integration of the most recent data with previous data contained in the files to present a comprehensive picture makes this an extremely effective technique. Intrauterine growth retardation is assessed by performing multiple examinations in which the head circumference and abdominal circumference are measured over a period of several weeks. Because the results from each examination are stored in a database management system, the computer can rapidly in-

---

■ **Basic program to calculate fetal age**

```
10 REM INITIALIZE
20 REM FETAL AGE CALCULATION
30 REM FEBRUARY 1990
40 DIM PTDATA$(10), MA(10)
50 KEY OFF
60 REM *****************************************
70 REM PATIENT DATA INPUT
80 CLS
90 PRINT:PRINT
100 PRINT "ENTER PATIENT'S FIRST NAME";
110 INPUT PTDATA$(1)
120 PRINT "ENTER PATIENT'S LAST NAME";
130 INPUT PTDATA$(2)
140 PRINT "ENTER PATIENT'S ID NUMBER";
150 INPUT PTDATA$(3)
160 PRINT "ENTER PATIENT'S AGE";
170 INPUT PTDATA$(4)
180 PRINT "ENTER REFERRING PHYSICIAN";
190 INPUT PTDATA$(5)
200 PRINT "ENTER RADIOLOGIST";
210 INPUT PTDATA$(6)
220 PRINT "ENTER SONOGRAPHER";
230 INPUT PTDATA$(7)
240 PRINT "ENTER HISTORY";
250 INPUT PTDATA$(8)
260 REM *****************************************
270 CLS
280 PRINT:PRINT
290 PRINT "ENTER BIPARIETAL DIAMETER MEA-
SUREMENT IN CM";
300 INPUT BPD
310 PRINT
320 PRINT "ENTER MEASUREMENTS FOR HEAD CIR-
CUMFERENCE"
330 PRINT "ENTER OCCIPITO-FRONTAL DIAMETER IN
CM";
340 INPUT OFD
350 PRINT "ENTER HEAD DIAMETER IN CM";
360 INPUT HD
370 PRINT
380 PRINT "ENTER MEASUREMENTS FOR ABDOMI-
NAL CIRCUMFERENCE"
390 PRINT "ENTER ABDOMINAL DIAMETER #1 IN
CM";
400 INPUT AD1
410 PRINT "ENTER ABDOMINAL DIAMETER #2 IN
CM";
420 INPUT AD2
430 PRINT
440 PRINT "ENTER FEMUR LENGTH MEASUREMENT";
450 INPUT FL
460 REM *****************************************
470 REM CALCULATE CIRCUMFERENCE
480 AC=3.1416*SQR( (AD1^2+AD2^2)/2)
490 HC=3.1416*SQR( (HD^2+OFD^2)/2)
500 REM *****************************************
510 REM CALCULATE FETAL AGE
520 REM REFERENCE HADLOCK ET AL., RADIOL-
OGY 152, 497-501, 1984
530 FOR I=1 TO 4
540 MA(I)=0
550 NEXT I
560 IF BPD<9.399999 OR BPD>1.7 THEN 580
570 MA(1)=9.54 + 1.482*BPD + .1676*BPD^2
580 IF HC>34.6 OR HC<6.8 THEN 600
590 MA(2)=8.96 + 0.54*HC + 0.0003*HC^3
600 IF AC>35.3 OR AC<4.6 THEN 620
610 MA(3)=8.140001 + 0.753*AC + 0.0036*AC^2
620 IF FL>7.7 OR FL<.7 THEN 640
630 MA(4)=10.35 + 2.46*FL + 0.17*FL^2
640 REM *****************************************
650 REM OUTPUT BEGINS HERE
```

Continued.

■ Basic program to calculate fetal age—cont'd

```
660 CLS
670 PRINT : PRINT
680 PRINT "SELECT OUTPUT DEVICE"
690 PRINT "0 TO QUIT"
700 PRINT "1 FOR PRINTER"
710 PRINT "2 FOR SCREEN"
720 INPUT FLAG
730 IF FLAG = 0 THEN 1320
740 IF FLAG = 1 THEN OPEN "LPT1:" FOR OUTPUT AS
#2
750 IF FLAG = 2 THEN OPEN "SCRN:" FOR OUTPUT AS
#2
760 PRINT #2,CHR$(12):PRINT #2," "
770 PRINT #2," "
780 PRINT #2,TAB(45);DATE$
790 PRINT #2," "
800 PRINT #2, TAB(22);"PATIENT LAST NAME: ";
810 PRINT #2, PTDATA$(2)
820 PRINT #2, TAB(21);"PATIENT FIRST NAME: ";
830 PRINT #2, PTDATA$(1)
840 PRINT #2,TAB(22);"PATIENT ID NUMBER: ";
850 PRINT #2, PTDATA$(3)
860 PRINT #2,TAB(28);"PATIENT AGE: ";
870 PRINT #2, PTDATA$(4)
880 PRINT #2,TAB(20);"REFERRING PHYSICIAN: ";
890 PRINT #2, PTDATA$(5)
900 PRINT #2,TAB(28);"RADIOLOGIST: ";
910 PRINT #2, PTDATA$(6)
920 PRINT #2,TAB(28);"SONOGRAPHER: ";
930 PRINT #2, PTDATA$(7)
940 PRINT #2, TAB(32);"HISTORY: ";
950 PRINT #2, PTDATA$(8)
960 PRINT #2," " :PRINT #2," "
970 REM FETAL AGE OUTPUT
980 IF MA(1) = 0 THEN 1050
990 PRINT #2, TAB(10);"For a BPD of";
1000 PRINT #2, USING "#.#";BPD;
1010 PRINT #2, " cm, the age is ";
1020 PRINT #2, USING "##.#";MA(1);
1030 PRINT #2, " weeks."
1040 PRINT #2," "
1050 IF MA(2) = 0 THEN 1120
1060 PRINT #2, TAB(10);"For a HC of ";
1070 PRINT #2, USING "##.#";HC;
1080 PRINT #2, " cm, the age is ";
1090 PRINT #2, USING "##.#";MA(2);
1100 PRINT #2, "weeks."
1110 PRINT #2," "
1120 IF MA(3) = 0 THEN 1190
1130 PRINT #2, TAB(10);"For a AC of ";
1140 PRINT #2, USING "##.#";AC;
1150 PRINT #2, " cm, the age is ";
1160 PRINT #2, USING "##.#";MA(3);
1170 PRINT #2, " weeks."
1180 PRINT #2," "
1190 IF MA(4) = 0 THEN 1260
1200 PRINT #2, TAB(10);"For a femur length of ";
1210 PRINT #2, USING "##.#";FL;
1220 PRINT #2, " cm, the age is ";
1230 PRINT #2, USING "##.#";MA(4)
1240 PRINT #2, " weeks."
1250 PRINT #2," "
1260 CLOSE #2
1270 IF FLAG = 1 THEN GOTO 660
1280 PRINT : PRINT
1290 PRINT "STRIKE ANY KEY TO CONTINUE"
1300 RES$ = INKEY$:IF RES$ = " " THEN 1300
1310 GOTO 660
1320 END
```

■ Sample report generated by sample Basic program

```
                                       04-27-1993
     PATIENT LAST NAME: JOHNSON
    PATIENT FIRST NAME: CATHY
    PATIENT ID NUMBER: 888888
           PATIENT AGE: 26
  REFERRING PHYSICIAN: JONES
           RADIOLOGIST: SMITH
          SONOGRAPHER: FINLEY
               HISTORY: FETAL AGE DETERMINA-
                        TION
For a BPD of 6 cm, the age is 24.5 weeks
For an HC of 20.1 cm, the age is 22.3 weeks
For an AC of 19.8 cm, the age is 24.5 weeks
For a femoral length of 3.8 cm, the age is 22.5 weeks
```

corporate the most recent results with previous measurements to generate growth curves. The age determined by the first ultrasound examination now becomes the basis for the age determination on subsequent examination dates and the rate of growth is evaluated easily.

A data file containing measured values for the head and abdominal circumferences for several examinations is shown in Table 10-7. Each record holds the results from one examination. For simplicity, only seven records are listed; in practice, the number of records can be several thousand. In addition, although only head circumference and abdominal circumference are included, the data associated with each record could be extended to contain multiple parameters. On command, the computer is able to examine the records in the data file to identify entries related to a search parameter (e.g., ID number). A request for information pertaining to C. Smith, ID number 123456, would result in record numbers 1, 3, and 6 being selected, as illustrated in Table 10-8. The first examination, conducted on October 5, 1992, establishes the fetal age as 15.2 weeks. This determination is used to project the fetal age for subsequent examinations conducted on November 25, 1992, and February 1, 1993, as 22.5 weeks and 32.1 weeks. An evaluation of both head circumference and abdominal circumference as a function of fetal age can now be performed to determine whether the rate of growth is within normal limits. For this fetus the

■ **Table 10-7**   Contents of Data File

Record No.	Patient	ID No.	HC (cm)	AC (cm)	Date
1	C. Smith	123456	10.8	9.2	10/05/92
2	P. Jones	111111	12.8	10.6	01/02/93
3	C. Smith	123456	20.0	17.3	11/25/92
4	A. Adams	222222	15.0	13.0	02/10/93
5	P. Jones	111111	20.9	19.6	02/19/93
6	C. Smith	123456	27.3	25.0	02/01/93
7	P. Smith	333333	17.0	14.7	02/15/93

HC, Head circumference; *AC*, abdominal circumference.

■ **Table 10-8**   Evaluation of Growth Rate*

Record No.	HC (cm)	AC (cm)	Date	Fetal Age† (weeks)
1	10.8	9.2	10/05/92	15.2
3	20.0	17.3	11/25/92	22.5
6	27.3	25.0	02/01/93	32.1

*Information from database pertaining to C. Smith.
†Fetal age established by examination on 10/05/92.

head circumference increased from 10.8 cm at 15.2 weeks to 20 cm at 22.5 weeks and finally to 27.3 cm at 32.1 weeks. Several published studies[8,9,16] have shown normal growth curves to which these values can be compared.

PACS

Imaging departments are anticipated to be using digitally formatted data extensively by the year 2000. To achieve this goal, computer systems must be developed that allow digitized images from a variety of imaging modalities to be stored for later retrieval, display, manipulation, and interpretation. In addition, text and patient demographic data must also be stored in such a manner as to allow the appropriate information to be associated with the corresponding images. The method of storing and transmitting digital images is called a picture archiving and communication system (PACS). Other names are digital imaging network (DIN) and information management archiving and communications systems (IMACS).

Topology

The acquisition, display, archiving, hardcopy, and computer components of PACS must be interconnected in the form of a local area network (LAN). The term *topology* is used to describe the configuration in which these components are linked together in a network. A *bus* topology employs a common communication path shared by every device in the network; that is, all devices are, in essence, connected to the same cable. Transmission is not continuous (information would become garbled) but is in the form of packets. Each packet contains the source and destination addresses in addition to the data for transfer. The components in the network monitor the communication medium for packets addressed to them and copy only these packets from the network. In *star* topology all devices are connected directly to a central computer through which all data must pass. In *ring* topology all components are linked together in a ring and each is restricted to communicating with the neighbor on each side only. Each position on the ring contains a repeater, which allows the information to be relayed to other components around the ring. Other topologies are also pos-

sible. Each configuration has advantages and disadvantages, although no single topology has yet emerged as the one of choice.[17]

Ultrasound scan data are communicated to the network by digitizing the analog video signal with a video frame grabber. Another method uses a digital interface, which transfers the image and demographics directly to the network from the scanner. Standards for encoding patient file information have recently been developed by the American College of Radiology and the National Electrical Manufacturers Association.

In the network scheme, redundancy of certain hardware devices can be reduced. Hardcopy cameras are not required at each scanner; rather, a single hardcopy camera can provide image recording for multiple imaging modalities. Image processing stations can also be centralized.

Data Storage

The PACS assemblage must be capable of storing enormous quantities of data for long periods while allowing the user rapid access to the stored information. As an example of the storage capacity required, one ultrasound study consisting of twenty images in the 512 × 512 × 8-bit format would use 5 megabytes of storage. The demographic data are not included in this calculation and would require additional storage allocation. For an average-size radiology department all imaging modalities could easily generate 1000 or more megabytes per day.

■ **Example 10-2**

Calculate the storage requirements in megabytes for a study consisting of 80 images in a 1024 × 1024 matrix with 256 gray levels.

One byte is required to represent a pixel with 256 gray levels. Each image has 1,048,576 pixels or 1,048,576 bytes (1 megabyte). A total of 80 megabytes is required to store 80 images of 1 megabyte each.

A combination of storage devices is used to meet the diversified storage and retrieval requirements. A computer with the imaging device provides rapid access of the recently acquired studies. After initial review the digitally formatted data are transferred to a fixed magnetic disk drive for temporary storage. Because the magnetic disk drive has limited capacity, the information must be transferred once more to a slower, but much higher-capacity, device (e.g., an optical laser disk) for permanent storage.

Data Transmission

Transmitting large quantities of data in a timely fashion within the clinical setting is also a limiting factor in the PACS methodology. The speed of transfer of information is characterized by the number of bits transmitted per second. Twisted-pair cable, coaxial cable, and optical fiber cable are commonly used as communication media. The first two pass electrical signals whereas the third allows one-way transmission with a light-emitting diode at one end and a photodiode receiver at the other. Two cables are necessary for two-way communication. The maximum speed at which information is transmitted varies over a wide range—1 to 10 megabits per second for twisted-pair cable, 10 to 50 megabits per second for coaxial cable, 100 to 250 megabits per second for optical fiber. The process of coordinating information transfers in the network greatly reduces transmission rates below these idealized values.

Data Compression

To reduce the storage requirements of a digital image, a technique called compression is applied to reformat the image into fewer bits. Typically an image is stored in a matrix format, wherein each byte holds one value that is associated with a particular pixel in the image. An image consisting of 1024 pixels requires 1024 bytes; images with more pixels use more bytes. If storage requirements are reduced by decreasing the number of pixels or the bit depth, spatial resolution or contrast is sacrificed. An alternative method is to code the pixel values in a new format. Often, many redundant pixel values occur in an image. Instead of repeating these values over and over in the matrix format, an instruction coding for the number of repetitive pixels and the pixel value can be substituted. A variety of coding methods is available. If the original image data can be regenerated from the reformatted data with no loss of information, the compression is said to be reversible.

A typical reversible compression ratio is 3:1, which means that the storage requirements have been reduced by a factor of three. A greater gain in compression (with some loss in image quality) is possible, if perfect reproduction of the original image is not necessary. An irreversible compression ratio of 7:1 to 10:1 is obtainable without significant image degradation. Compression techniques are critically important for reducing PACS design requirements for data storage and transmission rates.

Workstations

Image review and manipulation take place at workstations located throughout the network. A workstation is an interactive minicomputer with specialized graphics capabilities. The random access memory capacity is 16 to 32 megabytes. A high-resolution CRT is required for image display. These workstations each have access to any study stored in the PACS network. Previous studies are available for review and comparison with the current image data.

Displayed image quality, system speed, and image processing options are the primary considerations in workstation design. The spatial resolution, contrast resolution, distortion, noise, and viewing conditions imposed by the workstation should be such that the information content of the image data is not degraded significantly when displayed. System speed determines the time required to retrieve, display, and manipulate image data. Image processing can enhance the presentation of the image data to facilitate interpretation.

In a multimodality workstation the matrix size and gray-level requirements are established by chest radiography, CT, or MRI. A large-format, 21-inch, progressive raster-scanned CRT is used as the high-resolution display device. This unit displays an image matrix of 2560×2048 with 128 gray levels, corresponding to 200 dots per inch. Most high-resolution CRTs are limited to a matrix size of 1280×1024. Either type is acceptable for the display of ultrasound images, which typically consist of 512×512 pixels and each pixel coded in 8 bits.[1]

Compared with transparency film, CRTs have inferior spatial and contrast resolution. The luminance of the screen is much lower than that obtained from the viewbox. Visual acuity and perception of luminance differences depend on the luminance level. Veiling glare (scattering of light from regions of high luminance to regions of low luminance) also degrades perceived contrast. Light output from the phosphor decreases as the phosphor ages. Long persistent phosphors cause blurring when rapid updates of the screen occur.

The time for image retrieval is determined mainly by the speed of the storage device. To achieve a retrieval time of 1 to 2 seconds, workstations are usually equipped with a high-capacity (hundreds of megabytes) magnetic disk drive. Studies on the system storage device (optical disk) are transferred via the network to the magnetic disk at the workstation.

After a study is selected, the image data are loaded from the magnetic disk into a frame buffer and then modified by means of look-up tables before placement in the video buffer. Video RAM can accommodate 2560×2048 pixels with a bit depth of eight. Rapid readout of the video buffer enables the screen to be refreshed at a rate of 75 times per second. The frame buffer holds more image data than the video buffer, but the video buffer configuration allows rapid updating of the screen when other image data are viewed.

The selection, positioning, and sequencing of images displayed on the CRT are specified by the operator. Tile mode places the images side by side on the screen. Stack mode allows sequential viewing of images, one at a time. Dynamic studies can be displayed in cine mode, which is the sequential projection of temporally contiguous images. The type of study and the preferences of the interpreting physician usually dictate the viewing format. An automatic viewing scheme for a study consisting of a predetermined number of images and views can be defined. The workstation must have the capability of manipulating the displayed image. These image-processing techniques include window and level, gray-scale mapping, zoom, panning, smoothing, and edge enhancement. Volumetric display, contour extraction, and spatial measurements are available on some workstations. Interactive mode requires time-efficient image processing, and thus the system must meet the demand for high computational ability.

Operator instructions are communicated to the computer via a graphical user interface. Selectable tasks are each indicated by an icon or pictorial representation of the operation displayed on the screen. A mouse is used to move a cursor to the appropriate icon, which is then selected by depressing a mouse button.

Advantages and Disadvantages

A major disadvantage of the current film archiving methods is that the hardcopy cannot be readily viewed by several observers in various locations simultaneously. Accountability of the film file becomes problematical. In the PACS scheme simultaneous requests for the same study or same patient file can be accommodated with short retrieval times. The problem of lost films is also eliminated.

The electronic archiving of images is expected to decrease film costs. Communication between the imaging service and referring physicians can be improved by the electronic distribution of reports.

The primary disadvantages of PACS are high cost and limited spatial resolution. The lack of industry standards and the demand for instant access have also impeded the acceptance of PACS. Imaging specialists are often hesitant to replace transparency film, the image-recording standard for the past 100 years.

Computer performance versus cost is doubling every 2 years. The rapid development of computer capabilities will enhance the attractiveness of PACS. The PACS networks must be modular and upgradable, however, to adapt to these technological changes.

Mini-PACS in Ultrasonography

The incorporation of all imaging modalities into a PACS network is expensive and a technically complex endeavor. Ultrasound scan data are in digital format and easily adapted to a mini-PACS environment consisting of ultrasound scanners only. In Figure 10-35 four scanners are interfaced to the network. A laser camera, workstation, and disk storage device are also included in the network. The sonographer selects the images that comprise the patient study. Image review and processing for any study archived on the network are performed at the workstation.

Recently equipment manufacturers have introduced digital management systems for ultrasound. Image data, patient demographics, and instrument settings are recorded. The ability to interface scanners from different manufacturers, however, is limited. These information systems are expensive and currently undergoing technical developments.

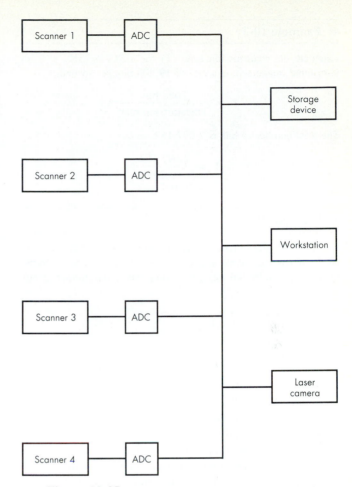

Figure 10-35 Configuration of a mini-PACS network.

TELERADIOLOGY

One application of the PACS technology is teleradiology, which is defined as the electronic transfer of images from one location to another.[2,3] Teleradiology allows multiple hospitals to have quick access to a radiologist's expertise. An increased use of teleradiology systems is expected because radiologists attain more efficient use of their time during evening and weekend coverage. Consulting with subspecialty radiologists at large academic institutions on difficult cases is also possible.

The time to transmit an image depends on the acquisition matrix, the extent of compression, and the method of transmission. Potential transmission methods include telephone lines, coaxial cables, fiber optic cables, microwave dishes, laser systems, satellites, and T-1 (multiple) telephone lines. For telephone lines the transmission rate is called the baud rate, which corresponds to the number of bits per second. If a system has a maximum rate of 19,200 baud (which is relatively slow compared with other methods), approximately 3 minutes will be required to transfer a $512 \times 512 \times 8$ bit image matrix. In practice, the actual transmission time is longer than anticipated because the maximum transmission rate is not attained. A decrease in transmission time can be achieved by sending a compressed image that is converted to matrix format at the receiving station.

■ Example 10-3

Calculate the transmission time (T) for a 512 × 512 × 8 bit ultrasound image sent at a rate of 19,200 bits per second.

$$T = \frac{\text{Total bits}}{\text{Transmission rate}}$$

The total number of bits is 2,097,152.

$$T = \frac{2,097,152}{19,200}$$
$$= 110 \text{ s}$$

■ Example 10-4

Calculate the transmission time (T) for a 512 × 512 × 8 bit ultrasound image that has undergone a 3:1 compression. The transmission rate is 19,200 bits per second. The total number of bits is 699,051.

$$T = \frac{699,051}{19,200}$$
$$= 37 \text{ s}$$

The T-1 telephone line system designed for digital data communication can achieve a transmission rate of 1.544 megabits per second. A 512-matrix image can thus be transferred in less than 2 seconds.

Most commercially available teleradiology systems are based on personal computer technology and use standard telephone lines. The film is placed on a uniformly illuminated light box and a television camera is focused on the image of interest. The television camera produces an output of 30 identical frames per second. A video frame grabber board performs the analog to digital conversion of the video signal, corresponding to a single frame. A matrix representation of the film image is created; the film image has been digitized. The digitized image is stored in computer memory. On the send command the image data are read from computer memory and transferred to the send modem, where the digital information is converted to pulsed tone signals for transmission over the telephone line. The modem at the remote site receives and decodes the transmitted information. The image data are placed in computer memory and displayed. If the image data had been compressed, the recovery algorithm must be applied before display. Various software packages are available to enhance the interpretation process. These include the ability to transmit text and images, real-time cursor interaction to denote areas of interest on the digitized image, voice communication, and image-manipulation techniques.

SUMMARY

In the near future, computer and digital manipulation of images will assume an expanding role in ultrasound imaging. The digitization of scan data provides the advantage of quantitative manipulation and analysis of echo data in very rapid fashion. Many manufacturers are incorporating special calculation options (e.g., fetal age based on measured parameters) as well as an array of postprocessing

features into their new scanners. The amount of information available from computerized ultrasound scanning will increase dramatically. The flexibility of user-selectable processing protocols is expected to further enhance this growth. The processing of information and images in a time-efficient manner to a form readily presentable for interpretation will be the responsibility of the sonographer. Consequently, sonographers must acquire a fundamental knowledge of computers and digital processing techniques.

■■■■■■ **REVIEW QUESTIONS** ■■■■■■

1. A binary digit is called a _____ .
   a. Bit
   b. Byte
   c. Word
   d. Pixel
2. In the binary number system, the decimal number 16 is represented by which of the following?
   a. 10101
   b. 10010
   c. 10000
   d. 10100
   e. 11000
3. Express decimal number 6 as a binary number.
   a. 110
   b. 0111
   c. 11
   d. 111
4. How many locations are available in memory in a 16K word computer?
   a. 131,072
   b. 32,786
   c. 16,000,000
   d. 16,000
   e. 16,384
5. Random access memory (RAM) is accessed
   a. Always in sequence, reading the contents of each location one after another.
   b. Directly, by location via a specific address.
   c. Directly, by pixel value.
   d. Randomly, by matrix size.
6. How many bits in a byte?
   a. 0
   b. 2
   c. 4
   d. 8
7. Which of the following statements is true regarding analog-to-digital converters?
   a. Accuracy of the digitization of the echo amplitude is improved by increasing the bit depth.
   b. Analog-to-digital converters provide continuously variable output.
   c. A bit depth of two is adequate for real-time imaging.
   d. All of the above.
8. If a word contains 3 bits, what is the maximum numerical value that can be represented by this word? Assume 0 to be the lowest number represented.
   a. 3
   b. 7
   c. 15
   d. 16

9. A pixel is a small square picture element in the matrix that denotes the intensity of the reflected echo generated at an interface within the area being scanned.
   a. True
   b. False

10. How many pixels are used to compose an image that is displayed in a matrix 256 × 256?
    a. 8192
    b. 1,048,576
    c. 65,536
    d. 256

11. The advantage of a 256 × 256 matrix format compared with a 64 × 64 matrix format is that
    a. Greater spatial detail is possible.
    b. A lower capacity memory is required.
    c. The number of shades of gray is increased.
    d. Contrast sensitivity is increased.

12. The processing technique to emphasize a change in signal level across an interface is called
    a. Selective enhancement.
    b. Edge enhancement.
    c. Contrast enhancement.
    d. Smoothing.

13. A magnification technique that is applied during data collection is called
    a. Freeze frame.
    b. Write zoom.
    c. Read zoom.
    d. Interpolation.

14. How many gray-scale levels may be displayed when using a 4-bit word?
    a. 2
    b. 4
    c. 8
    d. 16

15. A processing technique whereby values less or greater than a reference value are not displayed is known as
    a. Logarithmic compression
    b. Smoothing
    c. Filtering
    d. Thresholding

16. What is contrast enhancement as it pertains to digital images?
    a. A change in the digitization of the detector signals to alter pixel brightness
    b. Redistribution of gray scale to emphasize the difference in pixel values over a narrow range
    c. A filtering algorithm
    d. A technique of signal averaging

17. The postprocessing technique of smoothing is applied to image data to
    a. Reduce random noise.
    b. Decrease pixel size.
    c. Redistribute the gray scale.
    d. Enhance spatial resolution.

18. Database refers to
    a. A collection of data in a file that can be accessed and used for different applications.
    b. The address in memory that corresponds to the first pixel in the image matrix.
    c. The ability to convert a 64 × 64 matrix into a 256 × 256 matrix.
    d. A magnification processing technique.

19. Which programming language is used extensively in the personal computer environment?
    a. Basic
    b. Fortran
    c. Binary
    d. Kernel

20. A compiler is designed to
    a. Convert a high-level program into machine language instructions.
    b. Create a database.
    c. Test a hardware device for proper operation.
    d. Update the monitor (operating system).

21. The baud rate describes
    a. Storage capacity.
    b. The number of bytes per second that are transmitted.
    c. The number of bits per second that are transmitted.
    d. Program execution time.

22. Calculate the number of images that can be stored in 1 megabyte for an image format consisting of 256 shades of gray and 512 × 512 pixels. One megabyte is equal to 1,048,576 bytes. Determine the number of pixels in the image and then the number of bytes required for each pixel for the given shades of gray.
    a. 1
    b. 2
    c. 3
    d. 4

23. ROM is memory that can be
    a. Updated and changed as necessary.
    b. Read but not written to.
    c. Used only to store alphanumerical characters.
    d. Used for image storage only.

24. The term *block* in conjunction with *disk storage* refers to
    a. One track.
    b. One sector.
    c. A collection of words transferred in a group.
    d. A collection of images stored in a group.

25. Calculate the transmission time for a 512 × 512 × 8 bit ultrasound image that is transmitted at a rate of 1000 bits per second.
    a. 35 minutes
    b. 3 minutes
    c. 100 seconds
    d. 2 seconds

BIBLIOGRAPHY

1. Arenson RL, Chakaborty DP, Seshadri SB, Kundel HL: The digital imaging workstation, *Radiology* 176:303, 1990.

2. Barnes GT, Morin RL, Staab EV: Teleradiology: fundamental considerations and clinical applications, *Radiographics* 13:673, 1993.

3. Batnitzky S, Rosenthal SJ, Siegel EL, et al: Teleradiology: an assessment, *Radiology* 177:11, 1990.

4. Danielson K: Computers in ultrasound. In Hunter TB (ed): *The computer in radiology,* Rockville MD, 1986, Aspen Systems.

5. Enlander D: *Computers in medicine: an introduction,* St Louis, 1980, Mosby.

6. Gates SC, Becker J: *Laboratory automation using the IBM PC,* Englewood Cliffs NJ, 1989, Prentice Hall.

7. Hadlock FP, Deter RL, Harrist RB, Park SK: Estimating fetal age: computer-assisted analysis of multiple fetal growth parameters, *Radiology* 152:497, 1984.

8. Hadlock FP, Deter RL, Harrist RB, Park SK: Fetal abdominal circumference as a predictor of menstrual age, *AJR* 139:367, 1982.

9. Hadlock FP, Deter RL, Harrist RB, Park SK: Fetal head circumference: relation to menstrual age, *AJR* 138:649, 1982.

10. Hedrick WR, Hykes DL: Computer fundamentals in diagnostic ultrasound imaging, *J Diagn Med Sonogr* 5:293, 1989.

11. Hedrick WR, Hykes DL: Image and signal processing in diagnostic ultrasound imaging, *J Diagn Med Sonogr* 5:231, 1989.

12. Jeanty P: A simple reporting system for obstetrical ultrasonography, *J Ultrasound Med* 4:591, 1985.

13. Kuni CC: *Introduction to computers and digital processing in medical imaging*, Chicago, 1988, Year Book Medical Publishers.

14. Marateck SL: *BASIC*, ed 2, New York, 1982, Academic Press.

15. Ott WJ: The design and implementation of a computer-based ultrasound data system, *J Ultrasound Med* 5:25, 1986.

16. Robinson HP, Fleming JE: A critical evaluation of sonar crown-rump length measurements, *Br J Obstet Gynaecol* 82:702, 1975.

17. Templeton AW, Cox CC, Dwyer III SJ: Digital image management networks: current status, *Radiology* 169:1939, 1988.

18. Wolfman NT, Boehme JM, Choplin RH, Bechtold RE: Evaluation of PACS in ultrasonography, *J Ultrasound Med* 11:217, 1992.

CHAPTER 11

Image-Recording Devices

Color video printer
Dry processing
Film development
H and D curve
Laser camera
Multiformat camera

Optical density
Polaroid film
Transparency film
VHS and super VHS
Video cassette recorder

The two-dimensional scan produces an image that is normally displayed on a monitor. The screen is erased and updated with the most recent information each time a new scan is acquired. If the displayed image demonstrates relevant clinical findings, a hardcopy must be generated by an image-recording device interfaced to the scanner. The recorded image must render a faithful reproduction of the displayed image. A variety of image-recording devices—including multiformat cameras, laser cameras, and video printers—is available for this purpose.

The quality of the recorded image is primarily judged by the WYSIWYG—"what you see is what you get"—criterion. Repeatability, stability, ease of use, downtime, and cost are also considerations by which image-recording devices are evaluated.

The reasons for hardcopy recording are threefold. First, the physician who interprets the results of the study does not necessarily scan the patient. A means to communicate observations from the operator to the diagnostician must be included as part of the examination. Second, images from follow-up examinations can be compared with those obtained from previous examinations. And finally, documenting clinical findings for legal purposes is essential.

FILM CHARACTERISTICS

The most important recording medium is film. Based on previous experience with radiographic procedures, transparency film is well accepted by the medical community. The archival lifetime of film is several years, very likely longer than the clinical interest in the study. Storage space and retrieval problems are severe disadvantages, however, which has provided the impetus for alternative archiving methods.

Film is constructed by coating a polyester base with an emulsion layer, the active component. The emulsion consists of a large number of small silver halide grains suspended in a gelatin matrix. Gelatin maintains the distribution of silver halide grains and is porous to liquids used in processing. The transparent base provides physical support for the emulsion and resists warping with age.

To form an image, the film is first exposed to light and then processed in a series of chemical solutions. It is darkened where light was incident, the degree of darkening depending on the intensity of the light.

Absorption of light photons causes electrons to be released and move through the silver halide crystal, where they are trapped at sensitivity specks in the crystal lattice. A sensitivity speck is an imperfection in the crystalline structure (e.g., sulfur at a location where bromine normally is positioned). Negatively charged electrons migrate within the crystal to combine with the positively charged silver ions and form metallic silver. Deposits of silver atoms accumulate only in the exposed grains. The number of exposed grains increases with the intensity of the light. Information transmitted as variable light intensity applied across the film is captured by the distribution of metallic silver, which is referred to as the latent image. The latent image is not observable, but it does act as a template for visual image formation when subjected to chemical processing. The sensitivity speck acts as a catalyst for the conversion of additional silver ions to metallic silver during development. The silver halide crystal is transformed to a visible black particle in the emulsion. As the silver particles increase in concentration, the film becomes darker.

The amount of darkening is quantified by the optical density, which is defined as the logarithm of the ratio of incident to transmitted light. The relation between optical density and the percentage of light transmitted is shown in Table 11-1.

■ **Table 11-1** Relationship Between Optical Density and the Amount of Transmitted Light

Optical Density	Percent Transmitted
0	100
1	10
2	1
3	0.1

Film is generally characterized by a plot of optical density versus exposure or log exposure (Fig. 11-1). The resulting curve, called the H and D curve (named for Hurter and Driffield), describes the speed, latitude, and contrast of the film. Film speed determines the location of the curve with respect to the exposure scale and specifies the sensitivity (amount of exposure necessary to cause a particular optical density). Fast film requires less exposure for darkening. Speed is influenced by the number of sensitivity specks per grain, the concentration of grains, the size and shape of the grains, and the presence of chemical sensitizers in the emulsion. *Latitude* refers to the exposure range over which contrast is sufficient to be useful (e.g., optical density is between 0.25 and 2). The straight-line portion of the curve provides the highest contrast (change in gray level per increment of exposure). The maximum slope of the curve is the film gamma.

FILM PROCESSING

An automatic processor performs the chemical operations necessary to transform the latent image into a visual pattern of shades of gray. This four-step sequence involves development, fixing, washing, and drying. A roller system transports the film to the various chemical baths and to the drying chamber. The transport rate determines the time allowed for each processing step (established by the manufacturer). For 90-second processing the time for each step is partitioned as follows:

	Time in (seconds)
Development	22
Fixing	22
Washing	20
Drying	26

The developer solution consists of several chemical components. The primary task of the developing agent is to supply electrons so that silver ions can be reduced to metallic silver. Phenidone and hydroquinone, working in synergy, fulfill this requirement. Other chemical components include an accelerator (sodium carbonate) to control hydrogen ion concentration, a preservative (sodium sulfite) to inhibit oxidation of the developing agent by air, a restrainer (potassium bromide) to limit the reaction rate of the developing agent with unexposed grains, and a hardener (glutaraldehyde) to control emulsion swelling. At the conclusion of development, latent image grains have been converted to particles of metallic silver and unexposed grains remain distributed throughout the gelatin.

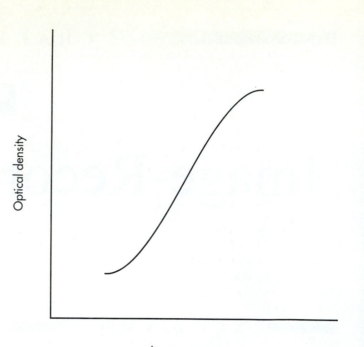

Figure 11-1 H and D curve to characterize a film.

The fixing solution contains acetic acid to stop the action of the developing agent and sodium thiosulfate to remove the undeveloped silver halide grains. A preservative (sodium sulfite) and hardener (aluminum chloride) are also present.

Fresh tap water washes the film to remove the fixer. If thiosulfate is retained, a yellow-brown stain is formed as the film ages. After washing, the film is transported to a drying chamber where hot circulating air dries the film.

Variations in film processing alter density and contrast. The composition of the processing solutions is different depending on the manufacturer. The chemical formulation must be compatible with the automatic processor and film. Developer concentration must be proper and uniform throughout the tank. A pump recirculates and agitates this solution. Contamination of the developer (a base) with the acidic fixing solution renders the developer inactive. Processing also consumes chemicals, which must be replaced. Replenishment of both developer and fixer is automatic based on the size of the film processed. Development time and temperature must be regulated within very narrow limits; otherwise, fluctuations in optical density will occur.

Automatic processors have increased efficiency (the processing time is reduced from 1 hour when done manually to 90 seconds) and provide rapid feedback of the recorded information. More important, consistent image quality is achieved by the tightly controlled processing conditions.

FILM SELECTION

A single-emulsion film, compatible with automatic processing, is recommended for hardcopy cameras. Image-recording devices have different operational characteristics, and these must be considered when selecting a film to be used with a specific device. For example, the light source may be blue or green (multiformat cameras) or red or infrared (laser cameras) and thus film with the appropriate spectral sensitivity is required. The polyester base may be clear or have a blue tint as preferred by the interpreting physician. The film gamma is typically 1.9 to 2.2. A light-absorbing antihalation layer, which prevents reflection from the base into the emulsion, improves the sharpness of the image. The recommendations of the manufacturer should be followed when selecting film and film processing chemicals.

MULTIFORMAT CAMERA

One or more images are recorded on a single sheet of transparency film (typically 8 × 10 inch size) by the multiformat camera. The number of images per sheet is usually fixed as 1, 2, 4, 6, or 9 depending on the model. Some devices have changeable formats, in which the size of the recorded image can be varied.

Transparency film exhibits good gray-scale characteristics (wide range of optical densities that are perceived as separate shades of gray). Development of the film is accomplished by the standard rapid processors common in radiology departments.

System Hardware

Information from the ultrasound scanner is communicated to an internal cathode ray tube (CRT) in the multiformat camera via an analog or digital interface. The analog form uses the 525- or 1050-line video signal. This type of multiformat camera is also called a video imager. Digital transmission consists of a series of 0s and 1s that encode the scan data. The digital interface has not been standardized, however, and several manufacturers have developed their own configurations.

The components of the multiformat camera include an ultrahigh-resolution monochrome CRT, optical system, photometer, and film cassette. The CRT produces a visible image for recording. Fine crystalline phosphors in the screen provide small dot size, homogeneous dot shape, and uniform light output. Different types of phosphors (green or blue) are used. Therefore the spectral response of the film must be matched to the emitted light to ensure proper contrast.

Light Output

The brightness of individual dots associated with different portions of the image is controlled by the incoming electronic signal. Light from the CRT is directed toward the film via a system of mirrors. A lens focuses the image in the film plane (the geometric relationship between CRT, lens, and film determines image size, and thus format), and a shutter controls the length of exposure (Fig. 11-2). The shutter is opened for a time ranging from a fraction of 1 second to several seconds. To record multiple images on a single sheet of film, the film cassette or optical system must move to a new position after each exposure. Double-sided film cassettes hold two sheets of film, which are individually exposed.

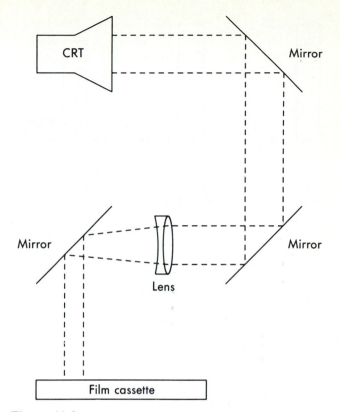

Figure 11-2 One possible configuration of a multiformat camera. A system of mirrors directs the light from the CRT to the film. A lens focuses the image in the film plane. Multiple images are placed on a single sheet of film by moving the film cassette after each exposure.

The light output from the CRT, given identical input signals, is not constant over time. A photometer is incorporated into the multiformat camera to maintain consistent optical density. A photocell measures the light emitted from a calibration pattern displayed on the CRT. The intensity of the light is converted to a voltage signal, which is compared with a reference level. The CRT brightness is automatically adjusted until it matches these values. The image is then displayed on the CRT; the proper brightness is based on monitoring of the calibration pattern, and exposure now takes place. This feedback circuit is designed to provide reproducible optical density. If the initial setup is in error and light or dark films are produced, this condition will be propagated until corrected by recalibrating the device.

Operator Controls

Adjustments for contrast, brightness, and exposure time can be manipulated to optimize the fidelity of the recording. The contrast control establishes the range of black and white levels of the gray scale. The brightness control changes the midpoint of the gray scale. The overall optical density is varied by shortening or lengthening the exposure time. The effect of improper brightness and contrast settings is illustrated in Figure 11-3. Signal levels from 0 to 255 are represented as various shades of gray by a properly calibrated device. Improper settings exclude some signal levels from

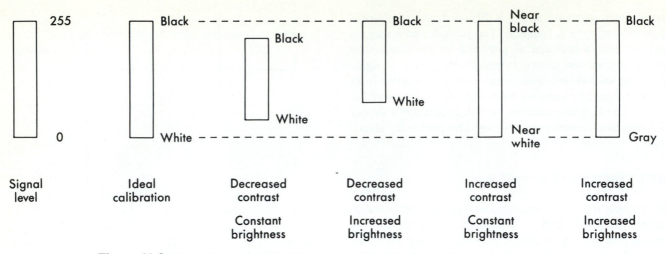

Figure 11-3 Effect of contrast and brightness controls on the gray scale. An ideal calibration allows the complete range of pixel values (0 to 255) to be expressed as various shades of gray from white to black. A change in brightness and/or contrast settings compared with the ideal calibration causes an incomplete use of all possible shades of gray (from white to black) or compresses the gray scale over a narrower range of pixel values.

being reproduced on film or prohibit the full extent of possible shades of gray from blacks to whites.

A common misconception is that proper gray-scale presentation on the display monitor is invariably reproduced on the film. The internal CRT in the multiformat camera is not controlled by the external monitor and must be adjusted independently. This becomes a practical problem in the clinical environment. To provide assurance that what is seen on the monitor is recorded on film, quality-control tests must be performed.

The operator selects a positive or negative mode for recording. The positive mode is described as white on black, which depicts strong echoes as white and weak echoes as black. This is the preferred mode for most applications in ultrasound. The negative mode displays strong echoes as black and weak echoes as white (the inverse of the positive mode).

Problem Areas

Multiformat cameras are not without their problems. If the phosphor is deposited on a curved face of the CRT, the image in the film plane is distorted because the depth of field is not constant. A nearly flat CRT (which is expensive) must be used. A uniform phosphor thickness is required to minimize the variation in light output across the screen.

The lens must be high quality and flat-field corrected. An aperture restricts the incident light to a small central area of the lens. For the best image quality a line drawn from the CRT to the center of the image on the film should pass through the center of the lens. This geometry is most easily maintained by moving the film cassette to change the image position.

Raster scanning with the video signal input interlaces two $\frac{1}{60}$-second fields to compose one frame (similar to tele-

vision). Distracting raster lines are sometimes present in the static images on film. To deemphasize this line structure, successive video fields are shifted slightly in the vertical direction to fill in the space between raster lines. Multiple video frames (at least eight) spread the raster lines over a larger area so each horizontal line merges with neighboring lines. The camera shutter must be synchronized with the start of a video frame; otherwise, a partial field included in the exposure will cause the optical density throughout the image to be inconsistent.

Some multiformat cameras contain density step patterns that can be printed on film and read with an internal densitometer after film development. The measured H and D curve is compared with the H and D standard curve stored in computer memory. Adjustment of the light intensity at each gray level is then made to achieve the desired optical density. This calibration corrects for film emulsion and processor variations and can be performed daily.

Spatial resolution is limited not by the film but by the video format (or pixel size in the digital format) and phosphor size.

CENTRALIZED MULTIFORMAT CAMERA

In a multiscanner facility the usual practice is to connect a multiformat camera to each scanner. Duplication of image-recording devices results in high equipment costs. An alternative method is to store patient images digitally on magnetic disk and then record the appropriate images on film at a central reader.

Each scanner is interfaced to a digital image manager computer, which includes a disk drive with a removable magnetic disk. The magnetic disk holds 65 to 80 images in a 512 × 512 matrix. Selected images acquired during the examination are transferred to the disk. At the conclusion of the study the disk is removed and carried to the reader for image recording. The reader contains a multiformat camera and the necessary computer hardware to retrieve the digital image information.

The image data are converted to a video signal, which modulates the light emitted from a CRT screen that exposes the film. Since flicker is not a consideration, consecutive rows are scanned over an extended time (15 seconds). Noninterlaced or progressive scanning improves the spatial detail compared with interlaced raster lines. After exposure to light the film is developed in the film processor. The format is 6:1.

LASER CAMERA

The major weakness of the multiformat camera is the cathode ray tube and optical system. Light-output variation related to phosphor nonuniformity and to electronic drift produces an inaccurate gray scale. Off-axis focusing (i.e., the light path is not through the center of lens) and the curved screen cause distortion. Phosphor dot size limits spatial detail.

System Components

A laser (*light amplification by stimulated emission of radiation*) replaces the CRT as the light source in the laser camera. The intensity and size of the laser beam are precisely controlled. Laser beam diameter is 0.1 mm or less. Two types of lasers are in common use: helium-neon and solid-state diode. The helium-neon laser emits light at a wavelength of 633 nm in the red region of the spectrum. The solid state diode emits light with a wavelength of 820 nm (infrared).

In one manufacturer's design the digital or video signal from the scanner is loaded in an image-storage memory. Multiple images can be stored simultaneously. Film is removed from the supply magazine and placed on a drum platen. The laser beam sweeps across the film, forming one line of the image. The intensity of the incident light is modulated according to the stored values in memory. A rotating mirror in the light path directs the laser beam to 4096 points along the line. Successive lines are formed by rotating the drum until 5120 lines are generated. When the exposure is completed, the film is transported to an attached film processor for immediate processing or to a receive magazine for remote processing.

An alternate scheme that does not use the revolving platen employs a series of rollers to maintain the film in a flat configuration while linearly advancing the film for line-by-line scanning by the laser beam.

In both methods many pixels compose the image (i.e., there is a potential for excellent spatial resolution). Each pixel can be represented in 256 to 4096 different shades of gray with a high degree of reproducibility (i.e., it provides excellent contrast solution). Also a wide dynamic range is achieved.

Image Presentation

When multiple images are recorded on a sheet of film, the area between images is exposed. The darkened borders around each image remove the glare of the viewbox light and improve the visual perception of contrast. Conventional multiformat film has unexposed areas adjacent to the recorded image that hinder contrast discrimination.

Adjustments for contrast, brightness, window width, window level, and gray-scale mapping are available to manipulate the recorded image. Controls for contrast and brightness operate in the same manner as described for the multiformat camera. Window width and level allow for contrast enhancement by defining the range of pixel values distributed throughout the gray scale. Gray scale maps specify the conversion of the pixel value to a particular shade of gray.

A single-emulsion film with antihalation backing is also used in a laser camera. However, red-sensitive or infrared-sensitive film is required to match the light produced by the laser. As a cautionary note, the usual safelight filter in most radiology darkrooms is not proper for use with laser camera film.

Quality Control

For purposes of quality control, several test patterns are available for imaging to evaluate uniformity, pixel registration, and gray-scale reproducibility. For example, the optical density of each step from a gray-scale bar test pattern recorded on film can be measured and then communicated to the laser camera via a keypad. The laser camera processes this information to adjust the exposure so the resulting optical density for each step is within certain tolerance limits.

Advantages and Disadvantages

The laser camera provides a fast and highly reliable method of recording hardcopy images on film. It can accommodate different film sizes, and the image format can be varied. In addition, multiple imaging devices can be interfaced to it and batch processing of examinations is possible. The expense of a laser camera dedicated to ultrasound, however, may be difficult to justify. If one has been purchased for another modality (e.g., MRI, CT, or DSA), consideration should possibly by given to interfacing the ultrasound scanner to it.

GRAY-SCALE MAPPING

Many image-recording devices using transparency film incorporate selectable gray-scale maps. The hardcopy camera can alter the translation of pixel values to a particular shade of gray to improve contrast. This manipulation of the recorded image is independent of the displayed image. Linear, logarithmic, inverse logarithmic, exponential, squared, and square root maps are available.

Figure 11-4 consists of three gray-scale maps. The linear map distributes gray levels equally throughout the range of

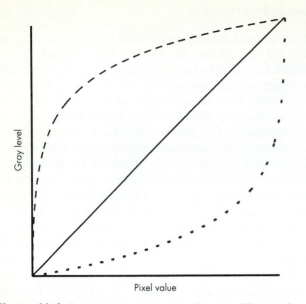

Figure 11-4 Hardcopy camera gray-scale maps. The translation of pixel values into gray level can be varied by selecting a linear *(solid line)*, logarithmic *(dashed line)*, or inverse logarithmic *(dotted line)* gray-scale map.

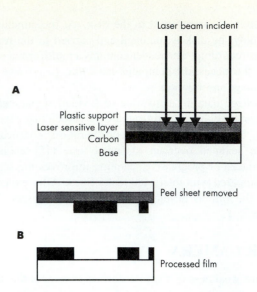

Figure 11-5 Dry processing of transparency film, cross-sectional view. **A,** The laser beam selectively scans across the film. Carbon particles attach to the laser-sensitive layer where the beam is incident. **B,** Removal of the peel sheet, consisting of a plastic support and a laser-sensitive layer, extracts the activated carbon. The processed film retains portions of the original carbon layer.

pixel values (echo strengths). The logarithmic map enhances the contrast of weak echoes. The inverse logarithmic map emphasizes variations in high-strength echoes. Usually these gray scale maps, available as postprocessing options in the scanner, are used to enhance contrast so its effect on the image can be visualized before recording.

Often a hardcopy camera gray-scale map is applied to compensate for differences in response between the monitor phosphor screen and the film. Matching displayed brightness levels with film optical densities is essential for the faithful reproduction of a displayed image.

TRANSPARENCY FILM WITH DRY PROCESSING

Recently a hardcopy imaging system using dry processing of transparency film has been introduced. The transfer of digital or analog video image information to film and the development of film are accomplished within the same unit. An 8 × 10 inch film is printed with 300 pixels per inch in 256 shades of gray. Pixel size is comparable to that from a laser camera. Variable film formats are possible. The processing time for a single film is 90 seconds, and the maximum processing rate is 40 films per hour. Dry film used in the system is insensitive to light. The archival lifetime is reported to be comparable to that of traditional transparency film.

The film consists of a 7 mil (i.e., 1/1000 inch) polyester base (clear or blue tint), an emulsion layer, and a laser sensitive layer contained in the peel sheet. The emulsion is a uniform coating of carbon instead of the silver halide crystals utilized in wet processing. A laser beam scans the film, selectively heating small regions of the laser-sensitive layer. When heat activates this layer, carbon from the emulsion adheres to the layer. The peel sheet acts as a carbon

receptor, which is removed after development. Carbon remains on the film only in regions not heated by the laser beam (Fig. 11-5).

The laser produces clear spots on the film a few microns in size. Over 4000 of these spots, called pels, compose a single pixel. A video frame grabber stores the image information in digital form in computer memory. The amount of carbon removed within each pixel is controlled by the digital image information. If all carbon is removed within the pixel, a white region results on the film. If all carbon is retained within the pixel, a black region results. Removal of carbon from multiple pels within the pixel creates intermediate shades of gray.

Video inputs and computer interfaces allow multiple scanners to be connected to a single image-recording unit with the capability of batch processing. Adjustments for brightness, contrast, gray-scale mapping, sharpness, and positive/negative mode are available.

Hardcopy image recording with dry processing offers many advantages—including consistent film quality, no need for a film processor, relative low cost, no darkroom requirement, no handling of chemicals, and no disposal of government-regulated effluents. The purchase price is similar to that for a laser camera. Lower cost is achieved by eliminating the expense of chemicals purchased for wet processing. However, film throughput rapidly becomes the limiting factor.

Hardcopy image recording with dry processing is particularly well suited for ultrasound departments or stand-alone clinics where wet processing of transparency film (e.g., in mammography) is not required. The lack of environmental constraints (no plumbing needed and small size) allows the image-recording system to be conveniently placed in the work area (next to an individual scanner or in a central location where quality control review of films takes place). Since dry processing of transparency film is relatively new, extensive clinical experience with it is lacking. Critical evaluation by clinical users will ultimately determine the utility of this image-recording device.

POLAROID FILM

Instant-print film or single-emulsion transparency film from Polaroid requires no special processing equipment, and development is complete within 10 to 30 seconds (black and white prints) or 60 seconds (color prints). Although capital costs are lower, the recording medium is relatively expensive compared to other film types.

Instant black-and-white print film is positive film in which increased exposure to light is depicted as white. Its characteristics are high speed, high resolution, and low contrast (film gamma is 1.3) with a limited dynamic range. Proper adjustment of light intensity and exposure time is critical.

The film consists of a negative emulsion in contact with a receptor. After exposure to light, the film is ejected through a pair of rollers, which break the chemical pods located on it and spread processing solution evenly between the layers. Unexposed silver halide grains dissolve and diffuse to the receptor layer, where they are converted to metallic silver (i.e., a positive image). Exposed silver halide grains are also converted to metallic silver but are retained in the negative. The process is called diffusion transfer reversal.

A dye-diffusion technique is used to develop color print film. Three emulsion layers are present, each sensitive to light in one of the primary colors (red, green, or blue). Following exposure, processing chemicals are spread over the multilayered film. Dye developer diffuses to each receptor layer, where a single-color dye is immobilized by the exposed silver halide crystals. Three patterns, one in each primary color, are formed and superimposed on each other to compose the color image. The development process is self-limiting and terminates automatically.

One method of transferring the displayed image on the monitor is to optically couple the screen and camera with a light-tight hood. Because the hood must be held steady during exposure, this technique may produce blurred images if motion is present. A relatively new device called a freeze-frame video-image recorder has been introduced to alleviate this problem. One frame or one field of the video signal is captured and stored in digital memory. However, the spatial resolution in the field mode is inferior because the number of raster lines is decreased by a factor of two. Raster lines from single-field video sources (e.g., tape recorders) are filled in to eliminate line structure. To compose the color image, light from a black-and-white monitor is directed through a green, blue, or red filter toward the film. The filter determines the color of light incident on the film. A total of three exposures takes place, one for each color. A separate light pattern is generated on the screen for each

color as dictated by the information stored in memory.

Adjustments for contrast, brightness color, tint, and sharpness can be manipulated to optimize the fidelity of the image recording. The contrast control changes the video-signal amplification and alters the translation of the video signal into the color level. The brightness control creates a lighter or darker print; the purity or shading of color is established by the color control; the tint control shifts the color balance toward red or green; and the definition of edges is altered by the sharpness control.

VIDEO PRINTER

The video printer (also called a video graphics printer) provides a black-and-white hardcopy recording of an image displayed on the monitor. Three methods have been developed to form a black-and-white image on a paper receptor—impact, photo, and heat.

In impact printing the print head strikes a ribbon, which places a black dot on the paper. The color of black is created by placing multiple dots within a small area on the paper. Impact printers are not used with ultrasound scanners because the gray level representation is poor.

Either light-sensitive or heat-sensitive paper acts as the receptor medium for video printers currently in use. The paper is supplied in long rolls of several hundred feet and is cut to size within the device. The thermal method has gained popularity because exposing heat-sensitive paper to light does not render it useless, as is the case with light-sensitive paper.

A video signal sent to the video printer is captured as one or two fields and stored in computer memory. The signal level in memory controls the exposure source (amount of light or heat applied to the paper).

In the photo method a dry silver-coated paper is pulled past the face of a CRT. A single scan line is illuminated on the CRT, and updated to correspond to successive lines of the image. As the paper moves past the CRT, it is exposed line by line. The exposed paper is heat developed by passage over a mechanical heater or by the application of an electrical current to the conductive back surface. Adjustments include contrast and brightness on the CRT and development temperature.

An alternative method for transferring the image data to paper employs a thermal print head instead of a CRT. This device scans chemically treated paper line by line. The heat generated by the print head is varied to correspond to changes in signal level. The application of heat cures the paper (forms deposits of black carbon). As more heat is applied, more carbon is created at that location and the area appears darker. The number of gray levels is typically 64 to 128. The dot density, indicative of spatial detail, is 3 to 7.7 dots per millimeter. A print is processed in approximately 10 seconds.

The operator selects how much of the video signal is stored in memory for printing by selecting the field or frame mode. Spatial resolution is sacrificed in the field mode because a reduced number of raster lines are available to compose the image. Consequently, the frame mode should be used if possible. Black-white reversal (also called positive-negative) inverts the gray scale to display blacks as whites and vice versa.

Adjustments for contrast, brightness, and sharpness are available. The contrast control changes the video-signal amplification and alters the translation of the video signal into gray level. The brightness control sets the overall optical density. Edges in the image are enhanced by the sharpness control.

Video printers offer several advantages compared with multiformat cameras. These include ease of processing, convenience, speed, and low cost. The paper print has a limited optical density range (maximum optical density is 1.6), however, and less archival stability.

COLOR VIDEO PRINTER

A color image on paper is viewed by sensing the reflected light from colored dyes distributed across the paper surface. The incident white light from a conventional light source, consisting of all colors, strikes the paper, and varying amounts of its constituent colors are selectively removed by the absorbing dyes. The color of the reflected light is altered. This process is repeated at every pixel throughout the printed image and results in the visual spatial pattern of colors.

Typical primary colors of the dyes are cyan, magenta, and yellow, which absorb red, green, and blue. Black is formed when all three primary colors are present. In some devices a separate black dye is used. The absence of dye yields white. A combination of the two primary colors magenta and yellow forms the reflected color red; all colors in the incident light are absorbed except red. Similarly, green and blue are produced by different combinations of two primary colors.

The color video printer provides a color hardcopy recording of the image displayed on the monitor. One or more images are printed on a paper sheet. Heat-activated dyes are transferred to the paper without the processor chemicals required for film. This device is used extensively for recording color-flow Doppler images.

A video signal sent to the color video printer is captured as one or two fields and stored in computer memory. One 512×512 color image requires 0.75 megabyte of computer memory. The video input can assume different formats to code for the color information (e.g., composite video, Y/C [luminescence and chrominance], and RGB analog). The colors yellow, magenta, and cyan are printed on the paper. A separate Mylar ribbon coated with dye is necessary for each color. The paper is printed three times—once for each color—which accounts for the increased printing time compared to black-and-white video printers.

The chemically treated paper with a smooth surface, is attached to a platen, which rolls around and is scanned line by line with a miniature thermal print head. A sublimation process (conversion of solid to gas) is used to transfer the dye from the ribbon to the paper. The dye on the ribbon is in solid form. When heated, the dye is converted to a gas.

The density of the gas and, consequently, the quantity of dye infused into the paper is increased as more heat is applied to the print head. The amount of heating at a particular location is controlled by the information stored in memory. During each rotation of the platen a different-colored dye ribbon is placed next to the thermal print head for transfer to the paper.

Color gradations are controlled by superimposing varying amounts of each dye on the paper. The number of color levels ranges up to several million. Each primary color is coded in 8 bits. A color selection table translates the video signal into various color levels. The number of lines printed is typically greater than 500 thus the video signal and not the device limits the spatial resolution. Three hundred dots per inch are printed. The printing time is usually less than 90 seconds.

The operator selects the number of images printed on a sheet (full or split mode) and how much of the video signal is stored in memory (field or frame mode). Spatial resolution is sacrificed in the field mode because a reduced number of video lines is available for image formation. Adjustments for contrast, brightness, color intensity, and tint can be manipulated to optimize the fidelity of the image recording. The contrast control changes the video signal amplification and alters the translation of the video signal into color level. The brightness control, in essence, determines the amount of dye used to print the image. The purity or shading of the color is established by the color control. The tint control adjusts the mixing of the three basic colors.

MAGNETIC TAPE RECORDER

Standard Video Home System

Recording a series of images for subsequent playback in real time is restricted to magnetic tape recorders. The video cassette recorder (VCR) has dominated the video home system (VHS) market. A ½-inch tape is enclosed in a cassette for ease of loading and unloading. The polyester tape is coated with a magnetic substance. Tiny regions called dipoles in this coating are aligned when subjected to an external magnetic field, and they maintain their induced orientation until a new magnetic force redirects them. During recording, the tape is mechanically driven past the writing head at a constant velocity. The writing head converts the input video signal to a rapidly changing magnetic field that extends beyond the head to the region of the tape. This fluctuating magnetic field varies the alignment of dipoles along the tape. During playback, the magnetic field associated with the aligned dipoles induces an electrical signal in the writing head as the tape moves past. The induced video signal, consisting of 525 lines, is sent to the television monitor for display. VHS, however, can preserve the spatial detail of only 240 lines; thus image quality is degraded.

Two writing heads mounted 180 degrees apart on a rapidly revolving drum (Fig. 11-6) each write a video field as an individual track with every revolution of the drum. In the VHS format a track width is 29 μm, with a gap between

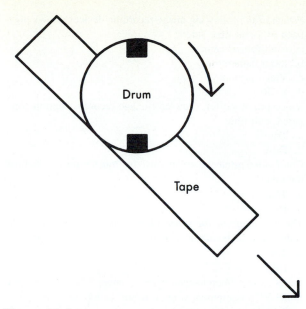

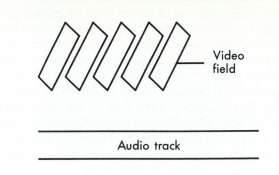

Figure 11-7 VHS format. Video tracks are narrow bands of aligned dipoles. To inhibit crossover, adjacent tracks are separated by a gap. An audio track allows sound recording.

Figure 11-6 Magnetic tape is moved past a revolving drum that contains two writing heads. Each head records one track corresponding to one video field.

adjacent tracks to reduce interference or cross-talk (Fig. 11-7). One or more linear sound tracks are included on the tape for audio capability.

The tracking control adjusts for small variations in tape speed caused by tape stretch or inconsistent tape transport. To reduce noise, only one head is active during playback. In the record mode, both heads are sent the video signal but only the head in contact with the tape writes the track to tape.

The amount of tape in the cassette can be increased 30 to 160 minutes to extend recording time. The physical size of the cassette is unchanged, but the diameter of the center hubs is made smaller to accommodate more tape. Longer recording times are also possible by reducing the tape speed. The fidelity of the recording is compromised, however, by slower tape speed.

Super Video Home System

The latest generation of video format, introduced in 1987, is super VHS. A high-density oxide tape in the standard cassette shell is used. The cassette is notched to identify the type of tape (standard or super). Super VHS videocassette recorders operate with a higher-frequency bandwidth, which allows 425 lines of horizontal resolution compared with 240 lines in standard VHS. Image quality is superior with super VHS because the information contained in the video signal is preserved.

Limited compatibility exists between super VHS and conventional units. A recording in the super VHS format cannot be played on a conventional VCR. Tapes in the standard format can be interchanged between super VHS and standard VHS equipment.

The low cost makes videotape recording very attractive. Voice commentary can be added to the audio track. Unfortunately, tape wear from contact with the writing head limits tape life to a few hundred plays. Also the recommended shelf life of 2 years prohibits long-term archiving. The freeze-frame option stops movement of the tape and a single track is repeatedly read for the video signal. This allows selected images consisting of one video field to be annotated and transferred to a multiformat camera or video printer for hardcopy recording. Measurements can be performed on the stop-framed image.

Cleaning Writing Heads

Dirt and magnetic particles from the tape collect on the writing head and must be removed periodically. The overuse of head cleaners, however, promotes head wear since cleaning is accomplished by scraping the head surface. Consequently, cleaning should be performed only when the playback picture becomes noisy.

The indirect method uses a special head-cleaning cassette that is loaded into the tape recorder. The cleaning material replaces the tape and is driven across the head surface. In the direct method a nonwoven, low-abrasive, lint-free cleaning pad is moved across the head in one direction only. Back-and-forth and up-and-down motions can damage the writing head. A Freon-base cleaning solution leaves no residue. Alcohol should be avoided because any remaining moisture will cause the tape to seize.

SUMMARY

The traditional image-storage medium is transparency film. Its cost, image quality, and long-term stability are the standards against which those features of alternative media are compared. Polaroid film is more expensive, has poorer contrast resolution, and fades more with age. Paper is less expensive, has slightly inferior spatial and contrast resolution, and is less stable with time. The most common image-recording device is the multiformat camera, although the laser camera (because of its excellent image quality) and the video printer (because of its low cost) are experiencing increased use. The newly developed hardcopy camera with dry-processed transparency film offers a promising alternative to the laser camera for high-quality image recording. Color video printers seem particularly well suited for recording color-flow Doppler images. VCRs offer a means of recording dynamic studies in real time for subsequent playback in real time. Magnetic tape cannot function as a permanent storage medium, and consequently appropriate frames from the video recording must be selected for hardcopy recording.

Quality assurance of the entire ultrasound system, including the recording devices must be monitored periodically to ensure that the recorded image matches that of the monitor.

■ **R E V I E W   Q U E S T I O N S** ■

1. What is the major disadvantage of transparency film as an image storage medium?
   a. Limited spatial resolution
   b. Limited contrast scale
   c. Bulk
   d. Poor long-term stability
2. What is the primary advantage of Polaroid film as an image-storage medium?
   a. Low cost
   b. Nearly instant presentation of the stored image
   c. Superb contrast scale
   d. Excellent long-term stability
3. The latent image is retained in which component of transparency film?
   a. Base
   b. Gelatin
   c. CRT phosphor
   d. Silver halide grains
4. The multiformat camera contains an internal CRT that is adjusted by the brightness and contrast controls on the display monitor.
   a. True
   b. False
5. In the laser camera a CRT is used as the light source.
   a. True
   b. False
6. Which of the following image-recording devices offers the best spatial resolution?
   a. Multiformat camera
   b. Laser camera
   c. Video printer
   d. VCR

7. Which of the following image-recording devices allows playback of a real-time study?
   a. Multiformat camera
   b. Laser camera
   c. Video printer
   d. VCR
8. Video printers offer a low-cost image-recording option compared with film.
   a. True
   b. False
9. Color video printers use a thermal dye-transfer process to form the image.
   a. True
   b. False
10. The advantage of the super VHS format compared with the standard VHS format is that spatial resolution is improved.
    a. True
    b. False
11. Tapes can be interchanged between super VHS and conventional VHS equipment without regard to format.
    a. True
    b. False
12. When image data transfer is accomplished with a video signal, the video signal provides an ultimate limit for spatial resolution regardless of the image-recording device.
    a. True
    b. False

BIBLIOGRAPHY

Bushong SC: *Radiologic science for technologists: physics, biology and protection,* ed 5, St Louis, 1993, Mosby.
Curry TS III, Dowdey JE, Murry RC Jr: *Christensen's Physics of diagnostic radiology,* ed 4, Philadelphia, 1990, Lea & Febiger.
Gray JE, Anderson WF, Shaw CC, et al: Multiformat video and laser cameras: history, design considerations, acceptance testing, and quality control. Report of AAPM Diagnostic X-ray Imaging Committee Task Group no 1, *Med Phys* 20:427, 1993.
Russ JC: The image processing handbook, Boca Raton, Fla, 1992, CRC Press.
Sorenson JA, Phelps ME: *Physics in nuclear medicine,* ed 2, Orlando Fla, 1987, Grune & Stratton.
Starkweather GK: Digital color printing, *Physics Today* 45:60, 1992.
Thompson TT: Laser applications in radiology, *Radiographics* 5:627, 1985.
Trefler M: Inside the multiformat camera, *Radiographics* 4:785, 1984.

▲

Biological Effects

AIUM statement on biologic
  effects
Benefits versus risks
Cavitation
Clinical imaging guidelines
Epidemiologic studies
Equipment output levels

Intensity
Intensity descriptors
Mechanical index
Mechanical interaction
Peak negative pressure
Thermal index
Thermal mechanism

The medical applications of ultrasound have experienced considerable growth during the past 20 years. The development and subsequent incorporation of new technology into reasonably priced, commercially available, devices have made ultrasound readily accessible. The increased acceptance of this modality, however, can be attributed in large part to one especially attractive feature—ultrasound does not use ionizing radiation. Obstetrics seems particularly well suited for ultrasonic techniques, which include amniocentesis, fetal heart monitoring, estimation of fetal age, determination of fetal position, diagnosis of multiple pregnancy, and placental localization. Indeed, ultrasound has almost completely replaced x-ray pelvimetry as a means of evaluating the maternal pelvis and fetal head before childbirth. Fetal exposure to ionizing radiation, which has the potential for latent biological injury at diagnostic x-ray levels according to current radiation protection philosophy, is completely eliminated in ultrasound.

Besides its applicability in obstetrics, ultrasound can be used in cardiology (for the detection of pericardial effusion, valvular dysfunction, or wall-motion abnormalities), in vascular studies, in ophthalmology (for the detection of vitreous hemorrhage, retinal detachment, or intraocular foreign bodies), and in gastroenterology (especially for the assessment of an abdominal mass).

AREAS OF RESEARCH

No acute harmful effects have been reported after diagnostic ultrasound examinations. Nevertheless, when large popu-

lations are exposed to any diagnostic technique, it is appropriate to investigate any potential long-term effects, which may not be evident on an individual case-by-case basis. Any risk (i.e., potential harmful effect) versus benefit (i.e., diagnostic information derived) analysis requires an assessment of the risk factors. Quantification of risk is not currently available and, most likely, will never be precisely known. Ethical considerations preclude experimentation on human subjects, although such studies would provide the necessary data. Instead, the potential harmful effects to the exposed human population must be inferred from other avenues of investigation. Several of these can contribute to an overall comprehensive picture:

Development of measurement techniques to quantify the ultrasonic dose received by a patient or test system

Identification of mechanisms by which ultrasound interacts with matter

In vitro studies of biologically significant molecules and various cell types

Animal studies with intensity levels comparable to those used in diagnostic ultrasound

Epidemiological studies of human populations that have undergone diagnostic ultrasound examination

Because of the observed bioeffects, most research has been conducted at higher intensity levels and with longer exposure times than those used clinically. The validity of results from these studies is limited when extrapolated to predict potential effects from medical exposures. The problem posed is not unique to ultrasound. If we wanted to know the hazard (or benefit) of the thermal effects resulting from taking a warm bath, the effect to $100°$ C could readily be measured using relatively few subjects. However, we would encounter some difficulty in constructing a model that permitted the extrapolation of resulting data to temperatures slightly above $37°$ C. To perform the study at $40°$ C, for example, would require an epidemiological comparison of possibly a million subjects in which the control and test populations were matched perfectly. For the study of any effect, as the probability of that effect approaches zero the number of individuals necessary to quantitate this probability approaches infinity. In most situations we attempt to avoid large risks and accept risks that may be nonzero but that are too small to measure accurately.

Intensity levels below a certain value may be incapable of inducing an effect if a threshold exists. Effects reported for high intensity levels will not be present at levels lower than the threshold. If the biologic response has no threshold, however, any exposure to the physical agent carries some risk; the question then becomes whether incidence rates per unit dose at low intensities are the same as those at high intensities for which the effects are observed. In addition, the dependency of the response on other factors such as frequency, pulse sequence, pulse width, and exposure time must be considered.

Unfortunately, much of the early work published in the scientific literature is seriously flawed. Many experiments have lacked proper controls; furthermore, the conditions of irradiation have not been specified, particularly with respect to defining the ultrasound field intensity. The term *irradiation* describes the process wherein ultrasonic energy is transmitted as a wave; it does not mean that the sound wave is ionizing. The early animal experiments were important for demonstrating acute functional or gross structural alterations at very high intensity levels (e.g., the production of lesions in the brain or the interruption of nervous conduction in the spinal cord). Recently, more research has been directed toward elucidating potential effects at intensity levels produced by diagnostic devices.

SPECIFICATION OF INTENSITY

To assess biological effects, we must know the dose of ultrasound. *Dose* in this instance has a meaning similar to that of *radiation absorbed dose* (rad). Therefore dose is the quantity of energy absorbed per unit mass of absorbing medium (e.g., tissue). Closely related to energy absorption throughout the medium is the point-by-point variation of intensity in the medium. Recall (from Chapter 1) that intensity is the rate of energy flow through a unit area. Unfortunately, state-of-the-art measurement techniques await a good method whereby the intensity (or some other parameter, such as pressure, from which intensity is calculated) could be ascertained at a particular point within tissue (classified as an in situ measurement). Typically the ultrasound device is characterized by using free-field experimental conditions in which the parameter of interest is determined in water without reflectors or other disturbances to the ultrasonic field. Free-field measurements do not assess the attenuation by tissue, focusing by anatomical structures, production of standing waves, or effect of reflecting boundaries. Nevertheless, free-field testing does provide measurable physical entities that characterize the ultrasound beam and allow comparisons between devices.

Because of the pulsing and scanning techniques employed, diagnostic ultrasound equipment produces complex and time-varying acoustic fields in space. Quantification of these patterns is impractical and difficult to correlate with the bioeffect potential of the ultrasound beam. Thus, characterization of the ultrasonic field is accomplished by a few select parameters, usually related to energy, such as acoustic power or intensity. Some researchers, however, have argued that other parameters (e.g., particle displacement, particle velocity, particle acceleration, or peak pressure amplitudes) are more indicative of potential damage. The spatial and temporal dependence of the intensity complicates this descriptive process. Several shorthand methods have been developed to describe intensity.

Temporal Dependence

As the transducer emits pulses, it causes large fluctuations of intensity in the region through which the pulses move. Each pulse consists of multiple cycles that produce intensity variations within the pulse itself—the maximum intensity designated temporal peak (TP), the intensity averaged over the duration of a single pulse designated pulse average (PA), and the intensity averaged over the longer interval of the PRP designated temporal average (TA). For a given pulse sequence TP has the highest value, followed by PA, and finally by TA (Fig. 12-1).

The TA intensity is related to the PA intensity by the duty factor (DF):

$$TA = DF \times PA \qquad \text{12-1}$$

or by the pulse duration (PD) and pulse repetition frequency (PRF):

$$TA = PD \times PRF \times PA \qquad \text{12-2}$$

For example, if the pulse duration is 1 μs and the pulse-repetition period is 1 ms, the duty factor is 0.001. The PA intensity is 1000 times greater than the TA intensity. A determination of the TP intensity from the PA intensity requires knowledge of the pulse shape. The ratio TP/PA is typically in the range of 2 to 10.

The relationship between intensity peak and intensity averaging is an important concept. The following analogy may help illustrate it: Suppose a row of sand castles has been built along the seashore, as in Figure 12-2. Each castle corresponds to a single pulse. The height of the tallest point of a castle represents the TP. If a castle is flattened so the sand is spread evenly over its base, the level of the sand will be lower than the original peak. This corresponds to the PA. If the sand is distributed over the area between castles, it will be even lower than the original height of the peak. This represents the TA.

Spatial Dependence

The additional factor of space must now be considered in the shorthand description of intensity. Once more, the peak or average value with respect to the variable (in this case space) is used. The TP intensity, PA intensity, or TA inten-

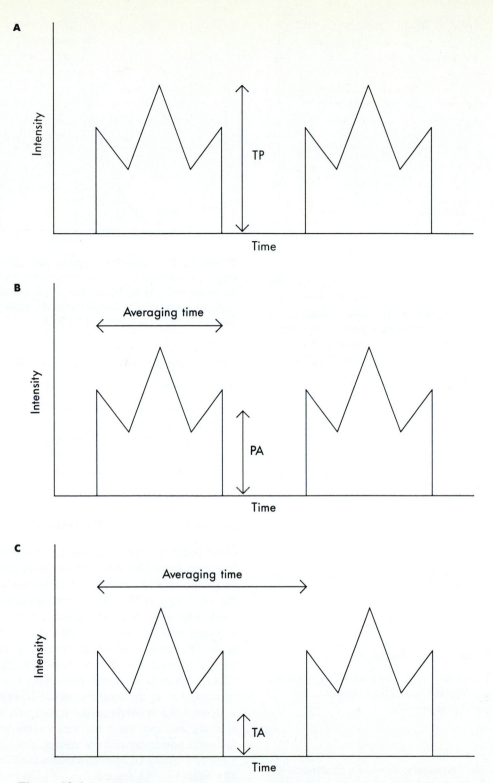

Figure 12-1 Specification of intensity with respect to time. **A,** Temporal peak (TP); **B,** pulse average (PA); **C,** temporal average (TA).

sity is mapped as a function of position. The variation in intensity along the axis of propagation is illustrated in Figure 12-3. The maximum intensity of all measured values within the sound field is designated as the spatial peak (SP). Thus three combinations are possible depending on which temporal intensity is mapped:

I(SPTP) — Spatial peak, temporal peak intensity
I(SPPA) — Spatial peak, pulse average intensity
I(SPTA) — Spatial peak, temporal average intensity

The designation SP is not clearly defined. In some applications it refers to the maximum intensity in a plane perpendicular to the beam axis at a particular distance from

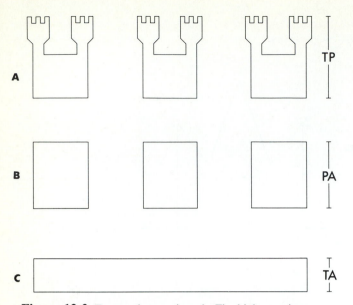

Figure 12-2 Temporal averaging. **A,** The highest points on the sand castles (turrets) correspond to the temporal peak *(TP).* **B,** Sand making up the turrets has been stacked on the base of each castle. This corresponds to the pulse average *(PA).* **C,** The sand has been flattened to cover the area between the castles. This corresponds to the temporal average *(TA).*

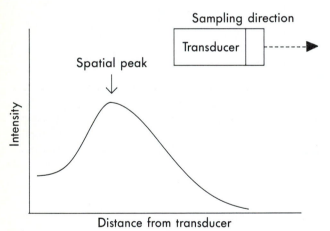

Figure 12-3 Axial intensity profile. The intensity is maximal at a particular distance from the face of the transducer. This point is called the spatial peak intensity.

the transducer. More commonly, however, it denotes the maximum intensity throughout the ultrasonic field, which usually occurs along the beam axis.

Spatial averaging (SA) over the cross-sectional area of the beam of one of the temporal intensities is also specified. A cutoff point of 0.25 times the SP intensity has been established to limit the area over which the intensity is averaged. Figure 12-4 shows the intensity profile through the cross section of the beam and the location at which the SA is obtained. Again, three combinations are possible:

I(SATP) —Spatial average, temporal peak intensity

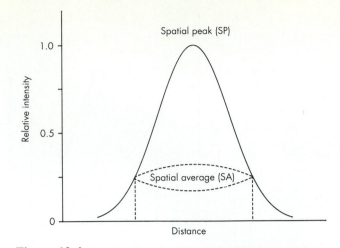

Figure 12-4 Relationship of spatial peak *(SP)* and spatial average *(SA)* intensities. The curve represents the intensity profile across the width of the beam. The spatial average intensity is found by averaging the intensity over the beam width. In this case the boundary is defined at 0.25 SP.

I(SAPA)—Spatial average, pulse average intensity

I(SATA)—Spatial average, temporal average intensity

For nonfocused transducers the SP is usually greater than the SA by a factor of 2 to 6. The SP intensity is often converted to an SA by multiplying the peak value by one third. In the case of focused transducers the degree of focusing influences this factor greatly. The ratio of SP to SA ranges from 5 to 50.

Alternative Intensity Descriptors

Other intensity descriptors have been used to specify the ultrasonic field. The instantaneous peak intensity (i_p) is the maximum intensity with respect to space and time and is the same as I(SPTP). The term *maximum intensity* (I_m), when used as a shorthand descriptor, refers to the time-averaged intensity over the largest half cycle in the pulse at the SP. For a perfect sine wave I_m equals I(SPPA), although generally for pulsed ultrasound I(SPTP) is greater than I_m, which is greater than I(SPPA). *Cycle-averaged intensity* (I_a) is an alternative term for I(SPPA). The symbol I_T denotes the I(SATA) at the transducer, which has been spatially averaged over the area of the radiating surface (acoustic power divided by area of the transducer equals I_T). The intensity (I) of continuous-wave (CW) devices usually refers to a TA intensity.

A summary of the various intensity descriptors is presented in Table 12-1.

Instantaneous Intensity

All the intensity parameters just discussed have been derived by averaging the instantaneous intensity (i) with respect to space, time, or both. The instantaneous intensity is determined from the measured acoustic pressure (p) using the equation

■ **Table 12-1** Intensity Descriptors

Parameter	Symbol
Instantaneous peak intensity (maximum intensity with respect to space and time)	I(SPTP) or i_p
Maximum intensity (at SP, time-averaged intensity over largest half cycle)	I_m
Pulse-averaged intensity at spatial peak (averaged over the duration of the pulse)	I(SPPA) or I_a
Spatial peak, temporal average intensity	I(SPTA)
Spatial average, temporal peak intensity	I(SATP)
Spatial average, pulse average intensity	I(SAPA)
Time averaged intensity at the transducer averaged over the area of the radiating surface	I_T
Spatial average, temporal average intensity	I(SATA)
Intensity of CW (time averaged intensity)	I
Instantaneous intensity	i

■ **Table 12-2** Relationships between Intensity and Pressure

Intensity (W/cm²)	Pressure	
	(MPa)	(atm)
0.001	0.004	0.04
0.01	0.0126	0.126
0.1	0.04	0.4
1	0.126	1.26
10	0.4	4
100	1.26	12.6

$$i = \frac{p^2}{\rho c}$$

12-3

where c is the speed of sound and ρ is the density of the medium.

Table 12-2 shows the conversion between instantaneous intensity (in W/cm²) and pressure (in megapascals, MPa, and atmospheres, atm). Frequently pulsed-wave (PW) ultrasound is characterized by a peak positive pressure or peak negative pressure (expressed in megapascals, MPa). The peak negative pressure is also called the peak rarefactional pressure (Fig. 12-5).

Clinical Usage

For continuous waveforms time averaging is usually employed with an intensity specification of I(SATA) or

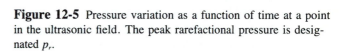

Figure 12-5 Pressure variation as a function of time at a point in the ultrasonic field. The peak rarefactional pressure is designated p_r.

I(SPTA). PA descriptors are not applicable for continuous-wave (CW) ultrasound.

These definitions of intensity descriptors must be modified slightly for real-time scanners. In autoscanning, consideration of the dwell time (i.e., time the ultrasound beam is directed toward a particular region) and the spatial sampling method must also be included in the averaging process.

The most frequently quoted intensity is the I(SATA), which is approximated by the ratio of ultrasonic power to beam cross-sectional area (scan cross-sectional area for autoscanning systems). In practice, the temporal average of the power is determined by placing a plane absorber or plane reflector in the beam and measuring the resultant force. The power and, subsequently, the I(SATA) are computed from the radiation force (see Chapter 13 for more information on the radiation force technique).

Approximate values of the intensity descriptors for an illustrative set of conditions are listed in Table 12-3.[77] The acoustic power is assumed to be 1 mW, and the beam cross-sectional area 1 cm². All the intensity descriptors are derived from I(SATA) using the SP/SA and TP/TA ratios defined previously. The duty factor is taken as 0.001. The ranking of intensity descriptors demonstrates that I(SPTP) has the highest value and I(SATA) the lowest. Although these parameters describe the same ultrasonic field, their values differ by a factor of 100,000 or more. The PA intensity can vary considerably depending on the ringdown characteristics

■ **Table 12-3** Calculated Intensity Parameter Values*

Descriptor	Nonfocused	Focused
SATA†	1 mW/cm²	1 mW/cm²
SAPA	1 W/cm²	1 W/cm²
SATP	2 to 10 W/cm²	2 to 10 W/cm²
SPTA	2 to 6 mW/cm²	5 to 50 mW/cm²
SPPA	2 to 6 W/cm²	5 to 50 W/cm²
SPTP	4 to 60 W/cm²	10 to 500 W/cm²

*Ultrasonic power of 1 mW and beam cross-sectional area of 1 cm².
PA/TA, 1000; TP/PA, 2 to 10; SP/SA for nonfocused transducers, 2 to 6; SP/SA for focused transducers, 5 to 50.
†Evaluated at the radiating surface.
Modified from O'Brien WD Jr: *Semin Ultrasound CT MR* 5:105, 1984.

of the transducer. The relative ranking of I(SPPA) and I(SATP) for a specific transducer is dictated by the pulse length and the degree of focusing.

OUTPUT LEVELS FROM DIAGNOSTIC EQUIPMENT

The intensity and power levels from commercial diagnostic instruments should also be examined. The output characteristics from diagnostic devices vary considerably depending on their designed application. Units are classified according to the major categories—static pulse-echo imaging systems, linear arrays, phased arrays, mechanical sector scanners, CW obstetric Doppler systems, CW peripheral vascular Doppler systems, CW fetal heart monitors, pulsed obstetric Doppler systems, pulsed peripheral vascular Doppler systems, and pulsed cardiac Doppler systems. In addition, among units of the same type, the intensity and power levels differ over a wide range of values.

Although many real-time pulse-echo imaging systems operate with an I(SPPA) in the range of 0.4 to 933 W/cm², most operate at less than 250 W/cm². Because the pulse duration is on the order of microseconds, with PRFs of approximately 1000 per second, the high intensity levels within a pulse are reached only a small fraction of the scan time. This produces an I(SPTA) in the 1 to 50 mW/cm² range. Acoustic power output is typically less than 50 mW.

PW Doppler units have the highest I(SPTA) values because the temporal pulse length is relatively long compared with those generated in real-time scanners. Also sensitivity (by increasing the power) must be improved to detect the weak scattering from RBCs. The I(SPTA) is usually less than 2 W/cm².

The acoustic power output and I(SPPA) of M-mode units are comparable to those found in real-time scanners. The I(SPTA) for M-mode equipment, however, is generally higher, with most devices operating in the range of 1 to 200 mW/cm².

The time-averaged intensity for CW peripheral vascular Doppler units is much higher than that obtained from CW obstetric Doppler units. The SATA intensities are typically 400 mW/cm² and 15 mW/cm², respectively. The pulsed Doppler units used in cardiology have SATA intensities of 3 to 32 mW/cm².

The various intensities produced by diagnostic devices are summarized in Table 12-4. The data represent a collection of the output levels reported by several investigators. The American Institute of Ultrasound in Medicine (AIUM),[3] the National Council on Radiation Protection and Measurements (NCRP),[72] and the Bureau of Radiological Health (Stewart and Stratmeyer)[89] have compiled similar tables. More recently, Duck[30] and Zagzebski[100] have surveyed the acoustic output levels of diagnostic ultrasound equipment (Table 12-5). The trend in the past few years is toward higher output intensity.

FDA Requirements

In the United States manufacturers and importers of diagnostic ultrasound equipment are required to submit to the Food and Drug Administration a report on the safety and testing of their products before the products are introduced on the market. This submission is called 510(k) notification, since section 510(k) of the Food, Drug, and Cosmetic Act established the requirement. The FDA has, in essence, set limits on the acoustic output intensity levels by stating that the intensity of diagnostic ultrasound equipment designed for a particular clinical use should be no greater than that measured in the past. Intensity measurements for each transducer are made under the worst-case condition of highest power setting. The FDA guidelines for acoustic output intensity levels are listed in Table 12-6.[35] CW fetal heart monitors have an I(SATA) limit of 20 mW/cm². By restriction of spatial-averaged pulse-averaged intensities to 20 mW/cm², PW fetal heart monitors are assured the same level of safety as CW fetal heart monitors.

Industry Standards

Manufacturers have an obligation to characterize their units with respect to standards established by scientific and industry organizations. The results of these measurements should be communicated to potential buyers. Unfortunately, these standards are currently not well defined and manufacturers are hesitant to provide test results. Nevertheless, frequency, pulse shape, pulse length, PRF, frame rate, power levels, and spatial profile of beam intensity should be specified.

INTERACTIONS OF ULTRASOUND WITH MATTER

Three mechanisms by which ultrasound interacts with matter have been identified: mechanical, thermal, and cavitation. These are microscopic effects as compared with the macroscopic interactions of ultrasound in tissue (Chapter 1). Other phenomena—microstreaming and altered chemical reaction rates—have been linked with experimental end points, but these are initiated by one of the aforementioned mechanisms of action.

■ Table 12-4   Intensity Ranges Produced by Diagnostic Ultrasonic Equipment*

Type	Acoustic Power (mW)	I(SATA) (mW/cm²)	I(SPTA) (mW/cm²)	I(SPTP) (W/cm²)
B-mode and M-mode	0.1 to 20	0.01 to 20	0.6 to 200	0.4 to 700
Phased arrays and wobblers	3 to 20	2.7 to 60	2 to 200	0.25 to 300
Sequenced linear arrays	0.1 to 33	0.06 to 10	0.1 to 12	0.2 to 120
Pulsed Doppler (cardiac work)	8 to 24	3 to 32	50 to 290	3 to 1400
Pulsed Doppler (obstetric work)	1 to 18	0.26 to 25	0.6 to 75	—
CW Doppler (peripheral vascular work)	6 to 105	38 to 840	110 to 2500	—
PW Doppler (peripheral vascular work)	6 to 10	87 to 175	350 to 700	1 to 12
CW Doppler (obstetric work)	1 to 37	0.2 to 20	0.6 to 80	—
CW Doppler (fetal monitor)	5 to 32	—	9 to 80	—

*Adapted from NCRP Report 74, *J Ultrasound Med Suppl* 2:532, 1983; and *HHS Publ* 82-8190, 1982.

■ Table 12-5   Survey of Maximum Acoustic Output Parameters in Diagnostic Ultrasound Equipment

Type	Power (mW)	I(SPPA) (W/cm²)	I(SPTA) (mW/cm²)	Peak negative pressure (MPa)
Real-time	360	933	560	3.9
PW Doppler	500	710	9500	6.3
M-mode	75	—	340	—

■ Table 12-6   FDA Guidelines for Acoustic Output Intensities of Diagnostic Ultrasound Equipment*

Clinical Application	I(SPTA) (mW/cm²)	I(SPPA) (W/cm²)
Adult		
Perpheral vessel	1500	350
Cardiac	730	350
Abdominal, small organ, cephalic	180	350
Ophthalmic	68	110
Pediatric and fetal	180	350

*All measurements in water.

Mechanical Interactions

The first mechanism by which damage can be induced, mechanical interactions, is sometimes called direct and generally includes all but thermal and cavitational effects. The ultrasound wave propagate through the medium by interactions between neighboring particles (see Chapter 1). The particles undergo considerable changes in velocity and acceleration. A discrete object with a density different from that of the surrounding medium experiences a force in the ultrasound field because acoustic pressure is applied over its surface. This causes translational or rotational motion of the object. The translational motion may transport biological particles (e.g., cells) to highly localized regions within the ultrasound field. The rotational motion may give rise to acoustic streaming (i.e., circulatory flow of the fluid), and spinning of intracellular particles may be induced. At high intensities, high-velocity gradients are formed near solid boundaries. The resulting microstreaming (i.e., rapid movement of fluid in a localized area) can fragment the macromolecules in these regions.

Thermal Interactions

The second mechanism by which damage can be induced is thermal. With the ultrasound beam propagation through the medium, its intensity decreases as the sonic energy is absorbed and converted to heat. The increased temperature has the potential to cause irreversible tissue damage. The rate of temperature rise depends on the temporal average intensity, the absorption coefficient of the medium, the cross-sectional area of the beam, the duration of exposure, and the heat-transport processes (thermal conductivity and blood flow). Within the frequency range of 1 to 10 MHz, the absorption coefficient increases with frequency.

Thermal effects dominate the low-megahertz frequencies and tend to mask other (nonthermal) effects. To observe cavitation and mechanical effects, it is necessary to minimize the thermal component by cooling the medium or by some other means (e.g., lowering the PRFs).

Cavitation Interactions

The third mechanism by which damage can be induced is cavitation. As the ultrasound wave propagates through the medium, regions of compression and rarefaction are created. Thus localized regions are subjected to increases and decreases in pressure in an alternating fashion and these cause gas bubbles to form and grow and to exhibit dynamic behavior. This phenomenon is known as cavitation, and it can be either stable or transient.

Stable cavitation. In stable cavitation microbubbles already present in the medium expand and contract during each cycle in response to the applied pressure oscillations. The bubbles may also grow as dissolved gas leaves the solution during the negative-pressure phase, a process called rectified diffusion. Each bubble oscillates about the expanding radius for many cycles without collapsing completely. At a characteristic frequency (which is a function of the size of the bubble) the vibration amplitude of neighboring liquid particles is maximized. This condition is called volume resonance. The action of the gas bubble in the liquid is analogous to a child's swinging on a swing. An external force (push) applied to the child at the proper point in the oscillatory path increases the height of the swing. If the force is repeated over and over at the proper frequency, the motion of the swing will be amplified. If the child is pushed opposite the direction of movement, the height of the swing will decrease. The interplay between the rate of pushing and the physical characteristic of the swing (e.g., length of rope between the pivot point and the seat) is essential for maximum effect. Similarly, in cavitation, the interaction between the size of the gas bubble (i.e., the swing) and the frequency becomes critically important. A free air bubble in water undergoes resonance at 1 MHz when its radius is 3.5 μm. At higher frequencies the size of the bubble required for resonance decreases. Bubbles somewhat smaller than resonance size tend to grow whereas those significantly larger than resonance size do not sustain stable cavitation. Oscillations of a gas bubble may produce high shearing forces in the nearby surrounding areas. Stable cavitation may also give rise to microstreaming. The radial oscillatory motion of the bubble is not always spherically symmetrical. An adjoining solid boundary may distort the motion of the bubble and cause eddies near the air-liquid interface. High-velocity gradients are created in the localized region of the oscillatory boundary layer. Biomolecules or membranes subjected to such gradients can fragment or rupture.

Stable cavitation has been reported[93] in mammalian tissue at the CW SP intensity of 80 mW/cm². O'Brien[76] has theorized that a CW SP intensity as low as 0.1 mW/cm² is sufficient to cause stable cavitation. The pulse sequence may have considerable importance and appears to be a resonant effect acting over several cycles.

Transient cavitation. Transient cavitation is a more violent form of microbubble dynamics in which short-lived bubbles undergo large size changes over a few acoustic cycles before completely collapsing.

During the rarefaction phase, bubbles may be formed by dissolved gases leaving the solution or bubbles of submicron dimensions may already exist in the medium. High viscosity and surface tension inhibit bubble growth. A rarefaction phase of long duration enhances bubble growth.

During the compression phase, changing pressure causes the bubbles to collapse and produce highly localized (within 1 μm³) shock waves. In addition, very high temperatures (up to 10,000° K) and pressures (10^8 pascals or higher) are created within the bubbles, resulting in the decomposition of water to free radicals. These pressures and temperature changes may also drive chemical reactions. The release of enzymes when shock waves rupture lysosomal membranes may also enhance DNA and protein synthesis.

The general consensus is that transient cavitation is a threshold effect. The intensity levels necessary for cavitation to develop in tissue are a matter of debate. The threshold for transient cavitation in water is 0.3 MPa at 1 MHz if gas bodies of optimal size are present (0.5 μm radius).[6] At higher frequencies increased pressure or intensity is required.[36] The threshold for transient cavitation in tissue without preexisting gas nuclei is most likely 1500 W/cm² I(SPTP) or greater.[42] Theoretical analysis[16] suggests that the I(SPTP) threshold for transient cavitation in tissue is in the range of 1 to 10 W/cm² for microsecond-pulsed ultrasound if gas bubbles of optimal size are present.

Apfel and Holland[6] have predicted that a negative peak pressure of 0.3 MPa at 1 MHz is sufficient to cause cavitation in blood under the conditions of short pulse length (5 μs) and low duty cycle (0.1%). The threshold of the peak negative pressure increases with frequency, exhibiting a p^2/f dependence. As the peak negative pressure is increased above the threshold value at a certain frequency, bubbles of different size can also undergo transient cavitation, which generally extends bubble activity to more sites. Transient cavitation has recently been demonstrated in mammalian systems at pressure levels generated by diagnostic imaging equipment.

Cavitation-Induced Effects

Organisms that contain small stable gas bodies are more likely to incur damage by cavitation when exposed to ultrasound. Cavitation has been demonstrated to be responsible for killing and for the abnormal development of *Drosophila* (fruit fly) larvae exposed to ultrasound. The contribution of thermal effects is eliminated by using very low TA intensities to prevent heating. The larvae contain air-filled tubes, which function as a respiratory apparatus. These naturally occurring gas bodies may serve as sites for cavitation. Peak intensity rather than TA intensity is the most important physical predictor of the effects induced by cavitation.

Attributing biological effects to cavitation in animals is more difficult because gaseous nuclei have not been identified and the associated heating in cavitation experiments interferes with the interpretation of data. Some evidence for the existence of gas bubbles in mammalian tissues has been presented in the literature. The intensity threshold for hind limb paralysis in neonatal mice was increased by raising the hydrostatic pressure.[37] Ter Haar and Daniels[93] observed stable bubbles in the hind limb of a guinea pig following exposure to a commercial ultrasound-therapy device operating at 0.75 MHz and 0.68 W/cm^2 I(SATA). In separate studies cavitation damage has been responsible for lung hemorrhage in dogs and mice exposed to a shock wave lithotripter.[27,44]

Hemorrhage in the mouse lung exposed to PW ultrasound demonstrated a sharply defined threshold for damage.[22] The pressure threshold at 1 MHz with 10 μs temporal pulse length was 1 MPa (instantaneous intensity of 62 W/cm^2). Beam diameter and temporal-averaged intensity did not influence the threshold. These findings are consistent with the cavitation phenomenon. The threshold showed a frequency dependence as predicted by Apfel and Holland,[6] which also supports the hypothesis of cavitation-induced damage in vivo.

Little damage has been observed in fetal lung exposed to a peak pressure of 20 MPa.[44] Mouse kidney showed essentially no damage at peak pressures almost 10 times greater than the threshold for lung hemorrhage.[17] The presence of appropriate-sized bubbles in the lung predisposes this organ to damage.

EFFECTS ON BIOMOLECULES

The observed biological effect on mammalian systems exposed to ultrasound is most likely the end product of a long chain of events involving physical, chemical, and physiological processes. The initial step is absorption of energy, generally considered to take place at the macromolecular level. Numerous studies on biomolecules in solution have identified the types of damage and elucidated the mechanisms by which damage is induced.

The in vitro experimental conditions have been extremely diverse. In many studies the physical aspects of ultrasound exposure and, consequently, the intensity field to which the biomolecules were exposed have not been well defined. The presence of reflecting boundaries distorts the ultrasonic field. Dissolved gas in solution, which cannot be controlled adequately, enhances cavitation.

Inactivation of enzymes in vitro has been demonstrated at very high intensities (e.g., 10^4 W/cm^2).[26] Cavitation appears necessary to produce damage in protein molecules. Certainly, most of the work has been directed toward DNA and its component parts (i.e., bases, nucleotides, and nucleosides). Base damage similar to that induced by ionizing radiation via free-radical formation has been identified. The bases appear to react with free radicals produced by cavitation. Degradation of DNA in solution is most often associated with intensities above 25 to 72 W/cm^2 as a result of cavitation.[25,46,48,78] One study,[41] however, reported partial degradation of DNA in solution for intensities as low as 200 mW/cm^2. Extrapolation to the in vivo case is difficult because the viscosity of cytoplasm necessitates higher intensity levels to produce comparable velocity gradients.[92] Also, DNA is not in a free state within the living organism but is part of an intricate structure that may protect it. Finally, the presence of gaseous bodies in solution may enhance damage.

In general, the damage to biomolecules in solution is associated with the cavitation type of mechanism.

EFFECTS ON CELLS

Cells are typically irradiated in an aqueous solution or monolayer state attached to the surface of a culture dish. An extremely diverse variety of cell types—including human red blood cells, human lymphocytes, human platelets, cells in culture, protozoa, amebae, and bacteria—has been investigated. The criticisms outlined in the previous section regarding biomolecules pertain to experiments involving cells.

Cell lysis is caused by cavitation at high intensity levels.[40] Cell killing has also been attributed to microstreaming near cavitating bubbles and to free radical production. In addition, altered morphology of cultured mammalian cells[50,54] has been observed. Both positive and negative neoplastic transformation of cultured cells has been reported,[43,54] although the studies with positive findings were criticized for low plating efficiency and a lack of certain types of transformed loci.

Survival and growth rate for some cell types are reduced following exposure to ultrasound. Cell-surface function as assessed by the transport of ions across membranes, by electrophoretic and phagocytic activity, and by attachment to surfaces is altered by shear forces generated from stable cavitation. Cell-cycle sensitivity has been reported, but researchers are not in agreement regarding the most sensitive phase of the cell cycle.

Few effects have been observed under conditions in which cavitation does not occur. The presence of gas nuclei is critical for damage to occur. In an experiment not involving cultured cells,[99] chick embryos in ovo were insonated with PW ultrasound. The exposure parameters were 1.1 MHz, PRF of 2000 per second, temporal pulse length of 75 μs, and exposure time of 10 minutes. No effect on cell proliferation and migration of chick motoneurons was observed.

EFFECTS ON MAMMALS

Focal lesions are observed in the brain following ultrasound exposure when the product of the I(SPTA) and the square root of the time for a single pulse exceeds a threshold of 200 W-s per square centimeter.[39] This relationship holds for a large range of exposures (100 μs to 10 minutes). The threshold for irreversible structural change is higher for other organs (e.g., liver, kidneys, and testes). When the spinal cords of neonatal mice were irradiated,[31] hind limb paralysis was induced at a threshold approximately 25% of that for brain lesions.

Accelerated tissue regeneration has been demonstrated[22] in some cases when the injured tissue was subjected to periodic exposure to ultrasound.

The combined application of ultrasound and ionizing radiation to solid tumors has produced a synergistic effect, reducing tumor volume and extending survival time.[53] Ultrasound heats the tumor site to approximately 43° C at the same time that ionizing radiation is delivered to the site. This treatment (called hyperthermia) has evolved into a highly specialized modality in radiation oncology.

Little evidence of biological effect exists for an I(SPTA) of less than 100 mW/cm², regardless of the duration of exposure. Few studies involving microsecond high-pressure pulses have been conducted. Recently lung damage in the mouse has been demonstrated at a TA intensity of 1 mW/cm². This finding has important ramifications regarding the clinical safety of ultrasound.

GENETIC EFFECTS

Mutations

In studies with yeast, bacteria, and fruit flies exposed to diagnostic levels of ultrasound, no evidence of increased mutations has been observed. Negative findings have also been reported for intensity levels greater than those used in clinical practice. Early work with *Drosophila,* presumably at high intensities, has shown that there is an induction of dominant lethal mutations. However, these mutations have been attributed to heat, which is mutagenic in *Drosophila.*[63]

Free radicals have been shown to cause DNA damage that may be expressed as a mutation. Hydroxyl radicals and hydrogen atoms are formed in aqueous solutions by transient cavitation. Free radical generation in aqueous solutions exposed to ultrasound pulses at diagnostic levels has also been reported.[12] If DNA is located near the site of free radical formation, mutations are possible.

The potential for DNA damage in cells exposed to ultrasound is unclear. Repair synthesis, an indirect indicator of DNA damage, has been shown to be both present[54] and absent[96] following insonation of intact cells. Thymine base damage in the DNA of cells has also been reported.[29]

Kaufman[50] observed mutations in cultured mammalian cells in suspension exposed to 1 MHz CW ultrasound at a spatial peak intensity of 35 W/cm². The mutation rate was very low but increased with exposure times ranging from 60 to 180 seconds. Another study involving hamster cells and human lymphoblasts[28] found that CW ultrasound at 35 W/cm² increased the mutation rate by a factor of approximately 2. Experiments with human-hamster hybrid cells containing human chromosome 11 following insonation with CW and PW ultrasound[80] failed to demonstrate mutagenic effects. The assay method used in the latter study is generally very sensitive to mutation caused by most agents.

Single-strand DNA breaks have been observed[66] in Chinese hamster ovary cells exposed to an I(SPTA) of 8 W/cm². Cell killing was extensive, however, and the breaks were in nonviable cells. Mutations cannot be propagated by nonviable cells.

Aberrations

During the early 1970s MacIntosh and Davey[61,62] reported an increase in the frequency of chromatid and chromosomal aberrations of human lymphocytes irradiated in vitro with a fetal heart monitor. These authors observed a threshold of 8.2 mW/cm² for a 1-hour exposure at 2.25 MHz. Their reports generated controversy as well as concern because this intensity level is in the diagnostic range and patients would definitely be at risk. Numerous investigations by other researchers have failed to support MacIntosh and Davey's observation of increased chromosomal aberrations at peak intensities of 300 W/cm². Indeed, MacIntosh et al.[60] subsequently repeated the experiments and found no evidence of chromosomal aberrations.

Several investigators[1,49,83] have tested for chromosomal aberrations in lymphocytes isolated from neonates exposed in utero. No significant differences in either type or number were found between the exposed and control groups.

Nonclassical chromosomal aberrations have been reported[19] for *Vicia faba* root tips exposed to ultrasound (8 W/cm² for 1 minute at 2 MHz). The chromosomal damage was in the form of bridged prophases and metaphases and agglomerated mitotics, which would not have been detected in the standard chromosomal aberration–scoring technique. The significance of this type of damage is unknown.

Lyon and Simpson[56] exposed the gonads of mice to approximately 1 W/cm² of either CW or PW ultrasound (pulse width 30 μs, duty factor 0.02) at 1.5 MHz. They tested for translocations in spermatocytes and dominant lethal mutations and found none. Only a small number of animals were examined, however. Mutation rates would have to have been high to be detected.

Sister Chromatid Exchange

During mitosis every chromosome must be replicated so each daughter cell receives identical genetic material. The chromosomes consist of two identical chromatids, which are joined together during the prophase and metaphase. Chromatids on the same chromosome can exchange DNA, generally at the same relative position. The process is called sister chromatid exchange (SCE). Although SCEs have been linked to mutagenic agents (e.g., ultraviolet radiation, x-rays, and certain drugs), their biological importance has not been established. Controversy regarding the potential of ultrasound at diagnostic levels to cause SCEs has evolved over the past several years.

An increased frequency of SCEs in human lymphocytes following exposure to a diagnostic ultrasound device has been observed by Liebeskind et al.[55] A different cell type (HeLa cells) from this same laboratory showed no difference in SCE frequency.[54] Additional studies by other researchers[9,88] have also found an increased frequency in SCEs following exposure to ultrasound. The majority of studies,* however, including those that attempted to replicate Liebeskind's work and those using much higher intensity levels, have demonstrated no effect on the frequency of SCEs. Because some researchers who reported positive results failed to include positive controls, the validity of their results remains in question. Nevertheless, the magnitude of the SCE effect is probably small, and the variability reported in the literature can be attributed to undefined experimental conditions in vitro.

Assays of DNA Damage

Other in vitro experiments have examined the effect on genetic material of exposure to ultrasound, with positive findings. As noted in the previous section, purified DNA is degraded by ultrasound. Transformation of cells, altered DNA synthesis, and formation of glycols have also been reported.[72] Unwinding of the DNA following exposure to diagnostic levels of ultrasound is suggested by the observation of increased immunoreactivity to antinucleoside antibodies in cultured cells. This is classified as an immune effect because the assay method involves an immune technique—not because a response of the immune system was evoked. Although they are not proof of a genetic effect, these results are suggestive of one.

Mutagenic Potential

The conflicting results obtained from mutagenicity studies of mammalian cells in culture remain unresolved. If ultrasound is a mutagen, its mutagenic action is relatively weak compared with that of x rays. Furthermore, intensity levels sufficient to produce cavitation are required. The site of cavitation must be close to the DNA so the free radicals produced can migrate to the DNA.

TERATOGENIC EFFECTS

The sensitivity of embryonic and fetal tissues to chemical and physical agents (e.g., ionizing radiation) is well documented. The extensive use of ultrasound in obstetrics combined with an anticipated increased sensitivity of tissues to ultrasound has led to the question whether diagnostic ultrasonic techniques can affect the developing embryo or fetus. The subject may be addressed from two approaches—one involving experiments with prenatal ultrasound exposure of animals, usually mammals, and the other involving epidemiological studies of human populations. These avenues are discussed in the following sections.

Experimental Observations

Much experimental work has been published regarding the possible effects following prenatal ultrasound exposure. Because of the diverse experimental conditions, these studies are difficult to consolidate in a consistent pattern. Single and multiple exposures to PW and CW ultrasound at different intensity levels have been used at various stages of gestation. Fetal deaths in rats and mice have been induced following such exposures. This effect is associated with a rise in temperature of the amniotic fluid. The initial rate of the temperature rise and the absolute evaluation in temperature are dependent on the intensity of the ultrasonic beam.

Some researchers[86] have reported on congenital malformations and fetal mortality rates. The type of malformation produced is a function of the developmental stage during which exposure occurred and is similar to that obtained with

*References 24, 67, 68, 71, 72, 77, 95.

ionizing radiation and thermal insult. Most of these studies, however, were conducted using intensities above diagnostic levels. In addition, there were many reports of negative findings, even at high intensities.[86]

In vivo exposure to CW ultrasound at intensities of less than 1 W/cm^2 during the preimplantation period does not appear to affect development in rodents.[86] When early rat embryos were exposed in vitro to CW ultrasound at 0.65 W/cm^2 for 1 hour, a retardation in development and abnormal morphological characteristics were observed.[2] These were attributed to a thermal mechanism, because embryos subjected to the same temperature increase without ultrasound exposure demonstrated similar results. Another study[79] reported embryolethality and weight reduction in rats exposed to pulsed ultrasound during the preimplantation period. Peak intensity has been estimated to be 1 W/cm^2, but the dosimetry aspects are questionable. Researchers from other laboratories[20] have been unable to replicate this finding for intensities as high as 10 W/cm^2.

Warwick et al.[94] found no significant differences in fetal weight, litter size, resorption rate, or number of abnormalities among groups of mice irradiated for 5 minutes on different gestational days with an I(SPTP) as high as 490 W/cm^2. Shoji et al., however, reported some very controversial findings: Pregnant mice were irradiated for 5 hours on the ninth day of gestation with CW ultrasound from a commercial fetal Doppler device, intensity level 40 mW/cm^2, had statistically significant increases in fetal mortality and congenital abnormalities. These observations have been attributed to the stress associated with physical restraint of the animals for 5 hours or to possible temperature elevation during the long exposure time. The results have not been confirmed by an independent research group.

Diagnostic Intensity Levels

Two studies have linked PW ultrasound exposure at diagnostic intensity levels with congenital abnormalities via a nonthermal mechanism. Takabayaski et al.[90] reported that pulsed ultrasound with an I(SATP) threshold of 60 W/cm^2 produced malformations in mice. (A repeat of this study by another laboratory, however, yielded completely negative results and additional experiments with microsecond PW ultrasound exposure to mouse fetuses under hyperbaric conditions[23] showed no malformations for an I[SAPA] of 100 W/cm^2.) Taylor and Dyson[91] observed congenital abnormalities following ultrasound exposure to chick embryos. The experimental conditions were 20 μs temporal pulse length, 5000 pulses per second, 1 MHz, intensity of 25 W/cm^2, and exposure time of 5 minutes. PW ultrasound provided a low TA intensity so the effects of heating were eliminated. At intensity levels of less than 10 W/cm^2 no congenital abnormalities occurred. A long temporal pulse length and high PRF are not characteristic of real-time instrumentation. Less controversial is the finding[45] that high-pressure shock waves from lithotripsers (10 MPa or greater) will induce malformations in chick embryos.

Thermal Damage

Thermal-induced damage is a threshold phenomenon; that is, no biological effects are observed unless the temperature elevation exceeds a particular value for a minimum time duration. The threshold for thermal bioeffects, including fetal abnormalities, is shown in Figure 12-6. A temperature increase of 2.5° C must be present for 2 hours to cause fetal abnormalities. At higher temperatures the time necessary to induce damage is shortened dramatically (e.g., at 43° C it is 1 minute).

Nonthermal Damage

Certainly exposure durations of 1 hour at TA intensities capable of increasing the temperature 3 to 4° C can induce fetal abnormalities in small mammals. Whether nonthermal mechanisms also contribute to fetal abnormalities is less certain. In an extensive research effort[77] fetal weight reduction in mice was linked to a dose parameter (intensity squared times the exposure time) for intensities greater than diagnostic levels. With this model, the fetal weight reduction predicted at diagnostic intensity levels was considered to be insignificant. Fetal weight reduction in rats has not been detected at SA intensities below 30 W/cm^2.

Subtle changes in some reflex responses for rodents after in utero exposure have been reported by a number of researchers. The effects were noted at or near diagnostic intensity levels. Such observations imply that in utero ultrasound exposure affects prenatal growth and development.

Beam Size

Most in vivo studies on mice and rats have been done using transducers from the clinical setting. Relatively speaking, these transducers produce large-sized beams for the animal

subject. The rodent fetus is usually completely enveloped by the beam whereas only part of the human fetus would be enveloped. The fraction of tissue exposed, which is much less for humans, may influence the amount of damage induced.

EPIDEMIOLOGICAL STUDIES

Although experimentation on animals has provided some insight into and reassurance regarding the potential effects from ultrasound exposure at diagnostic levels, the application of these data to human populations in limited. The ultimate assessment of biological effects induced in human populations exposed to ultrasound lies with epidemiological studies. Observational investigations of human populations attempt to answer the question whether individuals exposed to a particular agent have a higher risk of developing impaired health than nonexposed individuals do.

The major complication in epidemiological studies is the influence of other risk factors. The agent of interest is most likely not the sole determinant of an adverse effect; and, furthermore, the risk of a potential effect is not the same for all members of the population. Modification of the incidence of an adverse effect by other factors is called confounding.

If the additional risk to an exposed population is small, large sample sizes will be required to distinguish the agent-induced effects from disorders that occur spontaneously. Sample size limits the minimum level of excess risk detectable in a particular study.

Detection of Adverse Effects

The ability to identify an adverse effect in a population exposed to a particular agent (e.g., drug, x ray, or ultrasound) depends on the visibility of the effect and its probability in the exposed as well as unexposed population. The absence of a thumb at birth is readily observable; a small decrease in visual acuity at the age of 10 years is not.

For a new or very rare event (one whose occurrence in the unexposed population is highly unlikely) the risk can be quantified by surveying the exposed population for the number of times that the event has occurred. All events are attributable to the agent because the incidence rate in the unexposed population is zero or very nearly zero.

Consider, for example, the rare event of red eyes in humans. Assume that a 0.1% incidence rate of red eyes at birth is induced in a population exposed in utero to a particular agent. A survey of 100,000 neonates exposed to this agent would yield 100 cases of red eyes (or very nearly 100, based on the probability distribution of sampling 100,000 individuals with an incidence rate of 0.1% for the effect). If different researchers examined a different group of 1000 neonates exposed to the agent, however, at least one case of red eyes in a particular group might or might not be present. By random chance, different studies addressing the same question can obtain contradictory results. Absence of positive findings in an exposed population does not mean that a potential effect does not occur, but it does

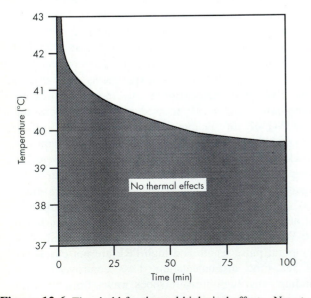

Figure 12-6 Threshold for thermal biological effects. No adverse effects are observed for time-temperature combinations in the shaded region.

establish an upper limit for the incidence rate of the effect. Obviously, surveys of increasingly larger populations with no positive findings reduce the upper boundary of the risk estimate. Very likely, the adverse effect attributed to a particular agent is an event that occurs naturally in the unexposed population. The exposed population is expected to have a higher incidence rate than the unexposed population. The ability to identify the adverse effect depends on the relative increase in incidence rate and the number of individuals observed. Epidemiological studies are designed to assess by statistical methods the occurrence of adverse effects in populations exposed to a particular agent.

Factors that may influence the relative incidence rates of a given outcome following in utero exposure include pregnancy complications, gestational age at the time of irradiation, maternal age, ethnic origin, diet, and geographic location. The selection of a control group with the same characteristics is essential. Ideally, the only difference between the exposed and unexposed groups would be the agent of interest. In practice, this is very difficult to achieve and is the major criticism of many epidemiological studies.

If the relative risk is small, a large sample size is required to distinguish the agent-induced effects from disorders that occur spontaneously in the population. Sample size limits the minimum level of relative risk detectable in a particular study.

The possibility of a long latent period (i.e., the delay between exposure and observable effect) must be considered. To assess risk factors accurately, it is necessary to examine these populations over a period of many years. Collecting data for a large population over a long time is an extremely expensive undertaking and subject to many difficulties.

Experimental Designs

Two commonly used experimental designs for assessing the association between exposure to an agent and its long-term effect are case-control (retrospective) and cohort (prospective) studies.

Case-control studies identify individuals with a particular health problem (cases) and research the histories of these individuals, particularly past exposure to the agent of interest. Past exposure to the agent is also examined for a reference group (control), which is free of the health problem. Ideally, the control group has similar attributes (e.g., socioeconomic status, age, ethnic origin, sex) as the case group. An excess of exposure to the agent by the case group compared with the control group indicates an association. Relative risk is estimated by the ratio of the fraction of subjects in each group exposed to the agent.[81] For example, a relative risk of five is assigned following a case-control study in which 50% of the case group and 10% of the control group were exposed to a particular agent.

Cohort studies identify a population that is initially free of the potential adverse effect. During the investigation observations regarding exposure to the agent, other potential etiological factors, and changes in health status are made. The occurrence of an adverse outcome is compared between the exposed and unexposed portions of the population. Many health end points can be assessed within the study and the absolute incidence rates can be determined. The major advantage of the prospective study is that the selection of individuals in the cohort is inherently unbiased because their disease status is not yet known, although bias in the diagnosis of health effect is possible.

Confounding factors may be present that modify the relative incidence rates between the two groups. In some studies attempts are made to eliminate the influence of these factors by matching the control and exposed groups initially with respect to several attributes (e.g., age, sex, race, and marital status). For large groups, however, this technique of matching is not feasible.

A different form of the cohort experimental design is the historical prospective study, which investigates events that have occurred during an earlier time. A cohort exposed to an agent in the past is identified and the health experience of this population over the ensuing years is examined. Rather than identifying subjects at the present time for future follow-up (spanning possibly many years), the investigators study consequences from past exposure to the agent in the population. The need for lengthy follow-up and the associated high costs of a prospective study are eliminated.

In a retrospective study the observations have been recorded in the past for some unrelated purpose and the investigators reexamine this collected information to test a particular hypothesis regarding exposure to the agent and its potential adverse effect. The data in many cases are incomplete because the original design of the information-gathering process did not specify the agent for special consideration. The possibility of biased recall of exposure to the agent exists. The selection of an appropriate control group is problematic. Case-control studies compared with cohort studies have certain advantages, however—including lower cost, smaller sample size, and shorter time interval to conduct the study (faster availability of results). For studying rare health effects, the case-control design is the method of choice.

Rarely does a single study become the definitive work regarding identification of an adverse effect and the level of risk from exposure to a particular agent. The overall assessment must be based on multiple studies conducted under diverse conditions involving different populations. Epidemiological studies are often flawed either in experimental design or by incompleteness of the data. To establish an agent as potentially harmful, a pattern must develop whereby the results from different studies associate the same biological effect(s) with prior exposure to the agent, produce a dose-dependent rate of occurrence, and demonstrate a similar time sequence with respect to onset of the adverse effect.

Clinical Surveys

Surveys of clinical ultrasound users incorporating over 400,000 patient examinations have shown no obvious increase in any anomalies that occur naturally, though rarely, in the general population.[33,101] These surveys, however, rely on the judgment of respondents who differ in scientific training and ability to perceive changes in patient status. The results nevertheless indicate that clinicians believe ultrasound to be safe for their patients. In another clinical study[52] passage of sonic energy through the skull of 20 neonates did not alter their cerebral activity patterns as monitored by electroencephalography.

Limitations of Exposure-in-Utero Studies

The most important issue that epidemiological studies must address is whether ultrasound exposure in utero at diagnostic intensity levels produces adverse effects. The current estimate is that over half of all pregnant women in the United States undergo an ultrasound examination during their pregnancies. Because large numbers of fetuses are exposed to ultrasound, the ability to demonstrate that the risk of adverse effects is extremely small becomes critically important.

Before reviewing reports of epidemiological studies of ultrasound exposure in utero, we must consider the limitations of these studies. Many retrospective clinical investigations contain methodological flaws—including small sample size, lack of controls, and limited information regarding characteristics of the population. The prevalence of in utero exposures creates difficulties in identifying a well-matched control group. The exposed group should be characterized by the following:

1. Reason for the examination
2. Gestational age at the time of the examination
3. Number of examinations
4. Exposure parameters

If an individual is not assigned to the exposed group at random, a biased selection process may lead to an invalid finding. A patient with a clinical problem is more likely to be assigned to the exposed group, because the diagnostic information obtained from the ultrasound examination is desirable for the management of that patient; patients with no clinical problems are preferentially assigned to the unexposed group. The suspected clinical problem may often result in an observed biological effect (e.g., low birth weight). Therefore an analysis of this end point would show a difference between the exposed and unexposed groups, but a question would still remain as to whether ultrasound exposure or the selection process was the cause of the adverse outcome.

For populations exposed in utero, the information gained from the ultrasound examination could be used clinically to alter patient health and distort the findings of the study. For example, fetuses with structural abnormalities could be identified and the pregnancy therapeutically terminated, thus selectively eliminating these fetuses from the analysis of biological end points evaluated at birth.

Experience with teratogenic agents (e.g., ionizing radiation) has shown that the induction of structural abnormalities is dependent on gestational age at the time of exposure. Negative findings from a study in which the exposure occurred at a gestational age of 32 weeks would not allow the conclusion to be made that exposure at any time during

pregnancy was without effect. If harm were caused by ultrasound, the probability and severity of the adverse effect would be expected to increase with the dose as monitored by the number of examinations and exposure parameters. Unfortunately, the exposure parameters are not well defined in most studies, and consequently, quantitative risk estimates have not been possible if a positive finding was obtained.

Results of Exposure-in-Utero Studies

Low birth weight, fetal chromosome abnormalities, structural fetal anomalies, altered neurological development, cancer, and hearing disorders have been investigated as possible adverse effects from fetal exposure to ultrasound. A summary of the findings from various studies is presented in Table 12-7.

Several studies, including three randomized clinical trials, have found no association between low birth weight and in utero exposure.[10,34,59,98] Moore et al.,[69,70] however, did report a positive correlation between low birth weight and insonation in utero. In their first study, 2135 births during the late 1960s and early 1970s in Denver were investigated. The reason for the examination, the physical size of the mother, and whether the mother smoked were not delineated, which could have introduced bias. An analysis of the Denver data by Stark et al.[87] contradicted Moore's conclusion by arguing that the complications affecting birth weight were not comparable in the exposed and control groups.

In a subsequent study Moore[70] acknowledged that the association of ultrasound with low birth weight was probably a result of confounding maternal and fetal factors. Women with problems during pregnancy are more likely to have an ultrasound examination, and complications are more likely to affect birth weight. In other words, intrauterine growth retardation would have been more prevalent in the group exposed to ultrasound even if the ultrasound exposure had not occurred. Thus designing a study to adjust for all potential confounding factors by matching exposed and unexposed infants is difficult.

The final conclusion regarding low birth weight and in utero exposure to ultrasound is based primarily on the three studies in which the subjects were randomly selected for exposure. No difference in birth weight was observed between the exposed and control groups. The finding of reduced birth weight in two retrospective studies has had little clinical importance.

Several other studies have found no association between ultrasound exposure in utero and fetal structural anomalies.* In 1969 Bernstine[11] compared the incidence of congenital anomalies in an ultrasound-exposed population with a U.S. Navy statistic for incidence of congenital anomalies. Presumably, this control incidence rate was derived from a reference population that was similar to the patient population identified by Bernstine. The study concluded that

---

*References 8, 11, 47, 57, 58, 82, 87.

■ **Table 12-7** Epidemiological Studies of Ultrasound Exposure in Utero

Study	Number of Subjects Exposed	Findings
Bernstine (1969)	720	Rate of congenital anomalies less than in reference population
Hellman (1970)	1079	Absence of dose-response relationship for fetal abnormalities
Serr (1971)	150	Suggested damage to chromosomes of fetal cells, but not statistically significant
Abdulla (1971)	35	No increase in chromosome abnormalities in fetal lymphocytes
Falus (1972)	171	Height and weight within normal range for age 6 mo to 3 yr; no developmental disorders
Ikeuchi (1973)	98	No chromosome damage
Scheidt (1978)	303 amniocentesis and ultrasound; 679 amniocentesis only (970 controls)	More abnormal grasp reflexes and abnormal tonic neck reflexes in amniocentesis with ultrasound group; 121 other outcomes negative, including low birth weight
Lyons (1979)	2428	No increased incidence of congenital malformations, chromosome abnormalities, neoplasms, speech disorders, hearing problems, development problems
Lyons (1980)	500	Increase in low–birth weight infants
Wladimiroff (1980)	341 (364 controls)	Negative findings for low–birth weight infants
Moore (1982)	2135	Association between ultrasound and low–birth weight infants
Stark (1984)	425 (381 controls)	Higher incidence of dyslexia, but not statistically significant
Bakketeig (1984)	510 (499 controls)	Negative findings for low birth weight, physical status, and mortality
Kinner Wilson (1984)	1731 cancer patients (1731 matched controls)	No difference in two populations with respect to exposure in utero
Cartwright (1984)	555 cancer patients (1110 controls)	No association between exposure in utero and childhood cancer
Moore (1988)	1594 (944 controls)	Association between exposure in utero and low–birth weight infants
Lyons (1988)	149 sibling pairs	Exposure in utero did not affect growth in childhood up to age 6 yr

examining pregnant women by Doppler ultrasound did not place the fetus at increased risk for structural anomalies. Hellman et al.[47] examined 1079 neonates for anatomical abnormalities following in utero ultrasound exposure. The gestational age at the time of examination varied from 10 weeks to 40 + weeks, and some patients had multiple examinations. Both continuous-wave and pulsed-wave regimens were used. The frequency of fetal abnormalities in this population was compared with the frequency in a large survey of 63,000 births. The number of abnormalities did not exceed that expected from the general population. In both of the above studies, however, the lack of well-matched control population casts doubt on the validity of the conclusions.

A study involving small groups of infants whose mothers had received either amniocentesis and ultrasound or amniocentesis alone[82] showed no association between ultrasound exposure and abnormalities. Lyons et al.[58] reported that the offspring of 10,000 women exposed to ultrasound during pregnancy showed no increased incidence of speech or hearing disorders, neoplasia, or congenital anomalies. This study is difficult to evaluate because many of the data underlying the conclusions were not included in the report.

No association between in utero ultrasound exposure and fetal chromosome abnormalities,[1,49,83] cancer,[18,51] and hearing disorders[82,87] has been demonstrated. The studies ex-

amining childhood cancer appear to be well-designed and involve large numbers of subjects.

Because migration of neurons within the developing brain takes place at a gestational age of 14 to 22 weeks, ultrasound delivered to the fetus during this period may affect neurological development. Scheidt et al.[82] reported abnormal grasp and tonic neck reflexes in infants exposed to ultrasound in utero. These results may be attributable to random chance, because 123 different end points were examined. Stark et al.[87] identified dyslexia as a possible learning disorder of children exposed in utero. All three hospitals in this study had higher incidence rates of dyslexia in the exposed population, although the increases were not statistically significant.

Assessment of Results

Results of the epidemiological studies have been generally negative, which indicates that damage, if any, is subtle, delayed, or infrequent. The number of subjects in a study reporting negative results places an upper limit on the incidence rate of an adverse effect, but it does not exclude the induction of the effect by ultrasound. The association of ultrasound exposure with a particular outcome does not absolutely establish ultrasound as the causative agent. The association may be the result of shared underlying factors.

Since ultrasonography is a rapidly developing technical field with new capabilities, past epidemiological studies have not investigated biological effects at the intensity levels associated with current medical practice. Well-designed epidemiological surveys involving large numbers of subjects are needed. The information derived from such studies is essential for assessing risk. The very nature of epidemiological surveys, which precludes the ability to control all factors, necessitates that numerous studies be undertaken, rather than a single study be relied on. It is hoped that this approach will reveal a consistent pattern of cause and effect.

AIUM EVALUATION OF BIOEFFECTS DATA

The Bioeffects Committee of the American Institute of Ultrasound in Medicine (AIUM) was established to examine the current knowledge concerning bioeffects and to assess the risk of clinical diagnostic ultrasound. This committee regularly publishes critiques of research reports and issues statements regarding the safety of diagnostic ultrasound. Its conclusions are acknowledged to be safety guidelines throughout the ultrasound community.

Statement on mammalion in vivo biological effects

In August 1976 the Bioeffects Committee reviewed all the data pertaining to biological effects attributable to ultrasound irradiation of mammalian tissue. Its evaluation of the scientific literature was summarized in a statement[5] that was subsequently revised in October 1978, reaffirmed in October 1982, and reassessed in October 1987. The statement is as follows:

In the low megahertz frequency range, there have been (as of this date) no independently confirmed significant biological effects in mammalian tissues exposed in vivo to unfocused ultrasound with intensities[a] below 100 mW/cm², or to focused[b] ultrasound with intensities below 1 W/cm². Furthermore, for exposure times[c] greater than 1 second and less than 500 seconds for unfocused ultrasound, or 50 seconds for focused ultrasound, such effects have not been demonstrated even at higher intensities, when the product of intensity and exposure time is less than 50 joules/cm².

a. Free-field spatial peak, temporal average (SPTA) for continuous-wave exposures, and for pulsed-mode exposures with pulses repeated at a frequency greater than 100 Hz.
b. Quarter-power (6 dB) beam width smaller than four wavelengths or 4 mm, whichever is less at the exposure frequency.
c. Total time includes off-time as well as on-time for repeated pulse regimes.

The low-megahertz frequency range is considered to be 0.5 to 10 MHz. CW and PW ultrasound, as well as focused and unfocused beams, are included. The intensity is designated SPTA, as measured under free-field conditions.

With the availability of later information the Committee statement has been modified to incorporate specifications that are more suitable for the clinical environment. In the most recent reassessment very low PRFs (less than 100 Hz) have been excluded and the intensity of focused beams has been evaluated explicitly. A diagnostic unit with high PRFs may produce an I(SPTA) above 100 mW/cm², the previous statement level for both focused and unfocused beams. Generally, bioeffects data have been obtained under the conditions of high-power, broad-beam, and continuous-wave irradiation. A focused beam is less damaging than an unfocused beam of equal I(SPTA). Most bioeffects are attributable to the thermal mechanism, and the temperature rise is a critical function of beam width. A small beam (less than 4 mm in diameter) transfers heat more rapidly from the irradiated volume than a large beam does, and the corresponding increase in temperature is only 1/10 to 1/100 that for a wide beam. The I(SPTA) estimate of 1 W/cm² for a focused beam is conservative, since this level is 10 times the level for an unfocused beam.

Figure 12-7 illustrates that, for intensities greater than 1 W/cm² (focused) or 100 mW/cm² (unfocused), damage appears to be dependent on the time integral of the intensity. Note in the figure, however, that the region below the dotted line for a focused beam and the solid line for an unfocused beam indicates not the "safe" levels but rather that no adverse effects have been observed for these combinations of intensities and exposure times.

Indeed, since 1987 several researchers have examined the effects of PW ultrasound with short temporal pulse lengths at diagnostic intensity levels. Most important of these has been the study of lung hemorrhage in mice with a threshold at 1 MHz and using low TA intensity (1 mW/cm²). These data are not included in the evaluation of the scientific literature on which the *Statement on Mammalian In Vivo Biological Effects* is predicated. TA intensity, however, is not the appropriate parameter for predicting cavitation. A new approach is necessary to correlate ultrasound exposure with potential biological effects. The observation of a cavitation threshold in mammalian tissue plays an essential role in the creation of a mechanical index as the risk indicator (discussed under "Clinical Safety" later in this chapter).

The AIUM Bioeffects Committee[5] also developed the *Statement of In Vitro Biological Effects* (October 1982, revised March 1988), the *Statement on Clinical Safety* (October 1982, revised March 1988), and the *Statement on Safety in Training and Research* (March 1983, revised March 1988).

Statement of in vitro biological effects

It is difficult to evaluate reports of ultrasonically induced *in vitro* biological effects with respect to their clinical significance. The predominant physical and biological interactions and mechanisms involved in an *in vitro* effect may not pertain to the *in vivo* situation. Nevertheless, an *in vitro* effect must be regarded as a real biological effect.

Results from *in vitro* experiments suggest new end-points and serve as a basis for design of *in vivo* experiments. *In vitro* studies provide the capability to control experimental variables and thus offer a means to explore and evaluate specific mechanisms. Al-

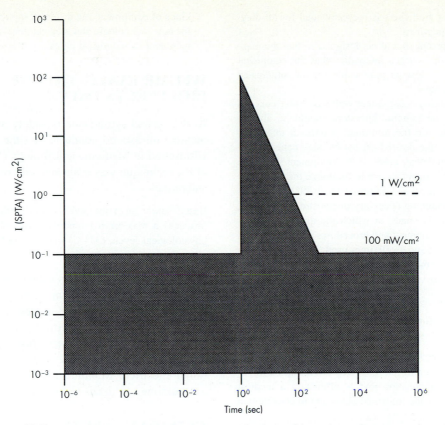

Figure 12-7 1987 AIUM statement indicating combinations of intensity and exposure times for which no effects have been observed as of that date. The *dotted line* for focused beams corresponds to an I(SPTA) of 1 W/cm². The *solid line* for unfocused beams corresponds to an I(SPTA) of 100 mW/cm².

though they may have limited applicability to *in vivo* biological effects, such studies can disclose fundamental intercellular or intracellular interactions.

While it is valid for authors to place their results in context and to suggest further relevant investigations, reports of *in vitro* studies which claim direct clinical significance should be viewed with caution.

Statement on clinical safety

Diagnostic ultrasound has been in use since the late 1950s. Given its known benefits and recognized efficacy for medical diagnosis, including use during human pregnancy, the American Institute of Ultrasound in Medicine herein addresses the clinical safety of such use:

No confirmed biological effects on patients or instrument operators caused by exposure at intensities typical of present diagnostic ultrasound instruments have ever been reported. Although the possibility exists that such biological effects may be identified in the future, current data indicate that the benefits to patients of the prudent use of diagnostic ultrasound outweigh the risks, if any, that may be present.

Statement on safety in training and research

Diagnostic ultrasound has been in use since the late 1950s. No confirmed adverse biological effects on patients resulting from this usage have ever been reported. Although no hazard has been identified that would preclude the prudent and conservative use of diagnostic ultrasound in education and research, experience from

normal diagnostic practice may or may not be relevant to extended exposure times and altered exposure conditions. It is therefore considered appropriate to make the following recommendation:

In those special situations in which examinations are to be carried out for purposes other than direct medical benefit to the individual being examined, the subject should be informed of the anticipated exposure conditions, and of how these compare with conditions for normal diagnostic practice.

NCRP EVALUATION OF BIOEFFECTS DATA

The National Council on Radiation Protection and Measurements (NCRP) was created by Congress in 1964 to promulgate information and recommendations in the public interest concerning protection against radiation. In 1983 it published a comprehensive work[72] detailing the biological effects of ultrasound. Contained within this document were specific recommendations regarding diagnostic equipment, clinical practice, and exposure guidelines—which are reproduced here in slightly edited form.

Recommendations regarding diagnostic equipment

1. Manufacturers of equipment for diagnostic ultrasound should make public their data on exposure parameters, including those specified by the industry standard.

2. The following set of guidelines is recommended for all diagnostic ultrasound equipment:
   a. Ultrasound equipment should be designed so that the maximum levels of the various intensities that the equipment can produce are as low as practicable for the anticipated uses of the equipment.
   b. Where such flexibility is consistent with reasonable cost and performance of the system, operators should be able to adjust controls to use the minimum acoustical intensities required to image the desired organs on each patient.
   c. As a matter of prudence, users of the equipment should be encouraged by the manufacturer to minimize the acoustical intensities to the patient and minimize the dwell times, within the limits of obtaining necessary diagnostic information.
3. Investigations should be made in which the diagnostic capabilities of ultrasonic equipment and procedures are assessed and related to the intensities and dwell times used. Such information is needed to guide manufacturers and users in choosing exposure parameters that yield maximum information with minimum risk.

Recommendations for clinical practice of diagnostic ultrasound

1. It should be recognized that the decision to use ultrasound clinically involves weighing the expected advantages and potential risks of any application and is ultimately a medical decision to be made by the informed physician in consultation with the patient.
2. In clinical practice, users should know the exposure parameters of the ultrasound equipment they employ. They should be thoroughly acquainted with the meaning and significance of these parameters.
3. Users should strive to obtain the most medically significant information possible, while producing the least ultrasonic exposure to the patient. By the latter is meant, specifically, that dwell times and total exposure times should be minimized and that, where adjustable, intensities should be minimized.
4. Routine maintenance and quality-assurance practices should be implemented. Specifically, clinical ultrasound instruments should be:
   a. Maintained and operated in accordance with the manufacturer's guidelines.
   b. Checked periodically and routinely for the maintenance of the system's performance and exposure parameters.

Exposure recommendations

1. Manufacturers and users should be guided by the following general principle: In a diagnostic examination, intensities, dwell times, and total exposure time should be no greater than these required to obtain the relevant clinical information.
2. Routine ultrasound examination of the human fetus should not be performed under exposure conditions in which a significant temperature elevation might be expected. (Because the normal diurnal temperature variation exceeds 1° C, temperature elevations of less than 1° C are usually not considered significant. It is highly unlikely that in clinical practice and using a currently available commercial diagnostic unit, the intrauterine temperature would be raised as much as 1° C.)
3. The establishment of a complete system of optimum exposure parameters for balancing benefit against risk should be accepted as a long-range goal, at least for those situations in which it is found that there is a reasonable expectation of significant risk. Such a system would have to distinguish between different kinds of equipment and different applications and would allow for new technologic and medical developments and for clinical judgment in individual cases.

WFUMB EVALUATION OF BIOEFFECTS DATA

At the second symposium on safety and standardization in medical ultrasound conducted by the World Federation of Ultrasound in Medicine and Biology (WFUMB), the safety of the technique was evaluated with respect to thermal considerations.

Based solely on a thermal criterion a diagnostic exposure that produces a maximum temperature rise of 1.5° C above normal physiological levels (37° C) may be used without reservation in clinical examinations.

The WFUMB[97] also has called for a voluntary standard for the real-time display of acoustic output information. Acoustic output would be expressed in terms of indices based on the instrument settings and on models describing thermal and mechanical interactions with tissue. These indices have recently been developed by AIUM and the National Electrical Manufacturers Association (NEMA) and are examined in detail in the following section.

CLINICAL SAFETY

We will now discuss several important concepts that have a bearing on the practice of diagnostic ultrasound: risks versus benefits, thermal considerations (including minimum threshold), indices of acoustic output, clinical efficacy in obstetrics, education and training, and potential exposure limits.

Risks Versus Benefits

Although harmful effects of ultrasound have not been demonstrated after exposure at diagnostic levels, the data are not sufficient to permit unquestioned acceptance of its safety. The potential for harm does exist. Interactions of ultrasound with biological tissue are not clearly understood; and until the risks are accurately defined the prudent course of action must be to apply objective criteria in the selection of patients for an ultrasound examination and to minimize exposure. Exposure in this sense consists of the intensity (or peak pressure) and the exposure time.

A diagnostic ultrasound examination should be conducted only when medically indicated. *Medically indicated* implies that some benefit can be expected from the information obtained. Furthermore, an intensity consistent with the objectives of the examination should be used. A low intensity that reduces the ultrasound dose but does not provide the desired diagnostic information exposes the patient unnecessarily. Although the dose is low, no benefit is gained. The same principles apply to an examination so limited in time as to compromise the validity of the study.

The selection process for new instruments should include consideration of the intensity specifications of the various units. If comparable units are available, then an instrument with the lowest intensity rating should be purchased.

If future work succeeds in quantifying risk factors for small animals exposed to diagnostic levels of ultrasound, the risk factors may not be readily extrapolated to human beings. The human in vivo situation likely provides some reduction in risk compared with that observed for small animals. The attenuation of an ultrasound beam by overlying tissues lowers the dose delivered to deeper structures. Also, since only part of an organ intercepts the beam only a fraction of it is at risk. During scanning, a particular volume of tissue is irradiated for only a portion of the examination time. In addition, focusing, reflections from body interfaces, and the formation of standing waves are all conditions that can increase the risk by creating locally intense ultrasound fields.

Damage induced by chronic exposure to ultrasound may be cumulative. The ability to repair the damage and thus reduce the overall effect must be investigated. Findings from such studies could have implications in the clinical setting with regard to the frequency of examination and the total number of procedures performed.

The identification of adverse effects attributable to diagnostic ultrasound would not necessarily preclude its medical application. A certain amount of risk is justified if morbidity and mortality can be reduced by the information gained thereby. An important example of this risk-versus-benefit concept in the healing arts is the use of ionizing radiation. Radiation doses are delivered to various organs during nuclear medicine, computed tomography, and radiographic procedures. If the dose-risk relationship is assumed to be linear, with no absolute dose threshold, a small increase in the cancer incidence rate can be expected for persons who have undergone such examinations. These high-technology specialty areas, however, provide such extensive diagnostic information that the small accompanying risk is overshadowed by the high standard of medical care. For example, if a study produces a mortality risk of one per million and a yield of 1% (in terms of saving life), the risk of not performing the procedure is 10,000 times greater than the risk of performing it.

When the risk factors become available, physicians must evaluate the risks associated with a particular procedure compared with the diagnostic information to be gained. Consideration must be given to the various types of examinations (e.g., ultrasound versus x-ray) that can provide the desired diagnostic information. The procedure with the lowest risk should be performed.

Thermal Considerations

For life processes to be maintained, the body temperature must stay within a narrow range. Although a variation of 1° C is tolerable (and indeed common), thermal-mediated fetal abnormalities can result from an elevation of 2.5° C for 2 hours. Avoiding a local rise in temperature above 1° C will ensure that no biological effects are induced.

Acoustic energy is converted to heat as the ultrasound beam passes through tissue. The heat production rate (q) in a small volume is determined by the absorption coefficient of the tissue (α) and the local time-averaged intensity of the ultrasound beam (I'):

12-4

$$q = 0.002\ \alpha I'$$

Heat production rate, absorption coefficient, and intensity are expressed in joules per cubic centimeter per second (J/cm³/s), nepers per centimeter (Np/cm), and milliwatts per square centimeter (mW/cm²). The rate of absorption for most tissues increases linearly with frequency. Variations in the heat production rate occur because of different tissue types and nonuniformity of the ultrasound field.

For example, the initial temperature rise caused by an ultrasound beam (3.5 MHz, 1000 mW/cm² TA intensity) incident on soft tissue is compared with one incident on bone. The heat capacity of a substance is the amount of energy required to raise the temperature 1° C. Dividing the heat production rate by the heat capacity yields the initial temperature rise. Table 12-8 lists the parameters necessary for this calculation. The initial temperature rise is approximately 50 times higher in bone.

The initial rate of temperature rise cannot be maintained. Heat removal by conduction and perfusion quickly slows it. Focused beams create small localized regions of heating. The removal of heat from small volumes is very rapid. Continuous insonation ultimately produces a steady-state condition in which the maximum temperature does not change (Fig. 12-8). Results of experiments quantifying the heating of rat skull bone exposed to a focused ultrasound beam form the basis for thermal models involving the insonation of bone.[15]

■ **Table 12-8** Initial Temperature Rise in Soft Tissue and in Bone*

Tissue Type	Absorption Coefficient (Np/cm/MHz)	Absorption Coefficient at 3.5 MHz (Np/cm)	q (J/cm³/s)	Heat Capacity (J/cm³/°C)	Initial Temperature Rise (°C/s)
Soft tissue	0.05	0.175	0.35	3.8	0.09
Bone	1.5	5.25	10.5	2.5	4.2

*Time averaged intensity is 1000 mW/cm². Transducer frequency is 3.5 MHz.

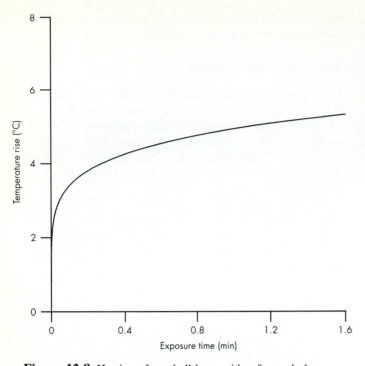

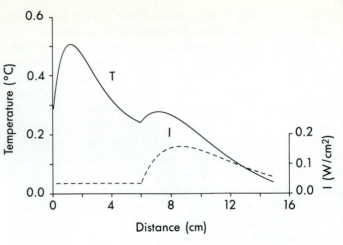

Figure 12-9 Temperature and intensity profiles along the axis of a focused beam. Exposure conditions include frequency 3 MHz, transducer diameter 2 cm, radius of curvature 10 cm, absorption coefficient 0.15 Np/cm, power 0.1 W. (Adapted from American Institute of Ultrasound in Medicine, *J Ultrasound Med* 7:S1, 1988.)

Figure 12-8 Heating of rat skull bone with a focused ultrasound beam. The temperature rise depends primarily on intensity and the cross-sectional area of the beam. The rapid initial rate of temperature rise is not sustained. After the ultrasound beam has been applied for some time, a steady-state condition of maximum temperature rise is approached.

■ **Table 12-9** Predicted In Situ Intensity in mW/cm² (Averaged Over the Focal Area) for Which the Temperature Rise is 1° C or Less

Focal Diameter (mm)	Frequency (MHz)			
	2	4	6	8
1	—	3500	2450	1900
2	—	1100	770	605
3	1070	570	405	320
4	680	365	260	205
5	480	260	185	145
6	365	200	140	115
7	290	160	115	91
8	240	130	94	76

Courtesy American Institute of Ultrasound in Medicine: *J Ultrasound Med* 7:S1, 1988.

By converting acoustic energy into heat, an absorbing object in the ultrasound beam becomes a heat source. Some fraction of the available acoustic energy (e.g., 0.3) is transformed into heat. As the total energy absorbed encompasses a larger and larger area, the efficiency of the beam in heating tissue becomes diminished. The total energy per unit time (the power) incident on an object is found by summing the intensity over the entire region where heat generation is taking place. More simply, in situ power (W') (in milliwatts) is determined by

12-5

$$W' = I'A$$

where A is the effective cross-sectional area (in cm²) of the ultrasound beam. Power then becomes a very important parameter that describes the heating of an object within the ultrasound beam.

Temperature profiles. Temperature profiles along the axis of a focused beam through a homogeneous medium can be generated for a given set of conditions: transducer diameter, frequency, intensity, absorption coefficient of tissue, and degree of perfusion (Fig. 12-9). From the temperature profiles for a wide range of parameters, a conservative estimate of the acoustic power output (W) (in milliwatts) necessary to maintain the maximum temperature rise to less than 1° C at any point along the ultrasonic path is given as

12-6

$$W = \frac{230 \, d}{f}$$

where d is the diameter of the transducer in centimeters, and f is the frequency (in MHz.).[4] Equation 12-6 is applicable for diameters of 1 to 2 cm and frequencies between 2 and 10 MHz. As the total energy absorbed encompasses a larger area, the effectiveness of heating tissue becomes less; therefore an increased diameter of the transducer raises the acoustic power limit (W is proportional to d). The energy of the sound beam is more readily converted to heat as the frequency is increased, which reduces the acoustic power limit (W is inversely proportional to f). The 1° C value of the I(SATA) at the transducer is calculated by dividing the acoustic power limit by the transducer area.

Figure 12-10 Focused transducer operating in the unscanned mode. Note the parameters of beam aperture diameter *(d)*, beam diameter *(w)*, and distance *(z)* from the transducer to the location of interest *(shaded region)*.

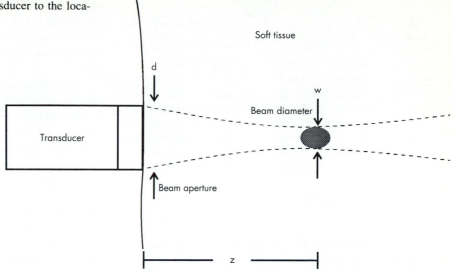

AIUM model to limit fetal temperature rise. For examinations of fetal soft tissues the AIUM[5] has estimated the in situ I(SATA) required to raise the temperature 1° C within the focal zone (Table 12-9). The model employed for these calculations assumes that the diameter of the focal zone is constant for several centimeters and that the absorption coefficient in the region before the focal zone is relatively low compared to the absorption coefficient within the focal zone. The latter condition is important for ensuring that heating in the intervening tissues does not contribute to the temperature rise within the focal zone. As shown in Table 12-9, the in situ I(SATA) decreases as the frequency and diameter of the focal zone increase; that is, the heating of tissue is more effective when high-frequency ultrasound is applied over a large area. The heat energy in a small volume of tissue traversed by the ultrasound beam is readily transferred to the surrounding region, which is at a lower temperature. When the irradiated volume is increased, removal of heat energy becomes less rapid and the local temperature rises.

The model, as presented by the AIUM, does not consider the thermal effect if fetal bone is present in the ultrasound beam. If fetal bone has a high absorption coefficient and exposure times are several seconds in duration, the local temperature rise may be greater than 1° C.

Currently the in situ I(SATA) cannot be measured. By correcting for attenuation along the path from the transducer to the focal zone, however, the in situ I(SATA) at the depth of interest can be estimated. This calculation depends on the thicknesses and attenuation coefficients of the intervening tissues. For example, consider a transducer operating at a frequency of 3 MHz with a focal diameter of 5 mm. Carson[13] has determined that attenuation by the overlying maternal tissues is a function of gestational age. A minimum value of 1.4 dB is obtained for the attenuation at 3 MHz. From Table 12-9, it can be seen that the 1° C in situ I(SATA) is 335 mW/cm², which when corrected for attenuation corresponds to an intensity in water of 462 mW/cm². If the measured free-field I(SATA) is not greater than 462 mW/cm², the temperature rise in vivo should not exceed 1° C.

Acoustic Output Indices

Derating acoustic output. Acoustic output is generally denoted by the power at the radiating source or by an intensity descriptor that characterizes the ultrasonic field. Peak pressure is also used as an output parameter. Intensity (or pressure) is measured at multiple points throughout the ultrasound field in a water medium. To quantify the tissue exposure to ultrasound, the free-field intensity or pressure must be converted to an in situ value.

When soft tissue replaces water along the ultrasonic pathway, a decrease in the intensity is expected because soft tissue has a much higher rate of attenuation. The fractional reduction in intensity caused by attenuation is denoted by the derating factor (R_F):

12-7

$$R_F = 10^{(-0.1 a f z)}$$

where a is the attenuation coefficient in dB/cm/MHz, f is the transducer frequency, and z is the distance along the beam axis between the source and the point of interest (Fig. 12-10). In Table 12-10 the derating factor is shown as a function of frequency and distance. The attenuation coefficient is assigned a value of 0.3 dB/cm/MHz in conjunction with the homogeneous soft tissue model, which is applied in later calculations of acoustic output indices. The derated intensity (I') represents the intensity in soft tissue and is calculated by

12-8

$$I' = I R_F$$

where I is the time-averaged intensity measured in water.

Power and peak pressure also decrease as the ultrasound beam penetrates tissue. A similar calculation can be per-

■ **Table 12-10**   Intensity Derating Factor

Distance (cm)	Frequency (MHz)			
	1	**3**	**5**	**7.5**
1	0.9332	0.8128	0.7080	0.5957
2	0.8710	0.6607	0.5012	0.3548
3	0.8128	0.5370	0.3548	0.2113
4	0.7586	0.4365	0.2512	0.1259
5	0.7080	0.3548	0.1778	0.0750
6	0.6607	0.2884	0.1259	0.0447
7	0.6166	0.2344	0.0891	0.0266
8	0.5754	0.1906	0.0631	0.0158

Attenuation coefficient equals 0.3 dB/cm/MHz.

formed to determine the derated power or peak pressure. The derating factor for power is identical to that specified for intensity in Equation 12-7. The derating factor for pressure is found by taking the square root of the intensity derating factor.

Thermal and mechanical mechanisms. Diagnostic ultrasound has well-established medical applications with known benefits and recognized efficacy. No acute harmful effects have been reported after its use. Two potential interactions through which it may induce biological effects, however, are thermal and mechanical mechanisms. Thermally produced teratological effects have been demonstrated in various laboratory animals, including nonhuman primates.[65,73,103] Mechanical mechanisms are considered to include cavitation. In vitro experiments and animal studies[22,27,44] suggest that cavitation may occur at peak pressures and frequencies used in some diagnostic equipment.

The *Statement on Clinical Safety* by the AIUM recommends prudent use of ultrasound in the clinical environment. The term *prudent use* is not clearly defined. Presumably, objective criteria are applied in the selection of patients for an ultrasound examination. Furthermore, knowledgeable users conduct the examination at minimum intensity levels and exposure times to obtain the desired diagnostic information. The principle of ALARA (as low as reasonably achievable) is applied in other areas, particularly x-ray imaging, to evaluate whether the conditions of use are prudent. If the sonographer is to practice ALARA, than an indication of exposure levels must be provided at the time of examination. Exposure of the patient may be minimized by adjusting acquisition parameters while maintaining the desired information content. Safety guidelines based on scientific knowledge concerning the interactions of ultrasound with tissue must be established to delineate prudent use.

In response to this need the AIUM and the National Electrical Manufacturers Association (NEMA)[4] adopted in 1992 the voluntary standard for display of acoustical output information. Two acoustic output parameters, called the thermal index (TI) and the mechanical index (MI), are defined as indicators of the potential for biological effects. The thermal index, in essence, gives the maximum tem-

perature rise in tissue that can be predicted as a result of the diagnostic examination, and the mechanical index describes the likelihood of cavitation. The agreement among manufacturers to standardize acoustic output information allows sonographers to apply the same safety principles to all diagnostic ultrasound equipment regardless of manufacturer.

Determining acoustic intensity distributions along various tissue paths for diverse equipment and operating modes in use today is an overwhelming task. Thermal and mechanical indices are generated from simplified models using conservative worst-case situations. The indices provide upper limits for the assessment of risk.

A homogeneous tissue model is assumed for soft tissue. Tissue in this model has low fat content and does not contain calcifications or large gas-filled spaces. Thermal conduction is the same as in water. The attenuation coefficient is uniform and equal to a value of 0.3 dB/cm/MHz. The probability of scatter is low, which allows the absorption rate to be represented by the attenuation coefficient. If bone is present, 60% of the incident energy is assumed to be absorbed within the volume of a thin disk.

Temperature elevation depends on power, tissue types, beam width, and scanning mode. *Scanned mode* or *autoscanning* refers to the steering of successive ultrasound pulses through the field of view. In the unscanned mode, emission of ultrasound pulses occurs along a single line of sight, which does not change until the transducer is moved to a new position.

Six thermal models have been developed to mimic possible clinical situations (Table 12-11). Figures 12-11 to 12-16 diagram these models. The homogeneous soft tissue model is used in determining the mechanical index.

The thermal index is defined as the ratio of the in situ acoustic power (W') to the acoustic power required to raise tissue temperature by 1° C (W_{deg}).

12-9

$$TI = \frac{W'}{W_{deg}}$$

Three thermal indices corresponding to soft tissue (TIS), bone (TIB), and cranial bone (TIC) have been developed for application to different examinations (e.g., TIS for abdominal, TIB for fetal and neonatal cephalic, TIC for pediatric and adult cephalic).

A conservative estimate of the acoustic power in milliwatts necessary to produce a 1° C temperature elevation in soft tissue is given by

12-10

$$W_{deg} = \frac{210}{f}$$

where f is the frequency in MHz. This reference power is used in the estimation of thermal indices for situations depicted by Models 1 through 4.

The power necessary to cause a 1° C temperature elevation in bone is considerably less, since acoustic energy

■ **Table 12-11** Thermal Models

Number	Composition	Mode	Specifications
1	Soft tissue	Unscanned	Large aperture
2	Soft tissue	Unscanned	Small aperture
3	Soft tissue	Scanned	Evaluated at surface
4	Soft tissue and bone	Scanned	Soft tissue at surface
5	Soft tissue and bone	Unscanned	Bone at focus
6	Soft tissue and bone	Unscanned or scanned	Bone at surface

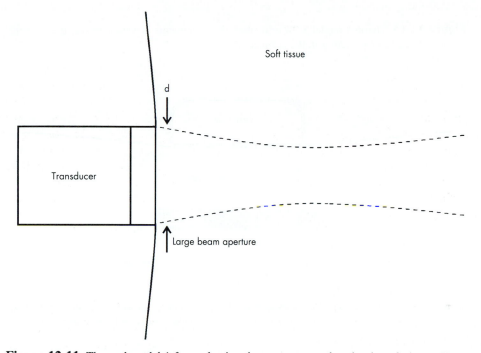

Figure 12-11 Thermal model 1 for evaluating the temperature elevation in soft tissue. Transducer operating in the unscanned mode with the entrance beam area greater than 1 cm².

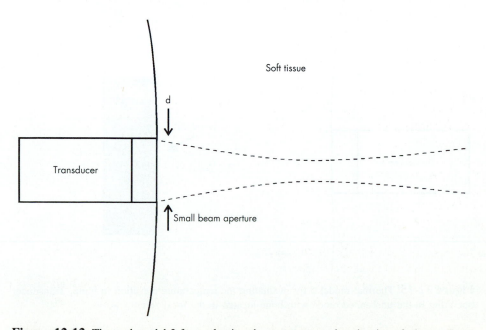

Figure 12-12 Thermal model 2 for evaluating the temperature elevation in soft tissue. Transducer operating in the unscanned mode with the entrance beam area less than 1 cm².

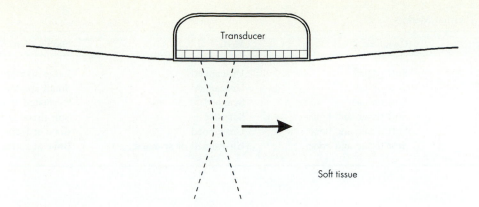

Figure 12-13 Thermal model 3 for evaluating the temperature elevation in soft tissue at the surface. Transducer operating in the scanned mode.

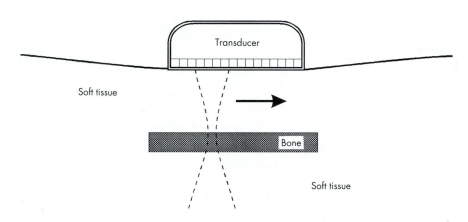

Figure 12-14 Thermal model 4 for evaluating the maximum temperature elevation in soft tissue at the surface. Transducer operating in the scanned mode with bone located in the focal zone.

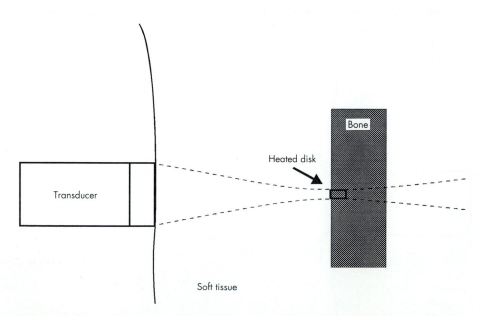

Figure 12-15 Thermal model 5 for evaluating the temperature elevation in bone. Transducer operating in the unscanned mode with bone located in the focal zone.

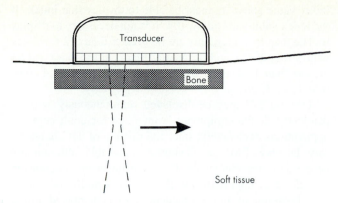

Figure 12-16 Thermal model 6 for evaluating the temperature elevation in bone. Transducer operating in the scanned mode with bone located near the surface.

absorption by bone is higher than by soft tissue. The equation for the reference power becomes

$$12\text{-}11$$

$$W_{deg} = 40\ Kw$$

where K is a beam shape factor that describes the radial nonuniformity of the intensity distribution and w is the beam diameter (in centimeters) at the depth of interest. The beam shape factor is set as 1.0 (uniform beam) or 1.1 (all other cases). For narrow nonautoscanning beams the beam diameter is considered to be no smaller than 0.1 cm. For autoscan systems, beam diameter is replaced by aperture diameter since the beam sweeps across the entrance surface. The reference power in Equation 12-11 is used in estimating the thermal index for situations depicted by Models 5 and 6.

Model 1 (soft tissue, unscanned, large aperture). The entrance area is more than 1 cm². At some distance from the transducer the beam may be focused. If the beam area is less than 1 cm², power controls the temperature rise. For broader beams, intensity controls the temperature rise. The derated intensity over a designated area (I′ × 1 cm²) and derated power (W′) are evaluated along the beam axis. At each point the minimum of these two functions, which determines the parameter responsible for heating, is designated the power parameter. The maximum power parameter for all points causes the maximum temperature increase and is used in Equation 12-9 to estimate the thermal index (TIS):

$$12\text{-}12$$

$$TIS = \frac{[(W'(z),\ I'(z)\ \times\ 1\ cm^2)min]max}{\dfrac{210}{f}}$$

The verbal explanation of this equation is difficult to express in clear and unencumbered language. A TIS calculation using profiles of the derated power and intensity functions is illustrated in Table 12-12.

Model 2 (soft tissue, unscanned, small aperture). For a small aperture in which the entrance area is less than 1 cm², the in situ power is maximal at the surface and equal to the

■ Table 12-12   Calculation of the Thermal Index (TIS) (Model 1)*

z (cm)	W′ (mW)	I′ × 1 cm² (mW)	Power Parameter (mW)
1	70.8	40	40
2	50.1	45	45†
3	35.5	40	35.5
4	25.1	60	25.1
5	17.8	150	17.8
6	12.6	125	12.6
7	8.9	60	8.9
8	6.3	6	6.0

*Focused transducer (weak focus); Transducer frequency is 5 MHz; acoustic source power equals 100 mW.
†Maximum power parameter is 45 mW.

$$TIS = \frac{45}{\dfrac{210}{5}} = 1.1$$

source acoustic power, W_0. The thermal index (TIS) is estimated as

$$12\text{-}13$$

$$TIS = \frac{W_0}{\dfrac{210}{f}}$$

Model 3 (soft tissue, scanned) and Model 4 (soft tissue and bone, scanned). Maximum temperature rise occurs at the surface for scanned modes such as real-time B-mode and color Doppler. The in situ power is set equal to the source acoustic power; however, if the active transmitting area is large (more than 1 cm²), a modification is applied to the measurement of source power. Power for the central portion of the radiating surface is determined over a scan width of 1 cm. In this measurement format, power is designated W_{01}. The thermal index for these models is

$$12\text{-}14$$

$$TIS\ (or\ TIB) = \frac{W_{01}}{\dfrac{210}{f}}$$

Model 5 (soft tissue, unscanned, bone at focus). Bone is assumed to be located in the focal region, where the product of the derated intensity and power is maximal (worst case situation). The diameter of the beam in the focal region is defined by the ratio of the derated power to the derated intensity:

$$12\text{-}15$$

$$w = \sqrt{\frac{4\ W'}{\pi\ I'}}$$

Substituting this expression for w and with 1.1 as the beam shape factor in Equation 12-11,

$$W_{deg} = 50 \sqrt{\frac{W'}{I'}}$$ 12-16

The in situ power at the focal region is the derated power, W'. Thus

$$TIB = \frac{\sqrt{W' I'}}{50}$$ 12-17

In the case of small-diameter beams a minimum value of 0.227 W' is assigned to TIB.

Model 6 (bone at surface, scanned or unscanned). The transducer is placed in contact with the head of an adult or infant. The sound beam crosses a thin layer of skin before striking bone. Because little attenuation occurs, R_F is essentially unity. The area of bone exposed is the same as the active area of the transducer (both scanned and unscanned modes). Summing the time averaged intensity over the active area yields the acoustic power at the source, W_o. The in situ power is considered equal to the transmitted power. The thermal index formula for this model is

$$TIC = \frac{W_o}{40 \, d}$$ 12-18

where d is the aperture diameter (in centimeters).

Mechanical index. The pulsed ultrasound wave, consisting of multiple cycles, causes large fluctuations in pressure as it moves through the medium (Fig. 12-5). Cavitation is more likely to occur at high pressures and low frequencies. The cavitation threshold under optimal conditions with pulsed ultrasound is predicted by the ratio of the peak pressure to the square root of the frequency.

For a specific transmit pattern the mechanical index (MI) is defined as

$$MI = \frac{P_r'}{\sqrt{f}}$$ 12-19

where p_r' is the derated peak rarefactional pressure (in megapascals, (MPa) and f is the frequency (in MHz). A factor of $(1 \text{ MHz})^{0.5}/(1 \text{ MPa})$ is implied; thus the mechanical index is expressed as a dimensionless quantity.

Measurement of peak rarefactional pressure is performed in water for the transducer under well-defined operating conditions. The location of measurement is specified at the point along the beam axis where the pulse intensity integral is a maximum. The pulse intensity integral is the total energy per unit area carried by the wave during the time duration of the pulse. Applying the homogeneous tissue model, the measured peak rarefactional pressure is derated using the factor R_F.

Display of output indices. The following display guidelines apply to all thermal and mechanical indices. Ultrasound equipment, which has the potential to produce an index value above 1, must be able to display that index. If the index value falls below 0.4, it is not necessary to display it. The display increments are no greater than 0.2 for index values less than 1 and no greater than 1.0 for index values greater than 1. Typical display index values are 0.4, 0.6, 0.8, 1, 2, 3, and 4.

TIS and TIB may be displayed simultaneously or independently. If the equipment is intended for adult cephalic applications exclusively, only the display of TIC is necessary. Display of MI and TI should be possible, although not necessarily simultaneously, for a transducer that operates in a mode other than real-time B-mode. For multimode ultrasound equipment, the mechanical index is displayed during real-time B-mode imaging and the thermal index during other modes—provided the above display criteria are met.

Output indices as risk indicators. The determination of thermal index is a conservative estimate based on a worst-case scenario. Although the calculated temperature elevation is subject to many uncertainties, it provides an upper limit of the actual temperature rise from typical clinical examinations. Insonation of long duration is necessary for achieving the steady-state temperature rise predicted by the thermal index.

Cavitation is generally believed to be a threshold phenomenon. No adverse effects caused by it have been observed in humans, including fetuses exposed to ultrasound at typical diagnostic output levels. By tracking peak rarefactional pressure and frequency the mechanical index provides an estimate of the potential for mechanical biological effects. Even if cavitation does occur at isolated sites, however, the affected area is extremely small and a small number of cells may be killed. The only situation in which the loss of a few cells would be of concern is when the subject is a fetus.

The acoustic output indices serve as risk indicators. If the index value is less than 1, the possibility of adverse effects or cavitation is low. If the index value is greater than 1, the physician must evaluate the risks associated with a particular ultrasound procedure against the diagnostic information to be gained.

An additional protective measure is to limit the exposure time when the thermal index exceeds 1. The maximum safe exposure duration is $4^{(6-TI)}$ minutes.[73,103] However, if the patient is febrile, the exposure time limit is reduced by incrementing TI by 1 for each degree centigrade the body temperature exceeds 37°.

Clinical Efficacy in Obstetrics

Because ultrasound yields excellent anatomical visualization and is generally considered to be without harmful effects, it has become widely used in the practice of obstetrics. Although it is assumed to contribute to the improved management and outcome of a pregnancy, its clinical efficacy has not been demonstrated in randomized research studies. This does not mean that no benefit is achieved, merely that proper clinical trials have yet to be conducted to assess the benefit.

■ Reasons for employing diagnostic ultrasound imaging in pregnancy

- Estimation of gestational age
- Evaluation of fetal growth
- Determination of placental location
- Detection of fetal death
- Location of pregnancy
- Determination of fetal presentation
- Determination of fetal number
- Detection of anomalies
- Adjunct to placement of cervical cerclage
- Suspected hydatidiform mole
- Adjunct to intrauterine transfusion
- Determination of source of vaginal bleeding
- Biophysical evaluation for fetal well-being after 28 weeks of gestational age
- Ajunct to amniocentesis
- Evaluation of pelvic mass
- Suspected polyhydramnios or oligohydramnios
- Suspected abruptio placenta
- Evaluation of fetal condition in late registrants for prenatal care

As a guide for practitioners, the National Institutes of Health (NIH)[74] reviewed the available scientific information and concluded that ultrasound has clinical benefit for certain applications, which are listed in the box. Although ultrasonography in these circumstances is not mandatory, it is appropriate when the information gained will influence prenatal care.

Currently the routine screening of every pregnancy is not recommended by the NIH. Ultrasonography during pregnancy should be performed for a specific medical indication and should be discouraged for the sole purpose of viewing the fetus by the mother or determining its sex (these are potential secondary benefits of a medically indicated examination). Additionally, feedback—in the form of viewing the monitor screen with explanation of the images—may improve maternal perception of the fetus and maternal-infant bonding. The maternal attitude can influence fetal outcome by causing prenatal behavioral changes (e.g., cessation of smoking). Education and commercial demonstrations of ultrasound imaging during pregnancy without medical benefit are inappropriate.[74]

Education and Training

In a perceptive editorial in the *Journal of Ultrasound in Medicine,* Ziskin[102] advocates educating physicians and sonographers as the major safeguard for patients. Well-designed instrumentation to limit exposure of the patient is an alternative measure. However, equipment safeguards can be bypassed by the operator. Knowledgeable users conduct the examination at the minimum intensity levels necessary to obtain the desired diagnostic information. In addition, the examination time is usually reduced. More important, misdiagnoses because of lack of education, inexperience, and poor examination technique are more likely to cause harm than is the potential damage from ultrasound itself.

The diagnostic efficacy of ultrasound is strongly operator dependent. Unfortunately, only about half of obstetric and gynecological sonographers are certified. The training and education requirements for physicians are not standardized. The ability of physicians to perform and interpret ultrasound examinations varies considerably. Minimum standards of education and training for clinical users of ultrasound (both physician and sonographer) must be established by regulatory agencies or by medical specialty societies.

Potential Exposure Limits

An assessment of risk facilitates the development of a safety program. When clinical studies are published, they must include a statement of the exposure conditions. These data will assist in the overall evaluation of risk. Lack of such information has in the past inhibited the development of a comprehensive theory of biological effects. It is to be hoped that the necessary parameters will become standardized; but in the meantime frequency, the I(SPTA) in water at maximum power, the attenuator setting, and the number of examinations and time duration of each examination should all be specified.

Developing equipment specifications may, in the future, limit intensity, PRF, and pulse duration for various types of scanners. Diagnostic units operating below the transient cavitation threshold will ensure that this type of cavitation does not occur. Such a restriction would be one possible consideration for an intensity limit on some types of diagnostic equipment, particularly obstetric units.

In the future it is also possible, though not probable, that permissible exposure levels for various ultrasound procedures will be established by regulatory agencies. (The diagnostic yield for these procedures is generally considered to be quite high, and the risk extremely low. If there were adverse effects, they would likely have become apparent as a result of the many millions of examinations that have already been performed.) Ill-conceived or inappropriately applied regulations, however, can easily interfere with the development of new procedures and instrumentation in this rapidly expanding field and must be avoided. Nevertheless, recommended intensity levels and exposure times for various examinations would be helpful for the physician in clinical practice, creating a performance standardization and reducing the overall risk of ultrasound on the population.

SUMMARY

Ultrasound is not a form of ionizing radiation. This attractive feature has resulted in its extensive use for the evaluation of pregnancy, fetal age, and fetal condition. Ultrasound also has demonstrated applications in abdominal and cardiac diagnostic studies. However, harmful effects are possible any time the human body is probed using energy that is ultimately deposited in the body, and ultrasound is no exception.

Characterization of the ultrasound beam is essential if the relationship between induced effects and the ultrasonic dose is to be described in a consistent and predictable manner. The most important beam parameters are intensity and pressure. Intensity exhibits wide spatial and temporal variation. Shorthand descriptors have been developed that designate a peak or average value with respect to both space and time. Although various combinations are possible, the most commonly used are SPTP, SPTA, and SATA. Pressure also fluctuates over a wide range, but ultrasound beams are usually denoted by a single pressure descriptor (called the peak negative pressure).

Three mechanisms for the interaction of ultrasound with matter have been identified: mechanical, thermal, and cavitation. These physical processes may give rise to the secondary actions of microstreaming and altered chemical reaction rates.

Early studies using high intensity levels and long exposure times reported numerous biological effects—including protein denaturation, changes in membrane permeability, membrane rupture, chromosomal breakage, nerve block, cataracts, brain lesions, and fetal developmental anomalies. Much of this work lacks the necessary dosimetric details.

During in vitro studies the particular molecule of interest is usually dissolved in aqueous media and then exposed to ultrasound. This experimental setup does not mimic the physical environment of the biomolecule in nature and thus creates the possibility of introducing microbubbles into the system, which may enhance cavitation. These types of studies are useful for identifying biomolecules sensitive to ultrasound, the type of damage induced, and the mechanisms of interaction; but their applicability to the assessment of risk is limited.

Although animal studies provide a good indication of potential damage and can aid in the establishment of reasonable levels of safety, they possess certain limitations when extrapolated to humans. Species sensitivity variation has been demonstrated, and there is no assurance that humans will respond in the same manner as certain species of animals. The amount of attenuation and the relative target size are also factors that must be considered. Nevertheless, dose-effect observations in animals are critically important to determining the mechanisms of interaction and assessing the risk in humans.

At current diagnostic intensity levels and scan times, no biological effects of ultrasound have been observed in humans. The AIUM has reviewed available data and (in essence) established intensity guidelines. A safe level of 100 mW/cm² I(SPTA) is often mentioned in the literature. The adoption of 1 W/cm² I(SPTA) as a safe level for focused beams by the AIUM has also become widely accepted. The recent observation of damage from cavitation at a peak pressure threshold of 1 MPa will necessitate a reevaluation of the AIUM statement. Newly developed thermal and mechanical acoustic output indices offer a new approach to controlling ultrasonic exposure of patients and providing assurance of safety.

Nevertheless, sufficient data do not exist to state categorically that ultrasound is absolutely safe. More complete risk assessment awaits epidemiological surveys involving large numbers of persons followed for many years. The continued use of diagnostic ultrasound examinations in obstetrics and other areas is justified, because the potential risk appears to be minimal and the benefit high. This does not imply that ultrasound should be employed indiscriminantly. The selection of patients should be a result of well-defined conscious processes, and steps should be taken to minimize exposure during the examination.

Both the NCRP and the AIUM have published reports summarizing the biological effects of ultrasound. In addition to these, the reader is referred to several review articles in the literature.*

*References 5, 7, 14, 38, 63, 72, 74, 75, 86, 103, 104.

■ ■ ■ **REVIEW QUESTIONS** ■ ■ ■

1. Rank the following intensity descriptors from highest to lowest: SPTP, SATP, SATA, SPTA.
2. Name the three mechanisms of interaction of ultrasound with matter.
3. Why should reports of experimental studies include irradiation conditions and specifications of beam parameters?
4. Why are epidemiological studies important for risk assessment?
5. Why is it essential to identify harmful effects and corresponding risk factors from fetal exposure?
6. According to the AIUM's evaluation of scientific data in 1987, no biological effects have been observed in mammalian systems below an intensity level of _____ for unfocused beams and _____ for focused beams. How is this intensity specified?
7. What are the units for peak negative pressure?
   a. Megapascal
   b. Watt/cm²
   c. Watt
   d. Megahertz
8. The thermal index indicates
   a. Maximum temperature rise in tissue
   b. Minutes of exposure time before heating is too great
   c. Seconds of exposure time before heating is too great
   d. Acoustic power in milliwatts
9. The mechanical index gives the likelihood of
   a. Beat frequency
   b. Cavitation
   c. Thermal damage
   d. Rotational motion
10. Damage induced by the thermal mechanism shows a threshold.
    a. True
    b. False
11. Routine screening of every pregnancy is recommended by the National Institutes of Health.
    a. True
    b. False
12. Suppose a patient asks you if a diagnostic ultrasound examination is "safe." What is your reply?

BIBLIOGRAPHY

1. Abdulla U, Dewhurst CJ, Campbell C, et al: Effects of diagnostic ultrasound on maternal and fetal chromosomes, *Lancet* 2:829, 1971.

2. Akamatsu N: Ultrasound irradiation effects on preimplantation embryos, *Acta Obstet Gynaecol Jpn* 33:969, 1981.

3. American Institute of Ultrasound in Medicine: Safety standard for diagnostic ultrasound equipment: Appendix B—Survey of exposure levels from current diagnostic ultrasound systems, *J Ultrasound Med* 2:S32, 1983.

4. American Institute of Ultrasound in Medicine and National Electrical Manufacturers Association: Standard for real-time display of thermal and mechanical indices on diagnostic ultrasound equipment, Rockville MD, 1992, AIUM-NEMA.

5. American Institute of Ultrasound in Medicine: Bioeffects considerations for the safety of diagnostic ultrasound, *J Ultrasound Med* 7:S1, 1988.

6. Apfel RE, Holland CK: Gauging the likelihood of cavitation from short pulse, low–duty cycle diagnostic ultrasound, *Ultrasound Med Biol* 17:179, 1991.

7. Baker ML, Dalrymple GV: Biological effects of diagnostic ultrasound: a review, *Radiology* 126:479, 1978.

8. Bakketeig LS, et al: Randomised controlled trial of ultrasonographic screening on pregnancy, *Lancet* 2:207, 1984.

9. Barnett SB, Miller MW, Cox C, Carstensen EL: Increased sister chromatid exchanges in Chinese hamster ovary cells exposed to high intensity pulsed ultrasound, *Ultrasound Med Biol* 14:397, 1988.

10. Bennett MJ, Little G, Dewhurst J: Predictive value of ultrasound measurement in early pregnancy: a randomized controlled trial, *Br J Obstet Gynecol* 89:338, 1982.

11. Bernstine RL: Safety studies with ultrasonic Doppler technic: a clinical follow-up of patients and tissue culture study, *Obstet Gynecol* 34:707, 1969.

12. Carmichael AJ, Mossoba MM, Riesz P, Christman CL: Free radical production in aqueous solutions exposed to simulated ultrasonic diagnostic conditions, *IEEE Trans UFFC* 33:148, 1986.

13. Carson PL: Medical ultrasound fields and exposure measurements. In *Proceedings of the twenty-second annual meeting of the National Council on Radiation Protection and Measurements*, Bethesda, Md, 1988, NCRP Publications.

14. Carstensen EL: Acoustic cavitation and the safety of diagnostic ultrasound, *Ultrasound Med Biol* 13:597, 1987.

15. Carstensen EL, Child SZ, Norton S, Nyborg WL: Ultrasonic heating of the skull, *J Acoust Soc Am* 87:1310, 1990.

16. Carstensen EL, Flynn HG: The potential for transient cavitation with microsecond pulses of ultrasound, *Ultrasound Med Biol* 8:L720, 1982.

17. Carstensen EL, Hartman C, Child SZ, et al: Test for kidney hemorrhage following exposure to intense, pulsed ultrasound, *Ultrasound Med Biol* 16:681, 1990.

18. Cartwright RA, et al: Ultrasound examinations in pregnancy and childhood cancer, *Lancet* 2:999, 1984.

19. Cataldo FL, Miller MW, Gregory WD, Carstensen EL: A description of ultrasonically induced chromosomal anomalies in *Vicia faba,* Radiat Biol 13:211, 1973.

20. Child SZ, Carstensen EL, David H: A test for the effects of low-temporal-average intensity, pulsed ultrasound on the rat fetus, *Exp Cell Biol* 52:207, 1984.

21. Child SZ, Carstensen EL, Gates AH, Hall WJ: Testing for the teratogenicity of pulsed ultrasound in mice, *Ultrasound Med Biol* 14:493, 1988.

22. Child SZ, Hartman CL, Schery LA, Carstensen EL: Lung damage from exposure to pulsed ultrasound, *Ultrasound Med Biol* 16:817, 1990.

23. Child SZ, Hoffman D, Norton S, et al: Pulsed ultrasound and the hyperbarically exposed mouse fetus, *Ultrasound Med Biol* 17:367, 1991.

24. Ciaravino V, Miller MW, Carstensen EL, Dalecki D: Lack of effect of high-intensity pulsed ultrasound on sister chromatid exchange and in vitro Chinese hamster ovary cell viability, *Ultrasound Med Biol* 11:491, 1985.

25. Coakley WT, Dunn F: Degradation of DNA in high intensity focused ultrasonic fields at 1 MHz, *J Acoust Soc Am* 50:1539, 1971.

26. Coakley WT, Dunn F: Interaction of megahertz ultrasound and biological polymers. In Reid JM, Sikov MR, editors: *Interaction of ultrasound and biological tissues,* HEW Publication (FDA) 73-8008:43, Washington, DC, 1972, Government Printing Office.

27. Delius M, Enders G, Heine C, et al: Biological effects of shock waves: lung hemorrhage by shock waves in dogs—pressure dependence, *Ultrasound Med Biol* 13:61, 1987.

28. Doida Y, Miller MW, Cox C, Church CC: Confirmation of an ultrasound-induced mutation in two in vitro mammalian cell lines, *Ultrasound Med Biol* 16:699, 1990.

29. Dooley DA, Sacks PG, Miller MW: Production of thymine base damage in ultrasound-exposed EMT6 mouse mammary sarcoma cells, *Radiation Res* 97:71, 1984.

30. Duck FA: Output data from European studies, *Ultrasound Med Biol* 15(Suppl 1):61, 1989.

31. Dunn F, Fry FJ: Ultrasonic threshold dosage for the mammalian central nervous system, *IEEE Trans Biomed Eng* 18:253, 1971.

32. Dyson M, Pond JB, Joseph J, Warwick R: The simulation of tissue regeneration by means of ultrasound, *Clin Sci* 35:273, 1968.

33. Environmental Health Directorate: *Safety code 23: Guidelines for the safe use of ultrasound, I, Medical and paramedical applications,* Report 8-EHD-59, Environmental Health Directorate of Canada, Health Protection Branch, Ottawa, 1981.

34. Falus M, Koranyi G, Sobel M, et al: Follow-up studies on infants examined by ultrasound during the fetal age, *Orv Hetil* 13:2119, 1972.

35. Federal Food and Drug Administration: *510(k) Guide for preparing reports on radiation safety of diagnostic ultrasound equipment,* Rockville Md, 1993, Center for Devices and Radiological Health.

36. Flynn HG: Physics of acoustic cavitation in liquids. In Mason WP, editor: *Physical acoustics,* New York, 1964, Academic Press.

37. Frizzel LA, Lee CS, Aschenbach PD, et al: Involvement of ultrasonically induced cavitation in the production of hind limb paralysis of the mouse neonate. *J Acoust Soc Am* 74:1062, 1983.

38. Fry FJ: Biological effects of ultrasound: a review, *IEEE Trans Biomed Eng* 67:604, 1979.

39. Fry FJ, Kossoff G, Eggleton RC, Dunn F: Threshold ultrasonic dosages for structural changes in mammalian brain, *J Acoust Soc Am* 48:1413, 1970.

40. Fu YK, Miller MW, Lange CS, et al: Ultrasound lethality to synchronous and asynchronous chinese hamster V-79 cells, *Ultrasound Med Biol* 6:39, 1980.

41. Galperin-Lemaitre H, Kirsch-Volders M, Levi S: Fragmentation of purified mammalian DNA molecules by ultrasound below human therapeutic doses, *Humangenetik* 29:61, 1975.

42. Gross DR, Miller DL, Williams AR: A search for ultrasonic cavitation within the canine cardiovascular system. *Ultrasound Med Biol* 11:85, 1985.

43. Harrison GH, Balcer-Kubiczek EK: Pulsed ultrasound and neoplastic transformation in vitro, *Ultrasound Med Biol* 17:627, 1991.

44. Hartman C, Child SZ, Mayer R, et al: Lung damage from exposure to the fields of an electrohydraulic lithotripter, *Ultrasound Med Biol* 16:675, 1990.

45. Hartman C, Cox CA, Brewer L, et al: Effects of lithotripter fields on development of chick embryos, *Ultrasound Med Biol* 16:581, 1990.

46. Hawley SA, Macleod RM, Dunn F: Degradation of DNA by intense, noncavitating ultrasound, *J Acoust Soc Am* 35:1285, 1963.

47. Hellman LM, Duffus GM, Donald I, Sunden B: Safety of diagnostic ultrasound in obstetrics, *Lancet* 1:1133, 1970.

48. Hill CR: Ultrasonic exposure thresholds for changes in cells and tissues, *J Acoust Soc Am* 52:667, 1972.

49. Ikeuchi T, Sasaki M, Oshimura M, et al: Ultrasound and embryonic chromosomes, *Br Med J* 1:112, 1973.

50. Kaufman GE: Mutagenicity of ultrasound in cultured mammalian cells, *Ultrasound Med Biol* 11:497, 1985.

51. Kinner Wilson LM, Waterhouse JAH: Obstetric ultrasound and childhood malignancies, *Lancet* 2:997, 1984.

52. Kohorn ET, Pritcheard JW, Hobbins JC: The safety of clinical ultrasound examination, *Obstet Gynecol* 29:272, 1967.

53. Kremkau FW: Cancer therapy with ultrasound: a historical review, *J Clin Ultrasound* 7:287, 1979.

54. Liebeskind D, et al: Diagnostic ultrasound: effects on the DNA and growth patterns of animal cells, *Radiology* 131:177, 1979.

55. Liebeskind D, Bases R, Mendez F, et al: Sister chromatid exchanges in human lymphocytes after exposure to diagnostic ultrasound, *Science* 205:1273, 1979.

56. Lyon MF, Simpson GM: An investigation into the possible genetic hazards of ultrasound, *Br J Radiol* 47:712, 1974.

57. Lyons EA, Coggrave-Toms M: Long-term follow-up study of children exposed to ultrasound in utero. *Proceedings of the twenty-fourth annual meeting of the American Institute of Ultrasound Medicine,* Montreal, August 1979.

58. Lyons EA, Coggrave M, Brown RE: Follow-up study in children exposed to ultrasound in utero: analysis of height and weight in the first six years of life, *Proceedings of the twenty-fifth annual meeting of the American Institute of Ultrasound in Medicine,* New Orleans, September 1980.

59. Lyons EA, Dyke C, Toms M, Cheang M: In utero exposure to diagnostic ultrasound: a six-year followup, *Radiology* 166:687, 1988.

60. MacIntosh IJC, Brown RC, Coakley WT: Ultrasound and in vitro chromosome abberrations, *Br J Radiol* 48:230, 1975.

61. MacIntosh IJC, Davey DA: Chromosome aberrations induced by an ultrasonic fetal pulse detector, *Br Med J* 4:92, 1970.

62. MacIntosh IJC, Davey DA: Relationship between intensity of ultrasound and induction of chromosome aberrations, *Br J Radiol* 45:320, 1972.

63. Martin AO: Can ultrasound cause genetic damage? *J Clin Ultrasound* 12:11, 1984.

64. Merritt CRB: Bioeffects and the safety of diagnostic ultrasound, *Appl Radiol* 22:50, 1993.

65. Miller DL: Update on safety of diagnostic ultrasonography, *J Clin Ultrasound* 19:531, 1991.

66. Miller DL, Thomas RM, Frazier ME: Single strand breaks in CHO cell DNA induced by ultrasonic cavitation in vitro, *Ultrasound Med Biol* 17:401, 1991.

67. Miller MW, Azadniv M, Cox C, Miller WM: Lack of induced increase in sister chromatid exchanges in human lymphocytes exposed to in vivo therapeutic ultrasound, *Ultrasound Med Biol* 17:81, 1991.

68. Miller MW, Azadniv M, Pettit SE, et al: Sister chromatid exchanges in Chinese hamster ovary cells exposed to high intensity pulsed ultrasound: inability to confirm previous positive results, *Ultrasound Med Biol* 15:255, 1989.

69. Moore R Jr, Barrick M, Hamilton P: Effects of sonic radiation on growth and development, *Am J Epidemiol* 116:571, 1982 (abstract).

70. Moore RM, Diamond EL, Cavalieri RL: The relationship of birth weight and intrauterine diagnostic ultrasound exposure, *Obstet Gynecol* 71:513, 1988.

71. Morris SM, Palmer CG, Fry FJ, Johnson LK: Effect of ultrasound on human leucocytes: sister chromatid exchange analysis, *Ultrasound Med Biol* 4:253, 1978.

72. *Biological effects of ultrasound: mechanisms and clinical implications,* NCRP Report 74, Bethesda Md, 1983, National Council on Radiation Protection and Measurements.

73. *Exposure criteria for medical diagnostic ultrasound. I. Criteria based on thermal mechanisms.* NCRP Report 113, Bethesda Md, 1992, National Council on Radiation Protection and Measurements.

74. National Institutes of Health: Diagnostic ultrasound in pregnancy: report of a consensus development conference, *DHHS, NIH Publ* 84-667, 1984.

75. Nyborg WL: Scientifically based safety criteria for ultrasonography, *J Ultrasound Med* 11:425, 1992.

76. O'Brien WD Jr: Biological effects of ultrasound. In Fullerton GD, Zagzebski JA (eds): *Medical physics of CT and ultrasound: tissue imaging and characterization.* New York, 1980, American Institute of Physics.

77. O'Brien WD Jr: Safety of ultrasound with selective emphasis for obstetrics, *Seminars in Ultrasound, CT, and MR* 5:105, 1984.

78. Peacock AR, Pritchard NJ: Some biophysical aspects of ultrasound, *Prog Biophys Mol Biol* 18:185, 1968.

79. Pizzarello DJ, Vivino A, Madden B, et al: The effect of pulsed low power ultrasound on growing tissues, I, Developing mammalian and insect tissue, *Exp Cell Biol* 46:179, 1978.

80. Ritenour ER, Braaton M, Harrison GH, et al: Absence of mutagenic effects of continuous and pulsed ultrasound in cultured A$_L$ human-hamster hybrid cells, *Ultrasound Med Biol* 17:921, 1991.

81. Savitz DA: Basic concepts of epidemiology. In Hendee WR (ed): *Health effects of low-level radiation,* East Norwalk Conn, 1984, Appleton-Century-Crofts, pp 47-56.

82. Scheidt PC, Stanley F, Bryla DA: One-year follow-up of infants exposed to ultrasound in utero, *Am J Obstet Gynecol* 131:743, 1978.

83. Serr DM, Padeh B, Zabat H, et al: Studies on the effect of ultrasonic waves on the fetus. In Huntington PJ, Beard RW, Hutten EE, Seapes JW (eds): *Proceedings of the second European congress on perinatal medicine,* London, 1971, The Congress.

84. Shoji R, Momma R, Shimizu T, Matsuda S: An experimental study on the effects of low-intensity ultrasound on developing mouse embryos, *Hokkaido Igaku Zasshi* 18:51, 1971.

85. Shoji R, Momma R, Shimizu T, Matsuda S: Experimental studies on the effect of ultrasound on mouse embryos, *Teratology* 6:119, 1972.

86. Sikov MR: Effects of ultrasound on development, II, Studies in mammalian species: an overview, *J Ultrasound Med* 5:651, 1986.

87. Stark CR, Orleans M, Haverkamp AD, Murphy J: Short- and long-term risks after exposure to diagnostic ultrasound in utero, *Obstet Gynecol* 63:194, 1984.

88. Stella M, Trevison L, Montaldi A, et al: Induction of sister chromatid exchanges in human lymphocytes exposed to in vitro and in vivo therapeutic ultrasound, *Mutation Res* 138:75, 1984.

89. Steward HF, Stratmeyer ME: An overview of ultrasound: theory, measurement, medical applications, and biological effects, *HHS Pub (FDA)* 82-8190, 1982.

90. Takabayashi YA, Sato S, Sato A, Suzuki M: Effects of pulse-wave ultrasonic irradiation on mouse embryo, *Cho-Onpa Igaku* 8:286, 1981.

91. Taylor KJW, Dyson M: Toxicity studies on the interaction of ultrasound on embryonic and adult tissues. In deVliger M, White DN, McCready VR (eds): Ultrasonics in medicine: Proceedings of the second world congress on ultrasound in Medicine (Amsterdam), *Excerpta Medica*, New York, 1974, American Elsevier, pp 353-359.

92. Thacker J: Ultrasound and mammalian DNA, *Lancet*, 2:770, 1975.

93. Ter Harr GR, Daniels S: Evidence for ultrasonically induced cavitation in vivo, *Phys Med Biol* 26:1145, 1981.

94. Warwick R, Pond JB, Woodward B, Connolly C: Hazards of diagnostic ultrasonography: a study with mice, *IEEE Trans Sonics Ultrasound* 5417:158, 1970.

95. Wegner RD, Meyenburg M: The effects of diagnostic ultrasonography on the frequencies of sister chromatid exchanges in Chinese hamster cells and human lymphocytes, *J Ultrasound Med* 1:355, 1982.

96. Wegner RD, Obe G, Meyenburg M: Has diagnostic ultrasound mutagenic effects? *Hum Genet* 56:95, 1980.

97. WFUMB: Second world federation of ultrasound in medicine and biology symposium on safety and standardization in medical ultrasound, *Ultrasound Med Biol* 15:S1, 1989.

98. Wladimiroff JW, Laar J: Ultrasonic measurement of fetal body size: a randomized controlled trial, *Acta Obstet Gynecol Scand* 59:177, 1980.

99. Yip YP, Capriotti C, Norbash SG, et al: Ultrasound effects on cell proliferation and migration of chick motoneutrons, *Ultrasound Med Biol* 17:55, 1991.

100. Zagzebski JA: Acoustic output of ultrasound equipment: summary of data reported to the AIUM, *Ultrasound Med Biol* 15:S55, 1989.

101. Ziskin MC: Survey of patient exposure to diagnostic ultrasound. In Reid JM, Sikov MR (eds): Interaction of ultrasound and biological tissues, *HEW Pub (FDA)* 73:8008, 1972.

102. Ziskin MC: The prudent use of diagnostic ultrasound, *J Ultrasound Med* 6:415, 1987.

103. Ziskin MC: Update on the safety of ultrasound in obstetrics, *Semin Roentgenol* 25:294, 1990.

104. Ziskin MC, Petitti DB: Epidemiology of human exposure to ultrasound: a critical review, *Ultrasound Med Biol* 14:91, 1988.

Quality Control and Acceptance Testing

■ K E Y   T E R M S ■

AIUM test object
Axial resolution
Belt phantom
Dead zone
Distortion
Feedback microbalance
Flow phantom
Focal zone
Gray scale adjustment
Horizontal distance
    measurement

Hydrophone
Lateral resolution
Pressure profile
Sensitivity
String phantom
Tissue equivalent
Uniformity
Vertical depth measurement

An effective quality-control (QC) program is essential for the proper operation of a medical diagnostic ultrasound imaging department. A comprehensive and routinely performed program is required to obtain high-quality images consistently and to ensure proper equipment performance. Cost efficiency is improved and patient inconvenience is reduced because fewer examinations are repeated. Earlier chapters in this text have discussed some of the important parameters (axial and lateral resolution, frequency, bandwidth, power, intensity, and sensitivity) that affect the overall performance of an ultrasound system. The purpose of this chapter is to discuss the ways in which these parameters and others can be measured to ensure proper functioning of equipment. Different phantoms and test objects are described. An example of a QC program that can be adapted to the needs of a particular institution is detailed.

Acceptance testing, another very important area of concern, is the initial evaluation of equipment after installation to determine whether it is operating properly and whether it meets specifications. Special-acceptance test procedures also are discussed but may be limited in application because of the cost or difficulty of using.

PURPOSE OF QUALITY CONTROL

A QC program is essential for the proper operation of ultrasound equipment on a long-term basis. It must be simple to implement and easy to maintain. One that is overambitious in terms of complexity or frequency of testing will often cease to be performed at all. At the same time, to be meaningful, it must be comprehensive and capable of thoroughly testing the equipment. This chapter describes a QC program for real-time ultrasound equipment. With slight modifications, it also can be used for other scanning modes. Special test procedures are included for the quality control of Doppler devices. Long-term performance is evaluated by periodically testing ultrasound equipment under well-defined conditions. The instrument settings must be maintained at the same values, and a standard must be used that mimics one or more properties of tissues. The properties of the standard must remain constant with respect to time. If changes do occur (e.g., because of temperature fluctuation), they must be quantified and the appropriate corrections applied to the test results.

A good QC program eliminates misdiagnoses because of improperly operating equipment and reduces patient exposure by decreasing the number of repeat examinations. There is also improved cost efficiency because fewer examinations are repeated. In recognition of the essential relationship between QC and correct diagnosis, the Joint Commission on Accreditation of Health Care Organization (JCAHO) requires periodical QC testing. Recommendations made by other agencies and organizations—the American Institute of Ultrasound in Medicine, the American Association of Physicists in Medicine, and the National Electronic Manufacturers Association—also include routine testing.

PERSONNEL

The QC procedures should be performed by the sonographer who routinely uses the equipment for patient examinations.

A more sensitive check on machine malfunction and technical error can thus be made. It requires administrative support to schedule the time necessary for that individual to conduct the QC testing. The time allotment must allow for access to the unit and for the analysis and documentation of results.

Results of the QC procedures should be reviewed on a quarterly basis by a QC review committee, which should include a radiologist, the diagnostic imaging supervisor (or ultrasound supervisor), the sonographer performing the QC procedures, and if possible a medical physicist. This committee determines the parameters to be tested, the results to be recorded, the performance limits for each parameter, and the corrective action to be taken. The QC review committee must also ensure the proper implementation of the program.

FREQUENCY OF QC PROCEDURES

The most frequently used transducers should be monitored on a monthly basis, and all other transducers should be tested at least quarterly. Testing initially on a weekly basis allows the sonographer to become proficient in the performance of QC procedures. With experience this person is more likely to perform them regularly over the long term. After a period of 6 months to a year, the QC committee may elect to change the frequency to once a quarter depending on the consistency of results.

When results outside the performance limits are obtained, further testing may identify the specific nature of the problem. QC procedures should be performed after the unit is serviced (preferably before the service representative leaves). Film processor checks should be completed once a day. Image-recording devices should be tested at least on a monthly basis for gray-scale contrast and at least quarterly for distortion.

The initiation of a QC program is very important because the results obtained serve as baseline values for future comparisons. The program must be continued even if the patient load becomes high, because a scanner operating under these conditions has an increased probability of failure. *The QC program may be able to identify problems before they become major, thus preventing excessive downtime, misdiagnoses, and repeat scans.*

DOCUMENTATION AND RECORD KEEPING

An important aspect of any QC program is documentation. QC test procedures are of little value without an effective means of recording the results for future reference. The primary concern is long-term operating performance of an imaging system, which this information provides. It is essential that all instrument settings (e.g., time gain compensation [TGC] and output) be specified for all future testing. To facilitate comparisons of results, they should be easily reproducible. Obviously, test results must be recorded. When abnormal values are obtained, further testing, the results of that testing, any corrective action (including service reports), and the results of that action should be documented.

Documentation provides potential solutions to problems that recur at a later date. Permanent records also aid in identifying problem areas in the system. Documentation of baseline values and abnormal values on a hardcopy format is extremely helpful. Film storage is bulky and time consuming, however; therefore appropriate test results can be recorded on special forms (see box on p. 282). Hardcopy images of results outside the specified limits are useful for proving malfunctions to service personnel, particularly for intermittent problems that disappear when the service representative arrives.

The minutes of the QC committee meetings should be recorded and maintained for the life of the unit. Documentation of machine or sonographer errors for both clinical and QC scans aids in identifying recurrent or systematic problems. Service records, including comments for specific problems, should be maintained as shown in the box on p. 283.

TEST OBJECTS AND TISSUE-EQUIVALENT PHANTOMS

A wide variety of test objects and phantoms has been developed to monitor the performance characteristics of ultrasound scanners on a routine basis. A test object must be differentiated from a tissue-equivalent phantom.

A *test object* usually consists of material in which the velocity of ultrasound is the same as in tissue (1540 m/s), but other properties with respect to ultrasound propagation vary from those of tissue. The AIUM test object uses a uniform liquid medium with poor scattering characteristics. Some test objects (e.g., the SUAR) do not mimic tissue at all but are designed to test performance under nonclinical conditions. The SUAR (sensitivity, uniformity, and axial resolution) is a rectangular block of acrylic with a wedge-shaped cavity that can be filled with water.

A *tissue-equivalent* (TE) *phantom* is a system that mimics all or most of the properties of tissue (velocity, scattering, and attenuation). The TE material is animal-hide gelatin or polysaccharide gel (agar) impregnated with graphite powder. The graphite particles act as nonspecular reflectors. Small strong reflectors are placed within the TE matrix in well-defined geometric patterns. Simulated cysts and masses may also be present. A simulated cyst consists of gel only without the scattering material whereas a simulated mass contains high concentrations of scattering material. A TE phantom is ideal for testing scanners under conditions that simulate the clinical environment.

Many excellent test objects and phantoms are available for the various types of scanners. Whereas some have specific applications (i.e., contrast resolution, beam shape determination, accommodation of endoscopic probes, and mimicking of breast tissue), others have multiple applications and are designed for comprehensive testing.

■ **Ultrasound quality-control form**

Date _____	Sonographer _____		
Parameter	MHz	MHz	MHz
Dead zone (Depth at which tissue pattern begins)			

Depth measurement
    Distance between top 2 rods
    Distance between bottom 2 rods
    Distance between top and bottom rods			

Lateral distance measurement
    Short
    Long			

Sensitivity (depth of maximum penetration)			
Uniformity (regularity of tissue pattern at maximum depth)			

Cysts
    No. sets seen (3 possible)
    No. sizes seen (3 possible)
    Shape (round, oval, rectangular)
    Fill-in
    Enhancement
    Sizes (make measurements with cursors)			

Axial resolution (separation of rods)
    Depth 1
    Depth 2
    Depth 3			

Lateral resolution (width of rods)
    Focal zone depth (if specified)
    Beam width near field
    Beam width focal zone
    Beam width far field
    (Specify depth for each position measured)			

Photography check
    Gray-scale contrast
    Distortion			

COMMENTS / SERVICE:

Tissue-equivalent phantoms have almost totally replaced test objects in QC testing. Indeed, in the AIUM test object now available the liquid medium has been replaced by tissue-equivalent material.

THE AIUM STANDARD TEST OBJECT

The American Institute of Ultrasound in Medicine 100×100 mm standard test object was originally designed for A-mode scanners, static B-mode imaging systems, and M-mode scanners. Special modifications have been incorporated for real-time scanning systems. Figure 13-1 diagrams the AIUM test object. Several groups of rods are contained within a 100×100 mm square. The rods are 0.75 mm diameter stainless steel wires placed at specific locations with an accuracy of ± 0.25 mm. The test object is not a perfect square, because one or two corners bordering on the top side have been cut away (B and D in Fig. 13-1). The test object is filled with a material in which the velocity of ultrasound is the same as in tissue. The material may be water at 37° C or an alcohol or saline solution at room temperature. Because the velocity of ultrasound changes with the temperature of the medium, various corrections of velocity must be made or the temperature must be kept within $\pm 3°$ C. The test object may be either an open (requires filling by the user) or a closed model.

Although the AIUM test object is designed for A-mode and static B-mode imaging systems, it can also be used to monitor the performance of real-time transducers. Sector scanners, however, are difficult to evaluate because of the

■ **Service record**

MACHINE Manufacturer					PAGE 1	
Date	**Initials**	**Brief description**	**Corrected**	**Date**	**Initials**
3/6/94	DLH	L538 missing scan lines on display, others also affected	Service replaced scan board, OK	3/9/94	DLH
5/17/94	WRH	No image for S228	Bent pin on connector, repaired	5/17/94	WRH
6/6/94	DLH	7.5 MHz endovaginal, no image	Service replaced transducer, OK	6/12/94	DLH

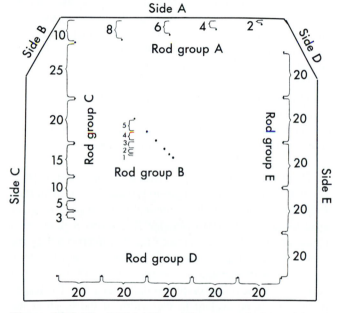

Figure 13-1 The AIUM 100 × 100 mm standard test object features specifically located and spaced rod groups.

inability to establish good surface contact throughout the arc of transducer movement. The major disadvantage of the AIUM test object is that it tests under nonclinical conditions (except for velocity measurements). It is useful for routine constancy checks, but scanner performance appears to be better in testing than can be achieved clinically.

The rods in the test object are arranged in five groups, each group configured to test a particular operating parameter or parameters. Specifically, the test object is designed to determine the dead zone, axial resolution, beam width or lateral resolution, accuracy of distance indicators, TGC characteristics, registration arm alignment, uniformity, and sensitivity.

Rod Group A

Rods in group A are located 2, 4, 6, 8, and 10 mm from the top surface of the test object. They determine the dead zone of the transducer. The dead zone corresponds to the region of material adjoining the transducer in which no useful information is collected, in part because of the pulse length (transducer ringing) and reverberations from the transducer test object (or patient) interface. To check the dead zone, the A-mode transducer is placed directly over each rod or the B-mode transducer (static or real time) is moved across the top (side A) of the test object. The depth of the rod that can be visualized closest to the surface indicates the depth of the dead zone.

Rod Group B

The axial resolution depends on pulse length, which in turn depends on the frequency bandwidth. If the integrity of the transducer is altered (cracked crystal, loose facing material, or loose backing material), a change in the pulse length and, hence, a degradation in resolution will result. Loss of transducer integrity may produce additional side lobes, which create image artifacts and influence the resolution.

Axial resolution is evaluated by using the six rods in group B, spaced 5, 4, 3, 2, and 1 mm apart in the vertical direction. To prevent shadowing from the rods above, they are situated at a 15-degree angle. The axial resolution is determined by scanning across the top (side A) of the test object. The smallest distance between any two rods in the group that can be differentiated yields the axial resolution. The pulse length (and therefore the axial resolution) also depends on gain, intensity, and transducer frequency. These parameters should be recorded when axial resolution measurements are made.

A problem with the closed version of the AIUM test object is that the axial resolution is measured at only one distance, which presents difficulties in evaluating focused transducers. The highest sensitivity of a focused transducer is in the focal zone. The position of the rods in the test object may not correspond to the focal zone, and thus the decreased sensitivity may alter the axial resolution (strong shadowing within the focal zone deteriorates the axial resolution). This test object is used primarily for consistency checks, and thus the single distance is satisfactory.

Rod Group C

The lateral resolution, which depends on beam width, can be measured several ways with the AIUM test object. The first method uses rod group C, scanning from side C. Typically, the distance from side C to group C is 5 cm. Note that this distance may vary among test objects from different manufacturers. The rods are spaced 25, 20, 15, 10, 5, and 3 mm apart in this group. The lateral resolution is expressed as the smallest distance between any two resolvable rods.

The lateral resolution is specified at a particular distance from the transducer. Often the position of the rods is not located within the focal zone of a focused transducer. Consequently, the rods in group C are scanned from a different direction (in this case using side E) to examine the resolution at a second distance (15 cm).

Rod Groups D and E

To facilitate the measurement of distance, area, and volume, most ultrasound systems are equipped with distance indicators, cursors, or both. These are usually timing marks superimposed on the image, and they must be properly calibrated to provide accurate values. The timing marks should be evaluated both near the face of the transducer and far from the face of the transducer. The total distance defined by the markers should also be varied for checking linearity. Scanning across rod group E (equally spaced vertical rods) from side A provides a check of the vertical distance indicators. The separation between rods corresponds to a distance of 2 cm. The orientation of the transducer may cause a change in the distance markers, which can be tested by scanning across rod group D (equally spaced horizontal rods) along side E. If the distance indicators and the rod

image separations do not correspond, either the instrument calibration is incorrect or the velocity of sound in the test object is not equal to the value assumed for distance measurements in the equipment (1540 m/s). A check of the test object temperature should be made to ensure that it is within the proper range. Scanning a second test object may also be helpful in determining the source of error.

An additional check of the test object velocity is possible. Some systems incorporate an electronic grid that can be superimposed on the image. The grid pattern represents a fixed spatial relationship (e.g., each side of the square corresponds to 2 cm). The distance between the rods is compared with the grid. A disparity between rod separations and the grid indicates that the velocity of sound in the test object is not the same as the calibrated velocity of the ultrasonic unit. Measurement of distance in the test object is, in reality, a measurement of the velocity of ultrasound. Because distance and velocity are directly proportional ($z = ct$), one is dictated by the other, given the time of the echo. If the rods are separated by a distance greater than that indicated by the grid, the velocity of sound in the test object is lower than the calibrated velocity. If the rods are separated by a distance less than that indicated by the grid, the velocity of sound in the test object is greater than the calibrated velocity of the unit. This provides an indication of the temperature and composition of the test object.

The photographic system may distort the image on the display when the image is recorded on film. The integrity of the hardcopy process is evaluated by comparing direct measurements of rod separation on film with those determined from the display. Photographic checks are discussed later in this chapter.

The beam pattern (i.e., the beam width at various depths) is obtained by scanning rod group E (equally spaced vertical rods) from side A or by scanning rod group D (equally spaced horizontal rods) from side E. An object produces a signal on the display the entire time it is intercepted by the beam. When a rod is scanned, it produces a signal as long as the rod is intercepted by the beam (Fig. 13-2). The rod appears as a line on the display rather than a dot. The length of the line is equivalent to the width of the beam at the depth of the rod. The beam pattern generated by scanning a set of rods at various depths permits measurements to be

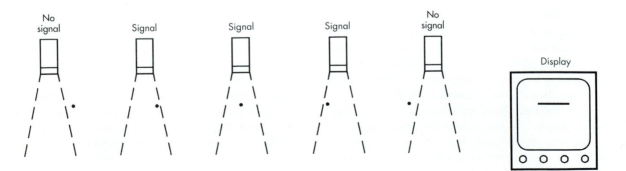

Figure 13-2 A rod scanned by the ultrasound beam produces a signal the entire time it is within the beam. It is thus represented as a *line* rather than a dot on the display.

made of the beam width as a function of distance from the transducer. This method also provides a means of visualizing the focal zone(s) of the transducer. The beam width is the major factor limiting the resolution of an ultrasonic image.

The sensitivity of the system is checked by noting the settings (gain, output, and TGC) needed to barely resolve the lowest rod in group E with the transducer positioned on side A. These settings should consistently result in a similar image when scanning group E over a period of time. An increase in the gain required to produce a comparable image indicates loss of sensitivity of the system. The uniformity is evaluated by scanning rod group D from side A with the same settings used to distinguish the lowest rod in group E. All rods should be displayed with equal brightness.

Rod groups D and E can also be used to study the TGC characteristics and gain settings of the system. All TGC controls are initially switched off. The gain (some units label this the output or dB) is adjusted to display each of the six rods in turn at a standard echo level (1 cm in height on an A-mode display or a certain gray level on the B-mode display). The gain setting is recorded for each rod. The process is repeated with the TGC control turned on. The TGC characteristic curve is obtained by plotting the difference between the two gain settings for each rod as a function of distance. Several TGC settings should be examined in this manner (Fig. 13-3).

All Rod Groups and All Sides

If interface locations are to be properly represented in the image, correct static B-mode registration is essential. In scanning an interface from many directions, the B-mode dot should be placed at the same position regardless of the orientation of the transducer. Misregistration is the positional dependence of the displayed interface on the location and angulation of the transducer. Misregistration causes sig-

nificant errors in distance measurement and the creation of a blurred image (the same interface is represented at multiple locations). B-mode registration is checked by scanning the AIUM test object from all sides of the test object. If registration is correct, each rod produces an asterisk (∗) on the display. If misregistration is present, each rod is depicted as multiple dissociated lines (Fig. 13-4). The center-to-center distance between the farthest lines represents the misregistration. Errors greater than 0.7 cm result in significant blurring of the image and inaccurate distance measurements. Consequently, units with values greater than 0.7 cm should be serviced.

TISSUE-EQUIVALENT PHANTOMS

Nylon fibers are placed at various locations within the tissue-equivalent (TE) material to evaluate the same parameters as discussed for the AIUM test object (Fig. 13-5). Because this test device consists of tissue-equivalent material, routine testing is performed under better simulated clinical conditions, as compared with the AIUM test object. Rubber-based phantoms have recently been developed to mimic the properties of tissue, except for velocity. These are more stable and have a longer life-span than the animal-hide or polysaccharide gel TE phantoms, but care must be taken when performing distance measurements using rubber-based phantoms.

Measured Parameters

The dead zone is visualized by scanning across the TE phantom surface. It corresponds to the region in which no useful information is obtained. The tissue scatter from parenchyma (individual graphite particle scattering) is not present in the dead zone. Beyond the dead zone the tissue texture pattern, similar to liver parenchyma, is observed.

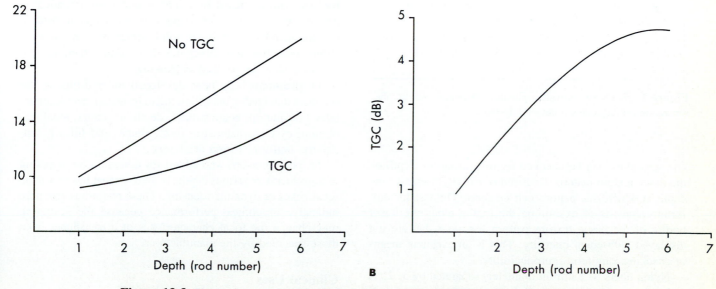

Figure 13-3 Time gain compensation characteristics with the AIUM test object. **A,** Gain setting (with and without TGC) to display the rods. **B,** The TGC curve obtained by taking the difference between the curves generated in **A.**

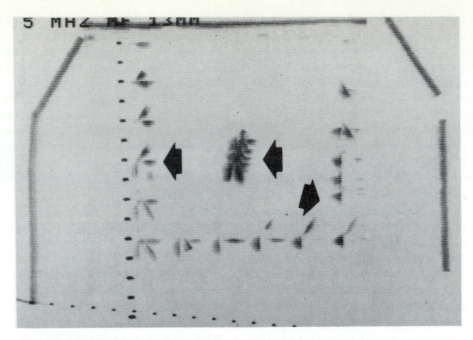

Figure 13-4 Image of the AIUM test object demonstrating misregistration.

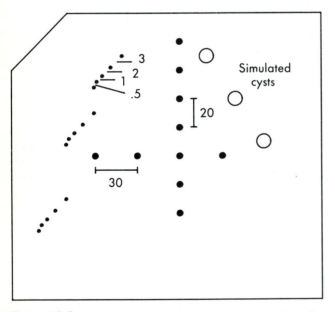

Figure 13-5 Tissue-equivalent phantom. *Numbers* indicate the separation (in millimeters) between rods.

The sensitivity can be checked by measuring the depth of the tissue texture pattern. Reduced sensitivity decreases the depth at which this pattern can be seen. The test for uniformity consists of examining the region along the lower border of the tissue texture pattern for areas that are not displayed with equal intensity. This is an excellent means of checking long-term reproducibility.

Nylon fibers (0.3 mm in diameter) separated by 3, 2, 1, and 0.5 mm (or the standard 5, 4, 3, 2, and 1 mm) and positioned at two or three different depths are used to measure the axial resolution. Two sets of nylon fibers (one along

the vertical direction and the other along the horizontal direction) have rods spaced 1, 2, or 3 cm apart. These fibers are used to evaluate the distance indicators and the beam pattern (focal zone and lateral resolution). All tests are performed under simulated clinical conditions that provide a more accurate indication of the system characteristics for imaging.

Some TE phantoms are so shaped that, by scanning from different directions, the B-mode registration error can be assessed. Often, cylinders, cones, or spheres of varying size are incorporated within the tissue matrix. These structures are weak reflectors compared with the background gel and usually appear anechoic. The simulated cysts are evaluated for size, fill-in caused by over- or undercompensation of gain or TGC, accuracy of shape, and enhancement distal to the simulated cyst. Similar solid structures consisting of strong reflectors are incorporated in some phantoms for checking size, shape, and shadowing.

TE phantoms have been developed for real-time sector scanners that enable the following to be tested: sector angle, lateral resolution, beam pattern, depth indicators, axial resolution, cyst characteristics (size, shape, and fill-in), sensitivity, uniformity, and dead zone.

TE phantoms are well suited for assessing the focusing of transducers at various depths in systems that have variable focal zones or dynamic focusing. These phantoms are more indicative of clinical performance because the scattering may change the focal characteristics of a transducer from those specified by the manufacturer.

Clinical Uses

Phantoms can be used for practice scanning to establish proper operation of TGC controls, gain settings, display settings, and output controls. They also are useful in the training of student sonographers.

Comparing instruments from different manufacturers is necessary to make rational equipment-purchase decisions. Ascertaining the performance characteristics of various scanners under the same conditions is highly desirable but often difficult. Phantoms offer a unique opportunity to evaluate units with a standard means of comparison.

Special-purpose TE phantoms have been developed to test almost any ultrasonic parameter. Some are used to measure tissue contrast and size resolvability. Others are designed to test small-parts transducers only. Still others are designed specifically for endosonography transducers, in which the probe is inserted into a cavity surrounded by tissue-equivalent material.

Typically a good TE phantom represents a small addition to the cost of an ultrasound system (1% to 2%), with special-purpose Doppler phantoms costing somewhat more. To preserve their acoustic properties, they should be maintained at a temperature of between 32° and 150° F in a dark place, preferably in an airtight plastic bag to inhibit moisture loss. Proper care will prolong their life, in some cases to 3 to 7 years, depending on conditions. Originally phantoms were refilled (at a cost of about 40% of their purchase price). Now they are replaced by the manufacturer at a cost usually around 60% of their current purchase price. In any case, the total cost for a phantom seldom exceeds a very small fraction of the revenue generated by the ultrasound system over the useful life of the scanner. Also a single phantom can be used to evaluate multiple ultrasound units, which tends to reduce its cost even further.

QUALITY-CONTROL PROGRAM FOR TWO-DIMENSIONAL IMAGING

QC tests provide objective assessment of instrument stability and performance. They have proved to be beneficial in diagnostic radiology and nuclear medicine facilities when conducted regularly. One of the most important advantages is the documentation of gradual degradation of system performance when compared with clinical impressions of image quality. The value of QC programs in these areas has extended to other imaging modalities; test objects and TE phantoms have been specifically designed for diagnostic ultrasound applications.

The goals of a QC program in diagnostic ultrasound are as follows:

1. To ensure proper operation of the different ultrasound systems to consistently produce high-quality images, thereby permitting correct diagnoses
2. To minimize the ultrasonic exposure to patients and personnel by reducing repeat studies
3. To minimize cost by reduction of repeat studies

Responsibility

Responsibility and authority for the overall ultrasound QC program and its monitoring, evaluation, and corrective measures should rest with the chairman of the department. Primary responsibility for implementing and maintaining the ultrasound QC program should be delegated to the ultrasound QC committee, consisting (preferably) of the chairman or director of the department, the supervisor of the department, the medical physicist, and one registered ultrasound technologist. The supervisor may delegate certain aspects of the program testing to a registered sonographer but should be responsible for ensuring that the program is executed, corrective actions are monitored, and appropriate people are contacted (i.e., service personnel or the medical physicist) when the need arises.

Purchase Specifications

Before the purchase of new equipment, the department chairman, supervisor, medical physicist, and other staff (as necessary) should determine the functions to be performed and the technical characteristics required to perform these functions. Based on requirements, the ultrasound QC committee should prepare objective technical specifications for bidding by qualified vendors.

The final purchase specifications should be in writing and include performance specifications. After the equipment is installed, the medical physicist or consulting physicist should conduct appropriate acceptance testing procedures to ensure that the equipment meets the agreed upon specifications, including federal and state equipment regulations. The equipment should not be accepted until any necessary corrections have been made by the vendor.

Performance Tests

Monitoring of each transducer should be conducted periodically (at least quarterly). The parameters listed in the box on p. 288 provide the best overall assessment of image quality.

In this section each parameter will be discussed individually—including its description, the reasons for testing it, the scanning and measurement procedures, and its performance limits. Although these parameters are all treated as separate scan procedures, multiple parameters can be evaluated from one image, especially for real-time imaging systems.

Dead zone
Description. The dead zone is the distance from the front face of the transducer to the first identifiable echo. No useful scan data are collected in this region. The dead zone is the result of transducer ringing and reverberations from the transducer–test object (phantom or patient) interface. Impedance matching between the transducer and the pulser/receiver is essential for prevention of electrical ringing (i.e., when part of the excitation pulse is reflected to the pulser). The transducer dead zone occurs because the system cannot send and receive at the same time. Thus performance is instrument dependent. As frequency is increased, the depth of the dead zone decreases, provided all other factors remain

constant. The acoustic output also influences the depth of the dead zone.

Reasons for testing. A shift in the depth of the transducer dead zone reflects changes in the transducer or pulsing system, or both. Specifically, an elongated pulse caused by a cracked crystal, a loose backing or facing material, a broken lens, or a longer excitation pulse deepens the dead zone. Artifacts in the dead zone may be indicative of input power fluctuations.

Scanning procedure. Coupling gel is used to place the transducer in contact with the AIUM test object or the TE phantom. Extra gel may be required when a sector transducer is used. The instrument settings (e.g., gain, TGC, and output) are adjusted to the established baseline values. For the AIUM test object these values are determined by scanning rod group E. The instrument settings are adjusted until the bottom rod is barely observable. A scan of the rods spaced 2, 4, 6, 8, and 10 mm from the top of the test object (rod group A) is then performed. The TE phantom is scanned from the top using a "normal liver" technique.

Measurement procedure. The depth of the rod that can be visualized closest to the surface indicates the extent of the dead zone (Fig. 13-6, *A*). Often, a real-time unit has a dead zone greater than 10 mm, which means the test object cannot evaluate the dead zone. The depth at which "normal tissue texture" begins to be seen determines the dead zone when a TE phantom is being used (Fig. 13-6, *B*). Electronic calipers or other distance indicators (marker dots) are used to quantitate the depth of the dead zone (Fig. 13-6, *C*).

Performance limits. If the depth of the dead zone exceeds 15 mm, an attempt should be made to correct the problem. Unfortunately, some units have dead zones in excess of 20 mm, which cannot be corrected. This poses difficulties when scanning shallow structures, as with neonatal patients. Special bolus material (similar to that used in radiation therapy) with appropriate coupling gel may enable the operator to position the structure of interest outside the dead zone. A water-filled balloon with appropriate coupling is also useful for this purpose. Careful consideration must be given to distance measurements in this case.

Depth measurement

Description. Depth is measured as the distance along the axis of the beam. The location of an acoustic interface with respect to the face of the transducer can be determined if the velocity of ultrasound in the medium and the time of flight of the ultrasonic pulse are known. In practice, the velocity of ultrasound in the test object, phantom, or patient is assumed to be constant (1540 m/s). The elapsed time between the transmitted pulse and the returning echo is

---

■ **Performance parameters to be tested**

Dead zone
Depth measurement
Lateral distance measurement
Lateral resolution
Focal zone
Axial resolution
Sensitivity
Uniformity
Cyst size, shape, and fill-in
Solid mass size, shape, and shadowing

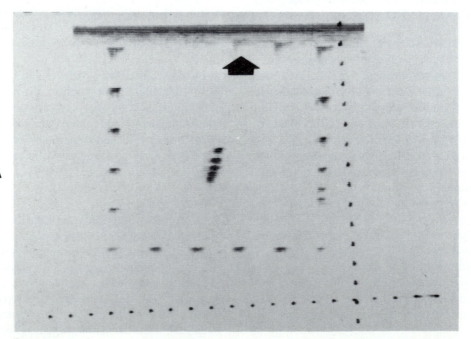

Figure 13-6 Dead zone measurement. **A,** 6 mm with the AIUM test object *(arrow)*; **B,** 15 mm with the tissue-equivalent phantom (distance from the face of the transducer to the beginning of the tissue-texture pattern); **C,** 3.0 mm in a TE phantom for a linear array transducer (cursors).

measured, which permits the calculation of the distance to the interface.

Reasons for testing. A major application of ultrasound scanning involves the measurement of length, area, or volume. Most ultrasound units employ depth markers to delineate distance on the monitor or hardcopy image. The proper diagnosis depends on the accurate representation of distance. Accuracy is checked by comparing distance indicators (markers or cursors) with the known separation between rods in the test object or phantom. Improper velocity calibration causes the scanner to fail this test.

Scanning procedure. The transducer is positioned over rod group E in the AIUM test object or over the vertical set of rods in the TE phantom, and scan data are acquired. Timing or depth markers are placed vertically near the imaged rods. To ensure that transducer position does not affect the distance measurements, the test object or phantom is also scanned from the side and the depth markers are placed along the imaged rods (rod group D of the test object and the horizontal rods of the TE phantom). Although the orientation is different, this is still a test of the marker calibration along the beam axis.

Measurement procedure. Assessment of depth accuracy involves comparing the known distance between rods with the distance indicated by the timing markers, electronic calipers, or both. The image is analyzed by determining the

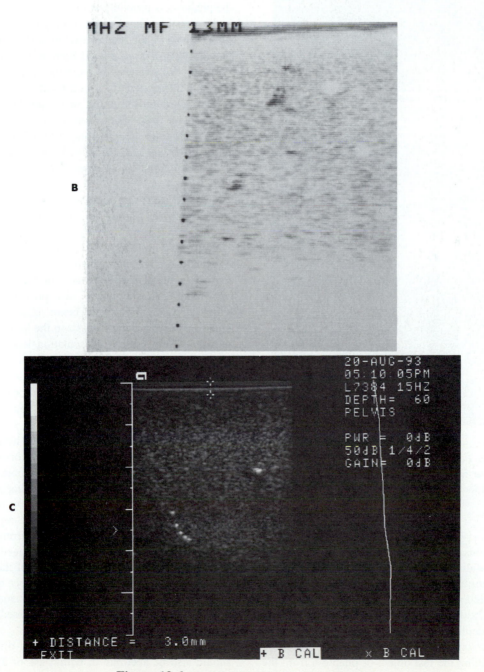

Figure 13-6, cont. For legend see opposite page.

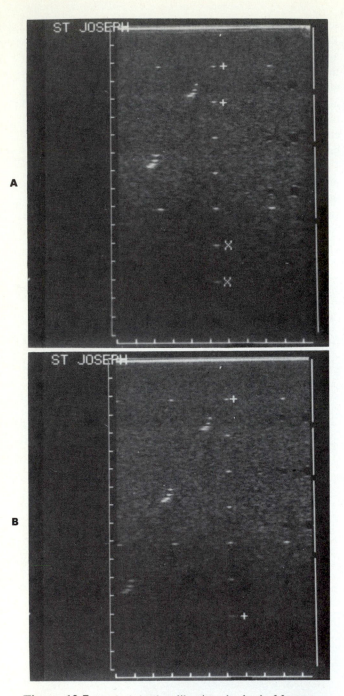

Figure 13-7 Vertical depth calibration check. **A,** Measurements of the distance between adjacent rods close to the face of the transducer and far from the transducer. **B,** Measurement when the separation includes several rods over the extremes of the scanning depth.

distance between rods located near the face of the transducer (Fig. 13-7, *A*), the distance between rods located far from the face of the transducer (Fig. 13-7, *A*), and the distance between rods located at the extremes of the scanning depth (Fig. 13-7, *B*). The latter measurement is most likely to identify vertical depth miscalibration because errors are compounded with longer distances. The same procedure applies when scanning the test object or phantom from the side, except that horizontal rods and markers are used. Some sector scanners have distance markers on the outside edges of the sector image with no other indicators available. Hand-held calipers must be used for distance measurements within the image on the monitor. They are also required for distance measurements on the hardcopy image.

Performance limits. The vertical distance indicators should be accurate to within 2% of the actual distance or 2 mm, whichever is less restrictive. Any discrepancy greater than this value is the result of either machine error or the fact that the velocity of ultrasound in the test object or phantom is not equal to that in soft tissue. A second phantom or test object is helpful in determining the source of the problem. If the distance measurements are erroneous for both phantoms, the ultrasound unit is likely at fault. If the distance measurements for only one phantom are erroneous, the phantom is probably at fault. The velocity of ultrasound in the test object or phantom is very sensitive to temperature fluctuations. A second ultrasound unit can be tested if only one phantom is available. If both units demonstrate similar behavior, the phantom is most likely at fault.

Some ultrasound units incorporate an electronic grid that can be superimposed on the image display. The grid pattern represents a fixed spatial relationship. The separations between rods should correspond within 2 or 3 mm to the grid lines. If they do not, the velocity of sound in the test object is different from the assumed value of 1540 m/s.

Lateral distance measurement

Description. Lateral distance is measured perpendicular to the beam axis.

Reasons for testing. The ultrasound image is a composite of many lines of sight, each representing the depth information gathered along the axis of the beam. The two-dimensional image, however, also provides spatial relationships perpendicular to the beam axis. Often information regarding the size of an object in the horizontal direction is desirable. This spatial representation depends on the number of lines of sight, output intensity, resolution of the scan converter (pixel size), resolution of the display, and beam width (lateral resolution). Changes in beam formation by a defective transducer (broken crystal, housing integrity) usually cause the scanner to fail this test.

Scanning procedure. A scan of the horizontal rods (rod group D in the AIUM test object and horizontal rods in the TE phantom) from the top of the test object or phantom is performed. Depth markers are placed horizontally near the imaged rods. To verify that the position of the transducer does not affect the horizontal distance representation, the test object or phantom is also scanned from the side and the depth markers are placed along the imaged rods (rod group E of the test object and vertical rods of the TE phantom).

Measurement procedure. The distance markers are compared with the rod echo positions in a manner similar to the vertical measurement procedure discussed in the previous section (Fig. 13-8).

Performance limits. The horizontal distance indicators should also be accurate to within 2% or 2 mm, whichever is less restrictive.

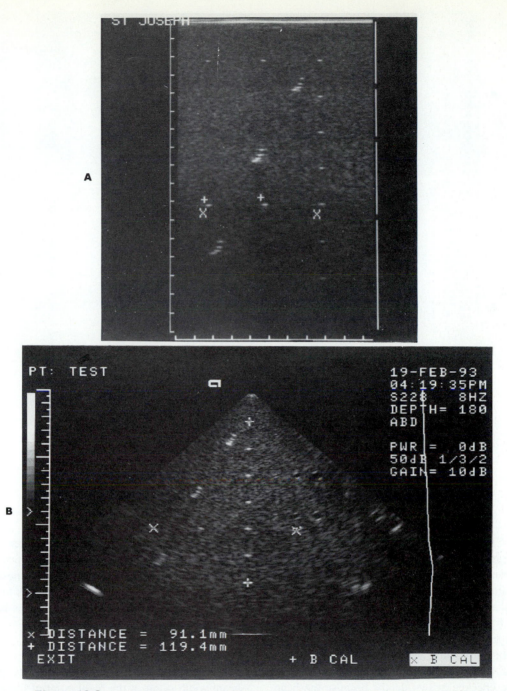

Figure 13-8 A, Horizontal distance calibration check over a short and a long separation. **B,** Horizontal and vertical measurements on one image.

Lateral resolution

Description. Lateral resolution is the ability to distinguish two objects adjacent to each other in a plane perpendicular to the beam axis. Decreasing the beam width improves the lateral resolution. A single object smaller than the ultrasound beam produces scattered echoes when intercepted by the beam; thus the object appears to be the same size as the width of the beam (Fig. 13-2). A small beam width enables small objects to become distinguishable.

Reasons for testing. The lateral resolution of ultrasound systems depends on the beam width, the number of scan lines (lines of sight) in the image, the resolution of the scan converter and display, and the reflection and scattering properties of the medium. The beam width is transducer dependent and is affected by the distance from the transducer, the geometric shape of the piezoelectric material, and the degree of focusing. As the focusing is made weaker (provided other factors remain constant), the beam width in the focal zone

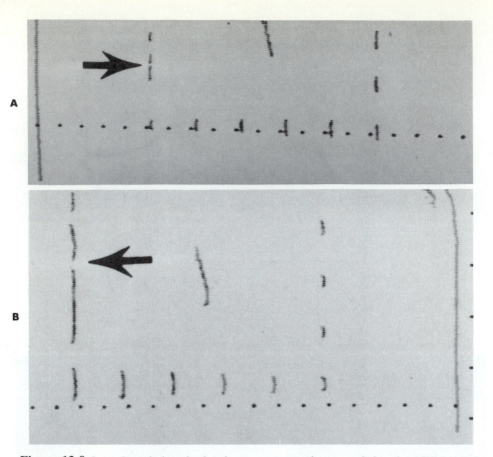

Figure 13-9 Lateral resolution check using a sector transducer coupled to the AIUM test object. **A,** At 5 cm depth, lateral resolution measures 10 mm; **B,** At 15 cm, it measures 15 mm.

becomes larger. Circular transducer elements produce beams that are cylindrical whereas rectangular elements (e.g., those used in linear and phased arrays) produce elliptical beams. In the latter case, lateral resolution is not constant for the in-plane and out-of-plane directions of the beam. High-frequency transducers have an extended near field and a less divergent far field.

Scanning procedure. Rod group C in the AIUM test object is scanned from sides C and E. This allows a focused transducer to be checked at two depths because the beam width varies with the distance from the face of the transducer. Lateral resolution is more difficult to measure with the TE phantom. The beam pattern is obtained by imaging a set of horizontal or vertical rods.

Measurement procedure. The rods in rod group C are spaced 25, 20, 15, 10, 5, and 3 mm apart. When the test object is scanned from the side (C or E), lateral resolution is determined by the smallest distance between any two separable rods. A sector transducer acquired the images in Figure 13-9. The lateral resolution is 10 mm at a depth of 5 cm and 15 mm at a depth of 15 cm. The TE phantom cannot give quantitative results unless the beam width is measured (see "Focal Zone," below).

Performance limits. The lateral resolution should be within manufacturer specifications. Typical values range from 5 to 20 mm for static B-mode systems and from 0.5 to 10 mm for the newer real-time systems, depending on the degree of focusing and the depth of measurement. Lateral resolution should not vary from week to week by more than 5 mm when the AIUM test object is being used or 1 mm when the TE phantom is used.

Focal zone

Description. The maximum intensity and narrowest beam width occur at the focal point of the transducer. The focal zone is the region surrounding the focal point in which the intensity is within 3 dB of maximum. This is also the region of the best lateral resolution.

Reasons for testing. Ultrasound can be focused either externally (by mirrors, lenses, or electronics) or internally (curved crystal) to reduce the beam width and improve lateral resolution at a certain depth. The manufacturer specifies the location of the focal zone of the transducer. When scanning a patient, it is important that the focal zone coincide with the depth of interest. Therefore the specified location of the focal zone must be verified. Any variation in output (due to broken lenses, mirrors, or crystals or to loose facing or backing material) will distort the focal zone. Because lateral resolution depends on beam width, any changes in the focal zone should be detected when they

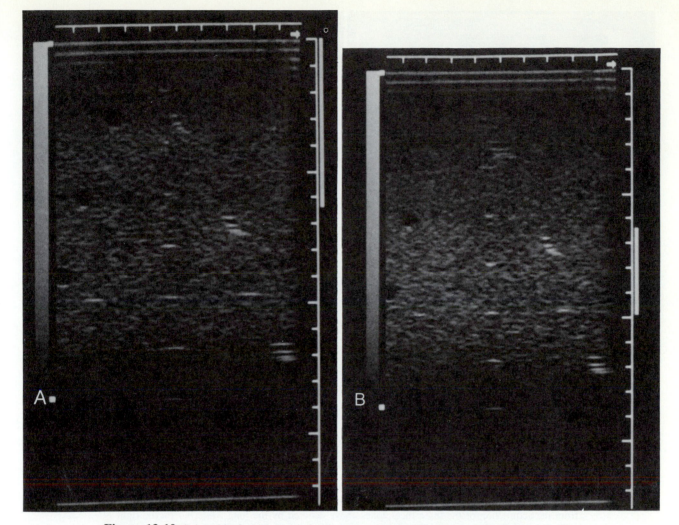

Figure 13-10 Selectable fixed transmit focal zones using the TE phantom. **A,** Short zone. The *white bar* on the right side denotes the focal zone. The vertical rods in this region are narrower than the rods below the focal zone. **B,** Medium focal zone denoted by the *white bar* on the right. The vertical rods in this region are narrower than the rods located above or below this focal zone.

Continued.

occur. Variable and dynamically focused transducers must be checked so the focal zone sweeps throughout the indicated range. The location of the focal zone can be changed by the properties of the reflective medium, which is outside the control of the sonographer.

Scanning procedure. A scan of either the vertical or the horizontal rods in the test object or phantom is performed.

Measurement procedure. Any small object creates an echo the entire time it is intercepted by the beam (Fig. 13-2). A line rather than a dot is produced on the display. The length of the line is indicative of the width of the beam, but it also varies with output and gain settings. The shape of the images of the rods determines the depth of the focal zone. Rods inside the focal zone form a shorter line than the rods above or below the focal zone. For a variable focused transducer, scans with several different focal zone settings should be performed. Figure 13-10 is four scans obtained with a transducer in which three focal zones were selected. Units that employ dynamic

receive focusing may not show a variable width of the rods on the display, but a change in intensity can be observed when the transmit focus of these transducers is adjusted (Fig. 13-11).

Performance limits. The location of the focal zone should agree with the manufacturer's specifications and should not change with time. Typically, the depth of the focal zone is indicated by labeling for static B-mode and mechanical real-time fixed focused transducers. Units employing dynamic receive focusing produce very narrow beam widths over a broad range of depths (Fig. 13-11).

Axial resolution

Description. Axial resolution describes the ability of an ultrasound system to resolve two closely spaced objects along the axis of the beam. (It also determines the smallest resolvable object along the beam axis.) The axial resolution is influenced by pulse length. A shorter pulse length improves the resolution.

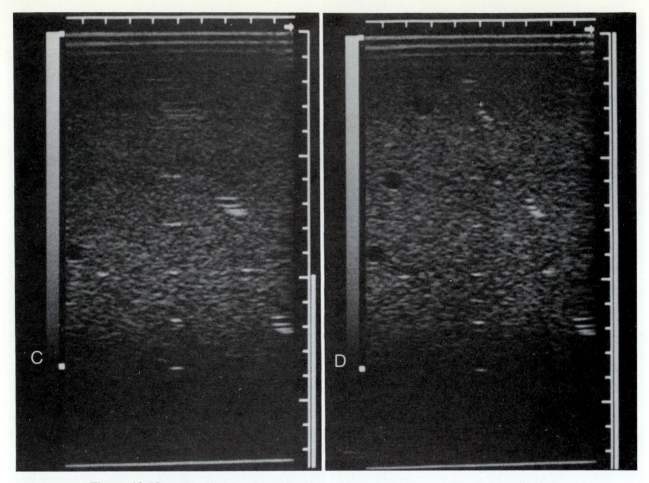

Figure 13-10, cont. **C,** Long focal zone denoted by the *white bar* on the right. The vertical rods in this region are narrower than the rods located above the focal zone. **D,** Composite image from the acquisition of the three focal zones above denoted by the long *white bar* on the right side of the image. This narrows the beam over the entire scanning depth. Note the small size of the vertical rods throughout the entire phantom.

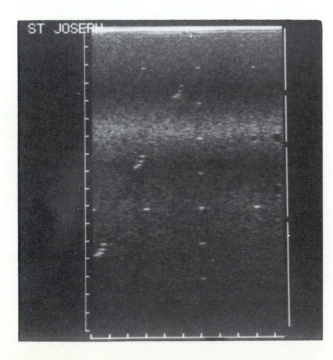

Figure 13-11 Dynamic receive focus transducer. Intensity banding is present in the fixed transmit focal zones, but narrow rods are maintained throughout the image.

Reasons for testing. Image quality is very dependent on the axial resolution. Damaged transducers (e.g., broken crystals, loose facing or backing material, or broken electrical connections) degrade the axial resolution because these conditions elongate the pulse length. The pulser characteristics may change, which also influences the pulse length.

Scanning procedure. A scan of rod group B in the AIUM test object is obtained. Measurement of axial resolution is possible only at a single depth, which is adequate for quality control (QC) but not for acceptance testing. Thus the AIUM test object is not ideal for variable focused transducers. Axial resolution is influenced by the beam intensity and consequently varies, depending on whether the point of measurement lies within the focal zone. Most TE phantoms allow testing of axial resolution at several depths (e.g., a commonly used phantom contains the axial resolution rod groups at three depths: 3, 7, and 12 cm).

Measurement procedure. The axial resolution is determined by measuring the smallest distance between any two rods that can be visualized as separate entities (i.e., a gap between rods). The spacing of the rods for the AIUM test object is 5, 4, 3, 2, and 1 mm. Figure 13-12, *A*, shows a scan obtained with a linear array transducer that has a resolution of 1 mm. An apparent degradation in axial resolution because of excessive shadowing is observed when high gain is used to scan the test object (Fig. 13-12, *B*). The importance of imaging at low gain is demonstrated by this gain-induced loss of image quality. The assessment of axial resolution should be repeated if a focused transducer has variable focal zone settings. The spacing for rods in the TE phantom are 3, 2, 1, and 0.5 mm. Figure 13-12, *C*, illustrates the axial resolution at various depths for a transducer with four fixed transmit focal zones and with dynamic receive focusing. For this transducer the axial resolution is uniform at all measured depths. Switching to a high-frequency transducer improves axial resolution (Fig. 13-12, *D*).

Performance limits. The axial resolution should be within the manufacturer's specifications. Typical values range from 0.5 to 2 mm. Determining whether a focused transducer is within specifications using the AIUM test object is difficult. The TE phantom is more appropriate because groups of the axial resolution rods are present at multiple depths. The consistency from week to week should not vary by more than 1 mm for the same instrument settings using either the test object or the TE phantom.

Sensitivity

Description. Sensitivity has no formal definition at the present time; rather, it refers to the ability of the scanning system to detect weak echoes from small scatterers located at specified depths in an attenuative medium. The weak signal is detected in the presence of noise, which is indicative of the system signal-to-noise ratio. Factors that influence the strength of the detected signal include the characteristics of the excitation pulse, degree of focusing, attenuation by the medium, distance to the reflector, and composition and geometry of the reflector. The signal-to-

noise ratio is maximal within the focal zone and decreases on each side. Typically, sensitivity is related to maximum penetration of the ultrasound beam under specified conditions.

Reasons for testing. The inability to detect weak echoes restricts the tissue volume that is probed. In addition, the internal detail of organs produced by weak echoes from nonspecular reflections is degraded with a loss in sensitivity. Variations of output intensity or receiver gain and loss of transducer integrity can cause the scanner to fail this test.

Scanning procedure. The transducer is coupled to the top of the AIUM test object or TE phantom. Instrument settings are adjusted to barely resolve the bottom rod in rod group E of the AIUM test object. Other rods may also be used (e.g., each rod in group E). In the case of the TE phantom, a "normal" liver scan is performed. Scans with the output set at extremely high and low values are also useful in testing sensitivity. This enables any changes in output to be more easily detected.

Measurement procedure. The settings required to barely display the bottom rod in rod group E of the AIUM test object are determined. The fading of the scattered echoes within the TE phantom indicates the depth of penetration. The maximum depths at which parenchymal scatterers are visualized for the various scanning techniques are measured. Figure 13-13 illustrates sensitivity testing using the TE phantom.

Performance limits. The maximum depth of visualization of parenchymal echoes is affected by transducer frequency, PRF, frame rate, and lines per frame. The latter three parameters are interdependent. The design of a particular unit incorporates trade-offs between frame rate, depth of penetration, and the number of lines of sight. Once the unit is selected, the limitations of the unit as imposed by the manufacturer must be accepted. Because consistency is important, any variation in sensitivity should be noted. A change of more than 6 dB in output when using the AIUM test object is unacceptable. For the TE phantom the depth of penetration for a particular transducer should not shift by more than 1 cm for identical settings.

Uniformity

Description. *Uniformity* refers to the ability of the ultrasound system to display echoes of equal magnitude with the same brightness on the monitor. Because TGC modifies the amplitude of the received signal, the echoes must originate at the same depth.

Reasons for testing. Testing for uniformity ensures that all lines of sight of a scanner contribute equally to the image. Digital scan converters and improper reception can change the uniformity of the signals from equal reflectors at the same depth.

Scanning procedure. The scanning procedure is the same as the procedure described for sensitivity.

Measurement procedure. All rods in rod group D in the AIUM test object should be displayed with equal brightness when scanned from the top surface. The air–test object interface should also be displayed with uniform intensity and equidistant from the top (Fig. 13-14). This is particu-

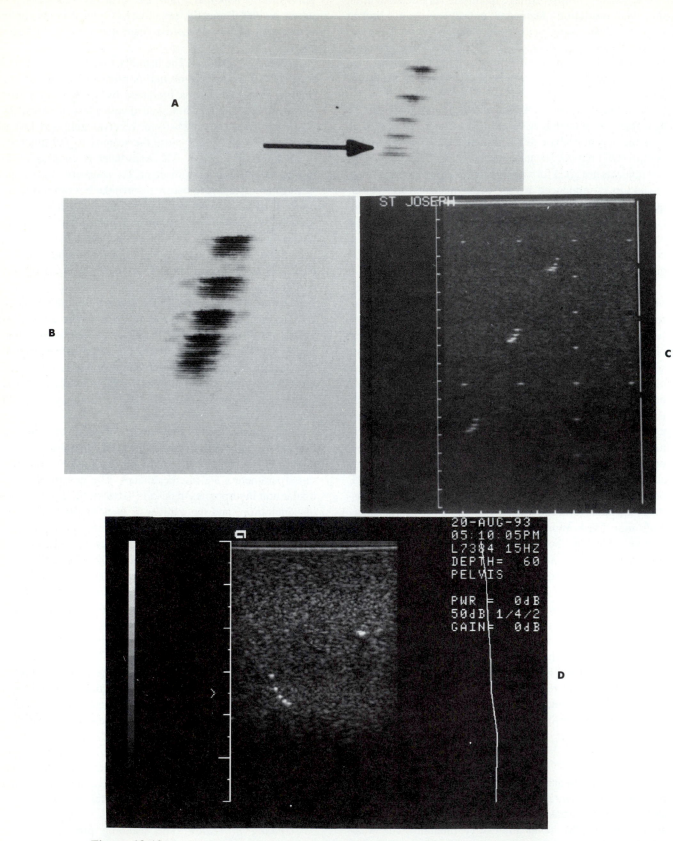

Figure 13-12 A, Axial resolution of 1 mm for a linear array transducer using the AIUM test object. **B,** Shadowing caused by high gain degrades the axial resolution. **C,** For a linear array using a TE phantom, axial resolution is 1 mm at 3 cm depth, 1 mm at 7 cm depth, and 1 mm at 12 cm depth. **D,** For a 7.5 MHz linear array, axial resolution of less than 0.5 mm.

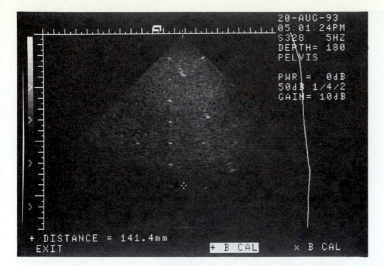

Figure 13-13 Sensitivity testing using the TE phantom. The fading of parenchymal scatterers indicates the maximum depth of penetration.

Figure 13-14 Uniformity testing using the bottom of the AIUM test object. The horizontal rods are displayed with uniform intensity and the air–test object interface is equidistant from the top of the phantom.

larly helpful in determining bad lines of sight resulting from broken crystals or improperly tuned electronics. The effect of shadowing from intervening rods must be taken into account. The tissue texture pattern of the TE phantom should be uniform in intensity at a particular depth of penetration. Sector scanners may not produce a uniform pattern at the edges of the sector (Fig. 13-15).

An alternative test method can also identify defective scan lines. The edge of the coin is coupled to the transducer with acoustic gel and then moved across the transducer face. Regions with decreased signal amplitude correspond to improper sampling along those lines of sight (Fig. 13-16).

Performance limits. This is a qualitative measurement, which is difficult to assess with any numerical limits. Figures 13-15 and 13-16 are scans obtained with units that demonstrate poor uniformity. These scanners require repair, adjustment, or both.

Cyst size, shape, and fill-in

Description. Cysts are fluid-filled structures that are anechoic and usually weakly attenuating. They also have slower velocities than the surrounding tissue. The acoustic image has a distinctive pattern that should represent the size, shape, and consistency of the cyst. A nonuniform echo pattern across the cyst is referred to as cyst fill-in. Changes in output and TGC can affect cyst fill-in. Because the reflector surface is curved, fill-in is expected to occur more readily outside the focal zone, where the beam width is greater. Multiple reflections may alter cyst shape and fill-in. When a cyst is scanned with few lines of sight, a smooth border is misrepresented as an irregular border. Cysts smaller than an individual pixel are displayed larger than actual size.

Reasons for testing. The scanner should be able to differentiate between cystic and solid structures. Contrast resolution characterizes a scanner's ability to distinguish struc-

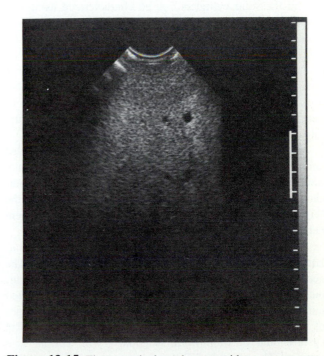

Figure 13-15 Tissue-equivalent phantom with a sector transducer. Nonuniformity occurs at the edges.

tures with similar reflection and attenuation properties. For the purpose of evaluating contrast resolution, some TE phantoms have multiple sets of simulated cysts in the form of solid cylinders with different diameters placed at varying depths. The ultrasound system should reproduce the size

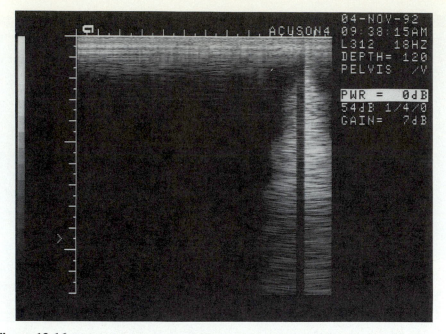

Figure 13-16 Defective scan lines in a real-time scanner. The image was acquired as a coin oriented edge-on was moved across the transducer surface.

and shape of the simulated cyst without fill-in. Enhancement behind the solid cylinders can be characterized using different TGC and output settings. The size of the observed simulated cyst also provides an indicator of spatial resolution. The AIUM test object *cannot* be used for this purpose.

Scanning procedure. An image of the simulated cysts is obtained by scanning from the top or side of the TE phantom. Some ultrasound units are limited in their depth of penetration and may not be able to image deep-lying structures.

Measurement procedure. The size of each displayed simulated cyst is measured in both vertical and horizontal directions by means of electronic calipers, distance indicators, or both. The shape of each simulated cyst and the brightness throughout the structure are noted. Enhancement behind the structures is also examined (Fig. 13-17).

Performance limits. The measured size of each simulated cyst should be within 1 mm of the actual size. The geometric shape of the solid cylinders should be circular, but often linear array transducers and systems with limited number of pixels or lines of sight tend to square the edges of the simulated cysts. This may not be correctable. The cysts should be of uniform brightness with normal scan settings. The effects of TGC and output on fill-in and enhancement behind the simulated cysts should be compared with the baseline results. Refraction may be observed at the edge of the simulated cyst.

Solid mass size, shape, and shadowing

Description. Some TE phantoms (i.e., Nuclear Associates model 84-317) have cylindrical structures that mimic solid tumors. These are normally more attenuating and produce more internal echoes (echoic) than soft tissue does.

The velocity of ultrasound is also usually faster in these structures than in normal tissues. Refraction at the edges of the simulated mass may be seen.

Reasons for testing. The scanner should be able to differentiate between solid masses and normal tissue structures. The correct size and shape of the mass should be reproduced. Shadowing behind the simulated solid mass can be characterized.

Scanning procedure. An image of the simulated solid masses is obtained by scanning from the top or side of the TE phantom.

Measurement procedure. The size of each observed simulated mass should be measured in both the vertical and horizontal directions using electronic calipers or distance markers. The shape of the structures should be round with uniform brightness. The shadowing beyond the simulated masses should be noted (Fig. 13-18).

Performance limits. The measured size of each simulated mass should be within 1 mm of the actual size. The simulated mass should appear round with uniform brightness.

Photography

The end product of an ultrasonic scan is typically a high-quality photographic reproduction of the display—a hardcopy visual representation of the interactions of ultrasound with tissue. The multiformat camera and laser camera both use transparency film as the recording medium. Transparency film exhibits a wide range of optical densities that are perceived as separate shades of gray. The image recorded on film must be a faithful reproduction of the image viewed on the display monitor. Gray levels must extend from black

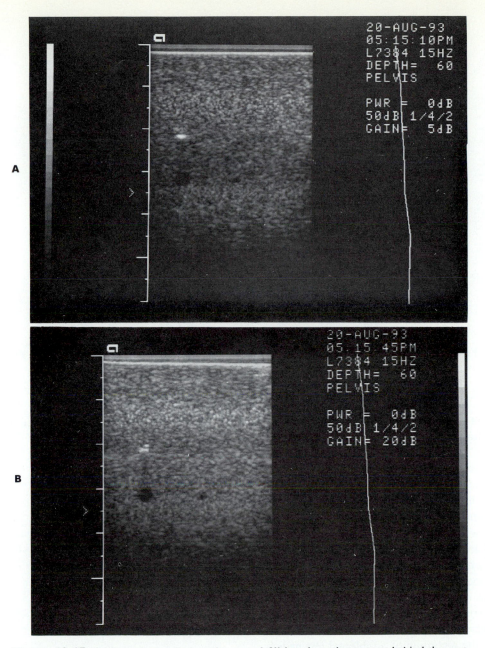

Figure 13-17 Evaluation of cyst size, shape, and fill-in, plus enhancement behind the cyst, using a tissue-equivalent phantom. **A,** Two simulated cysts showing enhancement but no fill-in. **B,** Same cysts showing fill-in.

to white with multiple intermediate shades. Hardcopy image quality depends on the matched response between display monitor and image-recording device as well as on proper film processing.

Photographic recording has a major impact on the quality of the final image. The fidelity of any recording with respect to resolution, distortion, and contrast is checked by comparing the display with the final hardcopy image.

Film processing. The assumption by some imaging departments has been that if a film processor does not develop radiographs a QC program for that film processor is not needed. The implication has been that films from another

imaging modality (e.g., ultrasound) are not susceptible to fluctuations in film processing. This is false. Variations in chemistry (replenishment rates, oxidation, and contamination), temperature, agitation, and cleanliness of the film processor all influence image quality. *Every ultrasound film processor requires **daily** monitoring of its performance.*

QC checks of the film processor should be conducted at the beginning of the workday, after processor warm-up, and before developing any patient films. This provides the opportunity to identify and correct problems before they impact on clinical practice.

The most important daily QC check is exposure, processing, and evaluation of a sensitometric strip. The sen-

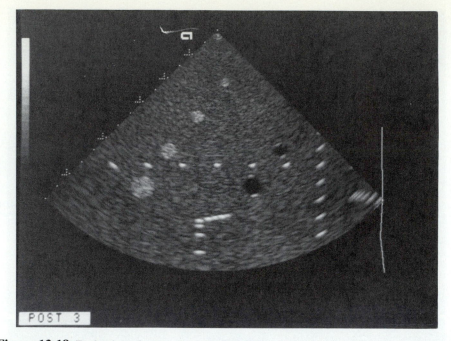

Figure 13-18 Evaluation of mass size and shape, plus shadowing behind the mass, using a tissue-equivalent phantom.

sitometer produces a highly stable and controlled light exposure to film that forms density variations in a step-wedge pattern (Fig. 13-19). The optical density (OD) of a particular step is measured with a densitometer, which detects the amount of transmitted light and expresses this on a logarithmic scale. The OD of various steps of the sensitometric strip shown in Figure 13-19 are listed in Table 13-1.

A sensitometer with an appropriate light source is not commercially available for laser camera film. An alternate method is used to generate density steps for monitoring film processor performance. Laser cameras are configured with internal test patterns containing various gray scales that can be selected for recording on film. Although this testing procedure does not completely isolate the laser camera from the film processor, the recording of an internal test pattern is very stable.

The three parameters base-plus-fog, speed index, and contrast index have been established for the assessment of film processor performance. Base-plus-fog is the optical density obtained from a clear area on the film where no exposure to light has occurred. Three steps in the sensitometric strip that have optical densities of approximately 0.45, 1.00, and 2.00 above the base-plus-fog are identified. The OD of 1.00 above base-plus-fog is classified as the speed index. The contrast index is calculated as the difference between the high-density (2.0) and low-density (0.45) steps.

With the data in Table 13-1 as an example, steps 9, 11, and 13 (with ODs of 0.36, 1.06, 2.16 above base-plus-fog) are selected for quality-control purposes. The OD of each step is measured whenever the sensitometric strip is processed. For this set of measurements the speed index is 1.06 and the contrast index 1.80.

■ **Table 13-1** Optical Densities of Sensitometric Steps

Step	OD	OD Minus Base-Plus-Fog
1*	0.16	0.00
2	0.17	0.01
3	0.17	0.01
4	0.18	0.02
5	0.18	0.02
6	0.20	0.04
7	0.24	0.08
8	0.33	0.17
9	0.52	0.36
10	0.82	0.66
11	1.22	1.06
12	1.72	1.56
13	2.32	2.16
14	2.72	2.56
15	3.00	2.84
16 and above	>3.00	—

*Denotes base-plug-fog.

The base-plus-fog, speed index, and contrast index must be determined and their values recorded daily. Furthermore, each parameter must be compared with the normal operating level to ensure that its current value falls within an acceptable variation (called control limit) from the normal operating level. Control limits for the speed index and contrast index are ±0.15. Base-plus-fog should not increase more than 0.05 the normal value.

It is advisable to reserve a box of film (same type as used clinically) exclusively for film processor QC. The sensitometer should produce a light spectrum similar to that of the image-recording device (blue or green light for multi-

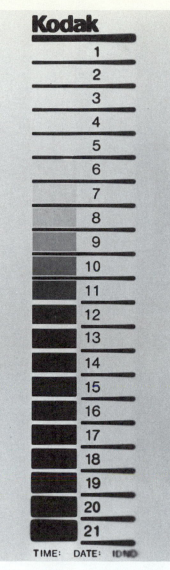

Figure 13-19 Sensitometric strip.

format cameras), and only the emulsion side of the film should be exposed. Generation of the sensitometric strip must be the same each day (i.e., less-exposed end inserted into the processor first, film edge next to the left [or right] guide, same time delay between exposure and processing, emulsion side oriented up [or down]).

The baseline levels for base-plus-fog, speed index, and contrast index are determined by averaging their respective values for 5 consecutive days. When a new box of processor QC film is opened, five sensitometric strips should be processed to ensure that the speed index and contrast index are unchanged (within 0.02 OD of the baseline level). Otherwise, new baseline levels must be established.

Film processors require regular cleaning. A typical cleaning schedule includes crossover racks daily, rack assemblies every 2 to 4 weeks, and tanks whenever chemical solutions are changed (usually monthly). Thorough cleaning of the processor is labor intensive and typically requires 1.5 hours.

A quality-control program that faithfully measures and records the sensitometric data will be ineffective if the data are not critically evaluated and corrective action taken when indicated.

Hardcopy recording. The photographic system should duplicate the structural detail of the displayed image. The display monitor and processed film must have the potential to exhibit a full range of shades from black to white. Also gray level variations on the display monitor must be reproduced on the film. Distortion should be minimal. A common problem is a lesion observed on the video monitor that is not present on the hardcopy image. This makes the diagnosis difficult to document. Often measurements are obtained by the physician from the film rather than from the displayed image. Hardcopy images derived from QC testing also provide documentation of properly functioning equipment.

Proper adjustment of the display monitor does not ensure similar gray-scale presentation by the processed film. The image-recording device is not controlled by manipulation of the display monitor. The translation of input signals to optical density by the hardcopy camera must be regulated independently via the controls of contrast, brightness, exposure time, and/or gray-scale map.

Manufacturers have incorporated a variety of test patterns in ultrasound scanners to aid in the setup and quality control of display monitors and hardcopy cameras. These test patterns usually include a gray-scale image in a set of 16 or more bars of varying brightness levels and a grid of equally spaced parallel horizontal and vertical lines. The gray-scale represents the entire dynamic range of potential signal levels. The grid allows an assessment of spatial distortion.

SMPTE test pattern. The Society of Motion Picture and Television Engineers (SMPTE) has developed a test pattern for use in the setup, acceptance testing, and quality control of display monitors and hardcopy cameras. It can be generated as an analog video signal or provided in digital form.

Figure 13-20 shows the SMPTE test pattern. Note that the background is a uniform gray at 50% video level. Low- and high-contrast bar patterns are placed at the center and at each corner. The size of the bars is varied, but the smallest bar is limited by the pixel size of the digital system (i.e., the width of the smallest bar is one pixel). The low-contrast bars are modulated in contrast from 1% to 5%. The high-contrast bars have maximum contrast of 100%. A crosshatch border defines the limit of the picture area to be displayed or recorded on film. Boxes with varying brightness levels are arranged in stepwise fashion throughout the central portion of the test pattern. The entire dynamic range of potential signal levels is represented in 11 steps from 0% to 100% with 10% increments. An incremental patch with 5% contrast is inset in each box. For example, a 95% patch is positioned within the 100% box.

Unfortunately, the standardized SMPTE video test pattern has not been adopted by ultrasound-equipment manufacturers. The ready accessibility of the test pattern as a display option in each scanner would improve setup and QC monitoring. In addition, more uniform image recording by equipment from different manufacturers would then be possible.

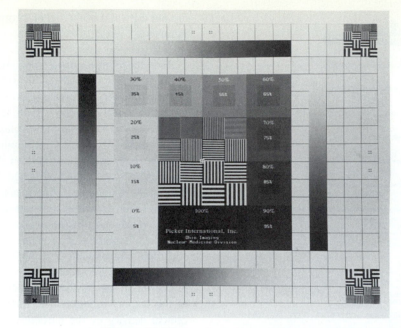

Figure 13-20 The SMPTE test pattern.

Gray-scale adjustment. Setup of the display monitor is accomplished by exhibiting the gray-scale test pattern and adjusting the brightness and contrast controls. Each bar in the test pattern should be distinguished as a separate shade of gray. The gray levels must range from black to white, with midscale bars depicted in gray tones. If tearing or blurring of letters in the text occurs, the brightness adjustment is too high. Once brightness and contrast controls have been adjusted to achieve the proper gray-scale presentation, the knobs can be taped in place (or at least labeled) to inhibit modifying the settings. A full sheet of gray-scale test pattern images is recorded in the format and size normally used clinically (i.e., a 6:1 format requires the pattern to be printed six times). The maximum optical density for film viewed on a conventional light box that allows differences in transmitted light to be discerned as separate gray levels is 2.5. Therefore the OD of black areas on recorded film should be no greater than 2.5. For laser cameras maximum density is usually set at 2.45, and for multiformat cameras at 1.7 to 2.1. The white area must have an optical density less than 0.1 above base-plus-fog. All bars in the test pattern should be distinguishable (Fig. 13-21).

Recording an image of the test pattern does not test all components of the ultrasound system (e.g., the transducer). A scan of the TE phantom can also serve as a photographic check and will indicate whether the entire system is functioning properly.

A simple technique can be used to generate an image with various shades of gray. A coin (nickel or quarter) is coupled flat side to the transducer (even a linear array), and a scan is performed. The coin creates a series of decaying reverberation echoes and produces an image with multiple shades of gray, which can be photographed (Fig. 13-22). Adjustments of output or TGC may be needed to optimize the gray-scale pattern. Pulse-burst generators or sine-wave

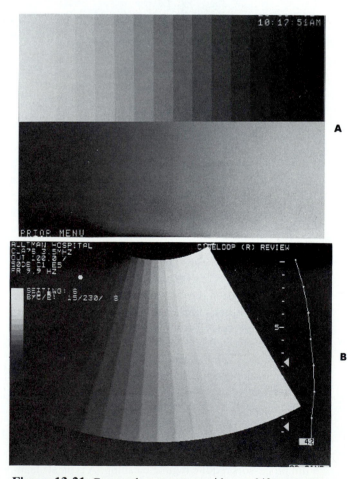

Figure 13-21 Gray-scale test pattern with a multiformat camera. **A,** Properly adjusted. All 16 bars are resolved. **B,** Improperly adjusted. The bars in the low–optical density range are not resolved.

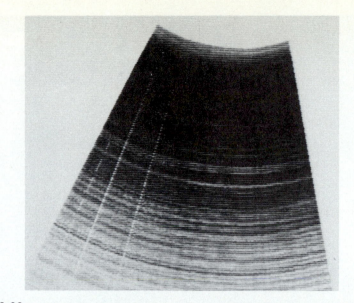

Figure 13-22 Reverberation pattern generated by a coin placed on the front of the transducer. This pattern is compared with that generated on the display.

generators are also used for producing gray-scale test patterns on the display device. They are calibrated to generate exponentially decaying signals to evaluate TGC characteristics of the system. Comparisons between the display and the film with these test patterns check for potential loss of contrast.

Distortion test methods. Size, shape, and relative positions of structures in the image should be accurately presented. *Distortion* is a parameter of image quality that describes the lack of adherence to original geometric relationships. Two common methods of testing for distortion include recording the electronic grid pattern and scanning a tissue-equivalent phantom. In addition, critically evaluating routine clinical images can identify distortion caused by the hardcopy device.

The first method evaluates the display and the image-recording device independent of the transducer and spatial mapping of the detected echoes. The grid pattern should appear symmetrical, with straight, equally spaced, parallel lines in both dimensions. The boxes formed by the intersection of horizontal and vertical parallel lines should be uniform in size throughout the recorded image (Fig. 13-23).

The second method is a total system approach that evaluates the entire imaging chain for proper operation, including distortion in the final recorded image. A distance-calibration scale for each direction is frequently included on the monitor screen and reproduced on the hardcopy, although many sector scanners contain only a vertical calibration scale. The assumption that this single calibration scale will be appropriate for any orientation within the image is valid only if the hardcopy device is properly adjusted.

When handheld calipers are used to measure distance, the measurement between any two points on the recorded image of the TE phantom should correspond to that obtained from the display. Also the scanner's internal calipers should yield distance values that agree with those measured from the film by the handheld calipers. Since the tissue-equivalent phantom has reflecting structures (rods) at known locations, every measured value obtained from the display and hardcopy image should agree with the actual separation between rods in the scanned phantom.

Figure 13-24 shows a sonogram of a breast containing a cyst recorded with a properly operating hardcopy camera. Distance measurements in the horizontal and vertical directions obtained by the internal calipers agree with measurements by handheld calipers. Furthermore, the graduated distance scales in both directions are equal; that is, the separation between any two points in the hardcopy image should be the same whether the horizontal or vertical calibration scale is used.

Hardcopy recording of the image, including the demographic information displayed on the monitor, requires data transfer to the image-recording device. To prevent geometric distortion, the aspect ratio of the monitor screen (ratio of width to height) must be maintained on the recording medium. The hardcopy image is often minified to accommodate various film formats (e.g., 15:1 on 14 × 17 inch film or 6:1 on 8 × 10 inch film). The aspect ratio of the recorded image is the same regardless of film format. The typical aspect ratio for ultrasound scanners is 4:3. A change in this ratio is accompanied by unequal magnification (or minification) in the horizontal and vertical directions.

Unequal magnification causes distortion. Circular shapes on the display monitor are elongated in the direction of higher magnification and appear elliptical on the hardcopy. For example, a fetal head that is round on the display monitor would be recorded as an oval. In addition, a distance measurement along any diagonal path through the hardcopy

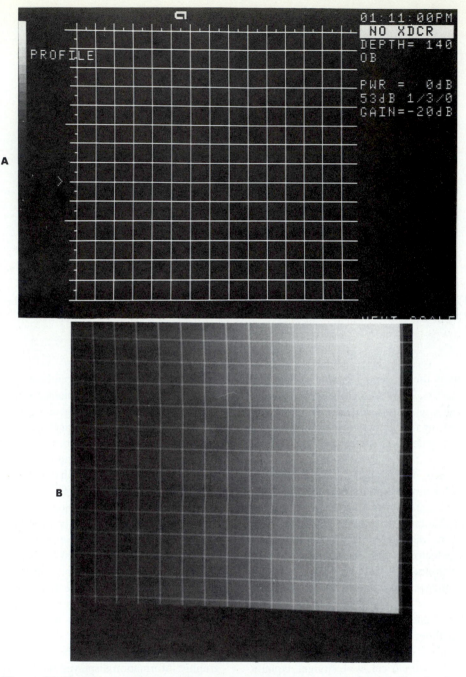

Figure 13-23 Grid test pattern. **A,** No spatial distortion is present. **B,** Spatial distortion introduced by the hardcopy camera.

image would yield an incorrect result. Figure 13-25 illustrates the effect of unequal magnification in the recording of a sonogram of the kidney. The size and shape of the kidney are distorted by being protracted in the horizontal direction. The calibration scale indicates that the distance between cursors is 145 mm instead of 108 mm as measured by the internal calipers. If distortion is introduced by the image-recording device, the internal calipers are unaffected by this malfunction and, consequently, the measured value for distance as designated by the cursors is correct.

The most likely circumstance for an improperly adjusted image-recording device is an incorrect initial setup (1) dur-

ing installation of the scanner or (2) during replacement of the hardcopy device (e.g., superseding the multiformat camera by interfacing the scanner to a laser camera). To ensure that the image recording device is functioning properly, acceptance testing following these events is essential. The test methods described previously are appropriate for evaluating distortion.

Frequency of testing. Initially, the gray-scale test pattern recorded on film should be monitored weekly. If consistency in quality is demonstrated, the monitoring frequency can be decreased to monthly. Optical density measurements of different gray-scale bars should be obtained as listed in Table

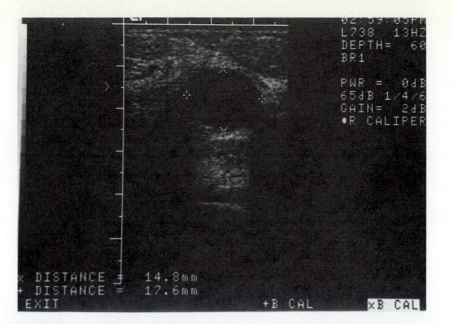

Figure 13-24 Sonogram of a breast containing a cyst. Cursors mark the dimensions of the cyst. A properly adjusted multiformat camera recorded the hardcopy image.

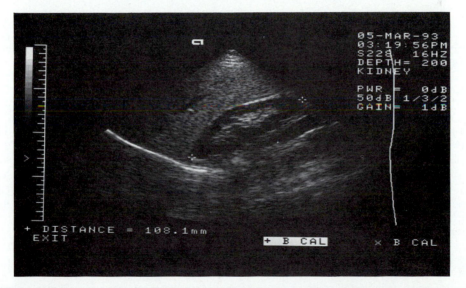

Figure 13-25 Sonogram of a kidney recorded with an improperly adjusted laser camera. Whereas internal calipers measure the craniocaudal dimension as 108 mm, the calibration scale indicates incorrectly that the distance (between cursors) is 145 mm.

■ **Table 13-2** Optical-Density Measurements for Film QC Using a Gray-Scale Test Pattern

Multiformat Camera	Laser Camera
Minimum OD bar	Minimum OD bar
0.45	0.45
1.2 to 1.5	1.8
Maximum OD bar	Maximum OD bar

13-2. The low-scale bar should maintain an OD less than 0.1 above base-plus-fog. The control limit for maximum density is suggested as 0.20. The OD difference between mid-scale bars denotes a contrast index for the processed film. Control limit is typically greater than that established for the sensitometric strip (by at least 0.05) depending on the stability of the hardcopy camera.

Distortion in the recorded image should be evaluated at least quarterly. Scans of the test patterns over a time provide the best means of identifying slow deterioration in image quality. This is particularly important for systems that have analog scan converters or multiformat cameras subject to drift. Various preprocessing and postprocessing algorithms can also be tested in this manner for consistency. New high-quality gray-tone paper printers are checked in a similar manner. If any discrepancies are present, the camera system should be adjusted until the two images appear to have no visual differences.

Record Keeping of QC Test Results

To help detect any degradation of image quality, whether rapid or gradual, records of performance must be maintained over a long period. An example of the results of performance testing on an ultrasound unit is shown in the box below.

■ **Ultrasound quality-control form**

Date _____ JUNE 6, 1994 _____ Sonographer _____ DLH

Parameter	Linear 5 MHz	Sector 5 MHz	Phased 5 MHz
Dead zone (depth tissue pattern begins)	1.5 cm artifacts	1.8 cm artifacts	0.8 cm
Depth measurement			
Distance between top 2 rods	20 mm	21 mm	20 mm
Distance between bottom 2 rods	21 mm	21 mm	20 mm
Distance between top and bottom rods	80 mm	60 mm	80 mm
Lateral distance measurement			
Short distance	30 mm	31 mm	30 mm
Long distance	60 mm	62 mm	60 mm
Sensitivity (depth of maximum penetration)	11 cm	10 cm	12.5 cm
Uniformity (regularity of tissue pattern at maximum depth)	Excellent	Good; edges cut	Good
Cysts			
No. sets seen (3 possible)	2 sets	2 sets	3 sets
No. sizes seen (3 possible)	2 sizes	2 sizes	3 sizes
Shape (round, oval, rectangular)	Top square	Round	Round
Fill-in	Top fill-in	None	None
Enhancement	OK	OK	OK
Sizes (make measurements with cursors)	5.8/4.2	5.5/3.5	6/4/2
Axial resolution (separation of rods)			
Depth 1	1 mm	2 mm	0.5 mm
Depth 2	1 mm	1 mm	0.5 mm
Depth 3	—	—	1 mm
Lateral resolution (width of rods)	Variable	Fixed	Variable
Focal zone depth (if specified)	NA	4-8 cm	NA
Beam width near field	3 mm @ 4 cm	5 mm @ 4 cm	2 mm @ 4 cm
Beam width focal zone	3 mm @ 6 cm	3 mm @ 6 cm	1.5 mm @ 6 cm
Beam width far field	4 mm @ 8 cm	5 mm @ 8 cm	1.8 mm @ 8 cm
(Specify depth for each position measured)		15 mm @ 10 cm	
Photography check			
Gray-scale contrast		OK	
Distortion		OK	

COMMENTS/SERVICE: All OK at present except problem with the 7.5 MHz.
Service called. 6/12/94—Service replaced. Now OK.

DOPPLER ULTRASOUND QUALITY CONTROL

QC and performance testing of stand-alone Doppler, duplex Doppler, and two-dimensional color-flow Doppler units have become increasingly important because of the dramatic increase in the clinical utility of these instruments. Most duplex Doppler and color-flow imaging systems combine real-time capabilities with Doppler. The tissue-mimicking test phantoms described previously are used to test the imaging component of these devices. The attenuation coefficient should be between 0.5 and 1 dB/cm/MHz. The velocity of ultrasound in the material should be 1540 m/s. To appropriately test the sensitivity of the imaging component, the velocity and attenuation values must be similar to those of normal tissue.

Additionally, the Doppler section of the unit must be tested. Three types of phantoms—flow, string, and belt—have been developed to evaluate velocity or flow measurements obtained with Doppler instruments.

Flow Phantoms

Flow phantoms contain simulated vessels (i.e., latex rubber tubing) through which a blood-mimicking fluid is propeled (Fig. 13-26). In this fluid (normally a degassed water and glycerol mixture) are polystyrene microspheres to simulate the backscattering properties of red blood cells. The attenuation coefficient is 0.1 dB/cm/MHz. The velocity of sound in the fluid is 1546 cm/s.

Special care is taken to prevent "clotting," which causes increased scattering. The blood-mimicking fluid is pumped through a closed-loop system by a variable-speed pump. Desirable characteristics of the pump include an accurate flow rate with maximum peak velocity of 1 m/s and the ability to produce steady flow, reverse flow, and physiological pulsatile waveforms. Gear, peristaltic, and piston pumps have been utilized. Gear pumps provide pulsed waveforms but also cause damage to suspended particles and produce cavitation within the fluid. Peristaltic and piston pumps cannot generate steady flow and have only limited ability to produce pulsatile waveforms. All these pumps require flow monitoring with feedback to the pump to maintain the selected flow characteristics. A new computer-controlled positive-displacement pump has achieved accurate flow rates between 0.1 and 40 ml per second without feedback circuitry. Care must be taken to avoid the production of cavitation air bubbles, particularly by centripetal pumps that many commercial companies use.

Variable speeds of continuous flow of the simulated blood provide a means of checking the accuracy of the Doppler shift. One of the problems with simulated tissue- and blood-mimicking phantoms, although "clinically" realistic, is that a single true calibration of peak flow velocity is not known. The velocity of simulated RBCs varies across the vessel, with maximum rates at the center of the vessels (i.e., the vessel walls tend to slow the "RBCs" just as in a true vessel). Flow phantoms are calibrated with respect to volume flow rate, not peak velocity. Peak velocity is based on calcula-

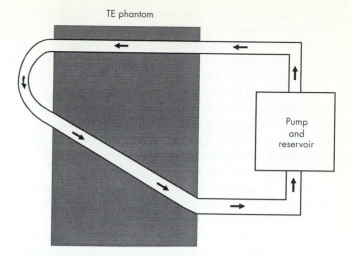

Figure 13-26 A tissue-equivalent Doppler phantom with simulated vessels and a variable-speed control pump.

tions using a volume flow rate in which the velocity profile (e.g., laminar) is assumed. The actual velocity profile depends on the compliance and resistance of the tubing.

The maximum depth of a detectable Doppler signal is evaluated by placing the simulated vessel diagonally across the phantom from the bottom corner on one side to the top corner on the other. This enables the Doppler sensitivity to be evaluated for different frequency probes. At maximum acoustic power the Doppler signal from blood-mimicking fluid is obtained near the transducer. The velocity of the moving fluid is set to be in the middle range of the instrument. The Doppler sample volume is adjusted until the maximum depth at which the signal can be detected is identified. Since the phantom attenuation is known (in dB/cm/MHz), sensitivity can be expressed in decibels by multiplying the attenuation rate times the depth times the transducer frequency.

By placing vessels at different angles through the tissue-mimicking material, it is possible to determine the accuracy of the Doppler angle indicator. The incorporation of various-sized vessels at different angles allows the accuracy of the sample volume cursor (position and size) to be evaluated. The phantom can also test the directional capability of the Doppler unit. Flow toward or away from the transducer is determined by reversing the pump or by routing the vessel with different orientations throughout the phantom. If the pump can be pulsed, various flow patterns are possible.

Not only are the Doppler tissue- and blood-mimicking phantoms valuable in testing the equipment under simulated clinical conditions, they are useful in the teaching of Doppler principles and in demonstrating instrumentation functions. Aliasing, sensitivity to slow flow, and color bleed beyond vessel walls are particularly well illustrated.

String Phantoms

String phantoms allow for accurate assessment of the flow velocity under nonclinical conditions. A loop of surgical thread (strong scatterer) or monofilament fishline (weak scatterer) is mounted on pulleys and driven at a known rate through a low–acoustic attenuating medium (degassed water or a 9% ethylene glycol–water mixture). The latter has an acoustic velocity of 1540 m/s, which allows a direct readout of velocity from the Doppler shift. Recall from Chapter 6 that the Doppler shift depends on the velocity of sound in the medium. The string can be moved at a constant speed ranging from 0.05 to 150 cm/s. A sequence of variable string speeds will produce pulsatile waveforms.

String phantoms can be used for evaluating flow angle indicators, Doppler sample volumes, wall filters, and sensitivity. When the angle of the string with respect to the fluid surface is varied, sampling is possible at different angles. The small physical size of the string, coupled with mechanical translation of the transducer, permits measurement of the Doppler sample volume in three dimensions. Removal of low-velocity components can be qualitatively checked when the wall filter setting is changed. Sensitivity is evaluated by placing additional attenuating material along the ultrasonic path.

In some designs the string is passed through air near the drive pulley. Air bubbles attach to the string and cause spectral broadening of the detected signal.

Belt Phantoms

The belt phantom contains a 2 cm thick layer of scattering material mounted on a belt that is moved at a constant but adjustable speed by drive pulleys. The belt assembly is placed in a water bath. The scattering material encompasses the entire Doppler sample volume. The accuracy, linearity, and precision of Doppler velocity measurements can all be assessed over a belt velocity range of 0 to 80 cm/s in both the forward and the reverse direction. No pulsatile waveforms are possible, however, since the belt velocity cannot be rapidly changed.

Clinical Use

Doppler phantoms cost somewhat more than tissue-equivalent phantoms. Another problem with them, as with normal TE phantoms, is that they eventually fail (i.e., both the latex tubing forming the simulated vessels and the TE material deteriorate). Flow phantoms also require periodical replacement. Their high cost and complex design, plus the lack of a single-phantom comprehensive test method, have restricted their use. None of the current commercially available phantom types has been adopted as the standard for Doppler testing. The most appropriate methods for evaluation of Doppler units are still evolving.

ACCEPTANCE TESTING

Test Objects and TE Phantoms

All of the above test objects and phantoms can be used on a routine basis to provide QC of ultrasonic systems. Some

also have applications as part of the acceptance testing of ultrasound instruments. Test objects are used for evaluating depth markers in the vertical and horizontal directions by scanning the appropriate rod groups. The accuracy of these distance indicators must be determined, however, before the unit is used to measure lengths, areas, or volumes. Evaluation of the dead zone specifies the minimum depth beyond which valid information can be obtained.

The focal zone of each transducer is determined by scanning the various rod groups. This helps establish whether the manufacturer has marked the transducer properly and defines the most useful depth of scanning for the transducer.

The B-mode registration evaluates the system's ability to correlate interface locations; it is crucial for establishing a high-quality image.

One of the best methods of testing the lateral resolution is to scan a rod target and determine the pulse-echo response profiles at several depths—at least at the focal point distance, at half the focal point distance, and at twice the focal distance—which specify the area within the focal zone. The profiles can be generated in TE attenuating media or non-attenuating media. Scanning the rod 6 dB above the just discernible level gives the 6 dB pulse-echo response profiles. Correspondingly, tests can be done at levels of 12 dB, 20 dB, and higher to produce the respective pulse-echo profiles. The width of these profiles at the various depths provides a measure of the beam width or lateral resolution. Beam shape phantoms have been developed that provide an image of the actual beam shape as a function of distance from the transducer. These phantoms are especially useful for comparing one transducer with another. The best method to test the axial resolution is to scan nylon monofilament lines or stainless steel wires placed at discrete locations in TE materials (TE phantoms) or nonattenuating media such as water (AIUM test object). The wires can be scanned at various output and TGC settings to determine the effects of various controls on the axial resolution. This provides a measure of total system performance with respect to the axial resolution.

Special phantoms with "cysts" and "tumors" (solids) embedded in TE material permit testing of the contrast and detail of the imaging system under simulated clinical conditions. A contrast-and-detail phantom with multiple conical targets having varying contrast (echoes vary by 20 dB) tests the system's ability to reproduce contrast and detail in quantitative terms. This evaluation is very helpful in comparing transducers on the same system and in comparing different systems for total performance. To provide a basis for comparison at a later date, baseline performance must be clearly established when the equipment is initially installed. Test objects and phantoms provide an easy means for baseline performance evaluation. Additional parameters (e.g., intensity, bandwidth, and beam profiles) should be evaluated, if possible. These parameters must be measured under more stringent conditions than normally associated with the test objects or phantoms.

This section of the chapter deals with the more expensive and more difficult acceptance test procedures, many of which must be done by the manufacturer before units are

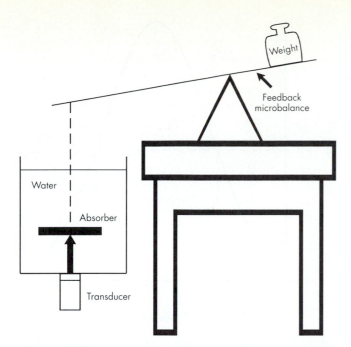

Figure 13-27 A feedback microbalance system for measuring the ultrasonic force on an absorber.

shipped to customers. Indeed, the customers should request documentation of the unit's performance, as indicated by the manufacturer's testing. It is often of value for the customer, either directly or through a physicist or physics consultant, to verify the performance of the unit, independent of the manufacturer.

Feedback Microbalance

Power and intensity are discussed in Chapter 12 relative to biological effects. The power is determined using a feedback microbalance system (Fig. 13-27). An absorber (rubber disk) placed in an ultrasound beam experiences a force arising from the pressure wave that strikes its surface. The radiation force on the absorber is measured by the balance. Because the response time of the balance is long compared with the period of the pressure wave, the reading represents the average force exerted on the disk. The radiation force (F_r) on a perfect absorber (with normal incidence) is related to the ultrasonic power (W) by the following equation:

$$F_r = \frac{W}{c}$$

where c is the velocity of ultrasound in the material surrounding the absorber.

A power of 1 mW corresponds to 68 μg.

Power Meters

Portable power meters have been developed, making the task of determining power easier and permitting (at least relative) calibration of output and gain settings. These controls can be marked in decibels to indicate the amount of power used for a particular scan. Various combinations of

TGC and gain controls may then be used to permit the best possible diagnostic image with the least patient exposure.

Hydrophone

Intensity is derived from measurements of acoustic pressure by means of a hydrophone placed in the ultrasonic field. The physical dimensions of the hydrophone are typically 0.5 to 1 mm in diameter; thus, to minimize spatial averaging, the measurements are performed over a very small area. The spatial variation in intensity is mapped by moving the hydrophone to different locations in the field.

The ultrasound wave incident on the hydrophone induces a voltage that is directly proportional to the acoustic pressure. Because the pressure is not constant but fluctuates as the pulse passes a point in space, a time-varying waveform of the voltage is obtained (Fig. 13-28, *A*). The maximum peak in the waveform corresponds to the temporal peak. This process is repeated so waveforms are collected throughout the ultrasonic field. The point that gives the highest temporal peak denotes I(SPTP).

Recall the relationship between instantaneous intensity and the acoustic pressure expressed by Equation 12-3. An analog-to-digital converter transforms the voltage signal from the pressure fluctuations into digital format for signal processing. The instantaneous intensity is calculated directly from the induced voltage by squaring this value and multiplying by a constant. To determine other intensity descriptors such as the pulse average intensity, the induced voltage waveform is squared and then integrated over time (Fig. 13-28, *B* and *C*). The resulting value is divided by the time duration of the pulse to yield the pulsed averaged intensity at the point of measurement. The maximum I(PA) obtained from all points throughout the ultrasonic field is the I(SPPA). Spatial averaging is applied by combining the results from multiple points in the region of interest.

Bandwidth Measurements

A frequency-calibrated hydrophone enables the transmitted frequency profile to be obtained when the output of the hydrophone is connected to a spectrum analyzer. The frequency profile provides the center frequency (f_c or f_0)—at which the amplitude frequency spectrum is maximal—and the transmitted bandwidth. The transmitted bandwidth is the difference between frequency values ($f_2 - f_1$), where the acoustic pressure magnitude is −3 dB below the maximum value (Fig. 13-29). A broad-band transducer (low Q) has a large frequency spread whereas a narrow-band transducer (high Q) has a small frequency spread. More precisely, a transducer is considered to be narrow band if its fractional bandwidth is less than 15%. Fractional bandwidth (BW) as a percentage is defined by the following:

$$BW = \frac{(f_2 - f_1)}{f_c} \times 100\%$$

In general, broadband transducers are superior for medical diagnostic ultrasound imaging.

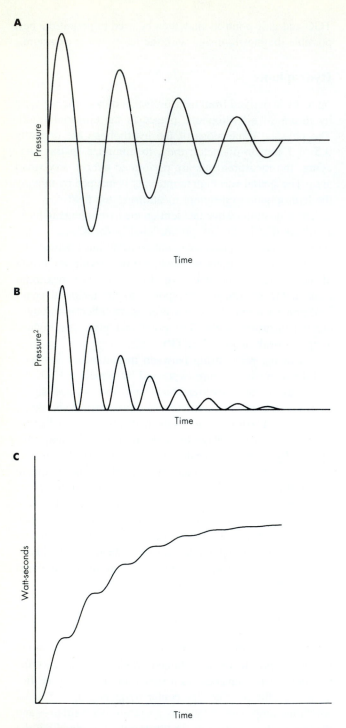

Figure 13-28 Data for calculation of various intensity parameters. **A,** Time-varying voltage waveform detected by a hydrophone. **B,** Squared time–varying voltage waveform. **C,** Integration of the squared time–varying voltage waveform in **B** over time.

The frequency spectrum, center frequency, and frequency bandwidth may be measured by testing the transducer separately from the rest of the ultrasound system. The transducer is normally connected to a broadband pulser (e.g., a pulse-burst generator), which is used to excite it. The voltage applied to the transducer from the pulser can be made to oscillate at any desired frequency. A long pulse drives the transducer at the applied frequency.

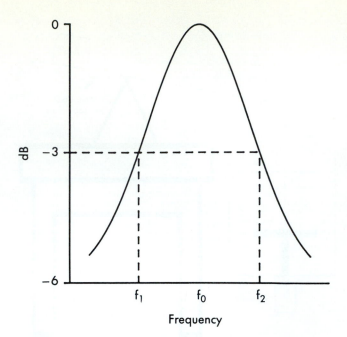

Figure 13-29 Acoustic pressure in decibels as a function of frequency. The transmitted bandwidth is given by $f_2 - f_1$.

The pulser is sequentially stepped at different frequencies throughout the bandwidth. Each ultrasound wave generated by the transducer with the pulser driven at a constant frequency is transmitted through water to a flat planar reflector. The echo from this reflector is detected by the transducer or by a hydrophone CW operation and sent to a spectrum analyzer, where a plot of signal strength versus frequency is made (Fig. 13-30). The signal strength increases as the match between driving voltage and the natural frequency of the transducer improves. The center frequency produces a signal with the greatest amplitude. Normally the excitation voltage waveform is continuous because a short pulse causes the transducer to resonate at a frequency specified by the thickness of the crystal. The resonant frequency (f_0) should be the same as the center frequency (f_c).

The bandwidth is determined from the amplitude-versus-frequency spectrum, by taking the differences in frequency at the points corresponding to half the maximum amplitude. The frequency spectrum depends on the transducer damping (Q value and backing material), the pulser, the transducer electrical and acoustic impedances, and the total system matching. This method evaluates only the transducer-related variables and not how well the transducer is matched with the rest of the ultrasound system. Testing the transducer frequency spectrum for a complete ultrasound system is more difficult and less accurate than evaluating the transducer by itself. Test devices are currently being developed to improve these system measurements.

Echo Amplitude Profiles

The combined transmit and receive characteristics of the transducer (i.e., the response to pulse echoes) is examined by moving a small target across the beam at various depths. The usual reflector is a sphere with a diameter of 3 to 10

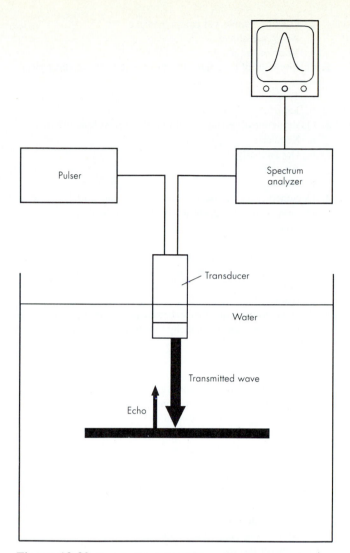

Figure 13-30 System for determining a frequency spectrum. The pulser excites the transducer, which sends an ultrasound wave toward a planar reflector. The wave is reflected, and the received echo signal is input into the spectrum analyzer, where the amplitude for each frequency is determined.

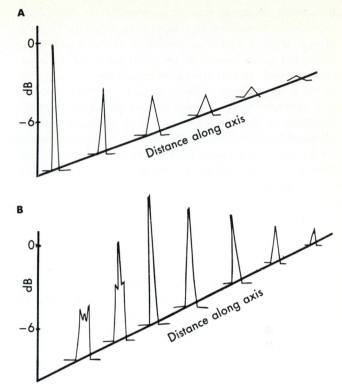

Figure 13-31 Echo amplitude patterns of a transducer. The received echo signals are measured as a small target moves across the beam at various distances from the transducer. **A,** High-frequency short-focused transducer. **B,** Medium-frequency medium-focused transducer.

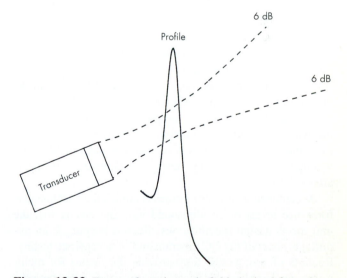

Figure 13-32 Extent of an ultrasonic field obtained from the analysis of pressure or echo amplitude profiles. The boundary *(dotted lines)* corresponds to a 6 dB reduction in intensity.

wavelengths. A large reflecting target may also be used. The target generates reflected ultrasound waves, which are detected and processed by the ultrasonic unit rather than by the spectrum analyzer alone. The echo-detection pattern at various depths is delineated for that particular unit (Fig. 13-31). These axial and transverse echo-amplitude profiles identify the focal zone and the extent of the ultrasonic field. The beam width and response with depth are illustrated. This information is obtained from the received echoes rather than from the induced voltage in a hydrophone from transmitted sound waves.

Pressure-amplitude or echo-amplitude profiles are consolidated to denote the limits of the ultrasonic field. The point on each side of the profile peak corresponding to a 6 dB reduction is identified, and then the points along each side of the transducer axis are connected to form a boundary of the ultrasonic field (Fig. 13-32). This is the common illustrative format to designate sound wave patterns produced by a transducer.

Test Generators

Test generators can be used to evaluate the dynamic range, TGC stability, gray-scale, linearity, depth marker accuracy, signal-to-noise ratio, photographic controls, and signal processing. These generators are connected at selected points throughout the unit to simulate scan conditions. In essence, well-known signals are introduced to ascertain the response of one or more system components. For example, when connected to the transducer, the generator furnishes an excitation pulse. Test signals can be sent to the scan converter or the display directly. Test generators normally produce exponentially decaying pulse bursts that can be triggered externally to the ultrasound system or internally with the ultrasound system transmitter. The test generators may be set for different frequencies, pulse rates, and decay rates. Information provided by the test generators is a valuable part of the acceptance procedures.

SUMMARY

The end product of an ultrasound scan is its image. The quality of the image depends largely on a properly functioning unit. Performance characteristics of the system are monitored via a QC program. Special test objects and TE phantoms measure resolution (axial and lateral), sensitivity, uniformity, dead zone, accuracy of distance markers (vertical and horizontal), and other parameters. Within well-defined limits, these parameters reflect properly functioning equipment.

The display monitor, hardcopy camera, and film processing all contribute to the image-recording process. To optimize photographic system performance, the recommendations of manufacturers of the image-recording device, film, and processing chemicals should be followed. The image-recording device should exhibit a full range of gray-scale contrast and an accurate portrayal of size, shape, and relative positions of structures in the displayed image. Matching the response of the display monitor and the hardcopy camera is necessary to ensure that what is seen on the monitor is recorded on film.

Flow, string, and belt phantoms are used for QC checks on Doppler instruments. Velocity (or flow), the Doppler angle indicator and Doppler sample volume, sensitivity, and the wall filter can be evaluated. An inexpensive, easy-to-use, and accurate Doppler test phantom has not been developed. Standards for QC testing of Doppler instruments are evolving.

Acceptance-testing procedures establish the baseline performance levels of an ultrasound unit and ensure that the unit meets design specifications. Record keeping is an important aspect of the QC program and of acceptance testing. Records of routine QC tests provide the means for monitoring performance levels of the unit over long periods. Service records should be included as part of this record-keeping process. The QC program must be structured so the testing is performed on a consistent basis. Often programs begin with an overambitious schedule that cannot be sustained in practice, and this can result in discontinuation of the entire QC program.

■■■■ **REVIEW QUESTIONS** ■■■■

1. A quality-control program
   a. Reduces patient exposures
   b. Monitors equipment performance
   c. Must be simple yet comprehensive
   d. All of the above
   e. None of the above
2. Quality-control tests must be performed by the medical physicist.
   a. True
   b. False
3. Quality-control testing should be performed how often?
   a. Regularly
   b. Occasionally
   c. Annually
   d. Never
4. Documentation of machine settings during initial testing is important for subsequent performance evaluations.
   a. True
   b. False
5. Service records do not need to be maintained because the scanner has been repaired and is currently working properly.
   a. True
   b. False
6. A tissue-equivalent (TE) phantom has properties similar to tissue, except that the velocity of ultrasound is approximately 4000 m/s.
   a. True
   b. False
7. The AIUM test object mimics
   a. The attenuation of ultrasound in tissue
   b. No properties of ultrasound in tissue
   c. The velocity of ultrasound in tissue
   d. The scattering of ultrasound in tissue
   e. None of the above
8. The AIUM test object or TE phantom measures registration arm error for a static B-mode scanner
   a. By scanning one side
   b. By scanning multiple sides
   c. By rotating the phantom and rescanning
   d. None of the above
9. Gray-scale contrast on the display monitor and film is evaluated using a
   a. Sensitometer
   b. Test pattern
   c. Hydrophone
   d. Microbalance
10. Tissue-equivalent phantoms are of value because they:
    a. Mimic the acoustic properties of tissue
    b. Have adjustable attenuation coefficients that are selected by the operator during scanning
    c. Are composed of materials that vary the velocity of ultrasound within the phantom
    d. None of the above
11. A hydrophone is a
    a. Test object
    b. Loudspeaker
    c. Tissue-equivalent (TE) phantom
    d. Miniature transducer with well-defined characteristics
    e. None of the above
12. Flow phantoms are established with respect to maximum peak velocity of the blood-mimicking fluid.
    a. True
    b. False
13. The AIUM test object consists of multiple rods in a well-defined pattern within an area that is
    a. 100 × 100 cm
    b. 100 × 100 m

c. 100 × 100 mm

d. 1 × 1 m

14. The velocity of ultrasound for the AIUM test object or tissue equivalent (TE) phantom is
    a. 4080 m/s
    b. 333 m/s
    c. 100 m/s
    d. 1540 m/s

15. The dead zone is the result of
    a. Attenuation
    b. Refraction
    c. Pulse length
    d. None of the above

16. Ultrasound phantoms are able to quantify beam-intensity profiles.
    a. True
    b. False

17. The accuracy of distance markers should be assessed along the beam axis and perpendicular to the beam axis.
    a. True
    b. False

18. If a multiformat camera introduces distortion in the recorded image, the internal calipers for distance measurements will also be in error.
    a. True
    b. False

19. Axial resolution is the ability of the ultrasound system to resolve objects that are perpendicular to the beam axis.
    a. True
    b. False

20. Daily QC checks of the film processor are not necessary.
    a. True
    b. False

21. Flow, string, and belt phantoms are used for quality-control and performance testing on Doppler ultrasound systems.
    a. True
    b. False

22. The frequency spectrum of a transducer is readily measured with tissue equivalent (TE) phantoms.
    a. True
    b. False

23. *Acceptance testing* is a term to describe the routine quality-control procedures to detect long-term deterioration in performance of an ultrasound system.
    a. True
    b. False

24. The rod groups in the AIUM test object or the tissue equivalent (TE) phantoms that measure axial resolution are offset at an angle to prevent
    a. Enhancement
    b. Penetration
    c. Shadowing
    d. Uniformity

25. The vertical rod group of the AIUM test object, which has separations of 25, 20, 15, 10, 5, and 3 mm, is designed to measure
    a. Accuracy of distance markers
    b. Dead zone
    c. Axial resolution
    d. Lateral resolution
    e. None of the above

BIBLIOGRAPHY

Banjavic RA: Design and maintenance of a quality assurance program for diagnostic ultrasound equipment, *Semin Ultrasound* 4:10, 1983.

Boote EJ, Zagzebski JA: Performance tests of Doppler ultrasound equipment with a tissue- and blood-mimicking phantom, *J Ultrasound Med* 7:137, 1988.

Carson PL, Dubuque GL (eds): *Ultrasound instrument quality control procedure, CRP Report Series 3,* Chevy Chase Md, 1979, AAPM-CRP.

Carson PL, Zagzebski JA: *Pulse echo ultrasound imaging systems: performance tests and criteria, AAPM Report 8,* New York, 1980, American Institute of Physics.

Goldstein A: *Quality assurance in diagnostic ultrasound: a manual for the clinical user, HHS Publ (FDA) 81-8139,* 1980.

Goldstein A: Performance tests of Doppler ultrasound equipment with a string phantom, *J Ultrasound Med* 10:125, 1991.

Gray JE, Winkler NT, Stears JG, Frank ED: *Quality control in diagnostic imaging,* Rockville, Md, 1983, Aspen Systems.

Gray JE, Lisk KG, Haddick DH, et al: Test pattern for video displays and hard-copy cameras, *Radiology* 154:519, 1985.

Hedrick WR, Hykes DL: Image recording devices, *J Diagn Med Sonogr* 7:56, 1991.

Hedrick WR, Hykes DL: Image distortion caused by an improperly adjusted hardcopy camera, *J Diagn Med Sonogr* 9:180, 1993.

Hedrick WR, Hykes DL: Photographic system quality control, *J Diagn Med Sonogr* 9:62, 1993.

Holdsworth DW, Rickey DW, Drangova M, et al: Computer-controlled positive displacement pump for physiological flow simulation, *Med Biol Eng Comput* 29:564, 1991.

Hoskins PR, Loupas T, McDicken WN: A comparison of the Doppler spectra from human blood and artificial blood used in a flow phantom, *Ultrasound Med Biol* 16:141, 1990.

Hykes DL, Hedrick WR, Milavickas LR, Starchman DE: Quality assurance for real time ultrasound equipment, *J Diagn Med Sonogr* 2:121, 1986.

Phillips DJ, Hossack J, Beach KW, Strandness DE: Testing ultrasonic pulsed Doppler instruments with a physiologic string phantom, *J Ultrasound Med* 9:429, 1990.

Rickey DW, Rankin R, Fenster A: A velocity evaluation phantom for colour and pulsed Doppler instruments, *Ultrasound Med Biol* 18:479. 1992.

Walker AR, Philpis DJ, Powers JE: Evaluating Doppler devices using a string target, *J Clin Ultrasound* 10:25, 1982.

▲

Image Artifacts

Assumptions for 2D echo mapping	Mirror image
Color aliasing	Misregistration
Color bleed	Partial volume
Color flash	Range ambiguity
Color noise	Reverberation
Comet tail	Shadowing
Enhancement	Velocity error
Ghost image	

The complexity of ultrasound equipment makes it difficult to isolate and understand the causes of ultrasonic imaging artifacts. Improper functioning or operation of equipment and limitations inherent in the ultrasound sampling process (i.e., the physical properties of ultrasound waves and their interactions with tissues) can contribute to the presence of artifacts. This chapter describes some imaging artifacts for both gray-scale and color Doppler.

DEFINITION OF ARTIFACTS

An ultrasound image is the portrayal of anatomy probed by an ultrasonic beam. An artifact is any structure in that image that does not correlate directly with actual tissue. Artifacts assume different forms—including perceived objects in the image that are not actually present, structures that should be represented in the image but are missing, and structures whose locations in the image are misregistered. These errors in acoustic presentation of the scanned subject are usually caused by technical limitations or anatomical factors.

CAUSES OF ARTIFACTS

The causes of artifacts in ultrasound imaging are many and varied. Equipment may not be functioning properly—including miscalibration of ultrasound velocity, broken or deformed crystals, broken or improperly assembled backing

or facing materials, faulty monitors, or defective recording devices. A defective recording device can introduce distortion, misrepresent the contrast scale, and cause a loss of image detail. An effective QC program should identify any malfunction of the scanner and recording device.

Improper operation of equipment can also play a role in the production of artifacts. This is particularly true with poorly trained or inexperienced personnel. The sonographer may not properly set gain, time gain compensation (TGC), or other controls for sensitivity and uniformity. The wrong area may be scanned (not a true artifact), or the right area scanned too rapidly.

The acoustic properties of tissues and the propagation of ultrasound waves through them can contribute to imaging artifacts. In addition, certain assumptions are necessary for the mapping of returning echoes into a composite picture, and when these are erroneous artifacts in the image are produced.

ASSUMPTIONS FOR TWO-DIMENSIONAL ECHO MAPPING

Ultrasound scanning techniques for the acquisition, processing, and display of ultrasonic data are based on several assumptions. The transmitted wave travels along a straight-line path from the transducer to the object and back to the transducer. Beam dimensions are infinitely small in both section thickness and lateral directions. All detected echoes originate from along the transducer axis only. All received echoes are derived from the most recently transmitted pulse. The ultrasound wave travels at the rate of 1540 m/s in tissue; thus the distance to the interface is determined from the time of flight (1 cm corresponds to 13 μs). The amplitude of the echo is directly related to the reflectivity of the object scanned. Violations of these assumptions produce artifacts in the image.

The foregoing assumptions are fundamental for imaging purposes. Each scanning mode, however, may also be based on additional assumptions that can lead to artifactual image formation. Technical limitations (temporal pulse length, scan line density, beam width, and PRF) restrict the fidelity of the overall imaging process.

GRAY-SCALE IMAGE ARTIFACTS

Some artifacts (i.e., enhancement behind a cystic structure and shadowing behind a solid structure) aid in diagnosis. Other undesirable artifacts should be identified because not recognizing them may result in a misdiagnosis.

The object's size, shape, and location can be misrepresented. Its brightness on the display may not correspond with the strength of the reflector. The most difficult artifact to recognize is, however, the missing structure.

Resolving Objects

The finite spatial pulse length limits the axial resolution. By increasing transducer frequency or minimizing ringing, it is possible to shorten the spatial pulse length and improve axial resolution. The best possible axial resolution is the spatial pulse length divided by 2 (as discussed in Chapter 2). Typical axial resolution of modern ultrasound systems is 0.5 to 2 mm. Objects smaller than this appear to be at least that size in the image (i.e., an object depicted with the incorrect size). Objects spaced closer together than the axial resolution merge together in the image (i.e., two objects appearing as one with the interface not shown).

The axial resolution remains fairly constant with depth. The lateral resolution, however, which depends on beam width, changes with depth. For circular single-element crystals, annular arrays, and rectangular arrays, the beam shape is symmetrical (in-plane and out-of-plane dimensions equal) at a given depth. Linear arrays (phased or segmental) produce a beam pattern that is mechanically focused in the out-of-plane direction and electronically focused in the in-plane direction. The in-plane and out-of-plane dimensions of the beam are not symmetrical. The beam width, and thus the lateral resolution, is best within the focal zone of the transducer. Two-dimensional imaging systems can achieve a lateral resolution of 1 to 3 mm if dynamic focusing is used. However, the same problem arises as with axial resolution:

a small object appears larger than it really is and two objects separated by less than the beam width appear as one on the display. These resolution artifacts contribute to an incorrect representation of the size and shape of interfaces and to missing interfaces. Objects as small as 0.5 to 1 mm in diameter can be resolved by modern real-time units.

Partial Volume

The finite beam width also can create a partial-volume artifact related to slice or section thickness. When the beam includes both a cystic structure (low attenuation, echo free) and a solid structure (high attenuation, echogenic), the scan line through that region consists of echoes that are characteristic of a partially solid and partially cystic structure (Fig. 14-1). An accumulation of scan lines of this nature produces fill-in of the cystic structure and may lead to misdiagnoses—such as debris in the gallbladder or a mass in the urinary bladder, which are actually not present. Improper machine settings (high gain or TGC) increase the visibility of this artifact (Fig. 14-2).

Acoustic Speckle

Although acoustic noise occurs throughout the image, it dominates near the face of the transducer. A tissue-texture pattern, finely structured and uniform, seemingly provides excellent resolution although, in fact, no direct relationship exists between image brightness and the strength of the scatterers. Acoustic speckle is often considered to be an artifact, because a one-to-one correspondence between image brightness and scanned objects does not exist. Speckle interferes with the ability of an ultrasound system to detect low-contrast objects—that is, objects with reflective properties similar to those of the surrounding tissue. Many manufacturers are using computers to help remove this speckle pattern so the low-contrast detectability and overall image quality can be improved. The primary speckle-reduction technique involves summing multiple images of the scan plane, a type of signal averaging. To optimize image quality improvement, scans are acquired from different scanning

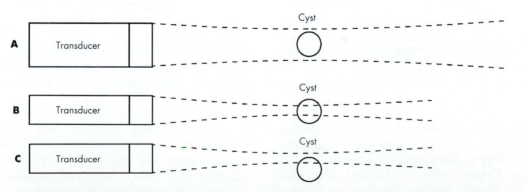

Figure 14-1 Partial volume effect. **A,** A large beam width extends beyond the boundary of the cyst, allowing echoes from surrounding tissue to contribute to the scan line. **B,** Reducing the beam width limits the sampling to the cyst through the central portion of the cyst. **C,** When sampling occurs at the edge of the cyst, a narrow beam may include echoes from surrounding tissue. This leads to fill-in near the border of the cystic structure in the image.

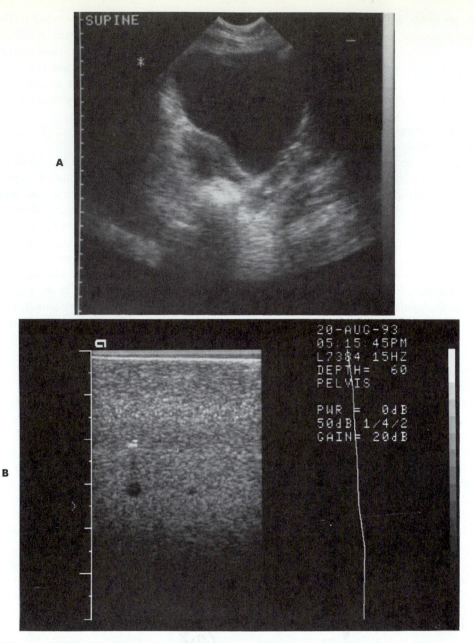

Figure 14-2 A, Slice thickness artifact illustrated as debris at the base of the bladder. **B,** Overcompensation of TGC causes fill-in of a simulated cyst in this TE phantom.

directions or obtained using different transducer frequencies.

Attenuation

The most easily recognizable and useful artifacts are related to attenuation of the ultrasound beam as it propagates through tissue. These artifacts affect the brightness of the displayed echoes. Cysts and other liquid-filled structures are normally less attenuating and are anechoic (no internal echoes) compared with surrounding soft tissues. The area distal to them is interrogated with a beam having greater intensity than is obtained when the beam travels an equivalent distance in tissue. Thus the region behind a liquid-filled structure produces brighter echoes than are observed from adjacent tissues (Fig. 14-3). For this reason the posterior wall of the bladder may appear thicker than the anterior wall.

Shadowing is the opposite effect; that is, solid masses are generally more attenuating and often more echoic, demonstrating more internal structural detail than the surrounding soft tissues. The area distal to the solid mass is interrogated with a beam of decreased intensity, and thus the displayed signals appear to be reduced in brightness compared with the adjacent tissue (Fig. 14-4).

The ability of ultrasound imaging to distinguish cystic and solid structures noninvasively has aided in its acceptance. However, anechoic masses that normally produce

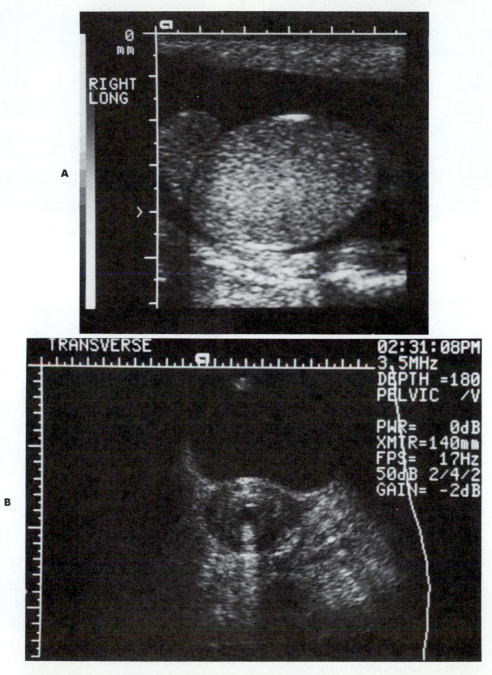

Figure 14-3 A, Enhancement behind fluid surrounding a testicle. **B,** Enhancement behind a nabothian cyst.

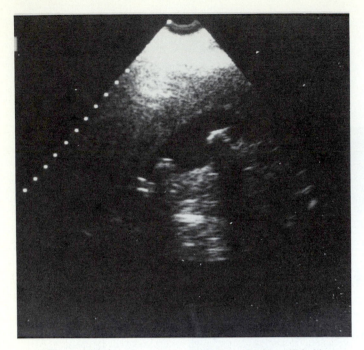

Figure 14-4 Shadowing behind stones in the gallbladder.

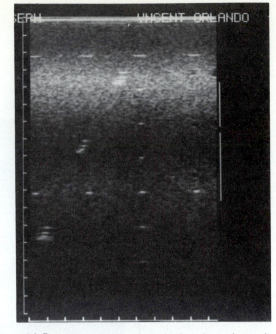

Figure 14-5 Banding artifact from both a dynamic receive–focused and a fixed transmit–focused transducer (*bright area* on the image).

shadowing rather than enhancement do exist. Hyperechoic cysts must be distinguished from slice-section fill-ins and solid masses. Scanning from different directions and using different planes may aid in the diagnosis. These special cases also indicate the need for a further workup with computed tomography (CT) or magnetic resonance imaging (MRI).

Banding

Focusing characteristics of the transducer may create a banding artifact (Fig. 14-5), which is a region of increased brightness caused by greater intensity in the focal zone. This is particularly noticeable with real-time systems that have fixed transmit focusing and dynamic receive focusing. Banding can also be created by improper TGC settings.

Refraction

Refraction of the ultrasound beam at a boundary between two media with different velocities causes two types of artifacts. As discussed in Chapter 1, refraction leads to improper placement of an interface. The assumption that all echoes originate along the straight line of sight is violated when refraction occurs. The interface lateral to the scan line is placed incorrectly along the scan line (see Fig. 1-18, *A*).

Refraction also produces shadowing at the edges of structures that are large (compared with the width of the ultrasound beam) and curved. After passing through such structures, the beams from multiple scan lines diverge or converge depending on the velocity within the structure. For a cyst the velocity is typically lower than in the surrounding tissue and a narrow-angle shadow projection is created (Fig. 14-6). A wide-angle shadow projection occurs when a rel-

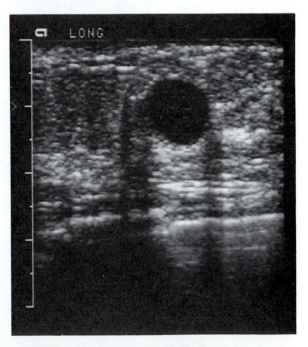

Figure 14-6 Refraction artifact at the edge of a cystic structure illustrating shadowing.

atively high-velocity structure, such as bone, is encountered (Fig. 14-7). Refraction may also distort the size and shape of structures. The incorrect positioning of interfaces is a major concern; but fortunately, this effect is minimized when tissues are scanned in which the ultrasound velocities are similar.

Side lobes and grating lobes (as discussed in Chapters 2

and 4) also induce positioning or range artifacts and false interfaces. These off-axis lobes interrogate structures outside the primary beam. If a highly reflective interface is encountered, it will be incorrectly positioned in the image along the path of the primary beam. This artifact is often observed during needle biopsy with ultrasound guidance (Fig. 14-8). Other examples of off-axis lobe artifacts are shown in Figure 14-9. High-frequency linear array and strongly convex curved linear array transducers are most likely to produce off-axis lobe artifacts.

Multipath Reflections

Incorrect axial placement of an interface is caused by multipath reflections. The ultrasound beam strikes an interface at an angle and is subsequently reflected from a second (or third) interface before being reflected to the transducer. The detected echo does not travel in a straight-line path. Specular scatterers reflect the beam at an angle that may not intercept the transducer, resulting in a "missing" interface in the image. Nonspecular reflectors scatter ultrasound in all directions, and therefore some ultrasonic energy is received from these reflectors.

Reverberation

When reverberations or multiple reflections from an interface are present, structures can be added to an image. The amount of sound energy reflected from an interface depends on the acoustic impedances of the two media. If the impedance mismatch is large (e.g., soft tissue–gas or fluid-gas) and the interface is oriented perpendicular to the direction of propagation, reverberations between the interface and the transducer can occur. A strong echo is created at the interface. On return to the transducer some of its energy is redirected into the patient where it can undergo a second reflection at the same interface. The second echo returns to

the transducer and the sequence is repeated. Since each succeeding echo is displaced in time, a series of bright bands of decreasing intensity and equidistant from each other is mapped in the image (Fig. 14-10). Clinical examples of reverberation artifacts are shown in Figure 14-11.

The loss of intensity is caused by the multiple reflections that take place at the strong reflector and the transducer. A fraction of the incident energy is transmitted through an interface each time one is encountered. Attenuation by the elongated path is compensated by TGC.

Reverberations can also occur between two strong reflectors along the ultrasound beam path; and, similarly, progressively weaker bands are depicted in the image. The

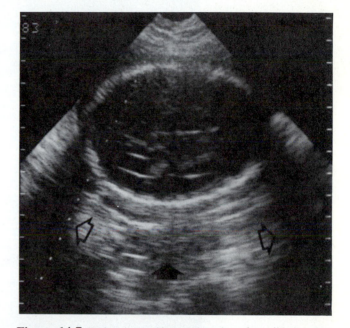

Figure 14-7 Refraction artifact at the edge of a solid structure illustrating shadowing.

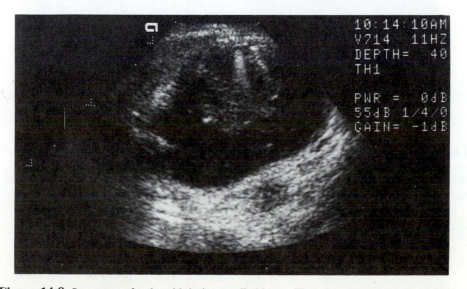

Figure 14-8 Sonogram of a thyroid during needle biopsy. The misregistered image of the needle is on the *left*.

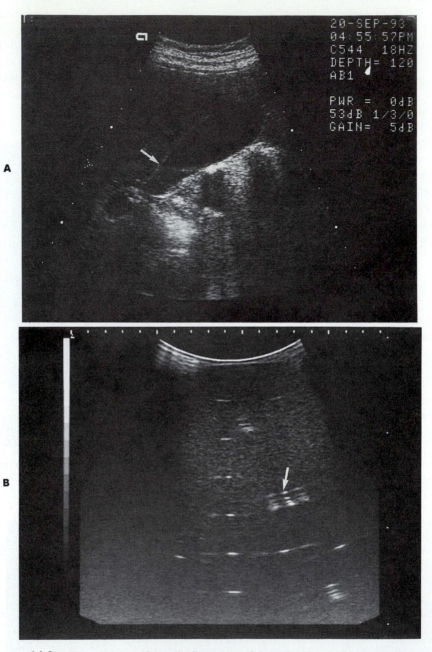

Figure 14-9 Off-axis lobe artifacts. **A,** Sonogram of the pelvis in which structures are misregistered in the anechoic region of the bladder *(arrow).* **B,** Sonogram of the TE phantom with a defective curvilinear array transducer. The resolution rod set at a depth of 7 cm is recorded at three different locations in the image *(arrow).*

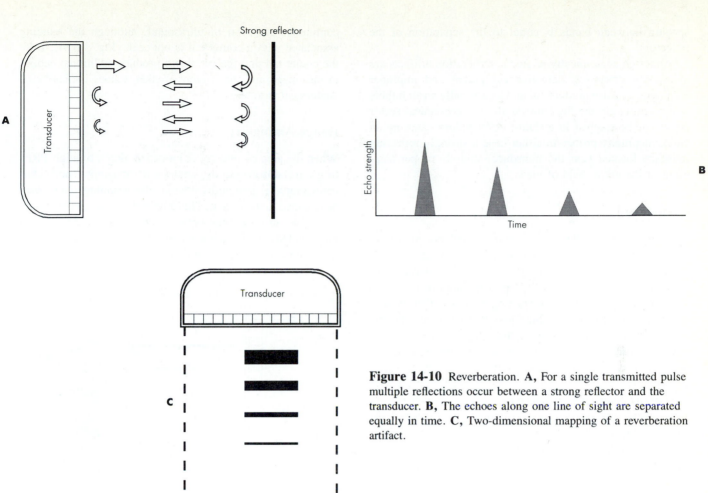

Figure 14-10 Reverberation. **A,** For a single transmitted pulse multiple reflections occur between a strong reflector and the transducer. **B,** The echoes along one line of sight are separated equally in time. **C,** Two-dimensional mapping of a reverberation artifact.

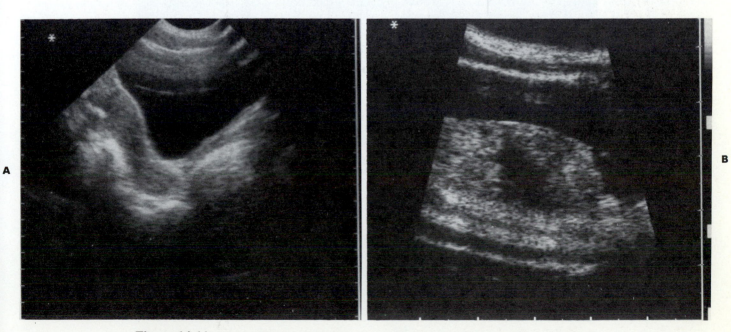

Figure 14-11 A, Reverberation artifacts in the bladder. **B,** Reverberation artifacts and fill-in simulating a carotid plaque.

spacing between bands is equal to the separation of the reflectors.

Although anatomically related reverberation artifacts are commonly observed, defective equipment and improper technique can also produce them. Occasionally an air bubble will form within the fluid surrounding a mechanical sector crystal or be trapped in a fluid-filled condom encasing an endosonography probe. In either case a strongly reflecting interface located near the transducer inhibits proper sampling of the entire field of view.

Comet Tail

Multiple internal reflections within a small but highly reflective object create a series of echoes. Compared with tissue, the object consists of high-Z or low-Z materials. The acoustic impedance mismatch at the boundary of the object forms two highly reflective opposing interfaces that produce short-path reverberations (Fig. 14-12). The time delay between echoes is short, because the sound wave travels the distance across the object and back between echoes. The series of echoes is expressed as multiple small bands, called comet tails, in the image (Fig. 14-13). The possibility of creating a comet tail is enhanced by the increasing difference in acoustic impedances. The complexity of a comet tail pattern depends on the shape, composition, and size of the object, as well as on the scan orientation and the distance from the transducer face. Comet tails are usually seen in relatively echo-free regions.

Resonance

A closely related phenomenon, called a ringdown artifact, occurs when a small gas bubble resonates, resulting in a continuous emission of ultrasound, although the banding associated with a comet tail is not seen (Fig. 14-14). Both the comet tail and the ringdown produce additional echoes in the image and mask other weaker echoes indicative of anatomical structures.

Range Ambiguity

When the area of interest is limited in depth by high PRFs (e.g., in endosonography, small parts sonography, and echocardiography), structures beyond the scanning range may be depicted in the image. This ambiguity in depth placement occurs because the time between the transmitted pulse and the detected echo is not measured properly. As stated earlier, ultrasound scanning assumes that all received echoes are

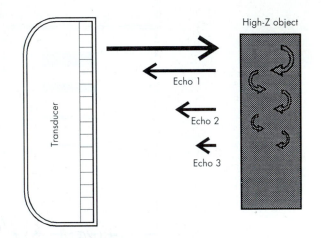

Figure 14-12 Comet tail artifact. Internal reflections give rise to multiple echoes from an object.

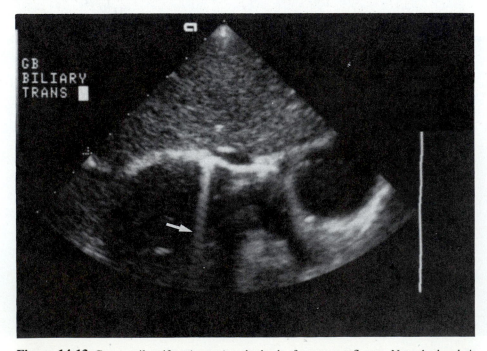

Figure 14-13 Comet tail artifact *(arrow)* at the back of a strong reflector. Note the bands in the comet tail.

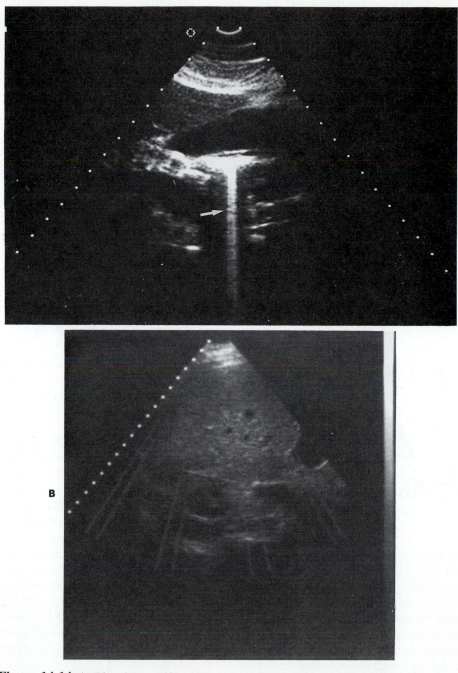

Figure 14-14 A, Ring-down artifact from a gas bubble resonating at its own frequency *(arrow)*. Note the lack of bands in the ring-down. **B,** Simulated ring-down artifacts caused by a defective transducer.

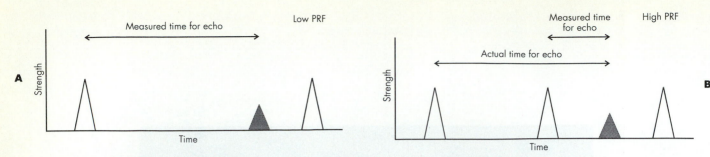

Figure 14-15 Timing between the transmitted pulse *(clear area)* and the echo *(shaded area)*. **A,** At low PRFs the measured time for the echo is proper. **B,** At high PRFs the time between the most recently transmitted pulse and the echo does not correspond to the actual depth.

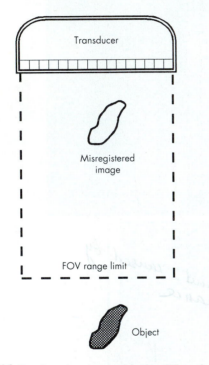

Figure 14-16 Depth assignment ambiguity. When the range of scanning is limited by a high PRF, deep-lying structures are incorrectly placed near the transducer in the image. *FOV,* Field of view.

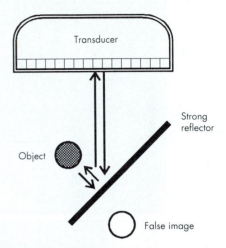

Figure 14-17 Mirror-image artifact. A strong reflector allows sampling of the object along lines of sight in which the sound beam does not follow a straight path.

formed from the most recently transmitted pulse. Normally a short pulse of ultrasound is sent out from the transducer, and the transducer is silent for a time to listen for returning echoes. All echoes received during this sampling period are assigned a depth based on the time interval between the transmitted pulse and the detected echo. A second pulse is then sent out, and the transducer again is silent to listen for returning echoes. At high PRFs echoes from deep structures interrogated by the first pulse arrive at the transducer after the second pulse has been transmitted. These echoes are interpreted as having originated from the most recent (second) transmitted pulse and are incorrectly placed near the transducer in the image (Figs. 14-15 and 14-16).

Mirror Image

Mirror-image artifacts are produced when an object is located in front of a highly reflective surface at which near-

total reflection occurs. Examples of strong reflectors include the diaphragm, pleura, and bowel. The object is imaged in the usual manner by scanning across it with multiple lines of sight. Along nearby lines (which normally would not interrogate the object) the ultrasound beam is reflected by the strong reflector toward the object. When the beam strikes the object, part of the energy is reflected back to the strong reflector, which then redirects the echo toward the transducer. The additional set of scan lines containing echoes from the object form a second image of the object located behind the strong reflector (Fig. 14-17). The time required for the sound wave to travel between the strong reflector and the object creates the mirroring effect so that the true image and false image are equidistant from the strong reflector (Fig. 14-18).

Ghost Image

A closely related phenomenon, called ghost-image artifact, is caused by refraction of the sound beam as it passes through tissues. It results in the duplication or triplication of an object, and its recognition is critical. The primary reason is that a single gestational sac could appear to be multiple (Fig. 14-19) because the rectus muscles (recti abdominales) act as lenses, causing refraction of the ultrasound beam that

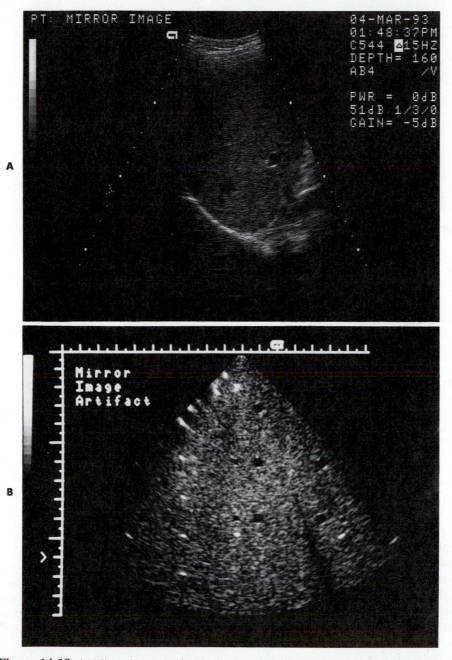

Figure 14-18 A, Mirror image artifact in the liver. The diaphragm acts as a strong reflector.
B, Mirror image of simulated cysts in a defective tissue-equivalent phantom.
(Courtesy Rob Steins, Acuson, Mountain View, CA.)

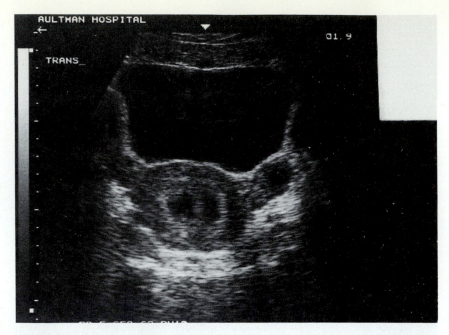

Figure 14-19 Ghost image artifact in which a single gestational sac is duplicated in the image.

leads to duplication of a small object separate from the muscles (Fig. 14-20). One common indication of ghost imaging is when the movement in unison of displayed fetuses actually turns out to be motion of just one mirrored. The ghosting may be eliminated by scanning from different angles or directions. Endosonography probes also may eliminate the problem.

Velocity Error

Measurements of distances, areas, and volumes are of particular importance in diagnostic ultrasound. They are based on the echo-ranging principle, in which the velocity of ultrasound is assumed to be 1540 m/s. Errors in calibration of the velocity or scanning through tissues (bone, lens of the eye, cartilage, fluid, and fat) that have different velocities of sound can cause an artifact called a velocity error, or propagation error. This artifact depends on the actual speed of ultrasound in the medium compared with the calibrated velocity. For small objects, a large velocity difference is necessary to observe a significant error. For large objects, however, a small deviation in velocity can introduce a large error in distance calculations, leading to the incorrect depth assignment of objects.

An interface is displaced toward the transducer and the size of the object is reduced if the actual speed is greater than the calibrated velocity. For example, consider a 10 cm diameter mass, in which the front face is 5 cm deep in tissue and the velocity of ultrasound is 2000 m/s. The front interface of the mass is properly located in the image because the velocity in the overlying tissue is correct; however, the back of the mass is displayed at a depth of 12.7 cm (rather

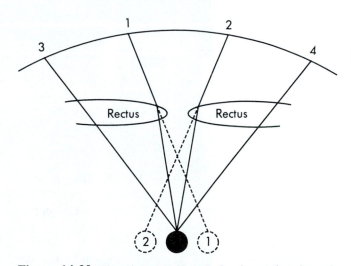

Figure 14-20 Ghost image artifact. Refraction at the edges of a strong reflector (the recti) causes misplacement of the gestational sac (sampling positions *1* and *2*). At sampling positions *3* and *4* the gestational sac is correctly registered in the image. (Adapted from Buttery B, Davison G: *J Ultrasound Med* 3:49, 1984.)

than the actual 15 cm). The calculation is illustrated in Example 14-1.

■ Example 14-1

Using z = ct, first convert the distance through the 10 cm mass to time (actual distance is 20 cm or 0.2 m because of the 10 cm down and 10 cm back).

$$z = ct \qquad 0.2 \text{ m} = (2000 \text{ m/s}) (t)$$
$$t = \frac{0.2 \text{ m}}{2000 \text{ m/s}}$$
$$= 1 \times 10^{-4} \text{ s}$$

Convert this time to the depth in tissue, assuming the unit is calibrated for 1540 m/s.

$$z = ct$$
$$= (1540 \text{ m/s}) (1 \times 10^{-4} \text{ s})$$
$$= 0.154 \text{ m or } 15.4 \text{ cm}$$

The actual diameter displayed is half this value, or 7.7 cm, rather than the true 10 cm.

Of course, the opposite effect (reflector position depicted further away from the transducer and the object magnified) occurs if the actual velocity is less than the calibrated velocity. Another scenario that produces similar results is when the actual velocity in tissue is 1540 m/s but the unit is calibrated for a different value.

Temporal Resolution

To adequately depict tissue motion, sampling must occur at frequent intervals during the motion. The frame rate determines the temporal resolution. Fast-moving structures (e.g., the fetal heart) require high frame rates (50 per second). Abdominal imaging may be satisfactory at a frame rate as low as 4 per second. At low frame rates scan data are placed in a buffer that continuously refreshes the display monitor to prevent flicker.

Limits of human visual perception cause the appearance of structural boundaries on real-time images, but the same boundaries disappear on static freeze-frame images.

Environmental Interference

Instrument noise caused by environmental electrical or radiofrequency interference also can create artifacts in the image. Normally, though not always, a repetitive pattern occurs across the face of the CRT display. Although these artifacts usually are easily recognizable, their actual source may be difficult to determine. If severe enough, they can cause the unit to be unusable where they are present. Manufacturers have improved the shielding design to reduce the effects of environmental interference; thus these siting problems are not frequently encountered.

COLOR DOPPLER IMAGING ARTIFACTS

Specific artifacts for the various scanning modes have been considered in other chapters—registration arm error for static B-mode in Chapter 3, aliasing and spectral broadening for pulsed-wave Doppler in Chapter 5. The subject of imaging artifacts with color Doppler will now be considered.

Because color Doppler (CD) imaging is a portrayal of the Doppler shifts in two dimensions, artifacts identified with imaging and PW Doppler are also possible in the color presentation. These potential artifacts include shadowing, reverberation, mirror image, misregistration from grating

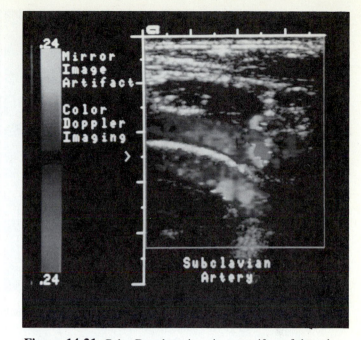

Figure 14-21 Color Doppler mirror image artifact of the subclavian artery. (Courtesy Rob Steins, Acuson, Mountain View, CA.) (See Color Plate 2F.)

lobes, depth ambiguity, and aliasing. In addition, artifacts such as color bleed, color flash, and color noise are unique to CD imaging.

Echo Mapping

Enhanced attenuation by overlying solid structures may cause no color to be displayed within the vessel although flow is present. In Figure 8-8 shadowing by a calcified plaque masks flow through the vessel.

When an anechoic wedge is used with a linear array to provide a more favorable angle of insonation, multiple reflections from interfaces formed by the wedge may introduce reverberation artifacts. Steering the linear array to improve the Doppler angle increases the number and intensity of the grating lobes, which can cause misregistration of interfaces.

Under conditions of high PRF, high gain, and low frequency, deep Doppler shifts may be depicted in a more superficial location. This depth ambiguity occurs because echoes originating beyond the set scanning depth are detected after the next pulse has been emitted. Flow can be portrayed in a region where no flow actually exists. Clinically this is not a common problem (except in cardiac scanning) because attenuation reduces the echo amplitudes from deep-lying reflectors and allows the color reject to exclude these signals from color encoding.

A mirror image of the color flow is produced when the vessel is in front of a highly reflective interface, resulting in the color's being placed at the wrong location. This type of artifact is also called ghosting. Spectral analyses of the real and virtual images are identical. For example, the lung acts as a strong reflector to form a mirror image of the subclavian artery (Fig. 14-21). Mirror images of the carotid and brachial arteries also can occur. This artifact is elimi-

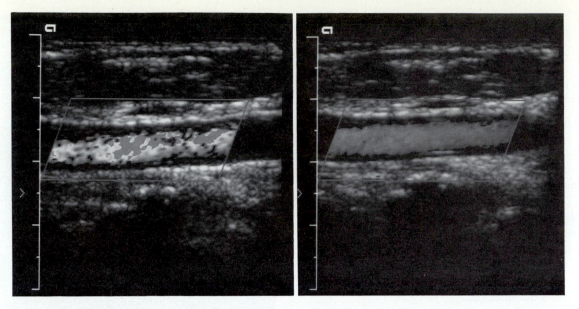

Figure 14-22 A, Color Doppler aliasing. Note the improper color progression of red to yellow to green to blue. If reverse flow were present, the two color directions would be separated by a black region. **B,** Increasing the velocity range removes the aliasing artifact. (See Color Plates 2G and 2H.)

nated by reducing the power, decreasing the color gain, changing the angle of insonation, or a combination of these.

Aliasing

Because moving reflectors are sampled intermittently along the color line of sight, aliasing occurs if the flow exceeds the velocity range set by the operator. A high-frequency shift above the Nyquist limit, but less than twice the Nyquist limit, is detected as a low-frequency shift with opposite phase. The reversal in phase is interpreted as flow in the opposite direction, and thus a color change is induced. Often, aliasing is readily identified as an inappropriate color progression in which a pale shade of red or blue is surrounded by a light shade of the contrasting color, or, in the case of the rainbow color map, contrasting colors representing flow in opposite directions are contiguous (Fig. 14-22). Aliasing is reduced by increasing the Doppler angle, decreasing the frequency of the transmitted pulse, expanding the velocity scale, or shortening the scanning depth. The latter two techniques act to raise the PRF.

Flow reversal must be distinguished from aliasing. The color filter removes low-frequency Doppler signals, thereby setting a velocity threshold below which color is not assigned to the image. Flow reversal is characterized as a black region separating areas with different color directions.

Misregistration of Color

The flashing artifact is a sudden burst of color that encompasses the frame. Cardiac motion, general pulsatility of the arteries, and respiratory movements are all responsible for a change in interface position, which is color encoded. The flashing artifact is suppressed by increasing the color filter,

decreasing the persistence, and reducing the width of the color field of view. Increasing the color filter removes a greater amount of low-velocity components associated with these motions. On a more limited basis, tissue movements are conveyed to nonvascular structures with low echogenicity, which are color encoded. Motion discriminators are less effective when the returning echoes are weak. Flow within dilated bile ducts, cysts, or the gallbladder may be incorrectly assigned. Doppler spectral analysis is necessary to distinguish these from flow areas.

Color bleed is the extension of color beyond the region of flow to the adjacent tissue. This artifact is eliminated by decreasing the transmit power and color gain.

Induced signal amplitude is often used to suppress color. Strong echoes are assigned a gray-scale value, but weak echoes are permitted a color assignment if other criteria are met (i.e., Doppler shift). If Doppler gain is set too high or the Doppler reject is set too low, random variations in echo measurements cause hypoechoic regions to fill with color. Fluid collections or thrombosed vessels may be color encoded by this color noise. Color noise can be differentiated from flow by spectral analysis.

SUMMARY

Sonographers and physicians must be aware that artifacts can lead to misdiagnosis. In addition to operator error and machine malfunction, scan conditions—including the finite size of the beam, the propagation properties of ultrasound in tissues, and the assumptions made concerning image formation—create potential artifacts. Among these artifacts are missing interfaces, wrongly placed interfaces, interfaces with misrepresented size or shape, interfaces with improper brightness, and false interfaces.

Some artifacts are inherent in the imaging process and cannot ever be totally eliminated. To interpret the study accurately, the diagnostician must be able to recognize them and modify the examination accordingly when appropriate.

■■■■■ **R E V I E W   Q U E S T I O N S** ■■■■■

1. Artifacts
   a. Can be completely eliminated by equipment that is operating properly.
   b. Are always detrimental to the proper diagnosis.
   c. Are inherent in the scanning process.
   d. Are easy to identify.

2. Which of the following statement(s) is (are) true?
   a. Artifacts may be caused by improper operation of equipment.
   b. The finite size of the ultrasound beam prevents artifact formation.
   c. Ultrasonic echoes originate from the main beam only.
   d. Ultrasonic echoes originate from the most recent transmitted pulse only.

3. The image artifact induced by the finite spatial pulse length include which of the following:
   a. Improper size of small objects
   b. Multiple false interfaces of small objects
   c. Cyst fill-in
   d. Reverberations

4. Image speckle
   a. Is induced by the finite beam size.
   b. Is not an important artifact.
   c. Influences low-contrast resolution.
   d. Is responsible for the display of small objects in the images.

5. Which statement is true about slice thickness artifacts?
   a. They are unimportant.
   b. They create debris in echogenic structures.
   c. They result from finite beam size.
   d. None of the above.

6. Shadowing
   a. Is an attenuation-related artifact.
   b. Is a propagation speed type of error.
   c. Results from finite beam size.
   d. None of the above.

7. Enhancement
   a. Is multiple reflections along the sampling path.
   b. Is a propagation type of error.
   c. Occurs behind cystic structures.
   d. None of the above.

8. The banding artifact
   a. Is due to reverberations.
   b. Is caused by a change in propagation speed.
   c. Is related to focusing.
   d. None of the above.

9. Lateral displacement of echoes from their true position is caused by which of the following:
   a. Reflection
   b. Refraction
   c. Attenuation
   d. None of these

10. The comet tail artifact is related to
    a. Multiple internal reflections
    b. Resonance of gas body
    c. Attenuation by high-Z objects
    d. None of these

11. Depth range ambiguity is caused by
    a. Reverberation
    b. Resonance
    c. Attenuation
    d. None of these

12. Mirror-image artifact occurs at
    a. Sites of refraction
    b. Compression surfaces
    c. Strongly reflective interfaces
    d. None of these

13. Which is not a possible artifact in color Doppler?
    a. Color flash
    b. Aliasing
    c. Mirror image
    d. Color banding

14. Propagation speed errors are caused by
    a. Improper calibration of equipment
    b. Actual velocities of tissue different than calibration velocity
    c. Highly attenuating tissue
    d. a and b
    e. b and c

15. Assume that the front of a cystic structure rests 3 cm from the face of the transducer and is 10 cm in diameter. If the velocity of ultrasound in the cyst is 1000 m/s, what is the actual size of the displayed cyst? Assume the calibration velocity is 1540 m/s.
    a. 7.7 cm
    b. 15.4 cm
    c. 30.8 cm
    d. 45 cm

16. Referring to Question 15, the position of _____ would be properly represented.
    a. The front surface
    b. The back surface
    c. Both the front and back surfaces
    d. Neither surface

BIBLIOGRAPHY

Avruch L, Cooperberg PL: The ring-down artifact, *J Ultrasound Med* 4:21, 1985.

Buttery B, Davison G: The ghost artifact, *J Ultrasound Med* 3:49, 1984.

Kremkau FW: *Diagnostic ultrasound: principles, instruments, and exercises,* ed 3, Philadelphia, 1989, WB Saunders.

Kremkau FW, Taylor KJW: Artifacts in ultrasound imaging: a review, *J Ultrasound Med* 5:227, 1986.

Laing FC, Kurtz AB: The importance of ultrasonic side-lobe artifacts, *Radiology* 145:763, 1982.

Pozniak MA, Zagzebski JA, Scanlan KA: Spectral and color Doppler artifacts, *Radiographics* 12:35, 1992.

Rose JL, Goldberg BB: *Basic physics in diagnostic ultrasound,* New York, 1979, John Wiley & Sons.

Scanlan KA: Sonographic artifacts and their origins, *AJR* 156:1267, 1991.

Thickman DI, Ziskin MC, Goldenberg NJ, Linder BE: Clinical manifestations of the comet tail artifact, *J Ultrasound Med* 2:225, 1983.

Ziskin MC, Thickman DI, Goldenberg NJ, et al: The comet tail artifact, *J Ultrasound Med* 1:1, 1982.

Review of Mathematics

In physics and mathematics, letters are often used to designate variables. They represent numbers and can be treated in the same manner as numbers. Often the value of a variable must be determined based on a given set of conditions (i.e., an alebraic equation must be solved). However, letters are also used to define various legitimate mathematical operations, which are necessary for the establishment of internal consistency. For example, a particular operation may be true for all positive integers. It is certainly more convenient to represent this set of numbers with a letter than to attempt to list all members of the set. In problem solving, as long as we obey the "rules," the final answer will always be correct, regardless of the order in which the mathematical operations are performed. This assumes that the logical interpretation of the problem, particularly a word problem, was correct.

EXPONENTS

The product of identical factors can be represented in exponential notation:

$$3^4 = 3 \cdot 3 \cdot 3 \cdot 3 = 81$$

or as

$$a^4 = a \cdot a \cdot a \cdot a$$

In this example, 3 (or a) is called the base. In the more general form, a represents any real number. The superscript 4 is the power, which indicates how many times the factor 3 (or a) is multiplied times itself. A more inclusive form would be

$$a^n = a \cdot a \cdots a \text{ (n factors)}$$

where n is a positive integer.

The use of exponents makes many operations faster and easier. The power can be extended to include negative integers if the relation between positive and negative exponents is defined:

$$a^{-n} = \frac{1}{a^n}$$

Examples of Negative Exponents

If a = 2 and n = 3, then

$$2^{-3} = \frac{1}{2^3} = \frac{1}{2 \cdot 2 \cdot 2} = \frac{1}{8} = 0.125$$

If a = 10 and n = 2, then

$$10^{-2} = \frac{1}{10^2} = \frac{1}{10 \cdot 10} = \frac{1}{100} = 0.01$$

Note that the final result is a positive number with a value between 0 and 1. Bases raised to negative powers provide a means of expressing small numbers.

Laws for manipulating exponents must be defined. When multiplying variables in exponential form, add the powers together and retain the base:

$$a^m + a^n = a^{m+n}$$

When dividing variables in exponential form, substract the power of the variable in the denominator from the power of the variable in the numerator and retain the base:

$$\frac{a^m}{a^n} = a^{m-n}$$

In both cases the bases must be the same for the exponents to be combined.

Examples of Multiplication Involving Exponents

$$2^2 \cdot 2^3 = 2^{2+3} = 2^5$$
$$x^4 \cdot x^3 = x^{4+3} = x^7$$
$$y \cdot y^3 \cdot y^5 = y^{1+3+5} = y^9$$
$$x^3 \cdot x^{-2} = x^{3-2} = x^1$$
$$(x^2y^3)(xy^2) = (x^2x^1)(y^3y^2) = x^{2+1}y^{3+2} = x^3y^5$$
$$(4x^2)(3x^3) = (4)(3)x^{2+3} = 12x^5$$

Examples of Division Involving Exponents

$$\frac{2^4}{2^2} = 2^{4-2} = 2^2$$

$$\frac{x^5}{x^3} = x^{5-3} = x^2$$

$$\frac{x^2y^4}{y} = x^2y^{4-1} = x^2y^3$$

$$\frac{10^3}{10^6} = 10^{3-6} = 10^{-3} \text{ or } \frac{1}{10^3}$$

The product of factors in which one of the factors has an exponent equal to zero is given by

$$a^0 \cdot a^n = a^{0+n} = a^n$$

Therefore, a^0 must be equal to 1 because only the product of the number 1 and any other number is the latter number. In general, any base raised to the 0 power is equal to 1. Consider

$$a^n \cdot a^{-n} = a^{n-n} = a^0 = 1$$

Or, substituting numbers

$$2^3 \cdot 2^{-3} = 2^3 \cdot \frac{1}{2^3} = \frac{2^3}{2^3} = 1$$

or

$$= 8 \cdot \frac{1}{8} = \frac{8}{8} = 1$$

or

$$= 2^{3-3} = 2^0 = 1$$

Other operations include raising a group of factors to the nth power.

$$(a^m)^n = a^{mn}$$

$$(ab)^n = a^nb^n$$

$$\left(\frac{a}{b}\right)^n = \frac{a^n}{b^n}$$

Examples of Factors Raised to Various Powers

$$(4^2)^3 = 4^6 = 4096$$

$$\text{or } (4^2)^3 = (4^2)(4^2)(4^2) = 4^{2+2+2} = 4^6 = 4096$$

$$(x^3)^3 = x^9$$

$$(y^2x^2)^4 = y^8x^8$$

$$\left(\frac{2x^3}{y}\right)^2 = \frac{2^2x^6}{y^2} = \frac{4x^6}{y^2}$$

The allowable values for exponents can be expanded to include exponents expressed in fractional form:

$$a^{1/n} \text{ (nth root of a)}$$

which indicates one of n equal factors of a. That is, a factor multiplied times itself n times equals a. If $n = 2$, then $a^{1/2}$ represents the square root of a; if $n = 3$, then $a^{1/3}$ represents the cube root of a, and so on.

Examples of Roots (Fractional Exponents)

$$4^{1/2} = 2 \text{ or } -2 \text{ because } 2 \cdot 2 = 4 \text{ or } -2 \cdot -2 = 4$$

$$8^{1/3} = 2 \text{ because } 2 \cdot 2 \cdot 2 = 8$$

$$27^{1/3} = 3 \text{ because } 3 \cdot 3 \cdot 3 = 27$$

$$16^{1/4} = 2 \text{ or } -2 \text{ because } 2 \cdot 2 \cdot 2 \cdot 2 = 16$$

$$\text{or } -2 \cdot -2 \cdot -2 \cdot -2 = 16$$

The previously defined rules for multiplication and division also apply to fractional exponents. In addition, operations with fractional exponents include

$$(a^{1/n})^m = a^{m/n} = (a^m)^{1/n}$$

where a = a nonnegative number

Further Examples of Fractional Exponents

$$(8^{1/3})^2 = 8^{2/3} = (8^2)^{1/3}$$

$$(8^{1/3})^2 = (2)^2 = 4$$

$$(8^2)^{1/3} = (64)^{1/3} = 4$$

$$(x^{1/2})^5 = x^{5/2} = (x^5)^{1/2}$$

SCIENTIFIC NOTATION

In physics we often deal with very large or very small numbers. For example, it is inconvenient to write the frequency of a 5 MHz transducer as 5,000,000 Hz. Fortunately, a method called scientific notation has been developed to represent and manipulate these numbers easily. In scientific notation the number if expressed as the product of a number between 1 and 10 and a power of 10 (base 10 with an integer exponent). If the exponent of the power of 10 is positive, the value of the power of 10 is greater than 1. If the exponent is negative, the value of the power of 10 is between 0 and 1. As with any base raised to the zero power, 10^0 is defined as being equal to 1. Numbers represented in powers of 10 are shown in the following table:

Number	Power of 10 notation
10,000	10^4
1000	10^3
100	10^2
10	10^1
1	10^0
0.1	10^{-1}
0.01	10^{-2}
0.001	10^{-3}

Note that, for positive exponents, the value of the exponent gives the number of zeros that follow the 1 in the decimal number. For example, 10^4 is equal to 10,000, and there are four zeros after the 1. In the case of negative exponents, the value of the exponent indicates the number of places to the right of the decimal point where the 1 is located. For example, in the case of 10^{-2}, the 1 is located in the second decimal place (0.01).

The numbers 3796 and 0.0214 converted to scientific notation are written as

$$3.796 \times 10^3$$

$$\text{and } 2.14 \times 10^{-2}$$

respectively. In each case the representation of the numeric value is identical. The scientific notation form is equal to 3.796×1000, which, in turn, is 3796. Similarly, 2.14×0.01 is 0.0214.

There are a few basic rules for converting a number into scientific notation. The first step is to determine the sign of the exponent. If the number is greater than 1, the exponent is positive. If the number is between 0 and 1, the exponent is negative. The second step is to count the number of decimal places that are moved to have a single digit to the left of the decimal point. This determines the integer value of the exponent. The number 3796 can be pictured with a decimal point after the 6 initially: 3796. The decimal point is moved three places to the left to give a number between 1 and 10 (i.e., 3.796).

The final task is to combine this number with a power of 10 so that the product equals the original number. The power of 10 has an exponent of $+3$ because the original number was greater than 1 and the decimal was moved three places to the left. The final result is 3.796×10^3.

In a similar fashion, a number less than 1 (e.g., 0.0214) is converted to scientific notation. The exponent 10 in this case is equal to -2 because the decimal point must be moved to the right two places to give 2.14. Combining this number with the power of 10 gives the final result 2.14×10^{-2}.

To convert a number expressed in scientific notation back into standard format, the process is essentially reversed; that is, a positive exponent indicates how many places to move the decimal point to the right and a negative exponent indicates how many places to move the decimal point to the left.

For the number 8.75×10^4 the decimal point must be moved four places to the right (to give 87,500) whereas 6.34×10^{-3} requires the decimal point to be moved to the left three places (to give 0.00634).

When multiplying or dividing numbers expressed in scientific notation, we treat the numerical factors as a group and the powers of 10 as another group. Manipulation of the powers of 10 follows all the laws of exponents. These operations are summarized by

$$(a \times 10^n)(b \times 10^m) = ab \times 10^{n+m}$$

and

$$\frac{(a \times 10^n)}{(b \times 10^m)} = \frac{a}{b} \times 10^{n-m}$$

EXAMPLES USING SCIENTIFIC NOTATION

$$(4.0 \times 10^2)(1.5 \times 10^3) = (4.0)(1.5) \times 10^2 \times 10^3$$
$$= 6.0 \times 10^{2+3}$$
$$= 6.0 \times 10^5$$
$$(2.2 \times 10^4)(3.0 \times 10^{-3}) = (2.2)(3.0) \times 10^4 \times 10^{-3}$$
$$= 6.6 \times 10^{4-3}$$
$$= 6.6 \times 10^1$$

$$\frac{4.0 \times 10^5}{2.0 \times 10^1} = 2.0 \times 10^{5-1} = 2.0 \times 10^4$$

$$\frac{248,000}{0.0124} = \frac{2.48 \times 10^5}{1.24 \times 10^{-2}}$$
$$= \frac{2.48}{1.24} \times 10^{5-(-2)}$$
$$= 2.00 \times 10^{5+2}$$
$$= 2.00 \times 10^7$$

SCIENTIFIC AND ENGINEERING PREFIXES

Another technique to facilitate communication of the very large and very small numbers encountered in ultrasound physics is the use of engineering prefixes. These prefixes correspond to various multiples of powers of 10 as shown in the table below.

Factor	Prefix	Symbol
10^9	giga	G
10^6	mega	M
10^3	kilo	k
10^{-2}	centi	c
10^{-3}	milli	m
10^{-6}	micro	μ
10^{-9}	nano	n
10^{-12}	pico	p

When a physical parameter is expressed in scientific notation that includes some standard unit (i.e., meter, second, hertz, watt, etc.), the prefix replaces the power of 10 and becomes a modifier of the unit.

Examples of Engineering Prefixes

$$3.5 \times 10^6 \text{ Hz} = 3.5 \text{ MHz}$$
$$2.0 \times 10^{-2} \text{ m} = 2.0 \text{ cm}$$
$$1.3 \times 10^{-5} \text{ s} = 13 \times 10^{-6} \text{ s} = 13 \text{ μs}$$
$$6.5 \times 10^{-3} \text{ W} = 6.5 \text{ mW}$$

In the above examples MHz, cm, μs, and mW are stated as *mega*hertz, *centi*meters, *micro*seconds, and *milli*watts. The prefix may also be replaced by the appropriate power of ten so the mathematical operations can be performed.

Examples of Numerical Conversions of Engineering Prefixes

$$7 \text{ μm} = 7 \times 10^{-6} \text{ m}$$
$$10 \text{ cm} = 10 \times 10^{-2} \text{ m} = 0.1 \text{ m}$$
$$1 \text{ kHz} = 1000 \text{ Hz}$$

SOLVING EQUATIONS

In algebra, equations are used to express relationships between a collection of variables. Each variable is usually denoted by a letter. When a set of conditions is given, a solution to the equation is sought by manipulating the equation according to well-defined mathematical principles. It is important to realize that the letter corresponding to a variable represents a number and therefore can be treated as a number; that is, the letter can be used in steps of addition, subtraction, multiplication, and division. Consider the equation

A-1

$$2x + 4 = 10$$

The equal sign separates one side of the equation from the other. The left-hand side has two terms (2x and 4) and the right-hand side one term (10). The terms are separated by minus ($-$) or plus ($+$) signs of operation. The term 2x consists of an unknown variable x and the number 2, which is the coefficient. A coefficient is a multiplication factor. In the absence of a coefficient, it is understood to be 1.

Because only one unknown (the variable x) is present in Equation A-1, the unknown can be isolated on one side of the equation and its value thus determined. This is the solution to the equation and represents a value that, when substituted for x, makes the statement, or equation, true. Two useful techniques are used to obtain the goal of isolating the unknown on one side of the equation:

1. Addition (or subtraction) of the same term to (or from) each side of the equation does not change the value of the unknown.
2. Multiplication or division of each side of the equation by the same factor does not change the value of the unknown. Division must be by a nonzero real number.

Let us apply the above techniques to solve for x in Equation A-1. All terms that do not contain x should be eliminated from the left-hand side. In this case, one term, the 4, must be removed by subtracting 4 from each side:

$$2x + 4 - 4 = 10 - 4$$
$$2x + 0 = 6$$
$$2x = 6$$

The process of solving the equation is not complete, because the coefficient of x is not 1 (x is not completely by itself on one side of the equation). If each side is divided by 2, then

$$\frac{2x}{2} = \frac{6}{2}$$
$$x = 3$$

The conditions of the original equation dictate that x must be equal to 3. The solution is tested by replacing x with 3 wherever x occurs in the original equation. Hence,

$$2 \cdot 3 + 4 = 10$$
$$6 + 4 = 10$$
$$10 = 10$$

which is obviously a true condition.

The order in which we apply the manipulation techniques is not fixed. Indeed, both sides can initially be divided by 2:

$$\frac{2x}{2} + \frac{4}{2} = \frac{10}{2}$$
$$x + 2 = 5$$

Note that each term on each side of the equation must be divided by the same number or variable. To isolate x, 2 is now subtracted from each side:

$$x + 2 - 2 = 5 - 2$$
$$x + 0 = 3$$
$$x = 3$$

Again, the solution of the equation is found to be x is equal to 3, which demonstrates internal consistency.

Another example may be useful. Suppose that

A-2

$$3x + 1 = 4x - 6$$

The variable x appears on both sides of the equation. Only like terms can be added or subtracted. Like terms are terms in which the variables, including their respective exponents, are the same. (Terms consisting entirely of numbers are also like terms.) To combine like terms, coefficients are added with coefficients. Begin to isolate x by adding 6 to each side:

$$3x + 1 + 6 = 4x - 6 + 6$$

The 6 and 3x as well as the 6 and 4x are unlike terms and cannot be combined:

$$3x + 7 = 4x$$

Next, subtract 3x from each side:

$$3x - 3x + 7 = 4x - 3x$$
$$0x + 7 = 1x$$
$$7 = x$$

This solution is tested by replacing every x in the original equation with a 7:

$$3 \cdot 7 + 1 = 4 \cdot 7 - 6$$
$$21 + 1 = 28 - 6$$
$$22 = 22$$

Once more, the operations have been applied properly to determine the unknown (x).

These techniques of manipulating equations can be summarized very concisely by remembering that whatever is done to one side of the equation must also be done to the other side.

Often the relationship between many variables is expressed in one equation. In ultrasound a very useful equation relates the properties of the ultrasound wave:

A-3

$$c = f\lambda$$

where c is the velocity, f the frequency, and λ the wavelength. It is possible to generate tables listing values for velocity, frequency, and wavelength, but this task would never be complete.

The limitation still exists; only one unknown in a given

situation can be determined by solving Equation A-3. This means, however, that if any two of the variables are given we can solve for the third. Rearranging Equation A-3 by dividing each side by λ yields

A-4

$$\frac{f\lambda}{\lambda} = \frac{c}{\lambda}$$

$$f = \frac{c}{\lambda}$$

Similarly, dividing each side by f gives

A-5

$$\frac{\lambda f}{f} = \frac{c}{f}$$

$$\lambda = \frac{c}{f}$$

Equations A-4 and A-5 express the same relation as Equation A-3 in different forms.

Problem A-1

What is the wavelength of the ultrasound wave in soft tissue with a frequency of 2.5 MHz? (Assume the velocity is 1540 m/s.)

Answer

$$f = 2.5 \text{ MHz} = 2.5 \times 10^6 \text{ Hz}$$
$$\text{or } 2.5 \times 10^6 \text{ c/s}$$
$$c = 1540 \text{ m/s} = 1.54 \times 10^3 \text{ m/s}$$

Solution: Using Equation A-5

$$\lambda = \frac{c}{f}$$

$$= \frac{1.54 \times 10^3 \text{ m/s}}{2.5 \times 10^6 \text{ c/s}}$$

$$= 6.16 \times 10^{-4} \text{ m}$$

$$= 6.16 \times 10^{-1} \text{ mm}$$

Problem A-2

The wavelength of ultrasound in a particular medium is 1 mm and the frequency is 5 MHz. What is the velocity of ultrasound in the medium?

Answer

$$\lambda = 1 \text{ mm} = 1 \times 10^{-3} \text{ m}$$
$$f = 5 \text{ MHz} = 5 \times 10^6 \text{ c/s}$$

Solution: Using Equation A-3

$$c = f\lambda$$

$$= (5 \times 10^6 \text{ c/s})(1 \times 10^{-3} \text{ m})$$

$$= 5 \times 10^3 \text{ m/s}$$

Problem A-3

The wavelength in tissue is 0.2 mm. What is the frequency of the transducer?

Answer

$$\lambda = 0.2 \text{ mm} = 2 \times 10^{-4} \text{ m}$$

Solution: The velocity in tissue is assumed to be 1540 m/s. Using Equation A-4

$$f = \frac{c}{\lambda}$$

$$= \frac{1.54 \times 10^3 \text{ m/s}}{2 \times 10^{-4} \text{ m}}$$

$$= 7.7 \times 10^6 \text{ c/s}$$

$$= 7.7 \text{ MHz}$$

It is not necessary to memorize all the forms of the relationship between velocity, wavelength, and frequency. The equation $c = f\lambda$ is sufficient. By substituting for the known variables and manipulating the equation, we can determine the remaining variable.

Problem A-4

See Problem A-3 using Equation A-3.

Answer

$$c = 1.54 \times 10^3 \text{ m/s}$$
$$\lambda = 2 \times 10^{-4} \text{ m}$$

Solution:

$$c = f\lambda$$

$$1.54 \times 10^3 \text{ m/s} = f (2 \times 10^{-4} \text{ m})$$

$$\frac{1.54 \times 10^3 \text{ m/s}}{2 \times 10^{-4} \text{ m}} = f$$

$$7.7 \times 10^6 \text{ c/s} = f$$

UNIT CONVERSIONS

A description of physical parameter is not complete unless the units also are specified. If someone were to ask how far Los Angeles is from New York City, the reply would most likely be 3000 miles. The unit "miles" is necessary for the answer to make sense.

Most physical parameters are expressed in units—some combination of length, mass, and time. Wavelength is expressed in terms of length, whereas velocity is in terms of length per time. Both 12 inches and 1 foot represent the same absolute measurement of length. The problem or traditional preference usually dictates which unit is to be used.

Note the importance of retaining units in the problems in the previous section. If this is done correctly, the solution for a particular unknown is always expressed in proper units (e.g., wavelength is found in units of length).

Sometimes unit conversions are necessary to maintain a

consistent set of units throughout the problem. Once the relationship between original units and desired units is known, this conversion factor is modified to a fractional form, which is equal to 1. The product of the fractional form of the conversion factor and the original units gives the desired units without changing the absolute value of the physical parameter.

Suppose 10 millimeters (mm) is to be expressed in terms of meters (m). The conversion factor is given by

$$1000 \text{ mm} = 1 \text{ m}$$

The problem can be viewed as

$$10 \text{ mm} \times \text{CF} = ? \text{ m}$$

where CF is the fractional form of the conversion factor. CF must be written so the unit m is in the numerator and mm is in the denominator. Dividing each side of the conversion factor by 1000 mm

$$1 = \frac{1 \text{ m}}{1000 \text{ mm}}$$

$$\text{CF} = \frac{1 \text{ m}}{1000 \text{ mm}}$$

Substituting for CF as the factor times 10 mm

$$10 \text{ mm} \times \frac{1 \text{ m}}{1000 \text{ mm}} = 0.01 \text{ m}$$

Note that millimeters in the numerator and the denominator cancel. We find that 0.01 m is the same as 10 mm. The fractional form of the conversion factor can be inverted to transform meters to millimeters.

To express 0.01 meters in terms of millimeters

$$0.01 \text{ m} \times \text{CF} = ? \text{ mm}$$

$$0.01 \text{ m} \times \frac{1000 \text{ mm}}{1 \text{ m}} = 10 \text{ mm}$$

Once again, the original unit cancels with the denominator in the conversion factor and the desired unit remains.

Problem A-5

A car is moving at a rate of 60 miles per hour. What is the velocity in terms of miles per minute?

Answer

The conversion factor is 60 min = 1 hr
Solution:

$$\frac{60 \text{ miles}}{\text{hr}} \times \text{CF} = \frac{? \text{ miles}}{\text{min}}$$

The fractional form (CF) must have hours in the numerator. Therefore

$$\text{CF} = \frac{1 \text{ hr}}{60 \text{ min}}$$

Substituting for CF

$$\frac{60 \text{ miles}}{\text{hr}} \times \frac{1 \text{ hr}}{60 \text{ min}} = 1 \text{ mile/min}$$

Common conversion factors

1000 mm	1 m
10 mm	1 cm
100 cm	1 m
1 MHz	10^6 Hz
1 μs	10^{-6} s
1 ms	10^{-3} s
1 gm/cm^3	1000 kg/m^3
1 gm/cm^2/s	10 kg/m^2/s
1 m/s	100 cm/s

TRIGONOMETRY

When two lines cross, they form an angle, which is usually specified in degrees. In Figure A-1, angle ϕ is larger than angle θ. A protractor is used to measure the angle. One complete revolution, a straight line, and a right angle correspond to 360 degrees, 180 degrees, and 90 degrees, respectively. The degree is divided into smaller divisions called minutes, and the minute into even smaller divisions called seconds:

$$1 \text{ degree} = 60 \text{ minutes}$$
$$1 \text{ minute} = 60 \text{ seconds}$$

This is similar to the relationship among hours, minutes, and seconds in timekeeping.

Degrees may also be expressed in decimal form, in which case the seconds and minutes must be converted into degrees via the conversion factors. For example

$$30° \, 45' = 30.75° \text{ because}$$

$$45 \text{ min} \times \frac{1°}{60 \text{ min}} = 0.75°$$

A unit called the radian is also used to describe the size of an angle. A complete revolution is equal to 2π radians, or identically, one radian is 57.3 degrees. The following tabulation shows various angles expressed in both radians and degrees.

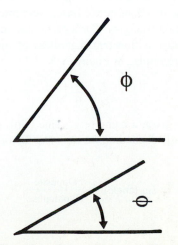

Figure A-1 Formation of an angle by two lines that cross. Angle ϕ is greater than angle θ.

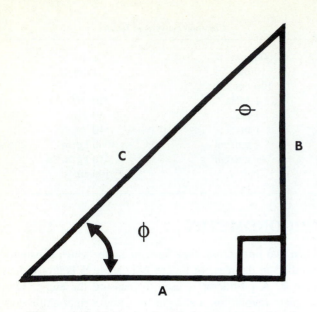

Figure A-2 Right triangle. The hypotenuse is side *C*.

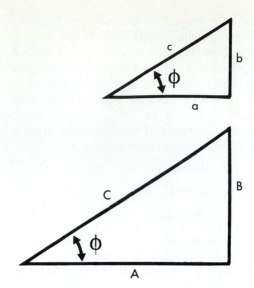

Figure A-3 Two triangles with equal angles but different lengths of sides.

Radians	Degrees
2π	360°
π	180°
$\pi/2$	90°
$\pi/4$	45°

A triangle is a three-sided geometric figure. If one of the angles is 90 degrees, the triangle is a right triangle (Fig. A-2). All the angles of the triangle, when added together, must equal 180 degrees. Therefore angle θ is calculated by subtracting angle ϕ from 90 degrees and vice versa.

The side opposite the right angle is the hypotenuse (side *C* in Figure A-2). The hypotenuse is always the longest side of the right triangle. An opposite side and an adjacent side are designated with respect to the angle of interest. For example, when the angle ϕ is considered, the adjacent side is side A and the opposite side is side B.

Early mathematicians noticed some very interesting properties about right triangles. For a particular angle, the ratio of any two sides is constant regardless of the size of the triangle. For example, in Figure A-3

$$\frac{a}{b} = \frac{A}{B}$$

The ratio was given a name (e.g., sine [sin], cosine [cos], or tangent [tan]) depending on the sides involved:

A-6

$$\sin (\text{angle}) = \frac{\text{Opposite}}{\text{Hypotenuse}}$$

A-7

$$\cos (\text{angle}) = \frac{\text{Adjacent}}{\text{Hypotenuse}}$$

A-8

$$\tan (\text{angle}) = \frac{\text{Opposite}}{\text{Adjacent}}$$

These are the most commonly used trigonometric functions. When problem solving with trigonometric functions, the angle must be identified, but the numeric value may be unknown. From Figure A-3, the trigonometric functions are found to equal:

$$\sin \phi = \frac{b}{c} = \frac{B}{C}$$

$$\cos \phi = \frac{a}{c} = \frac{A}{C}$$

$$\tan \phi = \frac{b}{a} = \frac{B}{A}$$

Values of the trigonometric functions have been collected in tables or they are readily obtainable from scientific calculators. Common trigonometric functions are shown in the following tabulation:

Angle	Sin	Tan	Cos
0°	0.000	0.000	1.000
30°	0.500	0.577	0.866
45°	0.707	1.000	0.707
60°	0.866	1.732	0.500
90°	1.000	—	0.000

Note that this tabulation is used in two ways. Given the ratio of the sides for the particular trigonometric function, read across to determine the angle; this procedure is referred to as taking the arc of the trigonometric function. Likewise, given the angle, read across to find the ratios of the various sides. Think of the trigonometric functions as equations with three variables. If any two of the variables are known, the equation can be solved for the third variable.

Problem A-6

In Figure A-2, assume that $\phi = 30°$ and that $A = 10$ cm. What is the length of side B?

Answer

$$\tan \phi = \frac{B}{A}$$

Solution:

$$\tan 30° = \frac{B}{10 \text{ cm}}$$

$$0.577 = \frac{B}{10 \text{ cm}}$$

$$5.77 \text{ cm} = B$$

Problem A-7

In Figure A-2, assume that side $B = 8$ cm and that side $C = 16$ cm. What is the angle θ?

Answer

$$\cos \theta = \frac{B}{C}$$

Solution:

$$\cos \theta = \frac{8 \text{ cm}}{16 \text{ cm}}$$

$$\cos \theta = 0.5$$

Examine the table for the angle that gives a value of 0.5 for the cosine trigonometric function:

$$\theta = 60°$$

Problem A-8

In Figure A-2, assume that θ is 60 degrees and that side A is 10 cm. What is the length of side C?

Answer

$$\sin \theta = \frac{A}{C}$$

Solution:

$$\sin 60° = \frac{10 \text{ cm}}{C}$$

$$0.866 = \frac{10 \text{ cm}}{C}$$

$$C = 11.5 \text{ cm}$$

LOGARITHMS

In essence, logarithms are a means to express numbers in terms of a base and an exponent, where the base is understood to be constant. Because the base is known, it does not have to be written explicitly. A number (x) can be represented in the form

$$x = b^y \quad (x \text{ is always greater than zero})$$

where b is the base and y the exponent.

The logarithm to the base b of x is an exponent. Thus

$$\log_b x = y$$

By taking the logarithm of a number, the exponent is found for which the number would be obtained if the base were raised to that exponent. Various types of logarithms exist depending on the base. The two types most frequently used are common logarithms (base 10) and natural logarithms (base e).

In common logarithms, the base is assigned a value of 10. Defining equations are

$$x = 10^y \quad \text{A-9}$$

and

$$\log_{10} x = y \quad \text{A-10}$$

A table of logarithms of the powers of 10 is as follows:

x	Power of 10	$\log_{10} x$
1000	10^3	3
100	10^2	2
10	10^1	1
1	10^0	0
0.1	10^{-1}	-1
0.01	10^{-2}	-2
0.001	10^{-3}	-3

Suppose the number x is not a power of 10; then log x is a decimal number. The number x is written in scientific notation, that is, the factor times a power of 10. The logarithm is found by adding the characteristic and the mantissa together. The exponent in the power of 10 is the characteristic, and the logarithm of the factor is the mantissa. Because the factor has a value between 1 and 10, the mantissa will have a value between 0 (the log of 1) and 1 (the log of 10). Mathematical tables list the logarithms of numbers between 1 and 10.

Although decimal exponents may be somewhat confusing initially, they can be understood simply as a combination of roots and powers. The square root of 10 can be written as fractional exponent ($10^{1/2}$), as a decimal exponent ($10^{.5}$), or as a number (3.16). For example, consider

$$10^{.25} = (10^{.5})^{1/2} = (3.16)^{1/2} = 1.78$$
$$10^{.67} = (10^{2/3}) = (10^2)^{1/3} = 100^{1/3} = 4.63$$

The following examples demonstrate the process of finding the logarithm of a number.

$$\log 42.5 = \log(4.25 \times 10^1)$$
$$= \log(4.25) + \log(10^1)$$

$$= 0.6284 \text{(mantissa)} + 1 \text{(characteristic)}$$

$$= 1.6284$$

$$\log 4250 = \log(4.25 \times 10^3)$$

$$= \log(4.25) + \log(10^3)$$

$$= 0.6284 + 3$$

$$= 3.6284$$

$$\log(0.00302) = \log(3.02 \times 10^{-3})$$

$$= \log(3.02) + \log(10^{-3})$$

$$= 0.4800 + (-3)$$

$$= -2.52$$

Numbers greater than 1 that differ only in their powers of 10 have the same mantissa. The logarithm of a number less than 1 but greater than zero is negative. The operation of finding the logarithm of a negative number is not defined.

Scientific calculators make the process of finding the logarithm of a number considerably easier. The number in standard format or scientific notation is entered into the display, and the log key is pressed. The logarithm is calculated and replaces the number in the display.

Suppose the log x is given; how do we determine the number x? That is, the exponent is known and x must be calculated. This process is the reverse of finding the logarithm and is called taking the antilogarithm (antilog). The antilog of y is the base 10 with an exponent of y:

A-11

$$\text{Antilog } y = 10^y = x$$

Examples of Antilogarithms

Given that log x = 1.6395, find x.

$$x = \text{Antilog } 1.6395$$

$$= 10^{1.6395}$$

$$= (10^{.6395})(10^1)$$

$$= (4.36)(10^1)$$

$$= 43.6$$

Given that log x = −2.52, find x.

$$x = \text{Antilog}(-2.52)$$

$$= 10^{-2.52}$$

$$= (10^{.48})(10^{-3})$$

$$= (3.02)(10^{-3})$$

$$= 0.00302$$

If tables are used, the mantissa must be a positive number between 0 and 1. That is the reason (-2.52) was rewritten as $(0.48 - 3)$ in this example. If one uses a calculator, this distinction does not have to be made because the base 10 raised to any power is calculated directly.

Because logarithms are exponents of bases, logarithms have properties similar to the operations defined for exponents. When two numbers are multiplied together, we can either take the logarithm of the product or add the logarithms of the individual factors:

A-12

$$\log(x_1 \cdot x_2) = \log(x_1) + \log(x_2)$$

For example,

$$\log(2 \cdot 3) = \log(2) + \log(3)$$

$$\log 6 = 0.3010 + 0.4771$$

$$0.7781 = 0.7781$$

This property has already been used in obtaining the logarithm of numbers expressed in scientific notation. In the case of one number divided by another, the logarithm of the divisor is subtracted from the logarithm of the dividend:

A-13

$$\log(x_1/x_2) = \log(x_1) - \log(x_2)$$

For example,

$$\log(8/2) = \log(8) - \log(2)$$

$$\log(4) = 0.9030 - 0.3010$$

$$0.6020 = 0.6020$$

The logarithm of a number raised to the mth power is the product of m and the logarithm of the number:

A-14

$$\log(x^m) = m \log x$$

For example,

$$\log(2)^3 = 3 \log 2$$

$$\log 8 = 3(0.3010)$$

$$0.9030 = 0.9030$$

The second type of logarithm, called natural logarithms, uses the base e, which has a numerical value of approximately 2.7183. The defining equations become

A-15

$$\log_e x = y$$

or

A-16

$$\ln x = y$$

and

A-17

$$e^y = x$$

The latter is called an exponential function and can be pictured as

$$2.7183^y = x$$

where the base (2.7183) is evaluated for y. The exponent y can be positive or negative or zero, but x is always greater than zero.

The natural logarithms of numbers have been compiled in mathematical tables. They are also readily available via scientific calculators. Natural logarithms do not use characteristics as do common logarithms. The inverse of the natural logarithm is the exponential function, which eliminates the need for the term antilogarithm when referring to natural logarithms. The relationship between e^y and ln x is shown in the following tabulation:

x or e^y	ln x or y
0.01	−4.6052
0.1	−2.3026
1	0
2.7183	1.0000
10	2.3026
100	4.6052

Scientific calculators provide values for exponential functions. The same properties defined for common logarithms apply to natural logarithms (ln). The relationship between the natural and common logarithms is given by

A-18

$$\ln x = 2.303 \log x$$

A-19

$$e^y = 10^{.4343y}$$

which permits easy conversion from one type to the other.

For example, the natural logarithm of x when x = 100 is solved by using the relationship between natural and common logarithms as follows:

$$x = 100$$
$$\ln 100 = 2.303 \log(100)$$
$$= 2.303(2)$$
$$= 4.606$$

To solve for e^y, when y = 2

$$e^2 = 10^{(.4343)(2)}$$
$$= 10^{.8686}$$
$$= 7.389$$

DECIBELS

In ultrasound the intensity at one point is compared with that at another. Relative rather than absolute values of the intensity are specified. Because many powers of 10 are involved, a logarithm scale is employed in which the change in intensity is given in decibels (dB). The level in dB is defined by:

A-20

$$\text{level (dB)} = 10 \log (I/I_0)$$

where I_0 is the intensity at the reference point and I the intensity at the point of interest. The ratio of I/I_0 must always be dimensionless; I_0 and I must be expressed in the same units.

Problem A-9

Determine the level in decibels if the ultrasound beam enters the material with an intensity of $1 \times 10^5 \text{ mW/cm}^2$ and exits with an intensity of $2 \times 10^2 \text{ mW/cm}^2$.

Answer

$$I_0 = 1 \times 10^5 \text{ mW/cm}^2$$
$$I = 2 \times 10^2 \text{ mW/cm}^2$$

Solution: Using Equation A-20

$$\text{Level (dB)} = 10 \log(I/I_0)$$
$$= 10 \log \frac{(2 \times 10^2)}{1 \times 10^5}$$
$$= 10 \log(2 \times 10^{-3})$$
$$= 10(-2.699)$$
$$= -26.99$$

The negative sign indicates the intensity decreased from the reference point to the point of interest.

Problem A-10

A 10 dB loss in intensity is observed at a certain depth (z) in the medium. If the intensity at the surface is $2.5 \times 10^3 \text{ mW/cm}^2$, what is the intensity at depth z?

Answer

$$I_0 = 2.5 \times 10^3 \text{ mW/cm}^2$$

Level (dB) = −10, because a loss in intensity occurred. Solution: Using Equation A-20

$$\text{Level (dB)} = 10 \log(I/I_0)$$
$$-10 = 10 \log(I/I_0)$$

Divide each side by 10:

$$-1 = \log(I/I_0)$$

Take the antilog of each side:

$$I/I_0 = \text{Antilog}(-1)$$
$$= 0.1$$

Substitute for I_0:

$$0.1 = \frac{I}{2.5 \times 10^3 \text{ mW/cm}^2}$$

Solve for I:

$$I = (2.5 \times 10^3 \text{ mW/cm}^2)(0.1)$$
$$= 2.5 \times 10^2 \text{ mW/cm}^2$$

Problem A-11

The surface intensity in Problem A-10 is raised to a new value. If the intensity at depth z is $8 \times 10^6 \text{ mW/cm}^2$, what is the intensity at the surface? Assume a 10 dB loss to depth z.

Answer

$$I = 8 \times 10^6 \text{ mW/cm}^2$$
$$\text{Level (dB)} = -10$$

Solution: From Problem A-10, the ratio of the intensities is 0.1:

$$0.1 = I/I_0$$

$$= \frac{8 \times 10^6 \text{ mW/cm}^2}{I_0}$$

$$I_0 = 8 \times 10^7 \text{ mW/cm}^2$$

Problem A-12

Determine the level in decibels if the intensity of interest is half the reference intensity.

Answer

$$I = 0.5 \, I_0$$

Solution: Using Equation A-20

$$\text{Level (dB)} = 10 \log(I/I_0)$$

$$= 10 \log \frac{0.5 \, I_0}{I_0}$$

$$= 10 \log(0.5)$$

$$= 10 \log(0.5)$$

$$= 10(-0.301)$$

$$= -3.01$$

If the intensity decreases by a factor of 2, a 3 dB loss results. Each half-value layer (HVL) of material causes a 3 dB reduction in intensity.

Problem A-13

The intensity at the surface is 5×10^6 mW/cm². What is the intensity after transversing a material four HVLs thick?

Answer

Determine the intensity level change caused by the absorbing material: -3 dB/HVL $\times$ 4 HVL $= -12$ dB

$$I_0 = 5 \times 10^6 \text{ mW/cm}^2$$

Solution:

$$\text{Level (dB)} = 10 \log(I/I_0)$$

$$-12 = 10 \log(I/I_0)$$

$$-1.2 = \log(I/I_0)$$

$$\text{Antilog}(-1.2) = I/I_0$$

$$0.063 = I/I_0$$

$$= \frac{I}{5 \times 10^6 \text{ mW/cm}^2}$$

$$I = 3.15 \times 10^5 \text{ mW/cm}^2$$

An alternative solution is to recognize that each HVL decreases the intensity by a factor of 2:

A-21

$$I = I_0/2^n = I_0(1/2)^n$$

where n is the number of HVLs.

$$I = 5 \times 10^6 \text{ mW/cm}^2(1/2)(1/2)(1/2)(1/2)$$

$$= 3.12 \times 10^5 \text{ mW/cm}^2$$

This does not agree exactly with the previous answer, because the decibel loss per HVL was rounded off to 3.

STATISTICS

Biological variations occur in populations. Heights of adult human females, birth weights of human fetuses, and mutation rates in mice are three examples of parameters that can be evaluated in the respective populations. Clearly, these parameters are not constant throughout a population. Statistics is the mathematical technique that describes and analyzes numerical data obtained from experimental observations of populations.

Since performing measurements on every member of a large population is not practical, a small representative sample is designated for study. The number of members investigated in this population is the sample size (N). Listing the individual measurements is time consuming and difficult to communicate. Statistical parameters (primarily the mean and the standard deviation) have been developed to characterize a set of measurements.

The mean ($\bar{x}$) is the arithmetical average, which is calculated by summing the individual measurements (x) and dividing by the number of measurements

A-22

$$\bar{x} = \frac{\Sigma x}{N}$$

The standard deviation (σ) indicates the amount of variability and is defined mathematically as

A-23

$$\sigma = \sqrt{\frac{\Sigma (x - \bar{x})^2}{N - 1}}$$

The standard deviation is expressed in the same units as the mean.

Suppose we have to record the height of women between the ages of 20 and 25 entering a building. The first five observations (in inches) are 64, 60, 64, 63, and 67. These data are presented as a histogram in Figure A-4. The horizontal axis represents the magnitude of measurement (height in inches) and the vertical axis shows the number of times each height is observed in the population. Graphical formats are useful in presenting large data sets in concise form.

As the sample size is increased, the distribution becomes centrally peaked, with falloff on each side of the peak (Fig. A-5). Irregularities become more smooth. The numerical data are depicted by a bell-shaped curve, called the normal distribution (Fig. A-6). The normal distribution is specified completely by the mean and the standard deviation. The mean corresponds to the horizontal value at the central peak and the standard deviation indicates the width of the distribution.

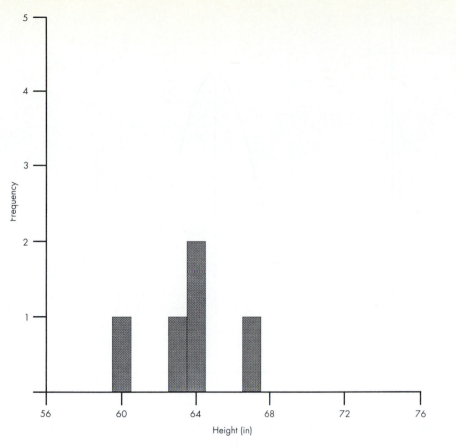

Figure A-4 Histogram of 5 observations of female height.

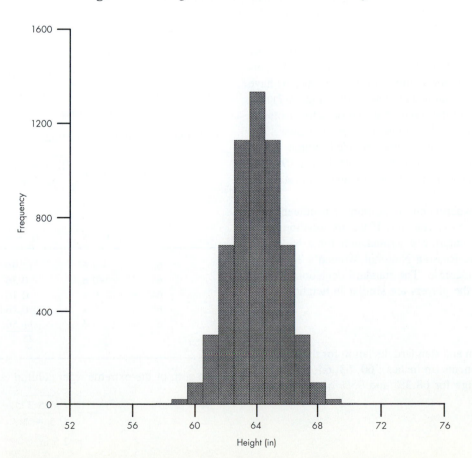

Figure A-5 Histogram of several thousand observations of female height. The mean is 64 inches, and the standard deviation is calculated to be 3 inches.

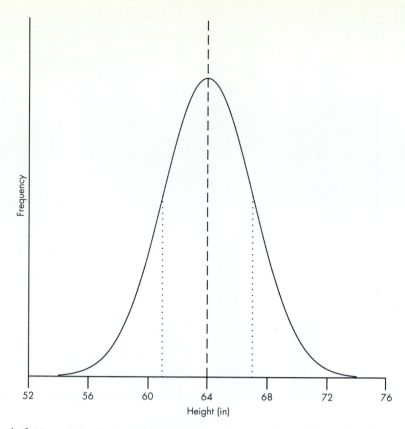

Frequency

Height (in)

52   56   60   64   68   72   76

Figure A-6 Normal distribution of female heights from the data in Figure A-5. The mean is 64 inches and is shown by the *dashed line*. The spread of the distribution is denoted by the *dotted lines* corresponding to one standard deviation on each side of the mean. In this numerical data set the standard deviation is equal to 3 inches.

Measurements that are fairly uniform yield a low value for the standard deviation and show little spread in the normal distribution. Another group of measurements may have the same mean but exhibit more variability (Fig. A-7). An important property of the standard deviation is to denote the fraction of measurements within a range of values. The percentage of all measurements included within $\pm 1\sigma$, $\pm 2\sigma$, and $\pm 3\sigma$ of the mean are 68.3%, 95.4%, and 99.7%. This is true regardless of the absolute value of the standard deviation.

Certainly the experimental conditions can influence the distribution of the measurements. If we are monitoring the heigth of women entering a gymnasium for a basketball game featuring the Russian National Women's Team, the mean height will increase. The standard deviation may actually decrease if the players are similar in height.

Problem A-14

Calculate the mean and standard deviation for the following series of measurements (in inches): 60, 63, 64, 64, and 67. Determine the range for 68.3% and 95% of the measurements.

Answer

Find the mean.

$$\bar{x} = \frac{\Sigma \, x}{N}$$

$$= \frac{60 + 63 + 64 + 64 + 67}{5}$$

$$= 63.6 \text{ inches}$$

Calculate the standard deviation.

$$\sigma = \sqrt{\frac{\Sigma \, (x - \bar{x})^2}{N - 1}}$$

x	$x - \bar{x}$	$(x - \bar{x})^2$
60	−3.6	12.96
63	−0.6	0.36
64	0.4	0.16
64	0.4	0.16
67	3.4	11.56
		25.2

The sum of the extreme right column equals $\Sigma \, (x - \bar{x})^2$.

$$\sigma = \sqrt{\frac{25.2}{5 - 1}}$$

$$= 2.5 \text{ in}$$

For the range 61.1 to 66.1 inches we would expect to find

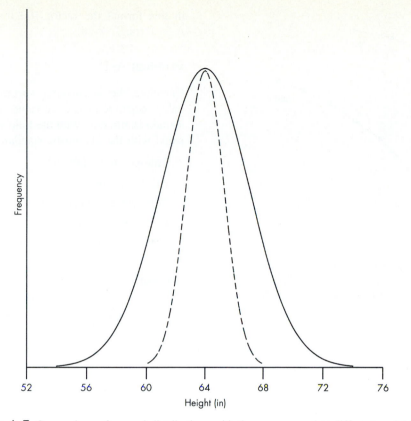

Figure A-7 Comparison of normal distributions with the same mean but different variability. The standard deviation associated with the distribution represented by the *dashed line* has a lower numerical value.

68.3% of the measurements. For the range 58.6 to 68.6 inches we expect to find 95.4%.

Two other statistics are often used to describe a collection of measurements. The median is the middle value when data are ranked from lowest to highest. The number of measurements is equally divided above and below the median value. The mode is the prevalent value in the collection of measurements. When presented in graphical format, it corresponds to the highest peak in the curve.

INDICES OF DIAGNOSTIC TEST PERFORMANCE

The growth of ultrasound can, in large part, be attributed to new clinical applications. Researchers must demonstrate that proposed applications selectively identify patients with specific disease. Statistical parameters (typically sensitivity, specificity, and accuracy) have been developed to judge the efficacy of diagnostic tests. The patient may or may not have disease and the ultrasound examination may or may not have positive findings. Four outcomes are possible:

1. True-positive (TP): the ultrasound findings are positive and the patient has disease.
2. False-positive (FP): the ultrasound findings are positive and the patient does not have disease.
3. True-negative (TN): the ultrasound findings are negative and the patient does not have disease.

4. False-negative (FN): the ultrasound findings are negative and the patient has disease.

The determination of disease is accomplished independently by using an established procedure (a surgical biopsy). The perfect diagnostic test would identify all diseased persons with positive findings and all nondiseased persons with negative findings. The sensitivity of the diagnostic test is the percentage of all subjects with disease that yield a positive test result. Mathematically

A-24

$$\text{Sensitivity} = \frac{\text{TP}}{\text{TP} + \text{FN}} \times 100$$

Sensitivity describes how well the diagnostic test identifies subjects with disease. Minimizing false-negatives improves the reliability of the diagnostic test. The specificity of a diagnostic test is the percentage of all subjects without disease that yield a negative test result. Mathematically

A-25

$$\text{Specificity} = \frac{\text{TN}}{\text{TN} + \text{FP}} \times 100$$

Specificity describes how well the diagnostic test excludes nondiseased subjects from having a positive test result. Minimizing false-positives also improves the reliability of the diagnostic test. Accuracy of the diagnostic test is the percentage of all subjects tested who are correctly assessed as

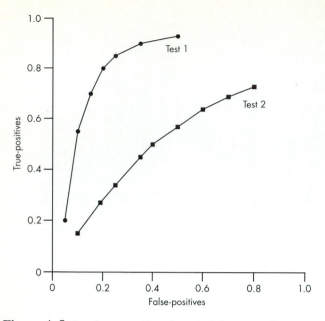

Figure A-8 Receiver operating characteristic curves for two diagnostic tests. *Test 1* is superior to *Test 2*.

having or not having disease. The equation for accuracy is

$$\text{Accuracy} = \frac{\text{TP} + \text{TN}}{\text{All subjects tested}} \times 100 \quad \text{A-26}$$

Positive predictive value (PPV) indicates the likelihood of disease if the test is positive and similarly, negative predictive value (NPV) indicates the likelihood of the subject being free of disease if the test is negative. The defining equations are

$$\text{PPV} = \frac{\text{TP}}{\text{TP} + \text{FP}} \times 100 \quad \text{A-27}$$

$$\text{NPV} = \frac{\text{TN}}{\text{TN} + \text{FN}} \times 100 \quad \text{A-28}$$

Sensitivity, specificity, accuracy, and positive and negative predictive values are also expressed by fractions between zero and 1 to indicate probability of various outcomes.

In this format the factor 100 is eliminated in Equations A-24 through A-28.

Problem A-15

Calculate the sensitivity, specificity, positive predictive value, negative predictive value, and accuracy for an ultrasound examination with the following outcomes when compared with the diagnostic standard.

True-positive (TP): 53

False-positive (FP): 18

True-negative (TN): 70

False-negative (FN): 4

Total number of subjects tested: 145

Answer

$$\text{Sensitivity} = \frac{53}{57} \times 100 = 93\%$$

$$\text{Specificity} = \frac{70}{88} \times 100 = 80\%$$

$$\text{Accuracy} = \frac{53 + 70}{145} \times 100 = 85\%$$

$$\text{PPV} = \frac{53}{71} \times 100 = 75\%$$

$$\text{NPV} = \frac{70}{74} \times 100 = 95\%$$

Imaging procedures are subject to interpretation by an observer. The observer may or may not correctly analyze the information content of the image. Sensitivity and specificity are dependent on the knowledge and experience of the observer. Consequently, the accuracy of the diagnostic test is expected to vary within a group of observers. A graphical method, called receiver operating characteristics (ROC) curve, summarizes the performance of multiple observers. The fraction of true-positives of all subjects with disease (sensitivity) is plotted against the fraction of false-positives of all subjects without disease (1 − specificity). Data points concentrated in the upper left portion of the graph indicate high sensitivity with a low rate of false-positives (the most desirable attributes of a diagnostic test). Example ROC curves are presented in Figure A-8.

Fourier Analysis

In physics, an entity often demonstrates a complex behavior that is difficult to describe mathematically. For example, the ultrasound wave produced by a piezoelectric crystal exhibits pressure (or intensity) fluctuations over time and space. Also the Doppler signal generated by interfaces moving at different velocities has multiple components that are not readily perceived. A simplified description of this complex variation (whether pulsed ultrasound wave or Doppler signal) is essential for understanding and analysis. One method, called Fourier analysis, identifies a series of sine wave constituents which, when added together, yield the original waveform. The technique of Fourier analysis has numerous applications in ultrasound physics, but the two most important are the determination of transducer Q value and Doppler spectral analysis.

A ball suspended from a string exhibits very nearly simple harmonic motion that can be described by a sine wave. When moved from its equilibrium position, it oscillates back and forth. The distance from the center for two starting positions is plotted with respect to time in Figure B-1. The rate of oscillatory movement can be increased by shortening the string (as demonstrated in Figure B-2).

Amplitude, frequency, and phase characterize sine waves. *Frequency* is the number of oscillations per unit time. *Amplitude* is the extent of the vibratory movement or, more generally, the range of values of the entity. *Phase* offsets or shifts the location of maxima and minima.

Figure B-1 shows sine waves of constant frequency with different amplitudes. In Figure B-2 the amplitude is kept constant while the frequency is varied. The appearance of the sine wave portraying the movement of the ball suspended from a string is modified by changing the starting position to the left of center, although the frequency and amplitude remain the same (Fig. B-3). This results in a phase shift of 180 degrees (the maxima of one wave correspond to the minima of the other). In another example a phase shift of 90 degrees moves the two-cycle sine wave a quarter cycle to the left in Figure B-4.

The mathematical description of the amplitude of the sine wave (A) is given by

$$A = A_o \sin(2\pi ft + \phi)$$

where A_o is the maximum amplitude, π is a constant with a vaue of 3.1416, f is the frequency, t is the variable of time, and ϕ is the phase. The amplitude at any point in time can be calculated using equation B-1. Consider the two-cycle wave generated in a time interval of 1 second with a maximum amplitude of 10 mm (Fig. B-5). The phase is zero. The amplitude (A) at 0.15 second is determined by substituting the appropriate parameters in equation B-1 and solving for A:

$$
\begin{aligned}
A &= (10\ \text{mm}) \sin(2\pi(2\ \text{cycles/s})(0.15\ \text{s})) \\
&= (10\ \text{mm}) \sin(1.884\ \text{radians}) \\
&= (10\ \text{mm})(0.95) \\
&= 9.5\ \text{mm}
\end{aligned}
$$

The amplitude at 0.15 second is 9.5 mm. Note that in this application the argument of the sine function is expressed in radians and not in degrees.

Sine waves can be algebraically added together to depict more complex variation. This superposition of sine waves is also called interference. Figure B-6 shows the result of combining a two-cycle sine wave with a three-cycle sine wave. The addition of sine waves is accomplished by summing the wave amplitudes at each point in time. At 0.15 second the amplitudes of the two-cycle and three-cycle waves are 9.5 mm and 3.1 mm. The resultant wave has an amplitude of 12.6 mm at 0.15 second. At a different time (0.22 second) the respective amplitudes (3.7 and -8.4 mm) combine to yield a value of -4.7 mm (as demonstrated in Figure B-7).

Multiple sine waves of varying frequency and amplitude can be combined to form a complex waveform. As an illustrative example, imagine viewing the shoreline from a distant cliff above the beach. The boundary between the water and sand form an intricate pattern (Figs. B-8 to B-10). This pattern of the idealized shoreline can be analyzed mathematically and then reproduced by combining sine waves; each component in the composite waveform has a

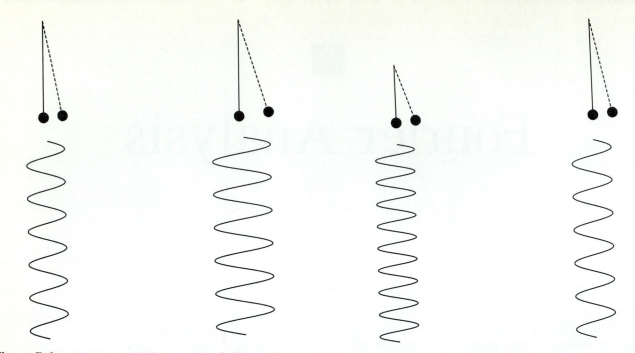

Figure B-1 A ball suspended from a string oscillates when released from its starting position (denoted by the *dotted line*). A sine wave describes the movement of the ball as a function of time. The ball on the right shows greater range of movement.

Figure B-2 The ball on the *left,* suspended from a shorter string, has a higher rate of oscillatory movement.

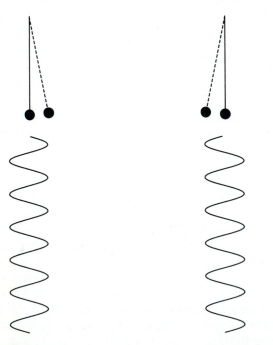

Figure B-3 Changing the starting position from the right to left side of center, but equidistant from center (denoted by *dashed lines*), produces sine waves with equal amplitude and equal frequency but different phase.

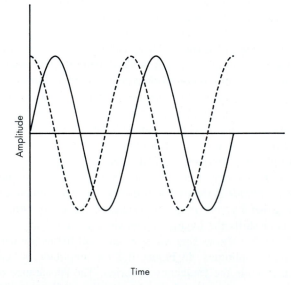

Figure B-4 Phase shift of 90 degrees. Two-cycle sine waves with a phase angle of 0 degrees *(solid line)* and offset one quarter cycle to the left *(dashed line).*

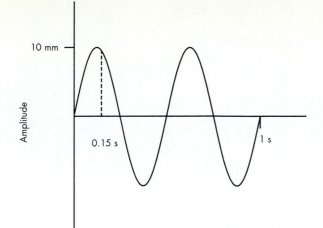

Figure B-5 The amplitude at 0.15 second is 9.5 mm for a sine wave with a frequency of 2 cycles/s and a maximum amplitude of 10 mm.

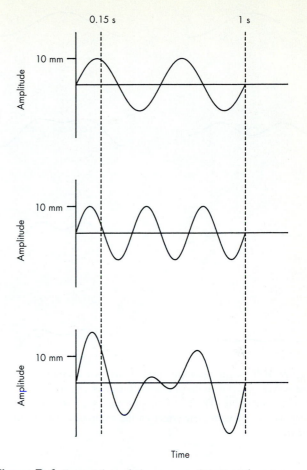

Figure B-6 Summation of sine waves. A two-cycle wave *(top)* is combined with a three-cycle wave *(middle)* to form the resultant wave *(bottom)*. The *vertical dashed line* on the left indicates the respective amplitudes at 0.15 second.

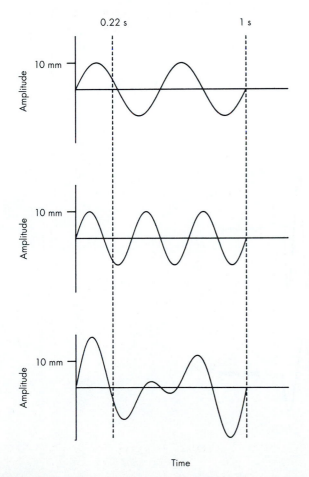

Figure B-7 Summation of sine waves. A two-cycle wave *(top)* is combined with a three-cycle wave *(middle)* to form the resultant wave *(bottom)*. The *vertical dashed line* on the left indicates the respective amplitudes at 0.22 second.

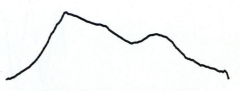

Figure B-8 Idealized shoreline.

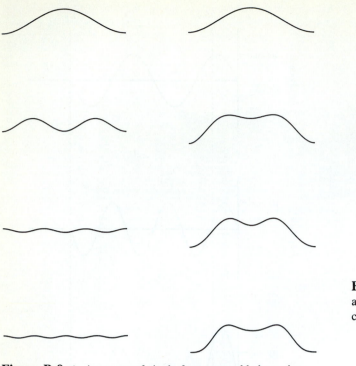

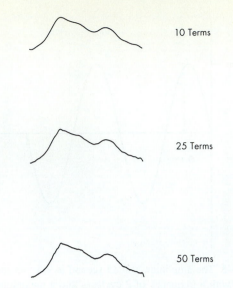

10 Terms

25 Terms

50 Terms

Figure B-10 As more sine waves with different frequencies and amplitudes are added together, the pattern generated more closely represents the idealized shoreline (10 to 50 sine waves).

Figure B-9 A sine wave of single frequency added to other sine waves yields a composite waveform that approximates the idealized shoreline. The first four sine waves are shown individually on the *left* with their effect on the composite waveform *(right)*.

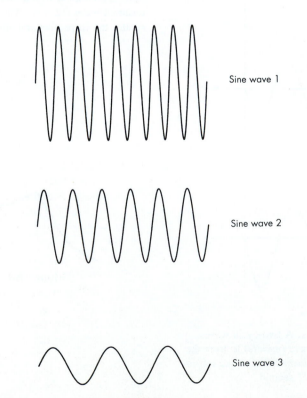

Sine wave 1

Sine wave 2

Sine wave 3

Figure B-11 Three separate sine waves. *Sine wave 1* has a frequency of 9 cycles/s and an amplitude of 0.75. *Sine wave 2* has a frequency of 6 cycles/s and an amplitude of 0.50. *Sine wave 3* has a frequency of 3 cycles/s and an amplitude of 0.25.

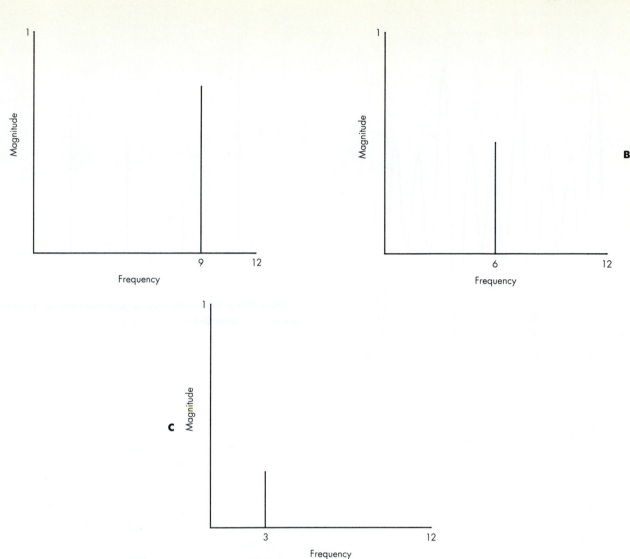

Figure B-12 Frequency domain representation of the sine waves in Figure B-11. Each sine wave consists of a single frequency denoted by the position of the peak along the horizontal axis. **A,** High frequency; **B,** middle frequency; **C,** low frequency.

well-defined amplitude and frequency based on the analysis the idealized shoreline. The composite waveform more closely represents the idealized shoreline as more sine waves are added together.

The presentation of sine waves in Figures B-1 to B-7 is in the time domain (the amplitude is plotted as a function of time). An alternative method, however, is to state the maximum amplitude (often in an abbreviated form as amplitude only) and frequency. The basis for comparison is frequency, which is described as the frequency domain. The identification of the frequency components is called *spectral analysis*. The frequency domain specification of the sine wave depicted in Figure B-5 has an amplitude of 10 mm with a frequency of two cycles per second. This information can be used to generate the sine wave in the time domain via equation B-1. The mathematical term for the process is *transformation*. It is important to recognize that the frequency domain gives an equivalent representation of the sine wave of interest in a simplified format.

Figure B-11 shows a time-domain presentation of three sine waves, each with a unique frequency and amplitude. Phase is constant and equal to zero. This same information can be presented concisely in a graphical format in the frequency domain. The amplitude of each wave (labeled as magnitude to indicate the spectral analysis) is plotted as a function of frequency (Fig. B-12).

When the three sine waves in Figure B-11 are added together, the complex pattern in Figure B-13 is generated. Fourier analysis of this pattern can be performed without previous knowledge of these individualized components and yields the frequency spectrum in Figure B-14. The magnitude at each frequency describes the relative contribution of that frequency to the original waveform. This recipe calls for a mixture in which we add 3 parts nine-cycle wave, 2 parts six-cycle wave, and 1 part three-cycle wave.

In the previous example the waveform consisted of three sine waves only. Often many sine waves of varying importance make up the waveform of interest. Upon Fourier

Sum of 3 sine waves

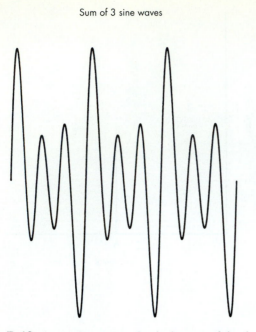

Figure B-13 A complex pattern that is the sum of the three sine waves in Figure B-11.

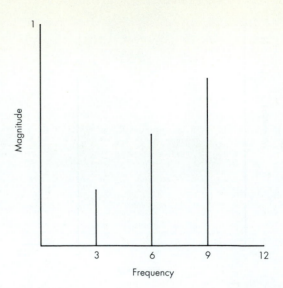

Figure B-14 Frequency domain representation of the complex pattern in Figure B-13.

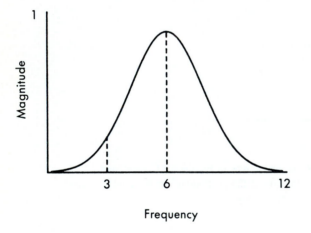

Figure B-15 Frequency domain representation in which broad range of frequency components contribute to the waveform of interest. The magnitude for 3 and 6 cycles per second is 0.22 and 0.88, respectively.

analysis a continuum of sine wave frequencies is obtained (Fig. B-15). The interpretation of this frequency spectrum is that a continuous range of frequency components from 0 to 12 cycles per second is present. The dominant frequency is six cycles per second. The contribution of the sine wave with frequency of three cycles per second is determined by finding the magnitude corresponding to this frequency on the graph. A similar procedure is followed for all other frequencies.

Mathematical algorithms have been developed that allow computers to quickly perform Fourier analysis on a data set. Personal computers can also be programmed to compute the sine wave components of functions.

Answers to Review Questions

CHAPTER 1
BASIC ULTRASOUND PHYSICS

1. b
2. a
3. b
4. b
5. b
6. a
7. a
8. b
9. b
10. b
11. b
12. a
13. b
14. a
15. b
16. 0.2 μs
17. 2.5 MHz
18. 0.44 mm
19. 3.2×10^6 kg/m²/s
20. 1.39×10^6 kg/m²/s
21. 13%
22. 1.1%
23. 99.31%
24. c
25. c
26. 65 degrees
27. 7.4 degrees
28. 0.8
29. 3.6 dB
30. −29 dB
31. 26.1 dB loss
32. 59.7 dB loss
33. 39.6 dB loss
34. 42.8 dB loss
35. 0.0032

36. 3 cm
37. 26 μs
38. c
39. b
40. b
41. a
42. b
43. c
44. b
45. ½, 2
46. d
47. Greater
48. a.　9
　　b.　6
　　c.　5
　　d.　3
　　e.　7
　　f.　2
　　g.　4
　　h.　8
　　i.　1
　　j.　10

CHAPTER 2
BASIC ULTRASOUND INSTRUMENTATION

1. c
2. d
3. b
4. a
5. b
6. b
7. a
8. a

9. a
10. b
11. b
12. a
13. a
14. b
15. a
16. b
17. c
18. c
19. b
20. a
21. a
22. b
23. b
24. a
25. c
26. b
27. b
28. a
29. a
30. b
31. c
32. c
33. a
34. b
35. a
36. b
37. b
38. a
39. a
40. a
41. a
42. d
43. a
44. b
45. a

CHAPTER 3
STATIC IMAGING PRINCIPLES AND INSTRUMENTATION

1. c
2. c
3. b
4. a
5. d
6. a
7. a
8. a
9. c
10. a
11. a
12. c
13. b
14. b
15. d
16. b
17. a
18. b
19. b
20. b

CHAPTER 4
REAL-TIME ULTRASOUND IMAGING PRINCIPLES AND INSTRUMENTATION

1. a
2. a
3. b
4. a
5. a
6. a
7. b
8. b
9. b
10. a
11. b
12. c
13. a
14. a
15. a
16. a
17. a
18. e
19. b
20. a
21. b
22. b
23. b
24. a
25. a
26. b
27. b
28. a
29. d
30. b
31. b
32. e
33. 42 fps
34. d
35. a
36. 1.67

CHAPTER 5
HEMODYNAMICS

1. Blood moves in concentric layers. Flow velocities vary across the vessel lumen, the slowest component near the vessel wall and progressively increasing toward the center of the lumen.
2. Pressure difference along the length of the vessel and luminal radius.
3. Hydrostatic pressure.
4. Bernouilli's equation. Conservation of energy from three sources: work, potential energy, and kinetic energy.
5. Frictional forces. Heat.
6. Inertia.
7. Acceleration, curvature of the vessel, branching, obstruction, and diverging cross section.
8. Fairly uniform distribution of flow velocities.
9. Localized slow rotation of concentric blood layers.
10. Velocity components are not coherent. Wide range is present. Cross flow and flow reversal occur.
11. 2650. Yes, since the Reynolds number exceeds 2000.
12. High-velocity jet at the stenosis, flow reversal and broadening

velocity distribution immediately distal, and turbulence more distal.

CHAPTER 6
DOPPLER ULTRASOUND PHYSICS AND INSTRUMENTATION

1. a
2. b
3. c
4. b
5. b
6. c
7. d
8. b
9. d
10. a
11. a
12. d
13. c
14. d
15. a
16. a

CHAPTER 7
COLOR FLOW IMAGING

1. d
2. c
3. c
4. c
5. a
6. a
7. b
8. c
9. c
10. a
11. b
12. d

CHAPTER 8
VASCULAR ULTRASOUND

1. Scattering from RBCs produces relatively weak echoes.
2. A time-dependent trace of the maximum velocity obtained in each Doppler spectral analysis.
3. Velocity profile, even insonation, assumed velocity profile, attenuation-compensated flow volume rate meter, time domain velocity profile.
4. Presence of plaque in the real-time image, high-velocity components and reduction of window in the Doppler waveform.
5. At angles greater than 60 degrees a small error in angle measurement introduces a large error in the velocity determination.
6. Loss of the triphasic pattern, increased maximum velocity, and spectral broadening.
7. Compression technique.
8. Global hemodynamics, imaging of tortuous vessels, proper placement of the Doppler sampling volume, and detection of low volume flow.

CHAPTER 9
M-MODE AND TWO-DIMENSIONAL ECHOCARDIOGRAPHY

1. a
2. b
3. a
4. a
5. b
6. a
7. b
8. a
9. a
10. a
11. b
12. a
13. a
14. b
15. a
16. a
17. a
18. b
19. a
20. b
21. b
22. a
23. a
24. a
25. a

CHAPTER 10
DIGITAL SIGNAL AND IMAGE PROCESSING

1. a
2. c
3. a
4. e
5. b
6. d
7. a
8. b
9. a
10. c
11. a
12. b
13. b
14. d
15. d
16. b
17. a
18. a
19. a
20. a
21. c
22. d
23. b
24. c
25. a

CHAPTER 11
IMAGE RECORDING DEVICES

1. c
2. b
3. d
4. b
5. b
6. b
7. d
8. a
9. a
10. a
11. b
12. a

CHAPTER 12
BIOLOGICAL EFFECTS

1. SPTP, SATP, SPTA, SATA
2. Mechanical, thermal, and cavitational
3. Collected works from many researchers combine to form an overall picture of the induced biological effects. The intensity descriptors, for example, provide a basis for comparison.
4. Biological effects in human populations exposed to the agent of interest are assessed under actual conditions of use.
5. An increasing number of individuals are exposed to ultrasonic examination in utero. Substantial damage can be manifested in large populations even if the probability of the effect is low.
6. 100 mW/cm^2, 1 W/cm^2, SPTA
7. a
8. a
9. b
10. a
11. b
12. There have been no demonstrated harmful effects at the intensity levels used in the examination. Numerous studies have been conducted to evaluate potential hazards and many more continue to be done. This examination was ordered by your physician because he or she believes it will provide diagnostic information important for your medical care that outweighs any risk associated with the ultrasonic exposure.

CHAPTER 13
QUALITY-CONTROL AND ACCEPTANCE TESTING

1. d
2. b
3. a
4. a
5. b
6. b
7. c
8. b
9. b
10. a
11. d
12. b
13. c
14. d
15. c
16. b
17. a
18. b
19. b
20. b
21. a
22. b
23. b
24. c
25. d

CHAPTER 14
IMAGE ARTIFACTS

1. c
2. a
3. a
4. c
5. c
6. a
7. c
8. c
9. b
10. a
11. d
12. c
13. d
14. d
15. b
16. a

Glossary

absorption   The process whereby energy is deposited in a medium by transforming of ultrasonic energy into other energy forms, primarily heat. It is an exponentially decreasing function and is the major factor in the total attenuation of the beam.

acceptance testing   The initial testing of equipment before acceptance that permits one to determine whether the equipment meets the specifications of the manufacturer, as well as the purchaser.

acoustic impedance (Z)   A measure of the resistance of a medium to the transmission of sound. The acoustic impedance is expressed as the product of acoustic velocity of the medium and the density of the medium ($Z = \rho c$). The acoustic impedance mismatch at the interface determines the amount of reflection that occurs. See *intensity reflection coefficient*.

address   The designator for the memory location corresponding to the X and Y position of the pixel in the image. The number stored in memory at that address represents the amplitude of the signal.

AIUM test object   The American Institute of Ultrasound in Medicine test object, composed of rods in a standard 100- × 100-mm square. This test object is used to test axial and lateral resolution, dead zone, distance indicators, registration arm alignment, sensitivity, and uniformity.

algorithm   A prescribed set of well-defined operations for the solution of a problem in a finite number of steps.

aliasing   An artifact in PW Doppler, in which a high-frequency Doppler shift is interpreted as a lower frequency.

alphanumeric   Alphabetic and numeric characters.

A-mode   Type of scanning mode in which the amplitude of the signal is plotted versus the depth of the interface. The strength of the reflected echo is represented by the height of a spike.

amplification   A technique in signal processing whereby a low-level signal (microvolt or millivolt) is increased to a higher level signal (volts).

amplitude   Normally used to refer to the particle displacement, particle velocity, or acoustic pressure of a sound wave. Amplitude also indicates the strength of the detected echo or the voltage induced in a crystal by a pressure wave.

analog   A continuously variable signal, as opposed to discrete values.

analog-to-digital converter (ADC)   A device that translates continuously variable signals into discrete values.

anechoic   The area in an image relatively free of echoes. This usually occurs within a fluid-filled structure or behind a very strong reflector.

angle of incidence   The angle from the normal at which the sound beam strikes the interface.

angle of reflection   The angle from the normal at which the beam of sound is reflected from an interface. The angle of reflection equals the angle of incidence.

aperture   The piezoelectric area of a transducer that is activated to form a transmitted beam.

apodization   A transmit and receive technique to reduce grating and side lobes. This process involves changing the excitation voltage pulse across the aperture of a segmented linear array to be maximum at the center and lower toward the boundary during transmission and changing the gain applied to each crystal of the segment during reception.

artifact   A false structure in the image of the scanned object created by the inherent nature of sound interactions (e.g., refraction, shadowing, and enhancement) or by the malfunction of equipment or by the improper operation of equipment.

asynchronous scanner   Flow and gray-scale scan data are acquired independently of each other.

attenuation   The decrease in intensity as a beam traverses a medium. Attenuation depends on all the interactions of ultrasound with tissues (i.e., macroscopic interactions), which include scattering, divergence, and absorption. Reflection may be included or treated separately as a component of beam intensity reduction.

attenuation compensated flow volume ratemeter   A device to measure volume flow rate that accounts for differences in path-length attenuation.

autocorrelation   A processing technique whereby a series of echoes from the same reflector are examined to assess motion. Very fast data-collection method in which the mean frequency of the Doppler signal is estimated.

axial pressure profile   A representation of the acoustic pressure along the axis of the beam. Measurements of acoustic pressure provide an indication of the variation in beam intensity.

axial resolution The ability to resolve two objects located near each other along the axis of the beam as separate entities. Axial resolution depends on the spatial pulse length.

backing material The material placed behind the crystal in the transducer to dampen ringing of the crystal. Air is used for therapeutic ultrasound where the difference between the acoustic impedances of the crystal and the backing material is large, resulting in maximum ringing and output. The acoustic impedance of the backing material and the acoustic impedance of the crystal are nearly the same for diagnostic systems to prevent ringing.

bandwidth A parameter that describes the distribution of frequency components in a wave.

baseline In flow detection a control that shifts the center of the velocity scale to display a greater range of velocities in one direction.

BASIC Beginner's All-Purpose Symbolic Instruction Code, a programming language used extensively with personal computers.

baud Data transmission rate of 1 bit per second.

beam cross-sectional area The area on the surface of a plane perpendicular to the beam axis consisting of all points at which the pulse intensity integral is greater than 25% of the maximum pulse intensity integral in that plane.

beam width The size of the beam at any location within the ultrasonic field. Beam width is smallest in the near field and increases with depth in the far field. Focusing reduces the beam width over part of the field and thus improves the lateral resolution.

beat frequency A phenomenon caused by wave interference in which waves of different frequencies, when added together, produce rhythmic cycles or beats. Beat frequencies in Doppler ultrasound obtained by combining the transmitted and received signals indicate the presence of motion.

bilinear interpolation An image manipulation technique in read zoom to increase the number of displayed pixels. Spatial resolution is not improved by bilinear interpolation.

binary The number system with a base of 2. Two possible conditions—either 1 or 0.

bistable scanning Storage of B-mode dots, which results in only a black and white image. The condition of the dot is either "on" or "off" (bright or dark).

bit A binary digit, either 1 or 0. The smallest unit of information in the binary system. Bits are the building blocks of computer words.

B-mode Brightness mode scanning, which modulates the brightness of a dot to indicate the amplitude of the signal displayed at the location of the interface.

broadband transducer A transducer with a wide frequency distribution. The fractional bandwidth is greater than or equal to 15%.

buffer A storage area where information is held temporarily until a device is ready to receive the information.

bulk modulus A physical parameter that quantifies the fractional change in volume when a pressure is applied to material. The bulk modulus is the reciprocal of the compressibility. The velocity of sound in the medium is directly proportional to the square root of the bulk modulus.

byte A group of 8 bits, usually handled together and treated as a unit by a computer.

capture function A color Doppler technique in which the maximum mean velocities detected during a sampling interval of 1 to several seconds are displayed.

cathode ray tube (CRT) A special display device that has a cathode (source of electrons) and an anode (phosphor screen) biased with a high potential difference. Electrons are accelerated across the tube to strike the phosphor screen. Focusing cups and magnetic or electronic deflection plates control the size and position of the electron beam on the phosphor screen.

cavitation Dynamic behavior of microbubbles in the medium exposed to an ultrasonic beam. Two types of cavitation are possible: stable and transient. An intensity threshold is associated with transient cavitation.

center frequency Transmitted frequency dictated by the thickness of the crystal. The frequency that has the highest magnitude in a graph of the frequency components of the transmitted sound wave.

clutter A type of acoustic noise. Signals induced by echoes created by secondary energy lobes striking off-axis structures.

C-mode scanning A gated-mode scanning technique that processes data from a specified depth only.

color aliasing An artifact in CD imaging, in which high-frequency Doppler shifts above the Nyquist limit are depicted by colors associated with slower flow.

color bleed An extension of color beyond the region of flow in CD imaging.

color Doppler (CD) imaging Motion encoded in color and stationary structures encoded in shades of gray are depicted throughout the field of view in real time.

color flash Sudden burst of color associated with tissue movement in CD imaging.

color flow imaging (real-time mode) Mapping of flow information on a gray scale image at a rate of several frames per second.

color flow imaging (static mode) Two-dimensional mapping of reflector velocity along different lines of sight as the transducer is mechanically translated across the region of interest.

color gain CD parameter that adjusts amplification of the Doppler signal.

color gate CD parameter that sets the axial length of the Doppler sampling volume.

color noise Random variations in signal detection cause areas with no flow to be color encoded in CD imaging.

color persistence   Frame averaging in CD imaging.

color reject   CD parameter that sets an amplitude threshold for the display of Doppler signals.

color threshold   CD parameter that sets the lower velocity limit for the display of moving reflectors.

color video printer   Color image recording device that receives the image data in the form of the video signal. The print medium is paper.

combined Doppler mode   The presentation of the color flow image in conjunction with the time display of the PW spectral analysis.

comet tail artifact   An artifact created from small, highly reflective interfaces. They originate from multiple internal reflections and are seen in normally echo-free areas.

compiler   A computer program that translates high-level language source code into machine language.

compound B-mode scanning   A set of B-mode dots indicates the origin and amplitude of the echoes. Special electrical components store the signals, and a registration arm is required to place the induced signals at the appropriate locations.

compound linear array   A linear array transducer that steers the beam via electronic phasing to extend the lateral field of view.

compressibility   The ease with which a medium can be compressed. The velocity of sound in a medium is inversely proportional to the square root of compressibility of the medium.

compression   A high-pressure region or a region of increased density of particles in a medium created by the action of the sound wave.

compression (digital processing)   A technique to reduce the dynamic range of signal values.

computer program   A series of coded instructions designed to solve a problem.

constructive interference   A process whereby two waves algebraically add together to produce a wave of greater amplitude than either of the original waves.

contrast agent   Material introduced to enhance tissue echogenicity.

contrast enhancement   An image-processing technique that changes the association between signal values and gray levels to display pixels with similar values as different shades of gray.

contrast resolution   The ability to resolve two objects with similar reflective properties as separate entities.

converse piezoelectric effect   A property of piezoelectric materials whereby an electric stimulus causes the dipolar material to expand and contract producing a pressure wave (sound wave). This property permits a material to be used as a transmitter of ultrasound. See *piezoelectric effect*.

convex linear array   A curved linear array that reduces side lobes and grating lobes. The lines of sight are always perpendicular to the array crystals. These systems are self-apodized by their curvature.

coprocessing   The computer processing of multiple lines of sight simultaneously to maintain high frame rates when multiple fixed transmit focal zones are used in real-time imaging.

Curie temperature   The temperature above which dipoles move about freely in a material.

curved linear array   See *convex linear array*.

cycle   A sequence of events recurring at regular intervals in time or space. As an example, particle density varies from a maximum in the compression zone to a minimum in the rarefaction zone and back to a maximum in the successive compression zone to complete one cycle. The distance for this cycle is the wavelength.

damping   The effect of reducing ringing or shortening the temporal pulse length after the excitation pulse. The damping is affected by the backing material and the Q value of the transducer.

database   A collection of interrelated data that can be accessed and used for one or more applications.

dead zone   The distance from the face of the transducer to the closest identifiable echo.

decibel   Relative measure of intensity or power: $dB = 10 \log I/I_0$, where I is the intensity at the point of interest and I_0 is the original or reference intensity.

deflection plates   Magnetic or electronic plates in a cathode ray tube or analog scan converter that control the horizontal and vertical position of the electron beam.

delay gain   A control of an ultrasound scanner to set the depth at which the time gain compensation slope begins.

demodulation   In signal processing, the technique of enveloping the components of the radiofrequency signal. Demodulation usually refers to isolating a signal that has undergone interference with a carrier wave. This procedure is often used in Doppler ultrasound, in which the "beat" frequency is separated from the sum of the reference and received signals.

density (ρ)   A physical parameter that describes the mass of a medium per unit volume. The velocity of sound is inversely proportional to the square root of density of the medium.

destructive interference   A process whereby waves add together algebraically to give a resultant wave of lower amplitude than either of the original waves.

dielectric constant (ε)   A transducer parameter that determines the electrical and mechanical matching of the transducer to the rest of the ultrasonic system.

differentiation   An electronic processing technique in which the slope of the video signal is represented as a voltage peak.

diffraction   The spreading out of the beam that results from the beam passing through a small aperture.

diffuse reflection   The reflection of an ultrasound beam in multiple directions from a large rough-surfaced object.

digital   A numerical representation of discrete values by a series of 1s and 0s.

digital filtering A computer technique designed to modify the value in each pixel throughout the image matrix based on the values in the surrounding pixels.

digitization The process of converting analog signals into digital signals.

dipole Positively and negatively charged regions on a molecule.

dispersion The dependence of the velocity of sound or other physical parameter on the frequency of the sound source.

distortion A parameter of image quality that describes the lack of adherence to the original geometric relationships.

divergence The spreading out of a beam that results from a source of small physical dimensions or diffraction or scattering. Divergence degrades the ultrasonic image by creating a loss of beam intensity.

Doppler angle The angle between the beam axis and the direction of travel for the moving reflector.

Doppler effect Relative motion between the sound source and sound receiver causes a change in the observed frequency.

Doppler scanning A scanning technique based on the Doppler effect to indicate the presence or absence of motion.

Doppler shift The frequency shift created between the transmitted frequency and received frequency by an interface moving with velocity (v) at an angle (φ) to the sound source:

$$\text{Doppler shift} = \frac{2\,fv\,\cos\phi}{c}$$

where c is the velocity of sound in the medium and f the transmitted frequency.

Doppler waveform The time display of the power spectrum of the Doppler signal.

duplex scanner Instrument that combines static B-mode or real-time imaging with Doppler flow detection.

duty factor The fraction of the time the beam is "on." The duty factor is found by dividing the pulse duration by the pulse repetition period. This factor is important when characterizing biologic effects of ultrasound.

dwell time The time required to interrogate one line of sight.

dynamic focusing An electronic focusing method that uses continuously variable delay lines to sweep the focal zone through all depths during reception of returning echoes.

dynamic range A measure of the range of signal magnitudes that can be represented or processed by the various components of a system.

echocardiography The branch of cardiology that uses ultrasound to study the function of the heart.

echoic The area of an ultrasound image that depicts strong echoes created by multiple interfaces.

echo-ranging A technique to determine the distance of an object from the transducer that relies on reflection. A sound beam is transmitted into a medium and reflected from the object back to the sound source. The elapsed time (t) between the transmitted pulse and the received echo is converted into distance (z) according to the formula z = ct. The velocity of sound in the medium (c) is assumed to be known. Half this total distance is the distance to the object.

echo wavetrain The succession of echoes detected along a line of sight following the transmitted pulse.

ECG-gated scanning A gated-scanning technique that processes information electronically during a specific portion of the heart cycle using the electrocardiographic wave as a trigger.

eddy flow A region of slowly swirling fluid motion.

edge enhancement A filtering technique to make the boundaries between structures more sharp.

electromagnetic radiation Waves consisting of alternating electrical and magnetic fields perpendicular to each other. Electromagnetic radiation such as light and x-rays can propagate through a vacuum.

electromechanical coupling coefficient (k) A transducer factor that describes how well the electrical stimulus is converted to acoustic energy and how well the returning echo is converted to an induced electrical signal in the crystal. Mathematically, the electromechanical coupling coefficient is equal to the product of the transmission and reception coefficient. This coefficient can be considered as the total conversion efficiency of the transducer.

electronic focusing Electronic delay lines connected to individual crystals of a segment are adjusted to cause the ultrasonic beam to reach the point of interest in phase (focus) or to reinforce the induced signal on reception of the echo.

electronic real-time scanner Automated (by electronic means) steering of the ultrasound beam through the area of interest to collect multiple lines of sight for each image at high frame rates.

endosonography Specialized real-time imaging with small probes that can be inserted into various body cavities (e.g., endovaginal and endorectal).

enhancement An image artifact created behind a low-attenuating medium such as a cyst. Interfaces distal to the low-attenuating medium appear to be greater in amplitude than identical interfaces located in the neighboring region.

ensemble length The number of pulses used to sample a color line of sight in CD imaging. Also called packet size.

enveloping The electronic process of surrounding the rectified radiofrequency signal.

facing material The material applied across the face of a transducer crystal to prevent damage to the crystal and to reduce the acoustic impedance mismatch between the crystal and tissue.

far gain Instrument time gain compensation setting that controls maximum amplification. Signals arising from this region decrease exponentially in strength with depth.

fast Fourier transform (FFT) Mathematical algorithm designed to break down a waveform into various frequency components. Spectral analysis of the Doppler signal identifies the Doppler shifts and their relative importance.

feedback microbalance A device that measures the average power over the beam cross-sectional area.

field of view (FOV) The physical region probed by the ultrasound beam that corresponds to the image.

flow phantom A Doppler scanner test device in which volume flow rate is regulated.

focal length (F) The distance from the front face of the transducer to the focal point.

focal point The point along the beam axis with minimum width and maximum intensity for a focused transducer.

focal zone For a focused transducer, the region defined by the pressure amplitude that is within 3 dB of the maximum pressure amplitude of the transmitted beam. The focal zone corresponds to the region of minimum beam width.

focusing A process whereby the beam width is reduced by mechanical or electronic means to improve the lateral resolution.

footprint The active piezoelectric area of a transducer which transmits ultrasound waves.

Fourier analysis The breaking down of a complex wave into a series of sine waves of different frequencies (component parts). This process changes the amplitude versus time domain to the amplitude versus frequency domain.

frame rate The number of images produced per second. The maximum frame rate (FR) is given as follows:

$$FR = \frac{c}{2\,RN}$$

where c is the velocity of ultrasound, R the sampling depth, and N the number of lines of sight per frame.

Fraunhofer zone (far field) The region beyond the near field for a nonfocused transducer in which the ultrasound beam diverges rapidly. In this region, lateral resolution becomes increasingly poor with depth. See *Fresnel zone*.

freeze frame A selected image in the real time acquisition is designated for continuous display until this mode is turned off.

frequency (f) The number of wave cycles passing a given point in a given increment of time. The unit is cycles/second or hertz. Frequency is the inverse of the period.

frequency domain processing Combined with quadrature phase detection to generate the spectrum of Doppler shifts.

Fresnel zone (near field) For the nonfocused transducer, the region from the front face extending to the beginning of divergence (corresponds to the last maximum). This is the area of best lateral resolution. See *Fraunhofer zone*.

gated-mode scanning A B-mode scanning technique that electronically processes selected received signals on command from a specific gated signal (i.e., depth or ECG cycle).

ghost-image artifact An artifact whereby a small object between two refractive structures is reproduced many times in the image.

ghosting A mirror image of the color flow produced when the vessel is located in front of a strong reflector.

grating lobes Secondary intensity lobes from linear arrays that are offset from the main intensity lobe. Grating lobes create artifacts in which a detected object is placed at the wrong location in the image.

gray bars The gray-scale test pattern present on most ultrasonic units that can be used to check the photographic system.

gray-scale imaging A B-mode scanning technique that permits the brightness of the B-mode dots to be displayed in various shades of gray to represent different echo amplitudes.

half-value layer (HVL) The amount of material required to reduce the intensity by one half of its original value. A half-value layer results in a 3 dB reduction in intensity.

hertz The unit of frequency that expresses the number of cycles per second. The kilohertz (kHz) is 1×10^3 Hz, and the megahertz (MHz) 1×10^6 Hz.

heterodyne Doppler detection method to identify the direction of motion. An offset signal is combined with the reference signal to place Doppler shifts corresponding to a particular direction within a well-defined frequency range.

high-pass filter A filter which removes the low frequency components of the signal.

Huygens' principle The division of a large sound source into a collection of small sources. Each individual source creates its own beam pattern, which interferes with those from the other sources to form a complex beam pattern.

hydrophone A device to measure pressure variations in the ultrasonic field.

infrasound Low-frequency (less than 20 Hz) mechanical waves that the human ear cannot detect.

in-line transducer A transducer that does not use an acoustic mirror to reflect the beam.

integration An electronic processing technique in which the area under the echo signal is represented as a spike or dot. The area is proportional to the amplitude of the returning echo; thus the height of the spike or brightness of the dot is also proportional to the echo amplitude.

intensity A physical parameter that describes the amount of energy flowing through a unit cross-sectional area of a beam each second. This is the rate at which the wave transmits the energy over a small area. The unit of intensity is the watt/cm² or the joule per second per square centimeter.

intensity reflection coefficient   The fraction of beam intensity reflected from an acoustic interface, given as

$$\frac{(Z_2 - Z_1)^2}{(Z_2 + Z_1)^2}$$

where Z is the acoustic impedance of the medium.

interelement coupling   The operation of one crystal element of an array affecting adjacent crystal elements. The coupling can be mechanical or electrical in nature.

interelement isolation   The process preventing mechanical and electrical coupling between crystal elements in an array.

interface   The junction of two media with different acoustic properties.

interference   The superposition or algebraic summation of waves. Constructive or destructive interference can occur.

kernel   A collection of weighting values used in a convolution operation, such as smoothing.

kilobyte (kB) 2^{10} (1024) bytes; generally denotes storage capacity.

laminar flow   Fluid flow in which neighboring layers are not mixed. The velocity profile incorporates slow-moving components near the vessel wall with faster-moving components toward the center of the lumen.

lateral resolution   The ability to resolve two adjacent objects that are perpendicular to the beam axis as separate entities. Lateral resolution depends on the beam width. Focusing the sound beam improves the lateral resolution.

leading edge detection   An electronic processing technique in which the front edge (leading edge) of the echo signal is represented as a spike.

length focusing (in-plane)   The focusing of a linear array along the in-plane or length direction of the array to reduce beam width in that direction. This type of focusing is normally accomplished electronically.

length-mode vibration   For a linear array, the expansion and contraction of the rectangular element along the length of the array that can cause interelement coupling, inducting artifacts in the final image.

linear array   A group of crystal elements placed one after another in a linear sequence.

line density   The concentration of lines of sight within a field of view.

line of sight   A line directed along the axis of the beam. B-mode scanners produce one line of sight at each position of the transducer. To collect multiple lines of sight, the data are stored at each location of the transducer by using the registration arm position sensors in conjunction with the analog or digital scan converter. Real-time images consist of multiple lines of sight collected by mechanically or electronically "sweeping" the beam through many directions.

liquid path   A nonattenuating liquid layer (usually water-alcohol mixture) added to the front of the transducer to permit better coupling to the patient. These systems typically use large radii transducers.

longitudinal wave   A wave in which the particle motion is along the same direction as the propagation of the wave energy (direction of travel of the wave).

low-pass filter   A filter that removes high-frequency components of the signal.

master synchronizer   A device that controls the timing sequence of all subsystems in the ultrasonic unit. The master synchronizer provides the "start" pulse to all the subsystem "clocks" at the time of the initial transmitted pulse.

matching layer   A layer of material placed next to the crystal in the transducer to facilitate the transmission of sound energy into the patient.

matrix size   The number of rows and columns of pixels composing the image. A 128 × 128 matrix consists of 16,384 elements.

maximum frequency   The Doppler shift associated with the most rapid motion. An upper cutoff limit between 1% and 5% is applied to the power spectrum in this determination.

maximum velocity waveform   The time display of the highest velocity component of the Doppler signal.

mean frequency   The average of all Doppler shifts in the power spectrum.

mechanical coefficient (Q)   The Q value of the transducer dictates the pulse length and frequency bandwidth. It is defined as either the energy stored per cycle divided by the energy lost per cycle or as the center frequency divided by the bandwidth.

mechanical focusing   The method of internally or externally narrowing the beam using acoustic lenses, acoustic mirrors, or curved crystals.

mechanical index   A parameter that describes the acoustic output in terms of the likelihood of cavitation. The cavitation threshold is predicted by the ratio of the peak rarefactional pressure to the square root of the frequency.

mechanical real-time scanner   A real-time imaging device in which a mechanical stepping motor sweeps the beam back and forth to collect the lines of sight.

median frequency   The middle frequency when all Doppler shifts in the power spectrum are ranked lowest to highest.

megabyte (MB) 2^{20} (1,048,576) bytes; generally denotes storage capacity. One MB equals 1024 kilobytes.

mirror-image artifact   An artifact produced when an object is located in front of a very strong reflector. A second representation of the object is placed at the incorrect location behind the strong reflector in the image.

misregistration   The improper placement of an interface in the image so the geometric relationships of the reflecting structures are misrepresented.

M-mode scanning   A scanning technique that depicts reflector position and velocity. The position of the reflector is plotted with respect to time. M-mode scanning was originally called time motion, or TM, scanning.

mode frequency   The prevalent Doppler shift in the power spectrum.

modem   A device that converts digital signals to analog signals for transmission over telephone lines.

multipath artifact   An image artifact that occurs when the beam strikes multiple interfaces before returning to the transducer. The interface is placed at the incorrect location with improper brightness.

narrowband transducer   A transducer with a narrow frequency spectrum. The fractional bandwidth is less than 15%.

near gain   Also called the mean gain. The instrument TGC setting that controls amplification in the region close to the transducer.

neper   A unit to describe a 1/e loss in amplitude (e.g., pressure amplitude) from absorption, scattering processes, or both. The defining equation is

$$neper = ln (p/p_0)$$

where p_0 is the initial pressure amplitude and p the pressure amplitude at the depth of interest. One neper equals -8.686 dB.

noise   Random variations in signal amplitude measurements of detected echoes.

nonfocused transducer   A transducer with no mechanical or electronic focusing. The beam is normally the width of the crystal in the near field and it diverges rapidly in the far field.

nonspecular reflector   An interface with small physical dimensions (i.e., less than several wavelengths in size).

Nyquist limit   The maximum frequency shift that can be measured in PW Doppler without aliasing.

offset transducer   A real-time transducer that uses a mirror to direct the ultrasound beam from the transducer to the patient and from the patient to the transducer. In Duplex scanning an offset transducer contains a crystal, separate from the imaging crystals, for acquiring the Doppler signal.

packet size   The number of pulses used to sample a color line of sight in CD imaging. Also called ensemble length.

PACS   A computer network for the acquisition, display, and storage of images.

panning   Translation of the write zoom field of view within the limits of the field of view imposed by the transducer.

parallel filter bank   Detector with multiple filters designed to separate the frequency shifts in the Doppler signal.

partial volume   The assignment of an intermediate signal level when the ultrasonic beam encompasses objects with different reflectivities.

particle displacement   The distance traveled by vibrating particles from their mean positions when acted on by a force.

particle velocity   The speed and direction at which the particles vibrate back and forth about their mean positions when acted on by a force. The particle velocity induced by a sound wave is not constant.

pascal   A unit of acoustic pressure in the MKS system of measurement one newton per meter squared (1×10^5 pascals equals 1 atmosphere).

peak detection   Electronic processing in which the peak (maximum amplitude) of the echo signal is represented as a spike.

peak negative pressure   The maximum rarefactional pressure produced by the sound wave.

percentage reflection   The percentage of the incident beam intensity reflected from an acoustic interface.

percentage transmission   The percentage of the incident beam intensity transmitted into a medium, which is calculated by subtracting the percentage reflection from 100.

period (τ)   The time for one complete wave cycle. The period is the inverse of the wave frequency.

persistence   A frame averaging technique to reduce noise. Temporal resolution is degraded when persistence is activated.

phantom   An object that mimics the properties of tissue with respect to sound transmission.

phased array   A linear array, rectangular array, or annular array system in which all the crystal elements are excited at or nearly at the same time. Short time delays (nanoseconds) are used to focus and sweep the beam.

phosphorescent material   A material that emits lights when electromagnetic radiation or particles (usually electrons) are incident on the material. The coating on the screen of a cathode ray tube (CRT) is composed of phosphorescent material.

photograph   The common end product of the ultrasound scan, which is a hardcopy of the image.

piezoelectric effect   An effect associated with dipolar molecules in which a pressure wave (sound wave) induces an electric signal in the material. This permits the material to be used as a receiver of sound waves. See *converse piezoelectric effect*.

pixel   A small square or rectangular picture element that represents a portion of the scanned area. The smallest component part of an image. Each pixel contains a value indicative of the intensity of the reflected echo. All the pixels are combined to form the image.

position generator   The component in a B-mode scanner that determines the displayed position of the interface.

position sensor   The device in the registration arm that measures the position of the transducer. Signals from the sensor are sent into the position generator, which controls the X and Y deflection plates of the analog scan converter and the address maker of the digital scan converter.

power   A measure of the total energy transmitted summed over the entire cross-sectional area of the beam per unit time (intensity $\times$ area). The unit of power is the watt (joule/second).

power map   Color assignment in CD imaging based on the intensity of the Doppler signal.

power spectrum   Graphic representation of the spectral analysis in which the magnitude of each frequency is plotted as a function of frequency.

P-QRS-T complex   The label given to the electrical currents that traverse the heart during each cardiac cycle.

propagation   The transmittal of sound energy to regions remote from the sound source.

pulsatility index (PI)   A means of quantifying the maximum velocity waveform with respect to shape. High values of PI indicate pulsatile flow.

pulse duration (temporal pulse length)   The time interval required for generating the transmitted pulse. The pulse duration is calculated by multiplying the number of cycles in the pulse times the period.

pulse repetition frequency (PRF)   The number of times the system is pulsed each second. The maximum PRF depends on the depth of interest (R) and the velocity of ultrasound (c):

$$PRF = \frac{c}{2\,R}$$

pulse repetition period (PRP)   The time needed to transmit a pulsed wave and detect the returning echoes. It is equal to the inverse of the pulse repetition frequency.

quadrature detection   The formation of an in-phase and a quadrature Doppler signal by dividing the received signal into two components, mixing with the phase-adjusted reference signal, and demodulating the resulting waveforms.

quadrature phase detection   Doppler detection method to identify the direction of motion. The Doppler signal is divided into two components, processed separately, and the relative phase between the two components is examined.

quality control (QC)   The routine testing of equipment to ensure proper functioning. An effective QC program is necessary to obtain high-quality images on a consistent basis.

quarter wavelength transducer   A transducer that uses a one-quarter wavelength matching layer in front of the crystal to reduce the crystal-tissue impedance mismatch.

Q value   A transducer parameter that characterizes the pulse length and bandwidth of the transducer.

radial mode vibration   For a circular or disc-shaped crystal, the expansion and contraction along the face of the crystal, which produces side lobes.

random access memory (RAM)   Information is written or read directly by location in computer memory.

range   The maximum depth from which a returning echo can be detected with the correct assignment of location of origin.

range ambiguity artifact   The misplacement of an interface when the assumption that each echo is derived from the most recent pulse is violated.

range gate   The selection of a time interval (time delay and time length) after pulsed wave transmission during which the detected echoes are processed for display. Since distance from the transducer is defined by the elapsed time, analysis is restricted to echoes originating from a specific depth.

rarefaction   A low-pressure region or a region of decreased density in a medium created by the action of the sound wave.

raster scan   A line-by-line output of information on the display device. The pattern is similar to the way in which we read a book.

rayl   The unit of acoustic impedance, which is equal to $kg/m^2/s$.

Rayleigh scattering   Scattering from small structures with dimensions less than the wavelength of the sound wave.

read mode   The process in the scan converter used to display the image in a continuous fashion. A new scan cannot be obtained while in the read only mode.

read only memory (ROM)   Special computer memory, which allows access to read only. No writing to ROM is permitted.

read zoom   During display, a method to magnify the image size on the monitor.

real-time scanning   An automated scanning techniqe in which a rapid series of images are acquired and displayed one after the other to depict motion.

receiver operating characteristics (ROC) curve   A graphical method of summarizing the performance of multiple observers.

reception coefficient (g)   A transducer factor that determines how efficiently the returning acoustic signal is converted to an electrical signal.

reception zone   The region within an ultrasonic field from which echoes can be detected.

records   Documentation of any clinical study or testing procedure using written reports or hardcopy images.

rectification   The electronic process of changing the negative component of the radiofrequency signal to positive.

reflection   An interaction that results in part of the sound being redirected into the medium from which it came after striking an acoustic interface. Reflection is the primary interaction used for all types of diagnostic scanning applications except transmission-mode scanning.

reflectivity   The combination of factors—including acoustic impedance mismatch, size, shape, and angle of incidence—that determine the intensity of a reflected echo from an interface.

refraction   A process whereby sound enters one medium from another, resulting in a bending or deviation of a sound beam from the expected straight-line path. Refraction obeys Snell's law, which is based on the ratio of the velocity of sound in the respective media. Refraction creates artifacts in the image by the misregistration of structures.

registration arm   A mechanical device on which the B-mode transducer is mounted. The position sensors in the registration arm provide the signals for the position generator, which controls the X and Y deflection plates of the analog scan converter or the address maker of the digital scan converter.

reject   Electronic processing that discards signals that are greater or less than a selected level.

relaxation time   A time indicative of the rate in which a molecule returns to its original position after being displaced by a force.

resistive index   A means of quantifying the maximum velocity waveform to evaluate downstream resistance to flow.

reverberation   An artifact created when an object is imaged more than once from repeated reflections by an interface nearer the transducer.

ring-down artifact   An image artifact created when an object vibrates at a characteristic resonance frequency. This artifact resembles a comet tail artifact without the specific banding seen with the comet tail.

ringing   The phenomenon of continued expansion and contraction of a crystal after being subjected to a short excitation pulse. A short ring time produces a short temporal pulse length and thus good axial resolution. Ringing depends on the Q value and the backing material used in the transducer.

scan converter   A device that stores scan data as echo signal strengths at the detected locations of the interfaces. This enables image formation using a gray scale.

scan cross-sectional area   For autoscanning systems, the area on the surface through which the beam passes during a scan.

scanning range   The maximum depth of the field of view.

scattering   The redirection of sound energy resulting from the sound beam striking an interface whose physical dimensions are less than several wavelengths. It is also called nonspecular reflection.

sector scanner   A real-time mechanical or phased electronic array that produces a pie-shaped field of view.

segmented linear array   An array of crystals in which groups of crystals are fired one after the other. The time delay between group activations is dictated by the depth of interest.

sensitivity   An index of diagnostic test performance denoting the percentage of all subjects with disease that yields a positive test result.

sensitivity (instrument performance)   The overall ability of the system to distinguish small, weak-reflecting objects at a specific distance from the transducer.

sequential linear array   An array of crystals in which each element is fired individually one after the other. The time delay between crystal activations is dictated by the depth of interest.

shadowing   The interfaces beyond a highly attenuating

object appear lower in signal strength than adjacent interfaces with similar reflectivities.

side lobes   Secondary intensity lobes displaced from the main beam, which are created by interference. Side lobes can misrepresent interface locations in the image. Side lobes are partially responsible for the formation of higher intensity grating lobes for linear arrays

signal   The voltage variation induced by a pressure wave incident on a piezoelectric crystal. The subsequent manipulation of a time-dependent voltage pattern is called signal processing.

signal processing   The manipulation of a received echo signal to enhance the presentation of scan data.

signal to noise ratio (SNR)   The strength of the echo signal as compared with the noise level. Contrast resolution and sensitivity improve as the SNR is increased.

single-sideband   Doppler detection method designed to identify the direction of motion. A filter technique to isolate the forward and reverse motions is employed.

slice thickness   See *width focusing*.

slope   A description of the amount of TGC amplification with depth.

smoothing   A filtering technique for reducing noise in the image.

Snell's law   A mathematical description of the principle of refraction:

$$\frac{\text{Sine incident angle}}{\text{Sine transmitted angle}} = \frac{\text{Velocity incident medium}}{\text{Velocity transmitted medium}}$$

sound   Mechanical vibrations or pressure waves that the human ear can detect. The frequency range is between 20 and 20,000 Hz. Sound waves require a medium for propagation. The term *sound* is used in the broad sense to include mechanical vibrations of all frequencies, including ultrasound.

spatial average intensity   The same as spatial average, temporal average intensity (SATA). Generally, this parameter is used when specifying the continuous waveform. NEMA standard.

spatial average, pulse average intensity (I[SAPA])   The pulse average intensity averaged over the beam cross-sectional area. (May be approximated as the ratio of ultrasonic power to the product of duty factor and beam cross-sectional area.) NEMA standard.

spatial average, temporal average intensity (I[SATA])   For autoscanning systems, the temporal average intensity averaged over the scan cross-sectional area on a surface specified. (May be approximated as the ratio of ultrasonic power to the scan cross-sectional area or as the mean value of that ratio if it is not the same on each scan.) For nonautoscanning systems, SATA is the temporal average intensity averaged over the beam cross-sectional area. (May be approximated as the ratio of ultrasonic power to the beam cross-sectional area.) NEMA standard.

spatial average, temporal peak intensity (I[SATP])   The value of the temporal peak intensity averaged over the beam cross-sectional area or scan cross-sectional area for autoscanning systems.

spatial filtering An image processing technique to reduce noise or enhance boundaries between structures. Spatial filtering describes CD applications in which pixels are color encoded only if the adjacent pixels are depicted in color.

spatial peak, pulse average intensity (I[SPPA]) The value of the pulse average intensity at the point in the acoustic field where the pulse average intensity is a maximum or a local maximum within a specified region. NEMA standard.

spatial peak, temporal average intensity (I[SPTA]) The value of the temporal average intensity at the point in the acoustic field where the temporal average intensity is a maximum or a local maximum within a specified region. NEMA standard.

spatial peak, temporal peak intensity (I[SPTP]) The value of the temporal peak intensity at the point in the acoustic field where the temporal peak intensity is a maximum or a local maximum within a specified region. NEMA standard.

spatial pulse length The spatial extent of an ultrasound pulse burst. The spatial pulse length is the product of the number of cycles in the pulse and the wavelength of the pulse.

specificity An index of diagnostic test performance denoting the percentage of all subjects without disease that yields a negative test result.

speckle Interference pattern incident on a transducer produced by echoes that have undergone multipath scattering. The signal does not exhibit a one-to-one correspondence with the scatters.

speckle tracking A two-dimensional time domain correlation technique for measuring reflector velocity in both the axial and the lateral direction.

spectral analysis The technique for identifying frequency components in a signal or waveform.

spectral broadening The presence of additional frequency components.

spectrum analyzer A device that identifies the frequency components of a signal.

specular reflector An interface larger than the width of the sound beam.

standard deviation A statistic that indicates the amount of variability in a collection of measurements.

step-down segmental array An electronic array in which a segment of crystals is excited to transmit a pulse and remains silent to listen for echoes before the next pulse is transmitted. The newest segment contains the same number of crystals, but it is offset from the previous segment by one crystal.

strip chart recorder An output device to record the M-mode tracing.

SUAR test object A test object used to measure the sensitivity, uniformity, and axial resolution of an ultrasonic system.

subdicing The normal crystal element of an array is divided into several smaller subelements. These subelements are electrically wired together to act conjointly. Subdicing helps reduce the intensity of the grating lobes.

synchronous scanner Flow and gray-scale scan data are acquired simultaneously along a line of sight.

temporal average intensity The time average of intensity at a point in space; equal to the mean value of the intensity at the point considered. For nonautoscanning systems the average is taken over one or more pulse-repetition periods. For autoscanning systems the intensity is averaged over one or more scan repetition periods for a specific operating mode. NEMA standard.

temporal peak intensity The peak value of the intensity at the point considered. NEMA standard.

test object A device that assesses system performance. It usually mimics the velocity of sound in a tissue.

thermal index The ratio of the in situ acoustic power to the acoustic power required to raise tissue temperature by 1° C.

thickness mode vibration The normal vibrational mode of the crystal that dictates the center frequency of sound transmitted from the transducer. The expansions and contractions of the crystal occur along the axis of the transducer.

time compression Doppler signal stored and then played back at an accelerated rate. A variable filter is swept through the frequency range of interest to identify Doppler shifts.

time domain correlation A processing technique whereby a series of echoes from the same reflector is examined to assess motion. Reflector velocity is obtained by measuring the time shift of the echoes.

time of flight The time required for an ultrasonic wave to leave the transducer, strike an interface, and return to the transducer.

time gain compensation (TGC) A method of increasing amplification of the signal with depth to compensate for losses from attenuation.

tissue characterization The identification of tissue type for a specific pathological diagnosis by noninvasive means.

tissue-equivalent (TE) phantom A phantom made of materials that permit the phantom to mimic the ultrasonic properties of tissue.

TM-mode scanning The original name of M-mode scanning, because the motion of the interface was plotted with respect to time.

total reflection A refraction process that prevents sound from entering a second medium from the first medium because the critical angle is reached or exceeded.

transducer Any device that converts one form of energy into another form. In ultrasound, a piezoelectric crystal converts an electrical stimulus into an ultrasound pulse and the returning echo into an electrical signal.

transit time broadening   Introduction of frequency components above and below the actual Doppler shift because of finite beam size.

transmission coefficient   A coefficient that describes the fraction of intensity of a beam transmitted through an acoustic interface. As a transducer factor, the term denotes the efficiency by which an excitation voltage pulse is converted to an ultrasound wave.

transmission-mode scanning   An ultrasonic scanning technique that records the ultrasound wave transmitted through a patient or phantom. This is the only diagnostic ultrasound imaging technique that does not rely on the echo-ranging principle.

transonography   Alternate term for endosonography.

transverse pressure profile   A measure of the acoustic pressure perpendicular to the axis of the beam.

transverse wave   The motion of the particles in the medium is perpendicular to the direction of wave propagation.

turbulence   A type of flow in a vessel characterized by cross currents and multiple velocity components.

ultrasonic field   The region over which sound energy is transmitted.

ultrasonic holography   A transmission-mode real-time imaging technique based on the principles of holography.

ultrasound   High-frequency (greater than 20 kHz) mechanical vibrations or pressure waves that the human ear cannot detect.

uniformity   Signals obtained for interfaces with similar reflective properties located at the same depth have the same amplitude.

variance map   Color assignment in CD imaging based on the spread of velocities within the sampling volume.

velocity (c)   The rate and direction at which sound propagates through a medium. The average velocity of sound in soft tissue is 1540 m/s.

velocity map   The assignment of various color hues or saturation to flow velocities in CD imaging.

velocity scale   In flow detection the range of velocities that can be displayed without aliasing.

velocity tag   CD parameter that allows a selected range of velocities to be depicted in a contrasting color (usually green or white).

VHS (video home system)   A ½-inch magnetic tape in a cassette for use with the videocassette recorder. VHS specifies a type of recording format.

videocassette recorder   A magnetic tape recorder that records a series of images in real time for subsequent playback.

video printer   An image-recording device that receives the image data in the form of a video signal. The print medium is paper.

video signal   The format consisting of 30 fps and 525 lpf for transmission of images to the output device.

viscosity   A parameter that describes the ability of molecules in a medium to move past each other.

volume flow rate   The quantity of blood per unit time flowing through a vessel.

wall filter   A high-pass filter that eliminates low-frequency Doppler shifts.

watt   A unit of ultrasonic power. One watt is equivalent to 1 joule per second.

wavefront   The compression zone within one wave cycle. Successive wavefronts illustrate the beam pattern generated by an ultrasound source.

wavelength (λ)   A physical characteristic of a wave that is the distance for one complete wave cycle.

width focusing   Focusing of the ultrasound beam in a plane perpendicular to both the beam axis and the direction in which the beam sweeps. Also called slice thickness or out-of-plane focusing.

width-mode vibration   For a linear array, the expansion and contraction of the rectangular element along the width (direction of mechanical focusing) of the array. This type of vibration can cause interelement coupling, thereby inducing artifacts in the final image.

word   A combination of bits treated as a single entity. The number of bits in the word dictates the number of different configurations (or values) that can be represented by the word.

word length   The number of bits in a computer word.

workstation   Computer with specialized graphics for the processing and display of digital images.

write mode   Collection of data by the scan converter during the scanning process. The scan converter places the echoes in the correct location as each line of sight is collected.

write zoom   Magnification technique applied during data collection to improve the spatial detail within the field of view.

zero-crossing detector   A device that monitors the rate of oscillation of the complex Doppler signal.

Index